Jones & Bartlett Learning's

COMPREHENSIVE MEDICAL ASSISTING

SIXTH EDITION

Judy Kronenberger, PhD, RN, CMA (AAMA)
President
Good Samaritan College of Nursing and Health Science
Cincinnati, Ohio

Julie Ledbetter, BS, CMA (AAMA), CMRS, CPC
Faculty, Medical Assistant Technology
Sinclair Community College
Dayton, Ohio

JONES & BARTLETT
LEARNING

World Headquarters
Jones & Bartlett Learning
25 Mall Road
Burlington, MA 01803
978-443-5000
info@jblearning.com
www.jblearning.com

Jones & Bartlett Learning books and products are available through most bookstores and online booksellers. To contact Jones & Bartlett Learning directly, call 800-832-0034, fax 978-443-8000, or visit our website, www.jblearning.com.

27556-8

Production Credits
Vice President, Product Management: Marisa R. Urbano
Vice President, Content Strategy and Implementation: Christine Emerton
Director, Product Management: Matthew Kane
Product Manager: Bill Lawrensen
Director, Content Management: Donna Gridley
Manager, Content Strategy: Carolyn Pershouse
Content Strategist: Ashley Malone
Content Coordinator: Jessica Covert
Director, Project Management and Content Services: Karen Scott
Manager, Project Management: Jackie Reynen
Project Manager: Brooke Haley
Digital Project Manager: Angela Dooley
Marketing Manager: Mark Adamiak

Content Services Manager: Colleen Lamy
Vice President, Manufacturing and Inventory Control: Therese Connell
Composition: Exela Technologies
Project Management: Exela Technologies
Cover Design: Briana Yates
Text Design: Briana Yates
Senior Media Development Editor: Troy Liston
Rights & Permissions Manager: John Rusk
Rights Specialist: Liz Kincaid
Cover Image (Title Page, Part Opener, Unit Opener, Chapter Opener): © YASNARADA/Shutterstock
Printing and Binding: McNaughton & Gunn

6048

Printed in the United States of America
27 26 25 24 23   10 9 8 7 6 5 4 3 2 1

Contents

Preface

Welcome to the *Study Guide for Jones & Bartlett Learning's Comprehensive Medical Assisting, Sixth Edition.* In this edition, we have aligned the exercises and activities with the most current curriculum standards published by the Medical Assisting Education Review Board (MAERB) and Accrediting Bureau of Health Education Schools (ABHES). Program directors, instructors, and students will know which activities in this *Study Guide* support comprehension of knowledge from the textbook (cognitive domain), which support the practice and skills needed to become a competent entry-level medical assistant (psychomotor domain), and which exercises encourage critical thinking and professional behaviors in the medical office (affective domain). This *Study Guide* is unique in a number of ways and offers features that are not found in most Medical Assisting study guides.

The *Study Guide* is divided into sections that coincide with the textbook: Administrative, Clinical, Laboratory, and Career Strategies. Parts I to IV include exercises that reinforce the knowledge and skills required of all Medical Assistants. Part V includes activities to "put it all together" as a potential medical office employee. All chapters have been updated and revised and we believe the extensive revision of the Clinical Laboratory chapters will be especially helpful.

Each chapter includes the following:

- **Learning Outcomes**—Learning outcomes are listed at the beginning of the chapter and are divided into AAMA/CAAHEP categories (Cognitive, Psychomotor, Affective) and ABHES competencies.
- **A Variety of Question Formats**—To meet the needs of a variety of learning styles and to reinforce content and knowledge, each chapter of the *Study Guide* includes multiple choice, matching, short answer, completion, and where applicable, calculation-type questions. These formats will

help you retain new information, reinforce previously learned content, and build confidence.

- **Case Studies for Critical Thinking**—These scenarios and questions are designed with real-world situations in mind and are intended to promote conversation about possible responses, not just one correct answer! These questions will be valuable to students who confront these types of situations during externships and graduates who encounter similar situations in their employment.
- **Procedure Skill Sheets**—Every procedure in the textbook has a procedure skill sheet in the *Study Guide*. These procedures have been updated and revised in this edition and include steps on interacting with diverse patients, such as those who are visually or hearing impaired, those who do not speak English or who speak English as a second language (ESL), and patients who may have developmental challenges.
- **Putting It All Together**—Chapter 47 in the textbook allows students in the final stages of their educational program to take a comprehensive examination, and Chapter 47 in the *Study Guide* gives students the opportunity to reinforce information learned throughout their program. This final *Study Guide* chapter includes documentation skills practice for a multitude of situations and active learning activities to engage students with previously learned knowledge.

This *Study Guide* has been developed in response to numerous requests from students and instructors for a concise, understandable, and interactive resource that covers the skills necessary to become a successful Medical Assistant. We hope you find the exercises and tools in this book productive and useful toward your goal of becoming the best Medical Assistant possible!

PART 1

Introduction to Medical Assisting

Understanding the Profession

CHAPTER 1

Medicine and Medical Assisting

LEARNING OUTCOMES

COG Cognitive Domain*

1. Spell and define the key terms
2. Summarize a brief history of modern medicine
3. Explain the system of health care in the United States
4. Discuss the typical medical office
5. List medical specialties a medical assistant may encounter
6. List settings in which medical assistants may be employed
7. List the duties of a medical assistant
8. Describe the desired characteristics of a medical assistant
9. *Identify scope of practice and standards of care for medical assistants*
10. *Identify the provider role in terms of standard of care*
11. Define a patient-centered medical home
12. *Identify the principles of self-boundaries*
13. *Identify the medical assistant's role in telehealth*
14. *Identify coping mechanisms*
15. Identify members of the healthcare team
16. Explain the pathways of education for medical assistants
17. Discuss the importance of program accreditation
18. Name and describe the two nationally recognized accrediting agencies for medical assisting education programs
19. Explain the benefits and avenues of certification for the medical assistant
20. *Identify licensure and certification as they apply to healthcare providers*
21. List the benefits of membership in a professional organization
22. *Identify potential effects of personal morals on professional performance*
23. *Identify professional behaviors of a medical assistant*

PSY Psychomotor Domain*

1. *Locate a state's legal scope of practice for medical assistants*
2. Perform within scope of practice
3. Practice within the standard of care for a medical assistant
4. *Demonstrate professional responses to ethical issues*

AFF Affective Domain*

1. Demonstrate awareness of the consequences of not working within the legal scope of practice
2. Apply ethical behaviors, including honesty and integrity in performance of medical assisting practice
3. *Recognize personal boundaries*

MAERB Standards are italicized.

ABHES Competencies

1. Describe the current employment outlook for the medical assistant
2. Compare and contrast the allied health professions and understand their relation to medical assisting
3. Describe and comprehend medical assistant credentialing requirements, the process to obtain the credential, and the importance of credentialing
4. Explain what continuing education is and how it is acquired
5. List the general responsibilities and skills of the medical assistant
6. Define scope of practice for the medical assistant within the state where employed
7. Describe what procedures can and cannot be delegated to the medical assistant and by whom within various employment settings
8. Demonstrate professional behaviors
9. Partner with healthcare teams to attain optimal patient health outcomes

Name: _____ Date: _____ Grade: _____

CCG MULTIPLE CHOICE

1. Julia is a student in her last year of a medical assisting program. What must she complete before graduating?
   a. Certification
   b. An associate degree
   c. A practicum
   d. Curriculum

2. Who is eligible to take the RMA examination? Circle all that apply.
   a. Medical assistants who have been employed as medical instructors for a minimum of 5 years
   b. Medical assistants who have been employed in the profession for a minimum of 5 years
   c. Graduates from ABHES-accredited medical assisting programs
   d. Graduates from CAAHEP-accredited medical assisting programs

3. Marie and Pierre Curie revolutionized the principles of:
   a. nursing.
   b. disease.
   c. infection.
   d. physics.
   e. radioactivity.

4. The medical assistant's role will expand over time because of:
   a. a growing population.
   b. the risk of disease and infection.
   c. advances in medicine and technology.
   d. a financial boom.
   e. more effective training programs.

5. What drives the management practices of the outpatient medical facility?
   a. The desire to compete with other medical facilities
   b. The need to adhere to government rules and regulations
   c. The attempt to fit into mainstream medical opinion
   d. The effort to retain medical employees
   e. The focus on hiring specialized healthcare workers

6. Which of the following tasks is the administrative team responsible for in the medical office?
   a. Physical examinations
   b. Financial aspects of the practice
   c. Laboratory test processing
   d. Minor office surgery
   e. Drawing blood

7. Which of the following is a clinical duty?
   a. Scheduling appointments
   b. Obtaining medical histories
   c. Handling telephone calls
   d. Filing insurance forms
   e. Implementing diagnostic and procedural coding for insurance claims

8. Empathy is the ability to:
   a. care deeply for the health and welfare of patients.
   b. keep your temper in check.
   c. show all patients good manners.
   d. remain calm in an emergency.
   e. feel pity for sick patients.

9. If a patient refers to you as a "nurse," you should:
   a. call the physician.
   b. ignore the mistake.
   c. politely correct them.
   d. send them home.
   e. ask the nurse to come into the room.

10. A group of specialized people who are brought together to meet the needs of the patient is called:
    a. multiskilled.
    b. multifaceted.
    c. multitasked.
    d. multidisciplinary.
    e. multitrained.

11. A medical assistant falls into the category of:
    a. nurse.
    b. physician assistant.
    c. medical office manager.
    d. allied health professional.
    e. all of the above.

12. The discovery of which vaccine opened the door to an emphasis on preventing disease rather than simply trying to cure preventable illnesses?
    a. Smallpox
    b. Cowpox
    c. Puerperal fever
    d. Typhoid
    e. Influenza

13. "Scope of practice" refers to:
    a. the tasks a person is trained to do.
    b. the tasks an employer allows an employee to perform.
    c. limitations placed on employees by law.
    d. a concept that varies from state to state.
    e. all of the above.

14. All accredited programs must include a:
   a. medical terminology course.
   b. computer course.
   c. practicum.
   d. certification examination.
   e. multidisciplinary program.

15. What is the requirement for admission to the CMA examination?
   a. Successful completion of 60 CEUs
   b. Successful completion of an externship
   c. Graduation from high school
   d. Graduation from an accredited medical assisting program
   e. Successful completion of a GED program

16. An oncologist diagnoses and treats:
   a. disorders of the musculoskeletal system.
   b. disorders of the ear, nose, and throat.
   c. pregnant women.
   d. the aging population.
   e. benign and malignant tumors.

17. A CMA is required to recertify every:
   a. 1 year.
   b. 2 years.
   c. 5 years.
   d. 10 years.
   e. 15 years.

18. Which organization offers the RMA examination?
   a. American Medical Technologists
   b. American Association of Medical Assistants
   c. American Academy of Professional Coders
   d. American Health Information Management Association
   e. American Board of Medical Specialties

19. Which of the following is a benefit of association membership?
   a. Time off from work
   b. Networking opportunities
   c. Hotel expenses
   d. Free health insurance
   e. Externship placement

20. Which specialist diagnoses and treats disorders of the stomach and intestines?
   a. Endocrinologist
   b. Gastroenterologist
   c. Gerontologist
   d. Podiatrist
   e. Internist

21. A goal of regenerative medicine is to:
   a. replace the need for organ donation.
   b. slow the healing process.
   c. provide more healthcare jobs.
   d. sell organs commercially.
   e. win the Nobel Prize in the medicine category.

22. "Standard of care" refers to:
   a. the focus of medicine.
   b. generally accepted guidelines and principles that healthcare practitioners follow in the practice of medicine.
   c. a physician's specialty.
   d. a concept that only applies to physicians.
   e. a policy that was written by Hippocrates.

23. Healthcare encounters that are conducted virtually require a:
   a. telephone
   b. wireless headset
   c. telecommunications platform
   d. computer
   e. digital blood pressure monitor

24. Medical assistants must have a basic understanding of healthcare reimbursement and the effects of the ACA for all of the following reasons except:
   a. an increase in patient access to health care
   b. managed care requirements that may affect healthcare delivery
   c. increasing healthcare costs
   d. to improve the quality in the delivery of health care
   e. decreasing healthcare costs

25. Which of the following medical assisting credentialing exams use the National Board of Medical Examiners as an exam consultant?
   a. CCMA
   b. NCMA
   c. CMAC
   d. CMA(AAMA)
   e. RMA

COG MATCHING

_____ Grade: _____

Match the following key terms to their definitions.

Key Terms

26. _____ caduceus
27. _____ medical assistant
28. _____ outpatient
29. _____ specialty
30. _____ clinical
31. _____ administrative
32. _____ laboratory
33. _____ multidisciplinary
34. _____ inpatient
35. _____ practicum
36. _____ accreditation
37. _____ certification
38. _____ recertification
39. _____ telemedicine
40. _____ PCMH

Definitions

a. Completed by a CMA every 5 years by either taking the examination again or by acquiring 60 CEU
b. Describing a medical facility where patients receive care but are not admitted overnight
c. A subcategory of medicine that a physician chooses to practice upon graduation from medical school
d. Referring to a team of specialized professionals who are brought together to meet the needs of the patient
e. Regarding a medical facility that treats patients and keeps them overnight, often accompanied by surgery or some other procedure
f. A medical symbol showing a wand or staff with two serpents coiled around it
g. Voluntary process that involves a testing procedure to prove an individual's baseline competency in a particular area
h. Regarding tasks that involve direct patient care
i. An educational course during which the student works in the field gaining hands-on experience
j. A multiskilled healthcare professional who performs a variety of tasks in a medical setting
k. A nongovernmental professional peer-review process that provides technical assistance and evaluates educational programs for quality based on preestablished academic and administrative standards
l. Regarding tasks that involve scientific testing
m. Regarding tasks that focus on office procedures
n. Encounters performed remotely using a telecommunications platform
o. A model of healthcare delivery that utilizes a team of providers to meet the needs of patients

COG SHORT ANSWER

_____ Grade: _____

41. What is the purpose of the Centers for Medicare and Medicaid Services?

_____

_____

_____

42. The following are three specialists who may employ medical assistants. Describe what each does.

a. Allergist: _____

b. Internist: _____

c. Gynecologist: _____

COG IDENTIFICATION

_____ Grade: _____

As a medical assistant, you must be "multiskilled," or skilled at completing many different tasks. Almost all of the tasks you will complete fall into one of two categories: administrative or clinical. But what is the difference between administrative and clinical tasks? Read each selection below and determine whether the task requires your clinical or administrative skills, then place a C or an A beside the task.

43. _____ preparing patients for examinations

44. _____ maintaining medical records

45. _____ ensuring good public relations

46. _____ obtaining medical histories

47. _____ preparing and sterilizing instruments

48. _____ screening sales representatives

AFF SHORT ANSWER _____ Grade: _____

49. What qualities do you possess that would make you a valuable member of your professional organization?

_____

_____

_____

50. List the characteristics that you possess that will make you a successful medical assistant.

_____

_____

_____

51. List any personal characteristics you believe you could improve.

_____

_____

_____

52. Describe the personal appearance of a professional medical assistant.

_____

_____

_____

53. What are the two accrediting bodies for the medical assisting education arena?

_____

_____

_____

54. What is the importance of having adaptive coping mechanisms in place? Give an example of a situation in which such tools would be helpful.

_____

_____

_____

55. How would you answer the question, "Legally, who is responsible for the actions of CMAs or RMAs as they perform their skills?"

_____

_____

_____

56. You are a CMA in a busy Ob/Gyn practice. You have been asked to orient a high school student who was hired to help up front and in medical records in the afternoons. She wants a career in health care but is unsure if she would be happier in a doctor's office or a hospital. She is debating between becoming a CMA and an RN but is confused about the difference. She asks for your help in deciding what profession to choose. How would you explain the difference in the two careers?

_____

_____

_____

57. Why is the ability to respect patient confidentiality essential to the role of the medical assistant?

_____

_____

_____

58. The medical office in which you work treats a variety of patients, from all ages and backgrounds. Why should you work with a multidisciplinary healthcare team? What are the benefits to the patients?

_____

_____

_____

WHAT WOULD YOU DO?

Grade: _____

59. You are preparing a patient for an examination, but the physician is running behind schedule. The patient is becoming anxious and asks you to perform the examination, instead of the physician. You comment that you will go check how much longer the physician will be, but the patient responds, "Can't you just perform the exam? Aren't you like a nurse?" How should you respond?

_____

_____

_____

60. The patient who asked you to perform the examination now refuses to wait for the physician. Even though they have a serious heart condition requiring monthly checkups, they leave without being treated by the physician. You need to write a note that will be included in their chart and in an incident report. What would you say?

_____

_____

_____

COG AFF PSY ACTIVE LEARNING

Grade: _____

61. Review the list of specialists who employ medical assistants in textbook Table 1-3. Choose one specialty that interests you. Perform research on the types of procedures the specialist performs. Then consider the tasks that a medical assistant employed by this specialist might perform. Write a letter to this specialist explaining why you would want to work in this kind of office. Be sure to include specific references to the tasks and procedures that interest you based on your research.

_____

_____

_____

62. Scope of practice for medical assistants can vary from state to state. In some states, CMAs are not allowed to perform invasive procedures, such as injections or phlebotomy. Go to the website for your state and research the laws in your state regarding the medical assistant's scope of practice. Why is it important to understand your scope of practice before beginning work in a new medical office?

_____

_____

_____

AFF CASE STUDIES FOR CRITICAL THINKING A

Grade: _____

You are a CMA in a family practice where many of your friends and neighbors are patients. One of them is being treated for breast cancer. It seems as though everywhere you go, someone asks about her condition. They are just concerned, and so are you. You really want to give them an update on her treatment, but you know that is prohibited.

63. What is your best action? Choose all appropriate actions from the list below.
    a. Ask the patient if she minds letting you give updates to their mutual friends.
    b. Tell them that you would be violating a federal law if you discuss her care, but they should call her to find out.
    c. Tell them what they want to know. After all, they are asking because they care.
    d. Offer to help your friend/patient join a website that will allow her to update her friends.

AFF CASE STUDIES FOR CRITICAL THINKING B

Grade: _____

You start your new position as a RMA for a busy pediatric practice. You are unsure of your job responsibilities, but the office manager expects you to "hit the ground running." Your first day is busy, and you are asked to handle the phones. Your first caller is a mother who is worried about their child's fever.

64. Your best response is:
    a. Don't worry. I'm sure they will be fine.
    b. Let me check the office protocol for children with fever. I will call you back.
    c. Today is my first day; I don't know, but I think they will be fine.
    d. You will need to make an appointment.
    e. I'll put you through to the doctor immediately.

65. What action could have prevented this uncomfortable situation?
   a. Having the opportunity to observe the office for a few weeks before starting
   b. Having read the policy and procedure manual before starting work
   c. Having more experience in the medical assisting field
   d. Paying better attention in class
   e. Refusing to answer the phone

66. You ask another medical assistant what you should do, and their response is, "I thought you were a RMA; you should know what to do." What is your next best action?
   a. Go immediately to your supervisor for guidance.
   b. Tell another coworker what she said and ask what she thinks you should do.
   c. Start looking for another job.
   d. Tell her that if the facility had trained you properly, you would have known what to do.
   e. Tell her that you are doing your best, and you are sure you will get up to speed soon.

AFF CASE STUDIES FOR CRITICAL THINKING C
Grade: _____

Mrs. Esposito approaches Jan, a medical assistant, at the front desk. Jan has recently treated Mrs. Esposito's son, Manuel, for a foot injury. Mrs. Esposito has just arrived in the United States and, with broken English, asks Jan if she may have her son's medical records to show Manuel's soccer coach that he will be unable to play for the rest of the season. Jan tries to explain to Mrs. Esposito that because her son is 18 years old and legally an adult, she must have his permission to release his medical records. Mrs. Esposito is frustrated and angry. Using Spanish translating software, Jan calmly attempts to explain that the physician would be happy to write a note for Manuel to give to his soccer coach explaining his injuries. After a great deal of time and effort, Mrs. Esposito thanks her for this information and apologizes for becoming angry.

67. From the list below, choose the characteristic of a professional medical assistant that Jan exhibited in the above scenario.
   a. Accuracy
   b. Proper hygiene
   c. The ability to respect patient confidentiality
   d. Honesty

68. What was the best action for Jan when she learned that Mrs. Esposito did not speak much English?
   a. Look in the Yellow Pages for a translator
   b. Try to find a Spanish translating software online
   c. Enlist the assistance of a fellow employee who speaks fluent Spanish
   d. Tell Mrs. Esposito to come back when she can bring a translator

69. When dealing with an angry person such as Mrs. Esposito, the most important action is to:
   a. raise your voice so they will hear you.
   b. treat them as they are treating you.
   c. remain calm.
   d. notify the office manager of a problem.

70. When responding to a request for the release of medical information, your first action should be to:
   a. explain the policy to the patient.
   b. check for the patient's signed authorization.
   c. ask the physician.
   d. copy the records.

PSY PROCEDURE 1-1 | **Locating a State's Legal Scope of Practice for Medical Assistants**

Name: _____ **Date:** _____ **Time:** _____ **Grade:** _____

EQUIPMENT: Computer, Internet connection, search engine, or website list

KEY: 4 = Satisfactory 0 = Unsatisfactory NA = This step is not counted

PROCEDURE STEPS	SELF	PARTNER	INSTRUCTOR
1. Using a search engine, locate your state's scope of practice law for medical assistants	❑	❑	❑
2. List some of the tasks within your state's scope of practice laws that can be delegated to medical assistants	❑	❑	❑
3. Identify tasks that are not permitted by your state's scope of practice laws to be delegated to medical assistants	❑	❑	❑
4. **AFF** Explain what you would say to a physician who asks you to perform a skill that you are not permitted by law to do.	❑	❑	❑

_____

_____

_____

_____

_____

CALCULATION

Total Possible Points: _____

Total Points Earned: _____ Multiplied by 100 = _____ Divided by Total Possible Points = _____ %

PASS **FAIL** **COMMENTS:**
❑ ❑

Student's signature _____ Date _____

Partner's signature _____ Date _____

Instructor's signature _____ Date _____

PSY PROCEDURE 1-2 **Demonstrate professional response(s) to ethical issues**

Name: _____ Date: _____ Time: _____ Grade: _____

EQUIPMENT: Computer with word processing software

KEY: 4 = Satisfactory 0 = Unsatisfactory NA = This step is not counted

The physician has ordered a blood transfusion for a patient with hemolytic anemia due to a chronic autoimmune disorder. While giving the patient instructions to receive the transfusion, the patient advises you that they cannot have the treatment for religious reasons.

PROCEDURE STEPS	SELF	PARTNER	INSTRUCTOR
1. Describe the medical ethical dilemma in the above scenario.	❏	❏	❏
2. Explain your personal beliefs about this medical dilemma.	❏	❏	❏
3. Identify professional ethics as a medical assistant with regard to this medical dilemma.	❏	❏	❏
4. Examine ways that your personal ethics may be in conflict with your chosen medical ethical situation.	❏	❏	❏
5. Demonstrate an appropriate response to the medical ethical situation based on your personal ethics.	❏	❏	❏
6. **AFF** Explain how you would respond to this scenario if the patient was a child and the parent refused the transfusion based on religious reasons.	❏	❏	❏

_____

_____

_____

_____

CALCULATION

Total Possible Points: _____

Total Points Earned: _____ Multiplied by 100 = _____ Divided by Total Possible Points = _____ %

PASS **FAIL** **COMMENTS:**
❏ ❏

Student's signature _____ Date _____

Partner's signature _____ Date _____

Instructor's signature _____ Date _____

CHAPTER 2

Law and Ethics

LEARNING OUTCOMES

COG Cognitive Domain*

1. Spell and define the key terms
2. Discuss all levels of governmental legislation and regulation as they apply to medical assisting practice, including the Food and Drug Administration (FDA) and the Drug Enforcement Agency (DEA)
3. *Identify licensure and certification as they apply to healthcare providers*
4. *Identify the standards outlined in the Patient Care Partnership*
5. *Identify criminal and civil law as they apply to the practicing medical assistant*
6. *Identify the purpose of medical malpractice insurance*
7. List the elements and types of contractual agreements and describe the difference between implied and express contracts
8. List four items that must be included in a contract termination or withdrawal letter
9. List six items that must be included in an informed consent form and explain who may sign consent forms
10. List five legally required disclosures that must be reported to specified authorities
11. Describe the four elements that must be proven in a medical legal lawsuit
12. Describe four possible defenses against litigation for the medical professional

13. Explain the theory of respondeat superior, or law of agency, and how it applies to the medical assistant
14. Outline the laws regarding employment and safety issues in the medical office
15. *Identify:*
    a. *Genetic Information Nondiscrimination Act of 2008 (GINA)*
    b. *Americans with Disabilities Act Amendments Act (ADAAA)*
16. *Define ethics and morals*
17. *Identify personal and professional ethics*
18. Differentiate between legal, ethical, and moral issues affecting health care
19. *Define:*
    a. *Negligence*
    b. *Malpractice*
    c. *Statute of Limitations*
    d. *Good Samaritan Act*
    e. *Uniform Anatomical Gift Act*
    f. *Living will/advance directives*
    g. *Medical durable power of attorney*
    h. *Patient Self-Determination Act (PSDA)*
20. *Identify compliance with public health statutes related to:*
    a. *communicable diseases*
    b. *abuse, neglect, and exploitation*
    c. *wounds of violence*
21. *Define the following medical legal terms*
    a. *Informed consent*
    b. *Implied consent*
    c. *Expressed consent*

    d. *Patient incompetence*
    e. *Emancipated minor*
    f. *Mature minor*
    g. *Subpoena duces tecum*
    h. *Respondeat superior*
    i. *Res ipsa loquitor*
    j. *Locum tenens*
    k. *Defendant-plaintiff*
    l. *Deposition*
    m. *Arbitration-mediation*
22. List the nine American Medical Association principles of ethics
23. List the five ethical principles of ethical and moral conduct outlined by the American Association of Medical Assistants
24. Identify the role of the medical assistant as the patient navigator
25. Describe the implications of the Health Insurance Portability and Accountability Act for the medical assistant in various medical settings

PSY Psychomotor Domain*

1. Monitor federal and state healthcare legislation (Procedure 2-1)
2. *Apply HIPAA rules in regard to privacy and release of information (Procedure 2-2)*
3. Apply local, state, and federal healthcare legislation and regulation appropriate to the medical assisting practice setting (Procedure 2-3)
4. *Perform compliance reporting based on public health statutes (Procedure 2-4)*

5. *Report an illegal activity in the healthcare setting following proper protocol* (Procedure 2-5)

AFF **Affective Domain***

1. Demonstrate sensitivity to patient rights
2. Recognize the importance of local, state, and federal legislation and regulations in the practice setting
3. Protect the integrity of the medical record

MAERB Standards are italicized.

ABHES Competencies

1. Comply with federal, state, and local health laws and regulations as they relate to healthcare settings
2. Institute federal and state guidelines when releasing medical records or information

3. Follow established policies when initiating or terminating medical treatment
4. Distinguish between employer and personal liability coverage
5. Display compliance with the Code of Ethics of the profession
6. Demonstrate compliance with HIPAA guidelines, the ADA Amendments Act
7. Demonstrate an understanding of the core competencies for Interprofessional Collaborative Practice., i.e., values/ethics; roles/responsibilities; interprofessional communication; teamwork

Name: _____ Date: _____ Grade: _____

OOG MULTIPLE CHOICE

1. The branch of law concerned with issues of citizen welfare and safety is:
   a. private law.
   b. criminal law.
   c. constitutional law.
   d. administrative law.
   e. civil law.

2. Which branch of law covers injuries suffered because of another person's wrongdoings resulting from a breach of legal duty?
   a. Tort law
   b. Contract law
   c. Property law
   d. Commercial law
   e. Administrative law

3. Choose all of the true statements below regarding the DEA.
   a. The DEA regulates the sale and use of drugs.
   b. The DEA regulates the quality of drugs manufactured in the United States.
   c. Providers who prescribe and/or dispense drugs are required to register with the DEA.
   d. Physicians must report inventory of narcotic medications on hand every month to the DEA.
   e. The DEA is a branch of the Department of Justice.
   f. Drug laws are federal and do not vary from state to state.

4. The Health Insurance Portability and Accountability Act of 1996 deals with the patient's right to:
   a. privacy.
   b. choose a physician.
   c. get information prior to a treatment.
   d. interrupt a treatment considered disadvantageous.
   e. refuse treatment

5. Which of the following can lead a patient to file a lawsuit for abandonment against a physician?
   a. The physician verbally asks to end the relationship with the patient.
   b. A suitable substitute is not available for care after termination of the contract.
   c. The patient disagrees with the reasons given by the physician for the termination.
   d. Termination happens 35 days after the physician's withdrawal letter is received.
   e. The physician transfers the patient's medical records to another physician of the patient's choice.

Scenario for questions 6 and 7: A man is found lying unconscious outside the physician's office. You alert several colleagues, who go outside to assess the man's condition. It is clear that he will be unable to sign a consent form for treatment.

6. How should the physician handle the unconscious man?
   a. Implied consent should be used until the man can give informed consent.
   b. A healthcare surrogate should be solicited to provide informed consent.
   c. The hospital administration should evaluate the situation and give consent.
   d. The physician should proceed with no-risk procedures until informed consent is given.
   e. The physician should wait for a friend or family member to give consent on the patient's behalf.

7. Once the man wakes up and gives his express consent to a treatment, this implies that he:
   a. No longer needs assistance.
   b. Verbally agrees in front of witnesses on an emergency treatment.
   c. Authorizes the physician to exchange the patient's information with other physicians.
   d. Trusts the physician with emergency procedures that can be deemed necessary at a later time.
   e. Is now familiar with the possible risks of the procedure.

8. A diagnosis of cancer must be reported to the Department of Health and Human Services to:
   a. Alert the closest family members.
   b. Protect the patient's right to treatment.
   c. Investigate possible carcinogens in the environment.
   d. Check coverage options with the insurance company.
   e. Provide research data for a national study.

9. What is the difference between licensure and certification?
   a. Licensure is accessible to medical assistants.
   b. Certification standards are recognized nationally.
   c. Licensure indicates that education requirements are met.
   d. Certification limits the scope of activity of a physician.
   e. Licensure allows a professional to practice in any state.

10. The Good Samaritan Act covers:
   a. Emergency care provided by a medical assistant.
   b. Compensated emergency care outside of the formal practice.
   c. Sensible emergency practice administered outside of the office.
   d. Emergency practice administered in the hospital to uninsured patients.
   e. Emergency care administered in the physician's office before the patient is registered.

11. The term *malfeasance* refers to:
   a. Failure to administer treatment in time.
   b. Administration of inappropriate treatment.
   c. Administration of treatment performed incorrectly.
   d. Failure to administer treatment in the best possible conditions.
   e. The physical touching of a patient without consent.

12. Which tort pertains to care administered without the patient's consent?
   a. Duress
   b. Assault
   c. Tort of outrage
   d. Undue influence
   e. Invasion of privacy

13. The statute of limitations indicates:
   a. The privacy rights of a minor receiving care.
   b. Risks that are presented to a patient before treatment.
   c. The responsibilities of a physician toward their patients.
   d. The right of a physician to have another physician care for their patients while out of the office.
   e. The time span during which a patient can file a lawsuit against a caregiver.

14. The court may assess contributory negligence when a:
   a. Team of physicians incorrectly diagnoses the patient.
   b. Physician's malpractice is aggravated by the patient.
   c. Patient does not follow the physician's prescribed treatment properly.
   d. Patient gives inaccurate information that leads to wrong treatment.
   e. Physician is entirely responsible for the patient's injury.

15. Which of these best describes the principle of patient advocacy?
   a. A medical assistant must adhere to their own code of conduct.
   b. A medical assistant must act first and foremost in the interest of the patient.
   c. A medical assistant must make sure the patient's information remains confidential.
   d. A medical assistant must make sure to act as a mediator between the physician and the patient.
   e. A medical assistant should only perform procedures that agree with their personal ethics.

16. Which of these is the basic principle of bioethics?
   a. All patients are entitled to the best possible treatment.
   b. Moral issues must be evaluated according to the patient's specific circumstances.
   c. Members of the medical community should never compromise their religious beliefs.
   d. The medical community must agree on a code of moral standards to apply to controversial cases.
   e. Moral issues are guidelines that the medical community is legally bound to follow.

17. What is the document created by the American Hospital Association that provides responsibilities and expectations to patients receiving healthcare services?
   a. Patient Care Partnership.
   b. HIPAA.
   c. Self-Determination Act.
   d. Patient Encounter Partnership.
   e. Americans with Disabilities Act.

18. What does the Self-Determination Act of 1991 establish?
   a. The physician has the last word on interruption of treatment.
   b. A person has the right to make end-of-life decisions in advance.
   c. The physician must follow advance directives from a patient verbatim.
   d. Family members cannot make decisions about terminating a patient's treatment.
   e. If a patient cannot make their own decision, a close family member can do so on their behalf.

19. Which of these patients would be unable to sign a consent form?
   a. A 17-year-old patient requesting information about a sexually transmitted disease
   b. A pregnant 15-year-old patient
   c. A 16-year-old boy who works full time
   d. A 17-year-old girl who requires knee surgery
   e. A married 21-year-old patient

20. In a comparative negligence case, how are damages awarded?
   a. The plaintiff receives damages based on a percentage of their contribution to the negligence.
   b. The defendant does not have to pay the plaintiff anything.
   c. The plaintiff and defendant share 50% of the court costs and receive no damages.
   d. The plaintiff has to pay damages to the defendant for defamation of character.
   e. The plaintiff receives 100% of the damages awarded.

21. Which of these laws protects you from exposure to bloodborne pathogens and other body fluids in the workplace?
   a. Civil Rights Act of 1964
   b. Self-Determination Act of 1991
   c. Occupational Safety and Health Act
   d. Americans with Disabilities Act
   e. Clinical Laboratory Improvement Act

22. The FDA is:
   a. not affiliated with the federal government.
   b. regulated by the Department of Health, Education, and Welfare.
   c. regulates the manufacture, sale, and distribution of drugs in the United States.
   d. charges with regulating drug quality and safety.
   e. divided among states.

23. A medical assistant performed venipuncture incorrectly, causing harm to a patient and resulting in a malpractice lawsuit.
   This type of negligence is called:
   a. Malfeasance
   b. A mistake
   c. Nonfeasance
   d. Intentional
   e. Misfeasance

ᴄᴏɢ **MATCHING**

Grade: _____

Match the following key terms to their definitions.

Key Terms

24. _____ abandonment
25. _____ slander
26. _____ assault
27. _____ battery
28. _____ ethics
29. _____ tort law
30. _____ civil law
31. _____ common law
32. _____ defamation of character
33. _____ defendant
34. _____ deposition
35. _____ durable power of attorney
36. _____ emancipated minor
37. _____ fee splitting
38. _____ fraud
39. _____ libel
40. _____ litigation
41. _____ locum tenens
42. _____ malpractice
43. _____ negligence
44. _____ plaintiff
45. _____ precedents
46. _____ res ipsa loquitur
47. _____ res judicata
48. _____ respondeat superior
49. _____ stare decisis

Definitions

a. A deceitful act with the intention to conceal the truth
b. Process of filing or contesting a lawsuit
c. Traditional laws outlined in the Constitution
d. A theory meaning that the previous decision stands
e. A person under the age of majority but married or self-supporting
f. Previous court decisions
g. A branch of law that focuses on issues among private citizens
h. Governs the righting of wrongs suffered as a result of another person's wrongdoing
i. A substitute physician
j. An arrangement that gives the patient's representative the ability to make healthcare decisions for the patient
k. Sharing fees for the referral of patients to certain colleagues
l. The accuser in a lawsuit
m. Failure to take reasonable precautions to prevent harm to a patient
n. The accused party in a lawsuit
o. A doctrine meaning "the thing speaks for itself"
p. The unauthorized attempt to threaten or touch another person without consent
q. The physical touching of a patient without consent
r. Malicious or false statements about a person's character or reputation
s. Written statements that damage a person's character or reputation
t. A process in which one party questions another party under oath
u. An action by a professional healthcare worker that harms a patient
v. A doctrine meaning "the thing has been decided"
w. A doctrine meaning "let the master answer"; also known as the *law of agency*
x. Guidelines specifying right or wrong that are enforced by peer review and professional organizations
y. Withdrawal by a physician from a contractual relationship with a patient without proper notification
z. Oral statements that damage a person's character or reputation

ᴄᴏɢ **SHORT ANSWER**

Grade: _____

50. List six items that must be included in an informed consent form and explain who may sign consent forms.

_____

_____

_____

51. List five legally required disclosures that must be reported to specified authorities.

_____

_____

_____

52. List nine principles cited in the American Medical Association's principles of ethics.

_____

_____

_____

53. List the five ethical principles of ethical and moral conduct outlined by the American Association of Medical Assistants.

_____

_____

_____

COG IDENTIFICATION
Grade: _____

The Americans with Disabilities Act Amendments Act (ADAAA) prohibits discrimination against people with disabilities in employment practice. Take a look at the scenarios in this chart and assess whether the ADA is being followed correctly. Place a check mark in the appropriate box.

Scenario	ADA-Compliance	ADA-Noncompliance
54. A physician's office extends an offer of employment to a man in a wheelchair but says that due to a shortage of parking, the office cannot offer him a parking space in the garage.		
55. A 46-year-old woman is refused a position on the basis that she is HIV positive.		
56. A mentally ill man with a history of violence is refused a job in a busy office.		
57. A small office with 10 employees chooses a healthy woman over a disabled woman because the office cannot afford to adapt the facilities in the workplace.		
58. A patient's wheelchair-bound husband cannot accompany her to her physician's visits because there is no handicap entrance for visitors.		
59. A job applicant with a severe speech impediment is rejected for a position as an emergency room receptionist.		

Some situations require a report to be filed with the Department of Health with or without the patient's consent. Read the scenarios in the chart below and decide which ones are legally required disclosures.

Scenario	Legally Required Disclosure	No Action Needed
60. A 35-year-old woman gives birth to a healthy baby girl.		
61. A physician diagnoses a patient with meningococcal meningitis.		
62. A 43-year-old man falls off a ladder and breaks his leg. He spends 3 weeks in the hospital.		
63. A teenager is involved in a hit-and-run accident. He is rushed to the hospital, but dies the next day.		
64. A 2-year-old girl is diagnosed with measles.		
65. A man is diagnosed with a sexually transmitted disease and asks the physician to keep the information confidential.		
66. A woman visits the physician's office and tells him she has mumps, but when he examines her, he discovers it is influenza.		

COG IDENTIFICATION

Grade: _____

67. Which of the following must be included in a patient consent form? Circle all that apply.

   a. Name of the physician performing the procedure

   b. Alternatives to the procedure and their risks

   c. Date the procedure will take place

   d. Probable effect on the patient's condition if the procedure is not performed

   e. Potential risks from the procedure

   f. Patient's next of kin

   g. Any exclusions that the patient requests

   h. Success rate of the procedure

68. Dr. Janeway has decided to terminate the relationship with his patient, Mrs. King. The office manager drafted the following letter to Mrs. King. However, when you review the letter, you find that there are errors. Read the letter below and then explain the three problems with this letter in the space below.

Dear Mrs. King,

Because you have consistently refused to follow the dietary restrictions and to take the medication necessary to control your high blood pressure, I feel I am no longer able to provide your medical care. This termination is effective immediately.

Because you do not seem to take your medical condition seriously, I'm not sure that any other physician would want to treat you either. I will hold on to your medical records for 30 days and then they will be destroyed.

Sincerely,
Anthony Janeway, MD

a. _____

b. _____

c. _____

COG PSY ACTIVE LEARNING

Grade: _____

69. Research two recent medical malpractice cases on the Internet. Write a brief outline of each case and make a record of whether the tort was intentional or unintentional, and what the outcome of the case was. Compare the cases to see if there is a common theme.

70. Visit a physician's office and make a list of steps that have been taken to comply with the law. For example, if the physician charges for canceling appointments without notice, there is probably a sign by the reception desk to warn patients of the fee. How many other legal requirements can you find? Are there any that are missing?

71. As technology develops, new laws have to be written to protect the rights of patients who use it. Stem cell research is a particularly gray area and has raised many interesting ethical dilemmas. Research some recent legal cases regarding stem cell research, and write a report on some of the ethical issues the cases have raised.

72. You are a medical assistant in a busy office, and the physician has been called away on an emergency. Some of the patients have been waiting for over 2 hours, and one of them urgently needs a physical checkup for a job application. Although you are not officially qualified, you feel confident that you are able to conduct the examination by yourself. Six months later, the patient files a malpractice suit because you failed to notice a lump in her throat that turned out to be cancerous. Describe the law of agency and explain whether it would help you in the lawsuit.

AFF WHAT WOULD YOU DO?

Grade: _____

73. A family member calls to inquire about a patient's condition. You know that the patient has not given written consent for information to be passed on, but you recognize the person's voice and remember that she came in with the patient the previous day. Explain what you would say and why.

OG IDENTIFICATION

Grade: _____

74. Mrs. Stevens visits Dr. Johnson's office with neck pain. Dr. Johnson examines her and recommends that she see a specialist. Several months later, Mrs. Stevens sues Dr. Johnson for malpractice, claiming that when he examined her, he made her neck pain worse. In court, she provides pictures of her neck that show severe bruising. A specialist confirms that muscle damage has restricted Mrs. Stevens from going about her daily life. Which of the four elements needed in a medical lawsuit has Mrs. Stevens failed to prove? Circle all that apply.

   a. Duty

   b. Dereliction of duty

   c. Direct cause

   d. Damage

AFF PATIENT EDUCATION

Grade: _____

75. You have a patient who has just been diagnosed with a sexually transmitted disease. After the physician leaves the office, the patient turns to you and begs you to keep the information confidential. It is obvious that the patient is worried and embarrassed. Explain how you would inform the patient about legally required disclosures and what you would say.

_____

_____

_____

_____

AFF CASE STUDIES FOR CRITICAL THINKING A

Grade: _____

Pamela Dorsett is a patient at Highland Oaks Family Practice. She is a 40-year-old woman who has five children and a house full of cats. She brings her children in for immunizations, but otherwise you rarely see them. She walks into the office on a busy Monday morning with all five children. They are surrounded by a pungent smell of cat feces. The children are dirty, and it appears are being neglected. All five of them have runny noses. She wants the doctor to see them now because she has transportation problems. You are the receptionist that day. Remember, pick the BEST answer.

76. The doctor is legally obligated to see the children at some point because:

   a. the children look neglected.

   b. there is a legal contract in place.

   c. medical ethics dictate it.

   d. all of the above.

77. If child neglect is suspected, the physician is required by federal law to:

    a. talk to the mother about her care.

    b. try to contact a family member.

    c. do nothing, as mandated by HIPAA.

    d. report the suspicions to authorities.

78. What would your first action be?

    a. Try to work the five children into the busy schedule.

    b. Consult with the providers.

    c. Make future appointments as soon as possible.

    d. Have them wait until the end of the day after all scheduled patients have been seen.

COG AFF CASE STUDIES FOR CRITICAL THINKING B

Grade: _____

As a medical assistant, you will be involved in some administrative issues. Read the following scenarios and assess whether the American Medical Association standards for office management are being met. Place a check mark in the appropriate box.

Scenario	Standards Met	Standards Not Met
79. Dr. Benson tells his medical assistant to cancel Mrs. Burke's tests because she recently lost her job and will be unable to pay for them.		
80. Mr. Grant canceled his appointment with less than 24 hours' notice. He was charged a fee as noted in a sign by the receptionist's desk.		
81. Mrs. O'Malley asks Dr. Jones to help her fill out an insurance form. The form is a four-page document that takes Dr. Jones an hour to fill out. Dr. Jones charges Mrs. O'Malley $15 for filling out the form.		
82. Dr. Harris dies suddenly, and his staff tell patients that the office will close and that copies of their medical records will be transferred to another physician.		
83. Mr. Davies owes the physician's office several thousand dollars. He is moving and asks the office to transfer his medical records to his new physician. The office refuses on the grounds that Mr. Davies has not paid his bill.		
84. Mrs. Jones comes into the office for a vaccination. The physician tells the medical assistant to charge her $10 less than other patients because she is elderly and cannot afford the standard charges.		

PSY PROCEDURE 2-1 | Obtaining an Informed Consent for Treatment

Name: _____ Date: _____ Time: _____ Grade: _____

EQUIPMENT: Computer, Internet connection, search engine, or website list

KEY: 4 = Satisfactory 0 = Unsatisfactory NA = This step is not counted

PROCEDURE STEPS	SELF	PARTNER	INSTRUCTOR
1. Using a search engine, go to the CDC's website to download and print the most recent Vaccine Information Statement for the inactivated influenza vaccine.	❏	❏	❏
2. Complete an Informed Consent form for the inactivated influenza vaccine.	❏	❏	❏
3. File the Informed Consent in the patient's medical record after obtaining the patient's signature.	❏	❏	❏
4. **AFF** Explain how you would respond to a patient who refused the vaccine after reading the risks in the VIS.	❏	❏	❏

_____

_____

_____

_____

CALCULATION

Total Possible Points: _____

Total Points Earned: _____ Multiplied by 100 = _____ Divided by Total Possible Points = _____ %

PASS   FAIL   COMMENTS:
❏   ❏

Student's signature _____ Date _____

Partner's signature _____ Date _____

Instructor's signature _____ Date _____

Great Falls Health System Physician Offices
INFORMED CONSENT FOR INACTIVATED INFLUENZA VACCINE

Complete **ALL** of the following information and sign the acknowledgment for consent to receive an inactivated influenza vaccine.

PATIENT INFORMATION:

Last name, First Name, Middle Initial	Date of Birth	Age:
Street Address:	Gender: M F (circle)	Email:
City, State, Zip	Cell Phone Number:	Work Phone Number:

INSURANCE/RESPONSIBLE PARTY INFORMATION:

Name of Financially Responsible Person:	Name of Policy Holder (Last, First, MI)	Date of Birth:
Address if different from patient:	Insurance Company:	
Relationship to Patient:	Member ID Number:	Group Number:

HEALTH QUESTIONNAIRE *(check yes or no):*

Place a check mark next to the questions below for the person receiving the vaccine:	Yes	No
1. Do you feel sick today or are you experiencing a high fever, vomiting, or diarrhea?		
2. Have you ever had a serious reaction after receiving an immunization?		
3. Do you have any allergies to **medication, latex, or food** including eggs, yeast, or gelatin?		
4. Do you have a weakened immune system due to a disease such as cancer, HIV/AIDS, etc.?		
5. Have you ever had a seizure disorder for which you are on medications?		
6. Have you ever had a nervous system problem?		
7. Do you have any chronic health condition such as a heart, lung, kidney, or blood disorder?		
8. Are you pregnant?		

CONSENT FOR TREATMENT:

A copy of the **most recent Vaccine Information Statement dated _____ has been provided to me about the inactivated influenza vaccine.**

I have read information and have been given an opportunity to ask questions that have been answered to my satisfaction about the disease and the vaccine to be administered. I understand the benefits and risks of the vaccine and hereby give **consent and authorization for the administration of the inactivated influenza vaccine.**

Signature of Patient *(Parent or Guardian, if minor)*	Date:

PSY | PROCEDURE 2-2 | Create an Office Policy to Report an Illegal Activity

Name: _____ Date: _____ Time: _____ Grade: _____

EQUIPMENT: Computer, Internet connection, search engine, or website list

KEY: 4 = Satisfactory   0 = Unsatisfactory   NA = This step is not counted

PROCEDURE STEPS	SELF	PARTNER	INSTRUCTOR
1. Using a search engine, locate your state's law that defines reportable child abuse and find your Health and Human Services Department for contact information to report cases of suspected child abuse and/or neglect.	❏	❏	❏
2. Write an office policy listing the steps for documenting the action taken and follow up as directed by the child welfare agency.	❏	❏	❏
3. Identify the name and title of the employee who will be responsible for contacting the child welfare or law enforcement member when directed by a physician in the office policy.	❏	❏	❏
4. Distribute the policy to every employee, obtaining signatures of acknowledgment of receipt and of their understanding of the policy and/or revisions.	❏	❏	❏

_____

_____

_____

_____

CALCULATION

Total Possible Points: _____

Total Points Earned: _____ Multiplied by 100 = _____ Divided by Total Possible Points = _____ %

PASS   FAIL   COMMENTS:
❏   ❏

Student's signature _____ Date _____

Partner's signature _____ Date _____

Instructor's signature _____ Date _____

PSY PROCEDURE 2-3 | **Monitoring Federal and State Regulations, Changes, and Updates**

Name: _____ Date: _____ Time: _____ Grade: _____

EQUIPMENT: Computer, Internet connection, search engine, or website list

KEY: 4 = Satisfactory   0 = Unsatisfactory   NA = This step is not counted

PROCEDURE STEPS	SELF	PARTNER	INSTRUCTOR
1. Using a search engine, go to the homepage for your state government (Example: http://www.nc.gov) and/or other related sites such as: Centers for Disease Control and Prevention (CDC), Occupational Safety and Health Act (OSHA), your state medical society, and the American Medical Association (AMA).	❏	❏	❏
2. Input keywords such as: Healthcare finances, allied health professionals, outpatient medical care, Medicare, etc.	❏	❏	❏
3. Create and enforce a policy for timely dissemination of information received by fax or e-mail from outside agencies.	❏	❏	❏
4. Circulate information gathered to all appropriate employees with an avenue for sharing information. Any information obtained should be shared.	❏	❏	❏
5. Post changes in policies and procedures in a designated area of the office.	❏	❏	❏
6. **AFF** Explain what you would say to a fellow employee who responds to a change in a current law with, "I will just keep doing it the old way. Who is going to care?"	❏	❏	❏

_____

_____

_____

_____

CALCULATION

Total Possible Points: _____

Total Points Earned: _____ Multiplied by 100 = _____ Divided by Total Possible Points = _____ %

PASS   FAIL   COMMENTS:
❏   ❏

Student's signature _____ Date _____

Partner's signature _____ Date _____

Instructor's signature _____ Date _____

PSY PROCEDURE 2-4 **Reporting an Infectious Disease**

Name: _____ Date: _____ Time: _____ Grade: _____

EQUIPMENT: Computer, Internet connection, search engine, or website list

KEY:　　　　4 = Satisfactory　　　　0 = Unsatisfactory　　　　NA = This step is not counted

PROCEDURE STEPS	SELF	PARTNER	INSTRUCTOR
1. Using a search engine, go to the Department of Health for your state and search for reporting requirements for hepatitis B.	❑	❑	❑
2. Input keywords such as: Reportable disease, hepatitis B, etc.	❑	❑	❑
3. Interpret your state's requirement and circulate information gathered to all appropriate employees with an avenue for sharing information.	❑	❑	❑
4. **AFF** Explain how you can protect the patient's private health information in the medical record from being accessed by others.	❑	❑	❑

_____

_____

_____

_____

CALCULATION

Total Possible Points: _____

Total Points Earned: _____ Multiplied by 100 = _____ Divided by Total Possible Points = _____ %

PASS　FAIL　COMMENTS:
❑　　❑

Student's signature _____ Date _____

Partner's signature _____ Date _____

Instructor's signature _____ Date _____

PSY PROCEDURE 2-5 | **Create an Office Policy to Protect Patient's Private Health Information**

Name: _____ Date: _____ Time: _____ Grade: _____

EQUIPMENT: Computer, Internet connection, search engine, or Web site list

KEY: 4 = Satisfactory 0 = Unsatisfactory NA = This step is not counted

PROCEDURE STEPS	SELF	PARTNER	INSTRUCTOR
1. Identify HIPAA's definition of *private health information (PHI)*.	❑	❑	❑
2. Research HIPAA privacy laws and patient rights regarding PHI in the medical record.	❑	❑	❑
3. Address how the Notice of Privacy Practices will be distributed and how refusal of acknowledgements will be handled.	❑	❑	❑
4. Address how the Notice of Privacy Practices will be distributed and how refusal of acknowledgements will be handled.	❑	❑	❑
5. Determine how the paper medical record will be protected and the responsibilities of the employees.	❑	❑	❑
6. Determine how the electronic health record will be protected and the responsibilities of the employees.	❑	❑	❑
7. Identify (by titles) employees who will have access to the various portions of the medical record.	❑	❑	❑
8. List the requirements for releasing medical records upon a patient's request including fees (search your state's statutes for permissible charges for copies of medical records).	❑	❑	❑
9. List the requirements for handling requests for medical records by individuals other than the patient.	❑	❑	❑
10. Indicate the title of the person responsible for updating and revising this policy as necessary.	❑	❑	❑
11. Provide the policy to all employees with an acknowledgement of receipt and their understanding of the policy and/or revisions.	❑	❑	❑

_____

_____

_____

_____

(continues)

PSY PROCEDURE 2-5 | **Create an Office Policy to Protect Patient's Private Health Information** (continued)

CALCULATION

Total Possible Points: _____

Total Points Earned: _____ Multiplied by 100 = _____ Divided by Total Possible Points = _____ %

PASS **FAIL** **COMMENTS:**
❏ ❏

Student's signature _____ Date _____

Partner's signature _____ Date _____

Instructor's signature _____ Date _____

CHAPTER 3

Communication Skills

LEARNING OUTCOMES

COG Cognitive Domain*

1. Spell and define the key terms
2. List two major forms of communication
3. *Identify types of verbal and nonverbal communication*
4. *Identify communication barriers*
5. *Identify techniques for overcoming communication barriers*
6. *Identify the steps in the sender–receiver process*
7. *Identify challenges in communication based on developmental stages*
8. *Identify steps in coaching a patient relevant to the individual patient's needs*
9. Identify resources and adaptations that are required based on individual needs, that is, culture and environment, developmental life stage, language, and physical threats to communication
10. *Identify issues associated with diversity as it relates to patient care*
11. *Identify the basic concepts of the following: Erikson and Kübler-Ross*
12. Explain how various components of communication can affect the meaning of verbal messages
13. Define active listening
14. List and describe the six interviewing techniques

15. Give an example of how cultural differences may affect communication
16. Discuss how to handle communication problems caused by language barriers
17. List two methods that you can use to promote communication among hearing-, sight-, and speech-impaired patients
18. Discuss how to handle an angry or distressed patient
19. List five actions that you can take to improve communication with a child
20. Discuss your role in communicating with a grieving patient or family member
21. Discuss the key elements of interdisciplinary communication
22. Explore the issue of confidentiality as it applies to the medical assistant

PSY Psychomotor Domain*

1. *Respond to nonverbal communication* (Procedure 3-1)
2. Use feedback techniques to obtain patient information, including reflection, restatement, and clarification (Procedure 3-1)
3. *Coach patients appropriately considering cultural diversity, developmental life stage, and communication barriers* (Procedure 3-2)

AFF Affective Domain*

1. *Demonstrate empathy for the patient's concern in responding to challenging patient communication*
2. *Demonstrate active listening in responding to challenging patient communication*
3. *Demonstrate respect for diversity when communicating with a patient*
4. Use appropriate body language and other nonverbal skills in communicating with patients, family, and staff
5. Demonstrate awareness of the territorial boundaries of the person with whom you are communicating
6. Demonstrate sensitivity appropriate to the message being delivered
7. Demonstrate awareness of how an individual's personal appearance affects anticipated responses
8. Demonstrate recognition of the patient's level of understanding in communications
9. Analyze communication in providing appropriate responses/feedback
10. Recognize personal boundaries

*MAERB Standards are italicized.

ABHES Competencies

1. Respond appropriately to patients with abnormal behavior patterns
2. Use empathy when communicating with terminally ill patients
3. Identify common stages that terminally ill patients experience
4. List organizations and support groups that can assist patients and family members of patients experiencing terminal illness
5. Display effective interpersonal skills with patients and healthcare team members
6. Demonstrate cultural awareness

Name: _____   Date: _____   Grade: _____

COG MULTIPLE CHOICE

Circle the letter preceding the correct answer.

1. Laughing, sobbing, and sighing are examples of:
   a. kinesics.
   b. proxemics.
   c. nonlanguage.
   d. paralanguage.
   e. clarification.

2. Hearing impairment that involves problems with either nerves or the cochlea is called:
   a. anacusis.
   b. conductive.
   c. presbyacusis.
   d. sensorineural.
   e. dysphasia.

3. Sally needs to obtain information from her patient about the medications he is taking. Which of the following open-ended questions is phrased in a way that will elicit the information that Sally needs?
   a. Are you taking your medications?
   b. What medications are you taking?
   c. Have you taken any medications?
   d. Did you take your medications today?
   e. Have you taken medications in the past?

4. Which of the following shows the proper sequence of the sender–receiver process?
   a. Person to send message, message to be sent, person to receive message
   b. Message to be received, person to send message, message to be sent
   c. Message to be sent, person to send message, person to receive message
   d. Person to receive message, person to send message, message to be sent
   e. Person to send message, person to receive message, message to be sent

5. "Those people always get head lice." This statement is an example of:
   a. culture.
   b. demeanor.
   c. discrimination.
   d. stereotyping.
   e. prejudice.

6. What can you do as a medical assistant to communicate effectively with a patient when there is a language barrier?
   a. Find an interpreter who can translate for the patient.
   b. Raise your voice so the patient can focus more on what you are saying.
   c. Give the patient the name and address of a physician who speaks the same language.
   d. Assess the patient and give the physician your best opinion about what is bothering the patient.
   e. Suggest that the patient find another physician who is better equipped to communicate with the patient.

7. When dealing with patients who present communication challenges, such as hearing-impaired or sight-impaired patients, it is best to:
   a. talk about the patient directly with a family member to find out what the problem is.
   b. conduct the interview alone with the patient because he needs to be able to take care of himself.
   c. address the patient's questions in the waiting room, where other people can try to help the patient communicate.
   d. refer the patient to a practice that specializes in working with hearing- and sight-impaired patients.
   e. make sure the patient feels like he is part of the process, even if his condition requires a family member's help.

8. A hearing-impaired patient's test results are in. It is important that the patient gets the results quickly. How should you get the results to the patient?
   a. Mail the test results via priority mail.
   b. Call the patient on a TDD/TTY phone and type in the results.
   c. Drive to the patient's house at lunchtime to deliver the results.
   d. Call an emergency contact of the patient and ask them to have the patient make an appointment.
   e. Send the patient a fax containing the test results.

9. Which of the following statements about grieving is true?
   a. The grieving period is approximately 30 days.
   b. Different cultures and individuals demonstrate grief in different ways.
   c. The best way to grieve is through wailing because it lets the emotion out.
   d. The five stages of grief must be followed in that specific order for healing to begin.
   e. Everyone grieves in their own way, but all of us go through the stages at the same time.

10. *Proxemics* refers to the:
    a. pitch of a person's voice.
    b. facial expressions a person makes.
    c. physical proximity that people tolerate.
    d. the combination of verbal and nonverbal communication.
    e. the ability of a patient to comprehend difficult messages.

11. Which of the following situations would result in a breach of patient confidentiality?
    a. Shredding unwanted notes that contain patient information
    b. Discussing a patient's lab results with a coworker in the hospital cafeteria
    c. Keeping the glass window between the waiting room and reception desk closed
    d. Shutting down your computer when you leave every night
    e. Paging the physician on an intercom to let them know a patient is waiting on the phone for results

12. "Those results can't be true. The doctor must have mixed me up with another patient." This statement reflects which of the following stages of grieving?
    a. Anger
    b. Denial
    c. Depression
    d. Bargaining
    e. Acceptance

13. Which of the following statements about communication is correct?
    a. Communication can be either verbal or nonverbal.
    b. Written messages can be interpreted through paralanguage.
    c. Verbal communication involves both oral communication and body language.
    d. Body language is the most important form of communication.
    e. Touch should be avoided in all forms of communication because it makes the recipient of the message uncomfortable.

14. During a patient interview, repeating what you have heard the patient say using an open-ended statement is called:
    a. clarifying.
    b. reflecting.
    c. summarizing.
    d. paraphrasing.
    e. allowing silences.

15. What should you do during a patient interview if there is silence?
    a. Silence should not be allowed during a patient interview.
    b. Immediately start talking so the patient does not feel awkward.
    c. Fill in charts that need to be completed until the patient is ready.
    d. Wait for the physician to arrive to speak with the patient.
    e. Gather your thoughts and think of any additional questions you have.

16. The physician is behind schedule, and a patient is angry that her appointment is late. The best way to deal with the patient is to:
    a. tell her anything that will calm her down.
    b. ignore her until the problem is solved.
    c. threaten that the physician will no longer treat her if she continues to complain.
    d. keep her informed of when the physician will be able to see her.
    e. ask her why it is such a big deal.

17. Why is it helpful to ask open-ended questions during a patient interview?
    a. They let the patient give yes or no answers.
    b. They let the patient develop an answer and explain it.
    c. They let the patient respond quickly using few words.
    d. They provide simple answers that are easy to note in the chart.
    e. They let the patient give their own feelings and opinions on the subject.

18. Difficulty with speech is called:
    a. dysphasia.
    b. dysphonia.
    c. nyctalopia.
    d. strabismus.
    e. myopia.

19. One particular physician runs behind schedule most of the time. His CMA has to work until he finishes seeing his patients, but her child must be picked up from daycare by 6:00 PM. Which statement below represents one of an assertive person?

    a. I won't work late another day! My hours are 8:00 AM to 5:00 PM.

    b. Sorry, doctor, I'm out of here to pick up my child. Someone else will have to stay.

    c. My daughter must be picked up by 6:00 every day. Could we look at the possibility of taking turns staying late? I could make arrangements for one day out of the week.

    d. Since you are the reason we run late, you should take care of the patients yourself.

    e. I can't believe you're asking me to stay late again. I am going to find another job.

20. The limit of personal space is generally considered to be a:

    a. 1-foot radius.

    b. 3-foot radius.

    c. 5-foot radius.

    d. 10-foot radius.

    e. 15-foot radius.

COG MATCHING

Grade: _____

Match the following key terms to their definitions.

Key Terms

21. _____ anacusis
22. _____ bias
23. _____ clarification
24. _____ cultures
25. _____ demeanor
26. _____ discrimination
27. _____ dysphasia
28. _____ dysphonia
29. _____ feedback
30. _____ grief
31. _____ messages
32. _____ mourning
33. _____ nonlanguage
34. _____ paralanguage
35. _____ paraphrasing
36. _____ presbyacusis
37. _____ reflecting
38. _____ stereotyping
39. _____ summarizing
40. _____ therapeutic

Definitions

a. Information
b. Something that is beneficial to a patient
c. A group of people who share a way of life and beliefs
d. Holding an opinion of all members of a particular culture, race, religion, or age group based on oversimplified or negative characterizations
e. Loss of hearing associated with aging
f. Difficulty speaking
g. Sounds that include laughing, sobbing, sighing, or grunting to convey information
h. The response to a message
i. Restating what a person said using your own words or phrases
j. Removal of confusion or uncertainty
k. Formation of an opinion without foundation or reason
l. A demonstration of the signs of grief
m. Complete hearing loss
n. Briefly reviewing information discussed to determine the patient's comprehension
o. Great sadness caused by a loss
p. Voice tone, quality, volume, pitch, and range
q. The way a person looks, behaves, and conducts himself
r. A voice impairment that is caused by a physical condition, such as oral surgery
s. The act of not treating a patient fairly or respectfully because of his cultural, social, or personal values
t. Repeating what one heard using open-ended questions

COG IDENTIFICATION

Grade: _____

41. The two main forms of communication are verbal communication and nonverbal communication. Read each form of communication below and place an "A" for verbal or a "B" for nonverbal in the space provided.
   a. _____ A patient sighs while explaining her symptoms.
   b. _____ A patient shrugs his shoulders after being told he needs to lose weight.
   c. _____ A patient's eyes dart around the room during the explanation of a procedure.
   d. _____ A physician writes "take two aspirin every 8 hours."
   e. _____ A mother is given a sheet of paper describing what to expect of her baby during months 6 to 9.
   f. _____ A physician puts her hand on a patient's shoulder before delivering test results.

COG PSY SHORT ANSWER

Grade: _____

42. List five local resources that can assist a grieving patient or family member. Include the name of the agency, type of help that it offers, and its phone number.

_____

_____

_____

43. Why is it important to respect cultural diversity?

_____

_____

_____

44. List the five stages of grief as outlined by Elisabeth Kübler-Ross.

_____

_____

_____

45. List five actions that you can take to improve communication with a child.

_____

_____

_____

46. List two methods that you can use to promote communication among hearing-, sight-, and speech-impaired patients.

_____

_____

_____

47. List and describe the six interviewing techniques.

_____

_____

_____

48. List two major forms of communication.

_____

_____

_____

49. What is the difference between aggressiveness and assertiveness?

_____

_____

_____

AFF WHAT WOULD YOU DO?

_____ Grade: _____

50. You are working in the reception area of a busy medical practice. Patients come and go all day long, and it is your responsibility to move the flow along. One particularly busy day, you are registering an 89-year-old man. You ask him to read and sign the Acknowledgment of Privacy Practices. He says that he cannot see the form and asks if his wife can sign. His nonverbal cues make you wonder if he can read and write. From the list below, choose all appropriate actions.
    a. Ask him if he would like the number for an adult literacy program.
    b. Tell him that his wife can sign for him, but she should also read the authorization for him.
    c. Have his wife initial the "signature" and then you sign as a witness.
    d. Tell him to make an "X" if he cannot write.
    e. Tell him to sign the form without reading it.

51. A patient calls the office with symptoms and a condition that you are not familiar with. She has used some terms that you do not understand. When you relay the message to the physician, how should you communicate the patient's problem?

    _____

    _____

    _____

COG IDENTIFICATION

_____ Grade: _____

52. Read the list of nonverbal communication cues below. Beside each one, list the problem or issue this action might indicate:

    a. Crossed arms _____

    b. Slumping in a chair _____

    c. A child hiding behind their mother _____

    d. Hand clenching _____

53. Physicians use the information obtained during a patient interview to help them assess the patient's health. Patients will be more willing to provide information during a professionally conducted interview. Read each of the following statements describing patient interviews. Answer "yes" if the statement describes a correct interview practice; answer "no" if it describes an incorrect interview practice. Explain how to correct the problem for all "no" answers.

    a. Patient interviews can be conducted in an exam room or in the waiting room. _____

    b. Answering a phone call in the middle of a new patient interview is acceptable if it is a call you have been waiting for. _____

    c. It is important to maintain eye contact with the patient, so you do not write any patient responses down until the interview is over. _____

    d. You confirm which blood pressure medication and what dosage the patient is taking.

    _____

    e. There is nothing wrong with skipping questions in a patient interview that may make the patient feel uncomfortable. _____

    f. Introducing yourself to the patient is a nice way to start an interview. _____

◆◆◆ TRUE OR FALSE?

Grade: _____

Determine whether the following statements are true or false. If false, explain why.

54. When the office is busy, it is okay to refer to patients by their medical conditions, for example, "stomach pain in room 1."

_____

55. If an older adult patient does not have a ride home, a staff member in the office should offer them one.

_____

56. When speaking with patients, do not reveal too many personal details about your life.

_____

57. It is inappropriate to carry on personal conversations with other staff members in front of a patient.

_____

PSY ACTIVE LEARNING

Grade: _____

58. Practice active listening with a partner. Have your partner tell you a detailed story that you have never heard before or explain a topic that you are unfamiliar with. After they have finished, wait silently for 2 minutes. Then, try to repeat the story or steps back to your partner. Next, reverse roles and let your partner listen while you tell a story or explain a concept.

_____

_____

_____

59. If you work in a pediatric office, you will certainly spend a good deal of time communicating with children. To help strengthen your communication skills with children, find a local preschool or elementary school teacher who has experience working with children. Interview this teacher about their communication techniques and write a list of 10 tips for communicating with children.

_____

_____

_____

AFF CASE STUDIES FOR CRITICAL THINKING A

Grade: _____

You are working in a geriatric office taking patients back, and one of your patients is a Spanish-speaking woman who comes into the office with her son and daughter. Her body language indicates fear and worry. She appears very shy and depends on her son and daughter for assistance. They speak a little bit of English, but it is difficult to communicate with them.

60. Your first duty is to interview the patient about her medical history. Of the following steps, circle the ones you should take to get information.
   a. Speak in a normal tone and volume.
   b. Speak directly to the son and daughter.
   c. When asking a question about eyesight, point to your eyes.
   d. Use abbreviations and slang terms for medical tests.
   e. Ask the woman's son to be the interpreter and her daughter to wait outside.
   f. Use complex medical language to explain procedures.
   g. Use a Spanish-to-English dictionary.

61. The physician will be doing a complete exam on the patient. She must change into a gown. You have everyone except her daughter leave the exam room and hand a gown to her daughter who starts toward her mother to help the patient change. The patient backs up into the corner of the room. Of the following actions, which ONE is the most appropriate?
   a. Take the gown from the daughter, give it to the patient, and use gestures as you explain that you want her to put on the gown.
   b. Leave the room and let the daughter handle it.
   c. Tell her that she will be covered and you have a blanket for her if she is cold.
   d. Tell the physician that the patient would not undress and let them handle it.
   e. Give the patient a big hug—that should make her feel better.

62. Following a difficult exam, the physician notes a suspicious mole on the patient's back. He instructs you to get her an appointment with a dermatologist. You explain to the three of them that you will make an appointment. You ask them if they have a preference, and they appear confused. Circle all appropriate actions in the list below.
   a. Give them a patient brochure on moles.
   b. Make an appointment in 2 weeks for them to return with a translator.
   c. Make the appointment, and write down the name and address of the facility.
   d. Give the patient a big hug and tell her what a brave woman she was.
   e. Use a Spanish-to-English dictionary to try to explain.

AFF CASE STUDIES FOR CRITICAL THINKING B

Grade: _____

63. Your physician is treating a 7-year-old girl who needs to have her tonsils removed. Her mother has 60% hearing loss and depends on lip reading to communicate. You need to have her sign paperwork and explain the child's need for a preanesthesia appointment at the hospital. Circle the suggestions below that will help you to communicate with her.
    a. Gently touch the patient to get her attention.
    b. Exaggerate your facial movements.
    c. Eliminate all distractions.
    d. Enunciate clearly.
    e. Use short sentences with short words.
    f. Speak loudly.
    g. Give the patient written instructions.
    h. Turn toward the light so your face is illuminated.
    i. Talk face-to-face with the patient, not at an angle.

64. Protocol dictates that the child has a history and physical exam before her surgery. She is obviously afraid and confused about what is happening. Circle the actions listed below that would be appropriate when communicating with the child.
    a. Tell the child when you need to touch them and what you are going to do.
    b. Speak loudly and sternly so the child will stay focused on you and not other distractions in the office.
    c. Work quickly and let them be surprised by what you do.
    d. Rephrase questions until the child understands.
    e. Be playful to help gain the child's cooperation.
    f. Try to speak to children at their eye level.

Additional procedure forms 3-1, "Recognizing Nonverbal Communication" and 3-2, "Understanding Barriers to Communication" are available on the following pages.

PSY PROCEDURE 3-1 **Recognizing Nonverbal Communication**

Name: _____ **Date:** _____ **Time:** _____ **Grade:** _____

EQUIPMENT/SUPPLIES: None

STANDARDS: Given the needed equipment and a place to work, the student will perform this skill with _____ % accuracy in a total of _____ minutes. *(Your instructor will tell you what the percentage and time limits will be before you begin.)*

KEY: 4 = Satisfactory 0 = Unsatisfactory NA = This step is not counted

PROCEDURE STEPS	SELF	PARTNER	INSTRUCTOR
1. Observe patient to determine if there is a problem.	❑	❑	❑
2. Take patient to a private area.	❑	❑	❑
3. Stay calm and maintain proper space between the patient and you.	❑	❑	❑
4. Gather information by using active listening and asking open-ended questions.	❑	❑	❑
5. Use *reflection* to gather additional information from the patient.	❑	❑	❑
6. Use *restatement* during the conversation with the patient.	❑	❑	❑
7. Ask a *clarification* question during the conversation.	❑	❑	❑
8. Allow *silence* during the conversation.	❑	❑	❑
9. Observe patient for signs of continued agitation.	❑	❑	❑
10. **AFF** Demonstrate the principles of self-boundaries.	❑	❑	❑

_____

_____

_____

_____

CALCULATION

Total Possible Points: _____

Total Points Earned: _____ Multiplied by 100 = _____ Divided by Total Possible Points = _____ %

PASS **FAIL** **COMMENTS:**
❑ ❑

Student's signature _____ Date _____

Partner's signature _____ Date _____

Instructor's signature _____ Date _____

PSY PROCEDURE 3-2 **Understanding Barriers to Communication**

Name: _____ Date: _____ Time: _____ Grade: _____

EQUIPMENT/SUPPLIES: Medical History Form

STANDARDS: Given the needed equipment and a place to work, the student will perform this skill with _____ % accuracy in a total of _____ minutes. *(Your instructor will tell you what the percentage and time limits will be before you begin.)*

KEY: 4 = Satisfactory 0 = Unsatisfactory NA = This step is not counted

PROCEDURE STEPS	SELF	PARTNER	INSTRUCTOR
1. Greet and identify the patient and explain what you need to ask.	❏	❏	❏
2. Take the patient to a private area.	❏	❏	❏
3. Sit facing the patient and maintain proper space between the patient and you. Observe the patient's comfort level with making eye contact.	❏	❏	❏
4. Note the patient's affirmative response to any of the health history questions.	❏	❏	❏
5. **AFF** Demonstrate respect for individual diversity including: a. gender, b. race, c. religion, d. age, e. economic status, f. appearance.	❏	❏	❏

_____

_____

_____

_____

CALCULATION

Total Possible Points: _____

Total Points Earned: _____ Multiplied by 100 = _____ Divided by Total Possible Points = _____ %

PASS   FAIL   COMMENTS:
❏   ❏

Student's signature _____ Date _____

Partner's signature _____ Date _____

Instructor's signature _____ Date _____

CHAPTER 4

Patient Education

LEARNING OUTCOMES

COG Cognitive Domain*

1. Spell and define the key terms
2. Explain the medical assistant's role in patient education
3. Define the five steps in the patient education process
4. Identify five conditions that are needed for patient education to occur
5. *Identify the basic concepts of the following theories: Maslow*
6. List five factors that may hinder patient education and at least two methods to compensate for each of these factors
7. Discuss five preventive medicine guidelines that you should teach your patients
8. Explain the kinds of information that should be included in patient teaching about medication therapy
9. Explain your role in teaching patients about alternative medicine therapies
10. List and explain relaxation techniques that you and patients can learn to help with stress management
11. Describe how to prepare a teaching plan
12. List potential sources of patient education materials
13. Locate community resources and list ways of organizing and disseminating information
14. *Identify communication barriers*
15. *Identify techniques for overcoming communication barriers*
16. Identify resources and adaptations that are required based on individual needs, that is, culture and environment, developmental life stage, language, and physical threats to communication

PSY Psychomotor Domain*

1. Document patient education (Procedure 4-1)
2. *Develop and maintain a current list of community resources related to the patient's healthcare needs (Procedure 4-2)*
3. *Coach patients regarding medical encounters (Procedure 4-1)*
4. *Use a list of community resources to facilitate referrals (Procedure 4-2)*

AFF Affective Domain*

1. *Reassure patients*
2. *Respect diversity*
3. *Demonstrate empathy for patients' concerns*
4. *Demonstrate active listening*
5. Demonstrate sensitivity appropriate to the message being delivered
6. Demonstrate recognition of the patient's level of understanding in communications

MAERB Standards are italicized.

ABHES Competencies

1. Assist the patient in navigating issues and concerns that may arise (i.e., insurance policy information, medical bills, and physician/provider orders)
2. Adapt care to address the developmental states of life
3. Display effective interpersonal skills with patients and healthcare team members
4. Display professionalism through written and verbal communications
5. Analyze the effect of heredity, cultural, and environmental influences on behavior
6. Teach self-examination, disease management, and health promotion
7. Identify community resources and Complementary and Alternative Medicine practices (CAM)
8. Make adaptions for patients with special needs (psychological or physical limitations)
9. Make adaptations to care for patients across their lifespans

Name: _____ Date: _____ Grade: _____

OOG MULTIPLE CHOICE

Circle the BEST answer.

1. During assessment, the most comprehensive source from which to obtain patient information is the:
   a. physician's notes.
   b. immunization record.
   c. medical record.
   d. family member.
   e. nurse.

2. When teaching a patient with many chronic health problems, it is important to:
   a. focus on each problem separately.
   b. tell them that your grandmother has many of the same problems.
   c. bond with them.
   d. have the patient come back another time with a family member.
   e. have the physician talk to them.

3. Which of the following is an example of a psychomotor skill that a patient may perform?
   a. Telling the physician about their symptoms
   b. Explaining how a part of the body is feeling
   c. Walking around with a crutch
   d. Watching television in the waiting room
   e. Listening to a physician's instructions

4. Which part of Maslow's pyramid is the point at which a patient has satisfied all basic needs and feels they have control over their life?
   a. Safety and security
   b. Esteem
   c. Self-actualization
   d. Affection
   e. Physiologic

5. Noncompliance occurs when the patient:
   a. experiences a decrease in symptoms healed.
   b. forgets to pay their bill.
   c. refuses to follow the physician's orders.
   d. requests a new medical assistant to assist the physician.
   e. agrees with the physician.

6. The power of believing that something will make you better when there is no chemical reaction that warrants such improvement is:
   a. self-relaxation.
   b. positive stress.
   c. acupuncture.
   d. placebo.
   e. visualization.

7. Patient education should consist of multiple techniques or approaches so:
   a. the patient can apply their new knowledge to real-life events.
   b. the patient will learn and retain more.
   c. the patient will understand that there are many ways to look at an issue.
   d. the patient will know where you stand on their healthcare options.
   e. the patient will have a wider choice of treatments.

8. One mental health illness that can hinder patient education is:
   a. diabetes.
   b. Lyme disease.
   c. obstructive pulmonary disease.
   d. Alzheimer's disease.
   e. anemia.

9. Health assessment forms that assess a patient's education level may also help you determine a patient's ability to:
   a. read.
   b. listen.
   c. communicate.
   d. respond.
   e. evaluate.

10. Before developing a medication schedule, you should evaluate the patient's:
    a. prescribed medication.
    b. side effects.
    c. changes in bodily functions.
    d. daily routine.
    e. bowel movements.

11. Which is an example of a recommended preventive procedure?
    a. Regular teeth whitening
    b. Childhood immunizations
    c. Daily exercise
    d. Yearly lung-cancer evaluations
    e. Occasional antibiotics

12. Which of the following is true of herbal supplements?
    a. A medical assistant can recommend that a patient start taking herbal supplements without the physician's approval.
    b. A health store clerk is a good source of information on supplements.
    c. Products that claim to detoxify the whole body are generally effective.
    d. Supplements will not interfere with blood sugar levels because they are not medication.
    e. Patients should be advised that because a product is natural does not mean it is safe.

13. One example of a physiologic response to negative stress is:
    a. elevated mood.
    b. hunger pangs.
    c. headache.
    d. profuse bleeding.
    e. energy boost.

14. In Maslow's hierarchy of needs, air, water, food, and rest are considered:
    a. affection needs.
    b. safety and security needs.
    c. esteem needs.
    d. self-actualization needs.
    e. physiologic needs.

15. When explaining the benefits and risks of a proposed treatment to a patient who uses American Sign Language to communicate, the physician must:
    a. be sure the patient is given the information in writing.
    b. provide a sign language interpreter if the patient does not bring one.
    c. make the patient feel comfortable.
    d. use a notepad to communicate.
    e. let the medical assistant handle it.

16. Humans use defense mechanisms to:
    a. cope with painful problems.
    b. increase their sense of accomplishment.
    c. decrease effects of chronic physical pain.
    d. learn to get along well with others.
    e. explain complicated emotions to medical staff.

17. Support groups give patients the opportunity to:
    a. exchange and compare medical records.
    b. meet and share ideas with others who are experiencing the same issues.
    c. spread the good word about the medical office.
    d. obtain their basic physiologic needs.
    e. learn more about malpractice suits.

18. When selecting teaching material, you should first:
    a. choose preprinted material.
    b. create your own material.
    c. assess your patient's general level of understanding.
    d. let the patient find a book from the clinic library.
    e. ask the patient to create a list of specific questions.

19. Acupressure is different from acupuncture because:
    a. it does not use needles.
    b. it is not an alternative medicine.
    c. it cannot be used with cancer patients.
    d. it does not require any licensure.
    e. it is less effective.

20. If your community does not have a central agency for information and resources, you should create a(n):
    a. hierarchy of needs.
    b. teaching plan.
    c. telephone directory.
    d. information sheet.
    e. flowchart.

21. Suppose you want to teach a patient about the need to adopt a low-sugar diet because of diabetes, but the patient doesn't believe that diabetes is a serious health problem. If education is to be effective, which of the following must the patient accept? Circle all that apply.
    a. Diabetes has to be managed.
    b. There is a correlation between high sugar intake and diabetes.
    c. Diabetes isn't as serious as other diseases.
    d. Diabetes management requires dietary changes.
    e. It is possible to consume large quantities of high-sugar foods, but only occasionally.

COG MATCHING

Grade: _____

Match the following key terms to their definitions.

Key Terms

22. _____ alternative treatment
23. _____ assessment
24. _____ coping mechanisms
25. _____ dissemination
26. _____ documentation
27. _____ evaluation
28. _____ implementation
29. _____ learning objectives
30. _____ noncompliance
31. _____ placebo effect
32. _____ planning
33. _____ psychomotor
34. _____ stress
35. _____ health literacy

Definitions

a. involves using the information you have gathered to determine how you will approach the patient's learning needs

b. skill that requires the patient to physically perform a task

c. the process that indicates how well patients are adapting or applying new information to their lives

d. produced by illness or injury and may result in physiologic and psychological effects

e. includes procedures or tasks that will be discussed or performed at various points in the program to help achieve the goal

f. the process of distributing information on community resources

g. includes recording of all teachings that occurred

h. the patient's inability or refusal to follow a prescribed order

i. involves gathering information about the patient's present healthcare needs and abilities

j. psychological defenses used to help deal with the painful and difficult problems life can bring

k. the power of believing that something will make you better when there is no chemical reaction that warrants such improvement

l. the expected outcomes for the teaching process

m. an option or substitute to the standard medical treatment such as acupuncture

n. an individual's ability to read and understand health information

SHORT ANSWER

Grade: _____

36. List three potential sources of patient education materials.

_____

_____

_____

37. List and explain three relaxation techniques that you and patients can learn to help with stress management.

_____

_____

_____

AFF WHAT WOULD YOU DO?

Grade: _____

38. You work in a pediatric practice. A mother brings her 6-month-old son in for a routine checkup. The child has a visible lump on the right side of his head, just above his ear. The mother states that the child fell off a twin bed when she was changing his diaper. After examining the child, the physician asks you to instruct the mother in safety and also have her watch the baby closely for the next few days for signs of concussion.

A. What resources might be available to you?

_____

_____

B. How might you evaluate the mother's barriers to communication and understanding?

_____

_____

C. What method of instruction would you use for this situation?

_____

_____

D. What would your teaching plan need to include?

_____

_____

E. What measures should be taken if the child's injuries were consistent with possible abuse?

_____

_____

F. Why is patient education important?

_____

_____

39. Write a sentence explaining why, as a medical assistant, you must set aside your own personal feelings and life experiences when educating patients.

_____

_____

_____

COG IDENTIFICATION

Grade: _____

List the five factors that can hinder patient education.

40. _____

41. _____

42. _____

43. _____

44. _____

COG PSY ACTIVE LEARNING

Grade: _____

45. Juggling school with other commitments may occasionally cause negative stress in your life. Make a list of how you experience stress in your daily life. Then choose one of the three relaxation techniques discussed in this chapter. Practice that technique and then write a paragraph describing the "pros" and "cons" of the chosen technique.

_____

_____

_____

46. Develop a teaching plan for a family member or friend. For example, if your mother has asthma, do research on the Internet to find information and resources about asthma. Remember to include all of the elements of a teaching plan. Practice your teaching techniques by educating a family member or friend about a particular illness or disease.

_____

_____

_____

47. Choose a health concern that may require external support. For example, a patient fighting cancer may wish to join a support group or other organization for help. Search the Internet for local, state, and national agencies that provide information, support, and services to patients with your chosen need. Then compile this information in an informative and creative brochure, pamphlet, or other learning tool.

_____

_____

_____

48. Research information on the *Healthy People 2030* website and list five of the social determinants of health that affect health, functioning, and quality-of-life outcomes and risks.

_____

_____

_____

COG PSY PATIENT EDUCATION

Grade: _____

49. A patient wants to use alternative medicine in addition to medicine prescribed by the physician. What should you do?

_____

_____

_____

50. A patient in your care is suffering physiologic effects from negative stress brought on by chronic back pain. What types of coping strategies would you recommend to the patient and why?

_____

_____

_____

51. Julia is an 8-year-old patient who has been diagnosed with type 1 diabetes. The medical office has a preprinted teaching plan titled, "Living with Type 2 Diabetes." Should you use this plan or develop your own? Explain.

_____

_____

_____

TRUE OR FALSE?

Grade: _____

Determine whether the following statements are true or false. If false, explain why.

52. Patients benefit from the use of teaching aids that they can take home and use as reference material.

_____

53. If a patient asks you a question and you are not sure of the answer, you should give your best guess.

_____

54. A patient must have his basic needs met before self-actualization may occur.

_____

55. Visualization is a relaxation technique that involves deep breathing and physical exercise.

_____

AFF CASE STUDIES FOR CRITICAL THINKING A

Grade: _____

A 5-year-old girl in your pediatric practice has just been diagnosed with juvenile diabetes. Your physician asks you to assist the patient's parents with resources available to them.

56. From the following list, circle the BEST resource.
   a. Materials from a pharmaceutical company
   b. Other patients who have this problem
   c. The official website of the American Diabetes Association
   d. Another pediatrician's office
   e. American Medical Technologists, Inc.

57. When developing a teaching plan, circle the most appropriate entry under Learning Objectives?
   a. The patient was not involved in training due to age.
   b. The patient's mother describes the body's use of insulin.
   c. See documentation of patient education in chart.
   d. Gave patient instructional video: "Your Child and Diabetes."
   e. The patient understands disease.

AFF CASE STUDIES FOR CRITICAL THINKING B

Grade: _____

Your physician instructs you to come up with a plan for Mr. Johns who has been diagnosed with hypercholesterolemia. He needs to change his eating habits and lifestyle drastically. You plan to help him form a plan for making these changes.

58. Patients should be encouraged to take an active approach to their health and healthcare education. To assist Mr. Johns effectively, which of the following must you do? Circle all that apply.
    a. Help Mr. Johns accept his illness.
    b. Expect Mr. Johns to follow your instructions without further explanation.
    c. Involve Mr. Johns in the process of gaining knowledge.
    d. Provide Mr. Johns with positive reinforcement.
    e. Give Mr. Johns the most in-depth professional textbooks you can find.

59. Your plan for Mr. Johns should include all of the following EXCEPT:
    a. a timeline for a gradually progressing walking program.
    b. recipes for low-fat dishes.
    c. pamphlets with information about his condition.
    d. documentation of your instruction.
    e. a list of his medications.

60. Ms. Jasinski is an older adult patient who has recently lost several relatives and friends. She lives alone, feels disconnected from others and, as a result, her health has begun to deteriorate. Brian, a medical assistant, gives Ms. Jasinski a friendly hug when he sees her during patient visits. He talks to her and listens to her stories. He has also encouraged her to join a senior citizens' group. Circle which of Maslow's hierarchy of needs has Brian helped fulfill for Ms. Jasinski?
    a. Physiologic
    b. Safety and security
    c. Affection and belonging
    d. Self-actualization

PROCEDURE 4-1   Document Patient Education

PSY

Name: _____ **Date:** _____ **Time:** _____ **Grade:** _____

EQUIPMENT/SUPPLIES: Patient's chart, pen

STANDARDS: Given the needed equipment and a place to work, the student will perform this skill with _____ % accuracy in a total of _____ minutes. *(Your instructor will tell you what the percentage and time limits will be before you begin.)*

KEY: 4 = Satisfactory   0 = Unsatisfactory   NA = This step is not counted

PROCEDURE STEPS	SELF	PARTNER	INSTRUCTOR
1. Record the date and time of teaching.	❏	❏	❏
2. Record the information taught.	❏	❏	❏
3. Record the manner in which the information was taught.	❏	❏	❏
4. Record your evaluation of your teaching.	❏	❏	❏
5. Record any additional teaching planned.	❏	❏	❏
6. **AFF** Explain what you would do if you forgot to document an action you took during the patient education process.	❏	❏	❏

_____

_____

_____

Note: The medical assistant may sign their name in the patient record using only the "CMA" credential if the office has a signature log denoting the entire credential as "CMA(AAMA)."

CALCULATION

Total Possible Points: _____

Total Points Earned: _____ Multiplied by 100 = _____ Divided by Total Possible Points = _____ %

PASS   **FAIL**   **COMMENTS:**
❏   ❏

Student's signature _____ Date _____

Partner's signature _____ Date _____

Instructor's signature _____ Date _____

PSY PROCEDURE 4-2 **Advocating on Behalf of Patients**

Name: _____ Date: _____ Time: _____ Grade: _____

EQUIPMENT/SUPPLIES: Computer with Internet access

STANDARDS: Given the needed equipment and a place to work, the student will perform this skill with _____ % accuracy in a total of _____ minutes. *(Your instructor will tell you what the percentage and time limits will be before you begin.)*

KEY: 4 = Satisfactory 0 = Unsatisfactory NA = This step is not counted

PROCEDURE STEPS	SELF	PARTNER	INSTRUCTOR
1. Assess the patient's needs for the following: a. Education b. Health insurance coverage c. Financial information d. Support groups e. Home health needs	❏	❏	❏
2. Using a search engine, research available resources to have them available for patients and to be prepared with materials on hand to give to patients.	❏	❏	❏
3. Give the patient the contact information in writing.	❏	❏	❏
4. Document actions and the information given to the patient.	❏	❏	❏
5. Instruct the patient to contact the office if they have any difficulty.	❏	❏	❏
6. **AFF** Explain what suggestions or assistance you would offer to a patient who would benefit from online patient education resources but does not own a computer.	❏	❏	❏

_____

_____

_____

CALCULATION

Total Possible Points: _____

Total Points Earned: _____ Multiplied by 100 = _____ Divided by Total Possible Points = _____ %

PASS **FAIL**   **COMMENTS:**
 ❏   ❏

Student's signature _____ Date _____

Partner's signature _____ Date _____

Instructor's signature _____ Date _____

PART 2

The Administrative Medical Assistant

UNIT TWO

Fundamentals of Administrative Medical Assisting

CHAPTER 5

The First Contact: Telephone and Reception

LEARNING OUTCOMES

OOG Cognitive Domain*

1. Spell and define the key terms
2. Explain the importance of displaying a professional image to all patients
3. List six duties of the medical office receptionist
4. List four sources from which messages can be retrieved
5. Discuss various steps that can be taken to promote good ergonomics
6. Describe the basic guidelines for waiting room environments
7. *Identify the following as practiced within an ambulatory care setting: medical asepsis*
8. Discuss the five basic guidelines for telephone use
9. Describe the types of incoming telephone calls received by the medical office
10. Discuss how to identify and handle callers with medical emergencies
11. Describe how to triage incoming calls
12. *Identify the physical manifestations and emotional behaviors of persons involved in an emergency*
13. List the information that should be given to an emergency medical service dispatcher
14. Describe the types of telephone services and special features

PSY Psychomotor Domain*

1. *Demonstrate professional telephone techniques (Procedures 5-1 and 5-2)*
2. *Document telephone messages accurately (Procedures 5-1 and 5-2)*
3. *Correctly use and pronounce medical terminology in healthcare interactions (Procedure 5-1)*
4. *Coach patients regarding office policies (Procedure 5-3)*

AFF Affective Domain*

1. *Demonstrate empathy for patients' concerns*
2. Implement time management principles to maintain effective office function
3. *Demonstrate active listening*
4. Demonstrate awareness of the consequences of not working within the legal scope of practice
5. *Respect diversity*
6. Demonstrate tactfulness

MAERB Standards are italicized.

ABHES Competencies

1. Follow documentation guidelines
2. Perform basic computer skills
3. Display effective interpersonal skills with patients and healthcare team members
4. Recognize and respond to medical office emergencies
5. Demonstrate professional behavior

Name: _____   Date: _____   Grade: _____

OOG **MULTIPLE CHOICE**

1. Which of the following creates a professional image?
   a. Arguing with a patient
   b. Clean, pressed clothing
   c. Brightly colored fingernails
   d. Referring to the physicians by their first names
   e. Expensive flowery perfume

2. How can you exercise diplomacy?
   a. Treat patients as they treat you.
   b. Treat patients as you would like to be treated.
   c. Ignore patients who complain about their illnesses.
   d. Answer patients' questions about other patients they see in the waiting room.
   e. Disclose confidential information if a patient or relative asks for it tactfully.

3. When preparing the charts for the day, they should be put in order by:
   a. age.
   b. last name.
   c. chart number.
   d. reason for visit.
   e. appointment time.

4. The receptionist should check phone messages:
   a. at night before leaving.
   b. in the morning when coming in.
   c. when on the phone and knowing a call has gone to voicemail.
   d. only after breaks, because each call coming in should be answered.
   e. when the office opens, after breaks, and periodically throughout the day.

5. Triaging calls is important because:
   a. it reduces the amount of time that callers wait.
   b. it places the calls in order of most urgent to least urgent.
   c. it lets the receptionist take care of the calls as quickly as possible.
   d. it puts the calls in time order so the receptionist knows who called first.
   e. it makes it easier for the receptionist to see which calls will be the easiest to handle.

6. There is a sign in the pediatrician's office that says "Do not throw dirty diapers in the garbage." Which of the following choices best explains the reason for the sign?
   a. Dirty diapers cannot be recycled.
   b. Dirty diapers are biohazardous waste.
   c. Dirty diapers could leave an offensive odor.
   d. Dirty diapers could make the garbage too heavy.
   e. Dirty diapers take up too much room in the garbage.

7. Chewing gum or eating while on the phone could interfere with a person's:
   a. diction.
   b. attitude.
   c. ergonomics.
   d. expression.
   e. pronunciation.

8. Which of the following activities should a receptionist do in the morning to prepare the office for patients?
   a. Vacuum the office.
   b. Complete an encounter form.
   c. Disinfect examination rooms.
   d. Turn on printers and copiers.
   e. Clean the patient restrooms.

9. Which of the following statements about telephone courtesy is correct?
   a. If two lines are ringing at once, answer one call and let the other go to voicemail.
   b. If you are on the other line, it is acceptable to let the phone ring until you can answer it.
   c. If a caller is upset, leaving them on hold will help improve the caller's attitude.
   d. If you need to answer another line, ask if the caller would mind holding and wait for a response.
   e. If someone is on hold for more than 90 seconds, they must leave a message and someone will call them back.

10. An ergonomic workstation is beneficial because it:
    a. prevents injuries to employees.
    b. educates patients about disease.
    c. maintains patients' confidentiality.
    d. creates a soothing, relaxed atmosphere.
    e. prevents the spread of contagious diseases.

11. Which feature fosters a positive waiting room environment?
    a. Abstract artwork on the walls
    b. Only sofas for patients to sit in
    c. Soap operas on the waiting room television
    d. Prominent display of the office fax machine
    e. Patient education materials in the reception area

12. When a patient calls the office and wants to be seen for chest pain, your first action should be
    a. Ask if they also have shortness of breath, nausea, and/or profuse sweating.
    b. Tell them to hang up and call 911.
    c. Asks the patient's name in case they lose consciousness.
    d. Tell the patient to make sure their front door is unlocked.
    e. Give the patient an appointment for the next day.

13. A 5-year-old girl has just come into the office with her mother. She has the flu and is vomiting into a plastic bag. Which of the following should the receptionist do?
    a. Get the patient into an examination room.
    b. Call the hospital and request an ambulance.
    c. Tell her to sit near the bathroom so she can vomit in the toilet.
    d. Place a new plastic bag in your garbage can and ask the girl to use it.
    e. Ask the patient to wait outside and you will get her when it is her turn.

14. An angry patient calls the office demanding to speak to the physician. The physician is not in the office. What should the receptionist do?
    a. Page the physician immediately.
    b. Try to calm the patient and take a message.
    c. Give the caller the physician's cell phone number.
    d. Tell the patient to calm down and call back in an hour.
    e. Place the patient on hold until they have calmed down.

15. Which of the following statements about e-mail is true?
    a. Precautions should be taken to prevent an accidental disclosure of PHI.
    b. The receptionist does not generally have access to e-mail.
    c. Actions taken in regard to e-mail do not need to be documented.
    d. Patients should not e-mail the office under any circumstances.
    e. E-mails should not be printed because the wrong person could view them.

16. The best technique for preventing the spread of disease is:
    a. washing your hands after any contact with patients.
    b. placing very sick patients immediately in an exam room.
    c. removing all reading materials or toys from the waiting room.
    d. keeping the window to the reception area closed at all times.
    e. preventing patients from changing channels on the TV in the waiting room.

17. One way to ensure patient privacy in the reception area is to:
    a. take all of the patient's information at the front desk.
    b. ask the patient's permission before writing her name on the sign-in sheet.
    c. use computers in examination rooms only.
    d. make telephone calls regarding referrals at the front desk.
    e. close the privacy window when you are not speaking with a patient.

18. When receiving a call from a lab regarding a patient's test results, you should post the information:
    a. as an e-mail to the physician.
    b. in the receptionist's notebook.
    c. in the front of the patient's chart.
    d. as an e-mail to the patient's insurance company.
    e. in the front of the physician's appointment book.

19. In case of an emergency in the physician's office, who is usually responsible for calling emergency medical services (EMS)?
    a. Physician
    b. Dispatcher
    c. Receptionist
    d. Clinical staff
    e. Patient's relatives

20. When calling EMS for a patient who has an abnormal EKG, which of the following should be given first?
    a. The patient's name and age
    b. Your location
    c. The patient's insurance carrier
    d. The patient's problem
    e. Where they will be taking the patient

OOG MATCHING

Grade: _____

Match the following key terms to their definitions.

Key Terms
21. _____ attitude
22. _____ closed captioning
23. _____ diction
24. _____ diplomacy
25. _____ emergency medical service (EMS)
26. _____ ergonomic
27. _____ receptionist
28. _____ teletypewriter (TTY)
29. _____ triage
30. _____ VRS

Definitions
a. a person who performs administrative tasks and greets patients as they arrive at an office
b. the art of handling people with tact and genuine concern
c. a group of healthcare workers who care for sick and injured patients on the way to a hospital
d. printed words displayed on a television screen to help people with hearing disabilities or impairments
e. describing a workstation designed to prevent work-related injuries
f. the style of speaking and enunciating words
g. the sorting of patients into categories based on their level of sickness or injury
h. a state of mind or feeling regarding some matter
i. a special machine that allows communication on a telephone with a hearing-impaired person
j. a system that allows deaf patients who know sign language to communicate via the Internet and video equipment

OOG SHORT ANSWER

Grade: _____

31. List the four sources of messages to be collected by the receptionist.

_____

_____

_____

32. Why is it important to keep the waiting area neat and clean?

_____

_____

_____

33. List the types of incoming calls received by the medical office.

_____

_____

_____

34. Infection control is important to prevent the spread of disease among patients. List three things a medical assistant can do to help with infection control.

_____

_____

_____

35. List four things you can do to maintain patient confidentiality within the reception area and waiting room.

_____

_____

_____

36. You are training a new receptionist. They do not understand why triaging calls is important. How would you explain this to them?

_____

_____

_____

PSY IDENTIFICATION

_____ Grade: _____

37. The waiting room should be a comfortable and safe place for patients to wait. Review the list of guidelines below and determine which contribute to a comfortable and safe waiting room environment. Place a check in the "Yes" column for those guidelines that contribute to a comfortable and safe waiting room and place a check in the "No" column for those that do not.

Task	Yes	No
a. Sofas are preferable because they fit more people.		
b. Provide only chairs without arms.		
c. Bright, primary colors are more suitable and cheery.		
d. The room should be well ventilated and kept at a comfortable temperature.		
e. Soothing background music is acceptable.		
f. Reading material, like current magazines, should be provided.		
g. Patients should be allowed to control the television.		
h. In an office for adults, anything can be watched on the television.		
i. Closed captioning should be offered to patients with hearing impairments who want to watch television.		

38. A patient comes into the office with a severe bloody nose. They left bloody tissues in the waiting room and got blood on a magazine and a chair. Your supervisor says to you, "Come on! Get some gloves. We've got to clean this right away." Why do you need gloves? Why is it important that the waiting room be cleaned immediately?

_____

_____

_____

COG TRUE OR FALSE?

Grade: _____

As a receptionist, you will be answering incoming calls. Review the statements below and place a check in the "True" column for those that are true and place a check in the "False" column for those that are false.

Incoming Calls	True	False
39. Always ask new patients for their phone numbers in case you need to call them back.		
40. Always give patients an exact quote for services if asked.		
41. Patient information cannot be given to anyone without the patient's consent.		
42. All laboratory results phoned into the office must be immediately brought to the physician's attention.		
43. When a nursing home calls with a satisfactory report about a patient, you should take the information down, record it in the patient's chart, and place it on the physician's desk for review.		
44. Never discuss unsatisfactory test results with a patient unless the doctor directs you to do so.		
45. Medical assistants are not allowed to take care of prescription refill requests.		

PSY TRIAGE

Grade: _____

46. Triage the following calls by writing the letters in the proper order.
   a. Line 1: A school nurse calls with a question about a medical form.
   b. Line 2: A mother calls about her child who is having an asthma attack.
   c. Line 3: A father calls with a question about his daughter's medication.
   d. Line 4: A patient calls complaining about a sore throat.

COG SHORT ANSWER

Grade: _____

47. A woman calls the office, frantic, because she thinks she is having a heart attack. What information should you try to get first from the caller?

_____

_____

_____

48. A patient in your office is having trouble breathing. You have been asked to call EMS. What five pieces of information will you need before you make the call?

_____

_____

_____

49. Dr. Porter is in a meeting, but he has instructed you to communicate with him via cell phone when you get the test results back for a certain patient. However, he does not like to have his cell phone ring while he is in meetings. How will you communicate with him?

_____

_____

_____

50. It is an exceptionally hot day in the spring. Because the air conditioner is not on yet, you take a chair from the waiting room and prop the door open with it. You also move the boxes that were delivered earlier away from the window so the air comes in. How is this a violation of the Americans with Disabilities Act?

_____

_____

_____

51. You receive a call from a patient who complains of being short of breath. What questions will you ask to determine whether this is an emergency?

_____

_____

_____

AFF PSY ACTIVE LEARNING

Grade: _____

52. Working with two classmates, role-play a medical emergency in the physician's office waiting room. Have one person play the role of the patient, the second person play the role of the receptionist, and the third person play the role of the EMS call operator. The patient should describe their condition, and the receptionist is responsible for conveying these details to EMS. Switch roles so that everyone gets a chance to play each role.

_____

_____

_____

WHAT WOULD YOU DO?

Grade: _____

53. Your office shows videos about healthy living, exercise, and nutrition throughout the day. It seems that most of the adults watch and enjoy the programming. One crowded afternoon, a patient comes up to the desk to complain that the programming is distracting and he would prefer having the television turned off. However, there are people in the room watching the television. What would you say to the upset patient?

_____

_____

_____

54. Mrs. Gonzalez calls to schedule her annual checkup. She is put on hold, and when the receptionist comes back to her call, she is upset that she was placed on hold. When she comes in for her appointment, she says that the receptionist should deal with every call individually and that no one should be placed on hold. How would you explain the phone call triage system to her?

_____

_____

_____

AFF CASE STUDIES FOR CRITICAL THINKING

Grade: _____

You are working for a pediatrician. A mother arrives carrying an 18-month-old child with symptoms of a respiratory illness. You ask for her insurance card and she yells, "take care of my child first." You are willing to rearrange the usual order of things, but when you direct her to sit in the sick-child area, as per office protocol, the mother refuses, stating, "I don't want my child to get sicker." Circle the appropriate response from the lists below each question.

55. What might you say to make the mother give you the insurance information?
   a. I am required to update your chart, including your insurance information, at each visit _before_ you see the physician.
   b. The physician will not see your child until I see your card.
   c. You are being very difficult. Can we start over?
   d. I'll hold the child while you get your card out.

56. What is your best action regarding the waiting area?
   a. Tell the physician.
   b. Calmly explain the policy and why you have it.
   c. Even though you will be putting her ahead of others, put the child in an open exam room.
   d. Ask the mother to leave.
   e. Tell her to take the child to the emergency room.

57. What is the most important thing you can do to make difficult situations like this better?
   a. Place signs in the waiting area about behavior.
   b. Make sure your work area is clean and neat.
   c. Make sure you always have someone else with you in the reception area.
   d. Remain calm and act professionally.
   e. Stand your ground with the angry person.

PROCEDURE 5-1 Demonstrate Professional Telephone Techniques

PSY

Name: _____ **Date:** _____ **Time:** _____ **Grade:** _____

EQUIPMENT/SUPPLIES: Telephone, telephone message pad, writing utensil (pen or pencil), headset (if applicable)

STANDARDS: Given the needed equipment and a place to work, the student will perform this skill with _____ % accuracy in a total of _____ minutes. *(Your instructor will tell you what the percentage and time limits will be before you begin.)*

KEY: 4 = Satisfactory   0 = Unsatisfactory   NA = This step is not counted

PROCEDURE STEPS	SELF	PARTNER	INSTRUCTOR
1. Gather the needed equipment.	❑	❑	❑
2. Answer the phone within three rings.	❑	❑	❑
3. Greet the caller with the proper identification (your name and the name of the office).	❑	❑	❑
4. Identify the nature or reason for the call in a timely manner.	❑	❑	❑
5. Triage the call appropriately.	❑	❑	❑
6. Communicate in a professional manner and with unhurried speech.	❑	❑	❑
7. Clarify information as needed.	❑	❑	❑
8. Record the message on a message pad. Include the name of the caller, date, time, telephone number where the caller can be reached, description of the caller's concerns, and person to whom the message is routed.	❑	❑	❑
9. Give the caller an approximate time for a return call.	❑	❑	❑
10. Ask the caller whether they have any additional questions or need any other help.	❑	❑	❑
11. Allow the caller to disconnect first.	❑	❑	❑
12. Put the message in an assigned place.	❑	❑	❑
13. Complete the task within 10 minutes.	❑	❑	❑
14. **AFF** Explain how you would respond to a patient who is obviously angry.	❑	❑	❑

_____

_____

_____

_____

(continues)

PSY PROCEDURE 5-1 **Demonstrate Professional Telephone Techniques** (continued)

CALCULATION

Total Possible Points: _____

Total Points Earned: _____ Multiplied by 100 = _____ Divided by Total Possible Points = _____ %

PASS **FAIL** **COMMENTS:**
❏ ❏

Student's signature _____ Date _____

Partner's signature _____ Date _____

Instructor's signature _____ Date _____

PROCEDURE 5-2 Calling Emergency Medical Services

PSY

Name: _____ Date: _____ Time: _____ Grade: _____

EQUIPMENT/SUPPLIES: Telephone, patient information, writing utensil (pen, pencil)

STANDARDS: Given the needed equipment and a place to work, the student will perform this skill with _____ % accuracy in a total of _____ minutes. *(Your instructor will tell you what the percentage and time limits will be before you begin.)*

KEY: 4 = Satisfactory   0 = Unsatisfactory   NA = This step is not counted

PROCEDURE STEPS	SELF	PARTNER	INSTRUCTOR
1. Obtain the following information before dialing: patient's name, age, sex, nature of medical condition, type of service the physician is requesting, any special instructions or requests the physician may have, your location, and any special information for access.	❏	❏	❏
2. Dial 911 or other EMS number.	❏	❏	❏
3. Calmly provide the dispatcher with the above information.	❏	❏	❏
4. Answer the dispatcher's questions calmly and professionally.	❏	❏	❏
5. Follow the dispatcher's instructions, if applicable.	❏	❏	❏
6. End the call per dispatcher instructions.	❏	❏	❏
7. Complete the task within 10 minutes.	❏	❏	❏
8. **AFF** Explain how you would respond to a family member who is getting in the way of performing this task.	❏	❏	❏

_____

_____

_____

_____

_____

CALCULATION

Total Possible Points: _____

Total Points Earned: _____ Multiplied by 100 = _____ Divided by Total Possible Points = _____ %

PASS   FAIL   COMMENTS:
❏   ❏

Student's signature _____ Date _____

Partner's signature _____ Date _____

Instructor's signature _____ Date _____

PSY PROCEDURE 5-3 — Coach Patients Regarding Office Policies

Name: _____ **Date:** _____ **Time:** _____ **Grade:** _____

EQUIPMENT/SUPPLIES: Patient's chart, office policy brochure

STANDARDS: Given the needed equipment and a place to work, the student will perform this skill with _____ % accuracy in a total of _____ minutes. *(Your instructor will tell you what the percentage and time limits will be before you begin.)*

KEY: 4 = Satisfactory   0 = Unsatisfactory   NA = This step is not counted

PROCEDURE STEPS	SELF	PARTNER	INSTRUCTOR
1. Assess the patient's level of understanding.	❏	❏	❏
2. Review important areas and highlight these in the office policy brochure.	❏	❏	❏
3. Ask the patient if they understand or have any questions.	❏	❏	❏
4. Give the patient the brochure to take home.	❏	❏	❏
5. Put in place a procedure for updating information and letting patients know of changes.	❏	❏	❏
6. **AFF** Explain how you would instruct a hearing-impaired patient about office procedures.	❏	❏	❏

_____

_____

_____

_____

_____

CALCULATION

Total Possible Points: _____

Total Points Earned: _____ Multiplied by 100 = _____ Divided by Total Possible Points = _____ %

PASS   FAIL   COMMENTS:
❏   ❏

Student's signature _____ Date _____

Partner's signature _____ Date _____

Instructor's signature _____ Date _____

CHAPTER 6

Managing Appointments

LEARNING OUTCOMES

COG Cognitive Domain*

1. Spell and define the key terms
2. *Identify different types of appointment scheduling methods*
3. Identify advantages and disadvantages of the following appointment systems: manual and electronic
4. Explain guidelines for scheduling appointments for new patients, return visits, inpatient admissions, and outpatient procedures
5. Recognize office policies and protocols for handling appointments
6. *Identify critical information required for scheduling patient procedures*
7. *Identify managed-care requirements for patient referrals*
8. List three ways to remind patients about appointments
9. Describe how to triage patient emergencies, acutely ill patients, and walk-in patients
10. Describe how to handle late patients
11. Explain what to do if the physician is delayed
12. Describe how to handle patients who miss their appointments
13. Describe how to handle appointment cancellations made by the office or by the patient

PSY Psychomotor Domain*

1. *Manage appointment schedule, using established priorities* (Procedure 6-1)
    a. Schedule an appointment for a new patient (Procedure 6-1)
    b. Schedule an appointment for a return visit (Procedure 6-2)
2. *Schedule a patient procedure* (Procedure 6-3)
    a. Schedule an appointment for a referral to an outpatient facility (Procedure 6-3)
    b. Arrange for admission to an inpatient facility (Procedure 6-4)
3. *Verify eligibility for services* (Procedure 6-3)
4. Apply third-party managed-care policies and procedures (Procedures 6-3 and 6-4)
5. *Coach patients regarding office policies* (Procedure 6-1)

AFF Affective Domain*

1. Implement time-management principles to maintain effective office functions
2. *Demonstrate empathy for patient's concerns*
3. *Demonstrate active listening*
4. *Demonstrate respect for individual diversity*

5. Communicate in language the patient can understand regarding managed care and insurance plans
6. Demonstrate recognition of the patient's level of understanding in communications
7. Display sensitivity when managing appointments

MAERB Standards are italicized.

ABHES Competencies

1. Display professionalism through verbal communications
2. Apply scheduling principles
3. Partner with healthcare teams to attain optimal patient health outcomes
4. Navigate electronic health record systems and practice management software
5. Assist the patient in navigating issues and concerns that may arise (i.e., insurance policy information, medical bills, and physician/provider orders)

Name: _____   Date: _____   Grade: _____

OOG MULTIPLE CHOICE

1. If your medical office uses a manual system of scheduled appointments for patient office visits, you will need a(n):
   a. toolbar.
   b. appointment book.
   c. computer.
   d. buffer time.
   e. fixed schedule.

2. How much time should be blocked off each morning and afternoon to accommodate emergencies, late arrivals, and other delays?
   a. 5 to 10 minutes
   b. 10 to 20 minutes
   c. 15 to 30 minutes
   d. 45 minutes to 1 hour
   e. 1 to 2 hours

3. When scheduling an appointment, why should you ask the patient the reason they need to see the doctor?
   a. To know the level of empathy to give the patient.
   b. To anticipate the time needed for the appointment.
   c. To confront the patient about their personal choices.
   d. To manipulate the patient's needs.
   e. To determine who should see the patient.

4. Which of the following is an advantage to clustering?
   a. Efficient use of the employee's time
   b. Increased patient time for the physician
   c. Reduced staff costs for the office
   d. Shorter patient appointments
   e. Greater need for specialists in the office

5. In fixed scheduling, the length of time reserved for each appointment is determined by the:
   a. physician's personal schedule.
   b. number of hours open on a given day.
   c. reason for the patient's visit.
   d. type of insurance provider.
   e. patient's age.

6. Double booking works well when patients are being sent for diagnostic testing because:
   a. it gives each patient enough time to prepare for testing.
   b. it leaves time to see both patients without keeping either one waiting unnecessarily.
   c. the physician enjoys seeing two patients at one time.
   d. it challenges the medical practice's resources.
   e. it gives the physician more "downtime."

7. Which of the following is a disadvantage to open hours?
   a. Patients with emergencies cannot be seen quickly.
   b. Scheduling patients is a challenge.
   c. Effective time management is almost impossible.
   d. Walk-ins are encouraged.
   e. Patient charts are not properly updated.

8. You should leave some time slots open during the schedule each day to:
   a. allow patients to make their own appointments online.
   b. make the schedule more well-rounded.
   c. leave some time for personal responsibilities.
   d. provide the staff with some flex time.
   e. make room for emergencies and delays.

9. Most return appointments are made:
   a. before the patient leaves the office.
   b. before the patient's appointment.
   c. after the patient leaves the office.
   d. during the patient's next visit.
   e. when the patient receives a mailed reminder.

10. Reminder cards should be mailed:
    a. the first day of every month.
    b. a week before the date of the appointment.
    c. the beginning of the year.
    d. with all billing statements.
    e. only when the patient requests one.

11. A condition that is abrupt in onset is described as:
    a. chronic.
    b. commonplace.
    c. lethal.
    d. acute.
    e. incurable.

12. Who is authorized to make the decision whether to see a walk-in patient or not?
    a. Medical assistant
    b. Emergency medical technician
    c. Provider
    d. Receptionist
    e. Nurse

13. If you reschedule an appointment, you should note the reason for the cancellation or rescheduling in:
    a. the patient's chart.
    b. the patient's immunization record.
    c. the patient's insurance card.
    d. the patient's billing form.
    e. the office's appointment book.

14. If you have to cancel on the day of an appointment because of a physician's illness:
    a. send the patient an apology letter.
    b. give the patient a detailed excuse.
    c. e-mail the patient a reminder.
    d. call the patient and explain.
    e. offer the patient a discount at their next appointment.

15. If you find that your schedule is chaotic nearly every day, you should:
    a. evaluate the schedule over time.
    b. keep that information private.
    c. tell your supervisor that you would like a new job.
    d. stop the old schedule and make a new one.
    e. let the patients know that the schedule is not working.

16. An instruction to transfer a patient's care to a specialist is a:
    a. precertification.
    b. consultation.
    c. transfer.
    d. referral.
    e. payback.

17. Established patients are:
    a. patients who are new to the practice.
    b. patients who have been to the practice before.
    c. patients who are over age 65 years.
    d. patients who are chronically ill.
    e. patients with insurance.

18. A flexible scheduling method that schedules patients for the first 30 minutes of an hour and leaves the second half of each hour open is called:
    a. clustering.
    b. modified wave
    c. streaming.
    d. fixed-schedule system.
    e. double booking.

19. A chronic problem is one that is:
    a. not very serious.
    b. occurring for a short period of time.
    c. longstanding.
    d. easily cured.
    e. difficult to diagnose.

20. Which of the following is true of a constellation of symptoms?
    a. It can only be assessed by a physician.
    b. It is only an emergency if a patient is having a heart attack.
    c. It means a patient is suffering from appendicitis.
    d. It is a group of clinical signs indicating a particular disease.
    e. It probably requires a call to emergency medical services.

21. When a patient calls with an emergency, your first responsibility is to:
    a. determine if the patient has an appointment.
    b. decide whether the problem can be treated in the office.
    c. verify that the physician can see the patient.
    d. identify the patient's constellation of symptoms.

22. What should you do if the physician decides not to see a walk-in patient?
    a. Ask the patient to schedule an appointment to return later.
    b. Explain that the physician is too busy.
    c. Tell the patient to try a different medical office.
    d. Tell the patient to go to the hospital.

23. When might you write a letter to a patient who has an appointment that you must cancel?
    a. When you cannot reach the patient by phone
    b. When the physician leaves the office abruptly
    c. When you do not have the patient's demographic information
    d. When you want to use written communication

COG MATCHING

Grade: _____

Match the following key terms to their definitions.

Key Terms

24. _____ acute
25. _____ buffer
26. _____ chronic
27. _____ clustering
28. _____ constellation of symptoms
29. _____ consultation
30. _____ double booking
31. _____ matrix
32. _____ precertification
33. _____ providers
34. _____ referral
35. _____ STAT
36. _____ streaming
37. _____ wave scheduling
38. _____ modified wave scheduling

Definitions

a. group of clinical signs indicating a particular disease process
b. the practice of booking two patients for the same period with the same physician
c. term used in the medical field to indicate that something should be done immediately
d. a system for blocking off unavailable patient appointment times
e. a flexible scheduling method that allows time for procedures of varying lengths and the addition of unscheduled patients, as needed
f. referring to a longstanding medical problem
g. grouping patients with similar problems or needs
h. a method of allotting time for appointments with several patients scheduled at the beginning of each hour and seen in the order of their arrival
i. extra time booked on the schedule to accommodate emergencies, walk-ins, and other demands on the provider's daily time schedule that are not considered direct patient care
j. healthcare workers who deliver medical care
k. referring to a medical problem with abrupt onset
l. request for assistance from one physician to another
m. approved documentation prior to referrals to specialists and other facilities
n. instructions to transfer a patient's care to a specialist
o. a method of allotting time for appointments with several patients scheduled at regular intervals for the first half of every hour

COG SHORT ANSWER

Grade: _____

39. List four advantages to clustering patients.

40. Name the three factors that can affect scheduling.

41. List the three ways to remind patients about appointments.

42. When calling another physician's office for an appointment for your patient, you will need to provide certain information. List the seven pieces of information that you should provide to another physician's office.

43. List three items usually included in preadmission testing for surgery.

_____

_____

_____

COG TRUE OR FALSE?

Grade: _____

Determine whether the following statements are true or false. If false, explain why.

44. Fixed scheduling is the most commonly used method.

_____

45. A medical office that operates with open hours for patient visits is open 24 hours a day, 7 days a week.

_____

46. Most appointments for new patients are made in person.

_____

47. Patients with medical emergencies need to be seen immediately.

_____

COG PSY ACTIVE LEARNING

Grade: _____

48. The appointment book below is divided into half-hour increments. The spaces below each time slot are empty. Fill in the appointment book with the following information: Dr. Brown has hospital rounds from 8:00 AM to 9:00 AM. He has the following appointments: Cindy Wallis at 9:30 AM; Bill Waters at 10:00 AM; Rodney Kingston at 10:30 AM.

8:00	8:30	9:00	9:30	10:00	10:30

Draw a line from the service to the appropriate time allotment.

Service	Estimated Time
49. blood pressure check	**a.** 5 minutes
50. complete physical exam	**b.** 10 minutes
51. dressing change	**c.** 15 minutes
52. recheck	**d.** 30 minutes
53. school physical	**e.** 1 hour

OG IDENTIFICATION

Grade: _____

Identify each type of scheduling system in the chart below.

Description	Type of Scheduling System
54. Several patients are scheduled for the first 30 minutes of each hour.	
55. Appointments are given based on the needs of individual patients.	
56. Each hour is divided into increments of 15, 30, 45, or 60 minutes for appointments, depending on the reason for the visit.	
57. Patients are grouped according to needs or problems.	
58. Two patients are scheduled for the same period with the same physician.	

OG PSY CORRECT OR INCORRECT?

Grade: _____

Below are the steps for making a return appointment. Some of the steps are false or incomplete. Review each step and decide if it is correct or incorrect. If incorrect, rewrite the statement to make it true and complete.

59. Carefully check your appointment book or screen before offering an appointment time. If a specific examination, test, or x-ray is to be performed on the return visit, avoid scheduling two patients for the same examination at the same time.

_____

60. Ask the patient when they would like to return.

_____

61. Write the patient's name and telephone number in the appointment book or enter the information in the computer.

_____

62. Transfer the information to an appointment card that you will mail out to the patient at a later date.

_____

63. Double-check your book or screen to be sure there are no errors.

_____

_____

64. End your conversation with a pleasant word and a smile.

_____

AFF WHAT WOULD YOU DO?

Grade: _____

65. An older adult patient walks into the medical office. His constellation of symptoms includes chest discomfort, shortness of breath, and nausea. He does not have an appointment. Explain what you would do.

_____

_____

_____

66. Sometimes, a patient may neglect to keep an appointment. When this happens, you should call the patient. What should you do if you are unable to reach the patient by phone?

_____

_____

_____

67. Maria has just called into the office to cancel her appointment for today. Explain what you should do.

_____

_____

_____

68. If diagnostic testing requires preparation from the patient, what should you do?

_____

_____

_____

AFF PATIENT EDUCATION

Grade: _____

69. Juan is consistently late for appointments. You have spoken with him several times. What should you do next? Explain what you will say to him and the information you will provide him with.

_____

_____

_____

AFF CASE STUDIES FOR CRITICAL THINKING A

Grade: _____

You are the RMA at the front desk of a busy family practice. The success of the day depends on how smoothly the schedule runs. It is your responsibility to check patients in as they arrive. Your office uses a sign-in sheet. Mr. Simpson is always late for his appointments and today is no exception.

70. Regarding the sign-in sheet, what other methods could you use that would limit the potential for invasion of patient privacy?
a. Have patients give their names to the receptionist as they arrive.
b. Periodically walk through the waiting area to see who is there.
c. Post a sign asking patients to whisper when they speak.
d. Use a sign-in clipboard that has a sliding shield to prevent seeing other names.

71. You notice that patients typically wait 30 to 45 minutes past their scheduled appointment times because the physician is chronically behind schedule. How would you handle the situation? Circle the best answer.
    a. Tell the office manager to talk to him or you will find other employment.
    b. Ask the office manager to put the issue of running behind on the next office meeting agenda.
    c. Ask to speak with the physician in private and explain how his running behind affects the entire office.
    d. Tease the physician about running behind in front of the patients and employees.

72. Circle the best strategy to handle Mr. Simpson's chronic tardiness.
    a. Schedule him for the last appointment of the day.
    b. Dismiss him from the physician's care.
    c. Call his family and ask if they can get him there on time.
    d. Tell him that he is messing up your whole day and he MUST stop being late.
    e. Do not worry about it. No matter what you do, he will still be late.

PSY PROCEDURE 6-1 | **Scheduling an Appointment for a New Patient**

Name: _____ Date: _____ Time: _____ Grade: _____

EQUIPMENT/Items needed: Patient's demographic information, patient's chief complaint, appointment book or computer with appointment software, information found in Activity #1.

STANDARDS: Given the needed equipment and a place to work, the student will perform this skill with _____ % accuracy in a total of _____ minutes. *(Your instructor will tell you what the percentage and time limits will be before you begin.)*

KEY: 4 = Satisfactory 0 = Unsatisfactory NA = This step is not counted

PROCEDURE STEPS	SELF	PARTNER	INSTRUCTOR
1. Obtain as much information as possible from the patient, such as: • Full name and correct spelling • Mailing address (not all offices require this) • Day and evening telephone numbers • Reason for the visit • Name of the referring person	❑	❑	❑
2. Determine the patient's chief complaint or the reason for seeing the physician.	❑	❑	❑
3. Enter the appointment on a date and for the amount of time established by office policies for a new patient appointment.	❑	❑	❑
4. Explain the cancellation and financial policies of the practice. Instruct patients to bring all pertinent insurance information.	❑	❑	❑
5. Give concise directions, if needed.	❑	❑	❑
6. Ask the patient if it is permissible to call at home or at work.	❑	❑	❑
7. Confirm the time and date of the appointment.	❑	❑	❑
8. Check your appointment book to be sure that you have placed the appointment on the correct day in the right time slot.	❑	❑	❑
9. If the patient was referred by another physician, call that physician's office before the appointment for copies of laboratory work, radiology, pathology reports, and so on. Give this information to the physician prior to the patient's appointment.	❑	❑	❑
10. **AFF** Explain how you would respond in a situation in which a patient does NOT give permission to phone them at work.	❑	❑	❑

_____
_____
_____
_____
_____

(continues)

PSY PROCEDURE 6-1 Scheduling an Appointment for a New Patient (continued)

CALCULATION

Total Possible Points: _____

Total Points Earned: _____ Multiplied by 100 = _____ Divided by Total Possible Points = _____ %

PASS **FAIL** **COMMENTS:**

❏ ❏

Student's signature _____ Date _____

Partner's signature _____ Date _____

Instructor's signature _____ Date _____

PSY PROCEDURE 6-2 Scheduling an Appointment for an Established Patient

Name: _____ Date: _____ Time: _____ Grade: _____

EQUIPMENT: Appointment book or computer with appointment software, appointment card, information found in Activity #1

STANDARDS: Given the needed equipment and a place to work, the student will perform this skill with _____ % accuracy in a total of _____ minutes. *(Your instructor will tell you what the percentage and time limits will be before you begin.)*

KEY: 4 = Satisfactory 0 = Unsatisfactory NA = This step is not counted

PROCEDURE STEPS	SELF	PARTNER	INSTRUCTOR
1. Determine what will be done at the return visit. Check your appointment book or computer system before offering an appointment.	❑	❑	❑
2. Offer the patient a specific time and date. Avoid asking the patient when they would like to return, as this can cause indecision.	❑	❑	❑
3. Write the patient's name and telephone number in the appointment book or enter it in the computer.	❑	❑	❑
4. Transfer the pertinent information to an appointment card and give it to the patient. Repeat aloud the appointment day, date, and time to the patient as you hand over the card.	❑	❑	❑
5. Double-check your book or computer to be sure you have not made an error.	❑	❑	❑
6. End your conversation with a pleasant word and a smile.	❑	❑	❑
7. **AFF** Explain how you would respond to a patient who insists on coming for a return appointment at a time when their doctor is in surgery.	❑	❑	❑

_____
_____
_____
_____

CALCULATION

Total Possible Points: _____

Total Points Earned: _____ Multiplied by 100 = _____ Divided by Total Possible Points = _____ %

PASS FAIL COMMENTS:
❑   ❑

Student's signature _____ Date _____

Partner's signature _____ Date _____

Instructor's signature _____ Date _____

PSY PROCEDURE 6-3 Scheduling an Appointment for a Referral to an Outpatient Facility

Name: _____ Date: _____ Time: _____ Grade: _____

Equipment: Patient's chart with demographic information; physician's order for services needed by the patient and reason for the services; patient's insurance card with referral information, referral form, and directions to office, information found in Activity #3.

Standards: Given the needed equipment and a place to work, the student will perform this skill with _____ % accuracy in a total of _____ minutes. *(Your instructor will tell you what the percentage and time limits will be before you begin.)*

KEY: 4 = Satisfactory 0 = Unsatisfactory NA = This step is not counted

PROCEDURE STEPS	SELF	PARTNER	INSTRUCTOR
1. Make certain that the requirements of any third-party payers are met.	❑	❑	❑
2. Refer to the patient's insurance to determine if the outpatient facility and the physician performing the procedure participate with the patient's insurance.	❑	❑	❑
3. Have the following information available when you make the call to schedule the procedure: • Physician's name and telephone number • Patient's name, address, and telephone number • Reason for the call • Degree of urgency • The patient's insurance information and precertification number, if necessary • Whether the patient is being sent for consultation or referral	❑	❑	❑
4. Advise the patient verbally and in writing of the following information as soon as possible: • The date, time, and location of the procedures • Insurance preauthorization information, if necessary, including any patient responsibility based on the plan benefits • Any specific restrictions or requirements to prepare for the procedure	❑	❑	❑
5. Record in the patient's chart the time and date of the call and the name of the person who received your call.	❑	❑	❑
6. Tell the person you are calling that you wish to be notified if your patient does not keep the appointment. If this occurs, be sure to tell your physician and enter this information in the patient's record.	❑	❑	❑
7. **AFF** Explain how you would handle the following situation: There are two physicians listed for a certain specialty in a patient's managed care's preferred provider list. The patient asks you who she should choose.	❑	❑	❑

_____

_____

_____

_____

PSY PROCEDURE 6-3 | **Scheduling an Appointment for a Referral to an Outpatient Facility** (continued)

CALCULATION

Total Possible Points: _____

Total Points Earned: _____ Multiplied by 100 = _____ Divided by Total Possible Points = _____ %

PASS **FAIL** **COMMENTS:**
❑   ❑

Student's signature _____ Date _____

Partner's signature _____ Date _____

Instructor's signature _____ Date _____

PSY PROCEDURE 6-4   **Arranging for Admission to an Inpatient Facility**

Name: _____ **Date:** _____ **Time:** _____ **Grade:** _____

Equipment: Physician's order with diagnosis, patient's chart with demographic information, contact information for inpatient facility, information found in Activity #2

Standards: Given the needed equipment and a place to work, the student will perform this skill with _____ % accuracy in a total of _____ minutes. *(Your instructor will tell you what the percentage and time limits will be before you begin.)*

KEY: 4 = Satisfactory   0 = Unsatisfactory   NA = This step is not counted

PROCEDURE STEPS	SELF	PARTNER	INSTRUCTOR
1. Determine the place where the patient and/or physician wants the admission arranged.	❑	❑	❑
2. Gather information for the other facility, including demographic and insurance information.	❑	❑	❑
3. Determine any precertification requirements. If needed, locate contact information on the back of the insurance card and call the insurance carrier to obtain a precertification number.	❑	❑	❑
4. Obtain from the physician the diagnosis and exact needs of the patient for an admission.	❑	❑	❑
5. Call the admissions department of the inpatient facility and give information from step 2.	❑	❑	❑
6. Obtain instructions for the patient and call or give the patient instructions and information.	❑	❑	❑
7. Provide the patient with the physician's orders for their hospital stay, including diet, medications, bed rest, etc.	❑	❑	❑
8. Document time, place, etc. in patient's chart, including any precertification requirements completed.	❑	❑	❑
9. Explain how you would respond to a patient who is visibly shaken about finding out that he is being admitted to the hospital.	❑	❑	❑

_____

_____

_____

_____

PSY PROCEDURE 6-4 **Arranging for Admission to an Inpatient Facility** (continued)

CALCULATION

Total Possible Points: _____

Total Points Earned: _____ Multiplied by 100 = _____ Divided by Total Possible Points = _____ %

PASS   FAIL   COMMENTS:
❑   ❑

Student's signature _____ Date _____

Partner's signature _____ Date _____

Instructor's signature _____ Date _____

Activity #1: Scheduling New and Returning Patients

Place the patients on the appointment book page provided. In order to make this activity more realistic, imagine that the patients are calling the office in the order they are listed. You will need to determine the time needed for the visit and the urgency of the patient's problem in assigning slots. Refer to **Box 6-1** in the textbook for suggested time allotment.

Set up the page and establish the matrix: Providers and availability:

Dr. Jones sees patients from 2:00 PM to 5:00 PM. In surgery until 12:00.
Dr. Smith sees patients from 8:00 AM to 3:00 PM. No lunch.
Dr. Stowe sees patients from 8:00 AM to 5:00 PM with lunch from 12:00 to 1:30 PM.

Jessica Marshall, CMA (AAMA), can give injections and do blood pressure checks. Lunch 1:00 to 2:00 PM. Use the lab column for patients who can see her.

Patient Name	Reason	Telephone #
1. Jeremy Cole	Stepped on rusty nail	937-570-7890
2. Cheryl Jennings (New)	Needs college physical	937-765-9087
3. Patty Cook	Sore throat	937-799-7225
4. Susan Stills	Woke up feeling dizzy	937-836-8765
5. Pamela Jones (New)	Wants to talk about weight reduction	937-765-0123
6. Steve Elliott	Hand laceration at work (supervisor called)	937-799-4391
7. Amy Quarrels	Vomiting and diarrhea × 3 days	937-571-5923
8. Layla Harris	Nosebleed that won't stop	937-799-0127
9. Sharon Morris	Needs refill on pain meds	937-836-2100
10. Jared Davis	Blood pressure check	937-792-8333
11. Ginger Parks	Knee injury last week, still swelling	937-791-4752
12. Landon Smythe	Coughing up blood	937-414-6787
13. Raymond Gray	Confused and foggy person	937-922-8641
14. Seth Etchison	Skin rash	937-266-0999
15. Raji Omar	Allergy injection	937-607-9125
16. Marilyn Easley	Shortness of breath and nausea	937-903-8957
17. Stephanie Lewis	Frequent urination and burning	937-792-1480
18. Shannon Mitchell	Pregnancy test	937-799-0731
19. Shantina Branch (New)	Kindergarten physical	937-792-4500
20. Lee Davis	Recheck on strep throat	937-799-4800

What might you do differently with the new patients?

_____

_____

_____

_____

Activity #2:   Scheduling Inpatient Admission

You work for Dr. James Gibbs, whose office is at 102 South Hawthorne Road, Winston-Salem, NC 27103. The office phone number is 336-760-4216.

Stella Walker is a 42-year-old female patient with diabetes. She has Blue Cross Blue Shield of NC. Her date of birth is 5/6/64. Her subscriber ID# is 260-21-5612. Her group # is 26178. She is the policyholder.

Dr. Gibbs instructs you to arrange admission to Forsyth Medical Center for Stella Walker for tomorrow. Her admitting diagnosis is uncontrolled diabetes. Her insurance requires that you precertify her for this admission. The doctor gives you his written orders and instructs you to give them to the patient to hand carry to the hospital.

You call the insurance company using the phone number on the back of her insurance card. The insurance company gives you the precertification number 1238952-1 and tells you that she is certified to stay in the hospital for 3 days. She has a $100.00 co-pay for a hospital stay.

Complete the form provided.

Hospital Admission

Patient Name: _____

Patient Insurance Company: _____

Patient Date of Birth: _____

Patient Subscriber ID#: _____

Patient Group #: _____

Insurance Policy Holder: _____

Precertification #: _____

Reason for Admission: _____

Admitting Physician Name and Address: _____

_____

Approved Length of Stay: _____

Inpatient Co-Pay: _____

Activity #3: Scheduling an Outpatient Procedure

Using the information on the physician's order below, record the dates and times for appointments made for Grace Woods to have arthroscopy of the left knee and physical therapy at Miracle Rehabilitation before and after surgery. Read the information carefully!

Physician's Order:

Hinged knee brace fitting for use after surgery at Miracle Rehabilitation.

Left knee arthroscopy with medial meniscal repair. Follow-up with me in office 5 days post-op.

Physical therapy at Miracle Rehabilitation for eight sessions beginning 1 week after surgery.

Date of surgery: _____

Date of Miracle Rehab appointment for fitting of brace: _____

Dates of Miracle Rehab physical therapy appointments: _____

_____

_____

Date of postoperative visit in your office: _____

CALCULATION

Total Possible Points: _____

Total Points Earned: _____ Multiplied by 100 = _____ Divided by Total Possible Points = _____ %

PASS   FAIL   COMMENTS:
❏   ❏

Student's signature _____   Date _____

Partner's signature _____   Date _____

Instructor's signature _____   Date _____

CHAPTER 7

Written Communications

LEARNING OUTCOMES

COG Cognitive Domain*

1. Spell and define the key terms
2. *Identify different types of electronic technology used in professional communication*
3. Discuss the basic guidelines for grammar, punctuation, and spelling in medical writing
4. Discuss the 11 key components of a business letter
5. Describe the process of writing a memorandum
6. List the items that must be included in an agenda
7. Identify the items that must be included when typing minutes
8. Cite the various services available for sending written information
9. Discuss the various mailing options
10. Identify the types of incoming written communication seen in a physician's office
11. Explain the guidelines for opening and sorting mail

PSY Psychomotor Domain*

1. *Using technology, compose clear and correct correspondence* (Procedure 7-1)
2. Gather and process documents (Procedure 7-2)

AFF Affective Domain*

1. *Demonstrate critical thinking skills*

2. Demonstrate sensitivity appropriate to the message being delivered
3. Demonstrate recognition of the patient's level of understanding in communications

MAERB Standards are italicized.

ABHES Competencies

1. Display professionalism through written communication
2. Perform basic computer skills
3. Define and use medical abbreviations when appropriate and acceptable
4. Gather and process documents

Name: _____ Date: _____ Grade: _____

OG MULTIPLE CHOICE

Choose the letter preceding the correct answer.

1. In a letter, the word "Enc." indicates the presence of a(n):
   a. summary.
   b. abstract.
   c. enclosure.
   d. review.
   e. invitation.

2. If you are instructed to write using the semiblock format, you should:
   a. indent the first line of each paragraph.
   b. use left justification for everything.
   c. use right justification for the date only.
   d. write the recipient's full name in the salutation.
   e. indent the first line of the first paragraph.

3. Which of the following items can be abbreviated in an inside address?
   a. City
   b. Town
   c. Recipient's name
   d. Business title
   e. State

4. Which sentence is written correctly?
   a. "We will have to do tests" said Doctor Mathis, "Then we will know what is wrong."
   b. "We will have to do tests" said Doctor Mathis. "Then we will know what is wrong."
   c. "We will have to do tests," said Doctor Mathis "Then we will know what is wrong."
   d. "We will have to do tests", said Doctor Mathis "Then we will know what is wrong."
   e. "We will have to do tests," said Doctor Mathis. "Then we will know what is wrong."

5. Which term should be capitalized?
   a. Morphine
   b. Fluoxetine
   c. Zithromax
   d. Antibiotic
   e. Catheter

6. If the fax machine is busy when sending an important fax, you should:
   a. mail the document instead.
   b. call the recipient and ask him to contact you when the machine is available.
   c. ask a coworker to send the document.
   d. make a note in the patient's chart.
   e. wait with the document until you receive confirmation that it was sent.

7. Which sentence is written correctly?
   a. The patient is 14 years old and is urinating 3 times more than normal.
   b. The patient is 14 years old and is urinating three times more than normal.
   c. The patient is fourteen years old and is urinating 3 times more than normal.
   d. The patient is fourteen years old and is urinating three times more than normal.
   e. The patient is fourteen years old and is urinating three times more than normally.

8. Which of the following always belongs on a fax cover sheet?
   a. The number of pages, not including the cover sheet
   b. A confidentiality statement
   c. A summary of the content of the message
   d. A summary of the content of the message, less confidential portions
   e. The name of the patient discussed in the message

9. The USPS permits imprint program:
   a. guarantees overnight delivery.
   b. provides receipt of delivery.
   c. offers physicians cheaper postage.
   d. deducts the postage charges from a prepaid account.
   e. addresses envelopes for no additional charge.

10. Which USPS service will allow you to send a parcel overnight?
   a. Registered mail
   b. First-class mail
   c. Presorted mail
   d. Priority mail
   e. Express mail

11. Which is the best way to highlight a list of key points in a business letter?
   a. Use boldface text
   b. Use a larger font
   c. Use bulleted text
   d. Use a highlighter
   e. Use italicized text

Scenario for questions 12–14: You are tasked with writing a letter to a patient on the basis of a chart from his last visit. Most important is a diagnosis listed as "HBV infection."

12. Which is an appropriate course of action?
    a. Including the words "HBV infection" in the letter
    b. Consulting the physician on the meaning of the term
    c. Omitting the diagnosis from the otherwise complete letter
    d. Guessing the meaning of the term and writing about that
    e. Asking the office manager what to do about the letter

13. Having learned that HBV means hepatitis B virus, you should:
    a. research HBV infection.
    b. give the patient your condolences.
    c. write a letter based on the physician's instructions.
    d. immediately schedule an appointment for the patient.
    e. ask the patient to visit the office to learn about their condition.

14. Who might receive a memorandum you have written?
    a. A nurse in your office
    b. A drug sales representative
    c. An insurance agent
    d. An outside specialist
    e. A recently admitted patient

15. Which closing is written correctly?
    a. Best Regards
    b. Sincerely Yours,
    c. Best regards,
    d. Sincerely yours
    e. Best Regards,

16. The purpose of an agenda is to:
    a. summarize the opinions expressed at a meeting.
    b. provide a brief outline for topics to be discussed at a meeting.
    c. inform participants of any changes since the last meeting.
    d. remind group members about an upcoming meeting.
    e. communicate key issues that should be addressed at future meetings.

17. Correspondence that contains information about a patient should be marked:
    a. personal.
    b. confidential.
    c. urgent.
    d. classified.
    e. top secret.

18. Which of these should be included in minutes?
    a. Individuals' statements
    b. Your opinion of the vote
    c. Names of those voting against
    d. Names of those voting in favor
    e. Date and time of the next meeting

19. Which type of mail provides the greatest protection for valuables?
    a. Certified mail
    b. International mail
    c. Registered mail
    d. Standard mail
    e. First class mail

20. Among these, which type of mail should be handled first?
    a. Medication samples
    b. Professional journals
    c. Insurance information
    d. Patient correspondence
    e. Waiting room magazines

21. Which charting note is written correctly?
    a. The patient is a 44-year-old Hispanic man with two sprained fingers.
    b. The patient is a 44-year-old hispanic man with 2 sprained fingers.
    c. The patient is a 44-year-old Hispanic man with 2 sprained fingers.
    d. The patient is a 44-year-old hispanic man with two sprained fingers.

22. Which of these statements is both clear and concise?
    a. Mr. Jensen entered the office in the early evening complaining of stomach pain unlike any he had felt before.
    b. Mr. Jensen complained of severe stomach pain.
    c. Mr. Jensen came to the office complaining about pain.
    d. Mr. Jensen complained about stomach pain before leaving the office.

COG MATCHING

_____ Grade: _____

Match the following key terms to their definitions.

Key Terms

23. _____ agenda
24. _____ annotation
25. _____ BiCaps/intercaps
26. _____ block
27. _____ enclosure
28. _____ font
29. _____ full block
30. _____ margin
31. _____ memorandum
32. _____ proofread
33. _____ salutation
34. _____ semiblock
35. _____ template
36. _____ transcription

Definitions

a. an informal intra-office communication, generally used to make brief announcements
b. a typographic style
c. a type of letter format in which the first sentence is indented
d. additional information intended to highlight key points in a document, typically written in margins
e. the process of reading a text to check grammatical and factual accuracy
f. a model used to ensure consistent format in writing
g. abbreviations, words, or phrases with unusual capitalization
h. a type of letter format in which all letter components are justified left
i. something that is included with a letter
j. the process of typing a dictated message
k. a brief outline of the topics discussed at a meeting
l. a type of letter format in which the date, subject line, closing, and signatures are justified right, and all other lines are justified left
m. the greeting of a letter
n. the blank space around the edges of a piece of paper that has been written on

SHORT ANSWER

_____ Grade: _____

37. List the items that are usually included in the minutes of a business meeting.

_____

_____

_____

38. What three things must be included on every piece of mail before sending it?

_____

_____

_____

39. Why is an agenda useful for meetings? What does it include?

_____

_____

_____

40. What should you do after composing a piece of written communication? Why?

_____

_____

_____

▲ WHAT WOULD YOU DO?

Grade: _____

41. Suppose the physician told you to read his e-mails while he was on vacation. In doing so, you come across a personal piece of information that you know he would not want you to see. How would you handle it? Would you tell anyone that you saw it? Would you question the physician about it?

_____

_____

_____

PSY ACTIVE LEARNING

Grade: _____

42. Compose a letter from Dr. Joseph Cohen, 321 Gasthaus Lane, Germantown, PA 87641, to Mr. Ligero Delgado, 888 La Sala Boulevard, Germantown, PA 87642.

The letter should inform Mr. Delgado of the following:

- The results of the biopsy taken during his sigmoidoscopy were negative.
- While these initial results are encouraging, his medical complaints need to be investigated further. Dr. Cohen would like to refer Mr. Delgado to a specialist, Dr. Douloureux.
- Dr. Douloureux's practice is in Suite 100 of the Atroce Medical Center, 132 West Broadway, Germantown, PA 87642.
- With Mr. Delgado's consent, his records can be forwarded to Dr. Douloureux and an appointment will be arranged.

Prepare the letter on a sheet of letterhead if available. If this is not available to you, print the letter on a standard 8 1/2 × 11 white paper and attach to this sheet. Proof your unedited copy and, using proofreader's marks, indicate your corrections. Make the corrections and reprint a final copy. Ask your instructor to review both copies.

43. Write 10 sentences using terms from Box 7-3. Use some terms correctly and others incorrectly. Exchange your sentences with another student. Correct your peer's sentences.

44. Collect five pieces of mail that you have received at home. What method of affixing postage did they use? Go to your local USPS office. Obtain either a priority mail or express mail envelope. Correctly address the envelope.

COG CORRECT OR INCORRECT?

Grade: _____

Read the following sentences. If the sentence is free of errors, write "correct" on the line. If the sentence contains errors, circle the problem and explain how you would fix the sentence.

45. The patient has a cold and is bothered by the postnasal drip.

_____

46. The patient complained of constipation and has not had a bowl movement in 3 days.

_____

47. The patient, Mrs. Philips, sought weight-loss advise from the physician.

_____

48. The nurse applied antiseptic to the wounded elbow.

_____

COG IDENTIFICATION

Grade: _____

Review the list of terms below and place a check mark to indicate whether each term must always be capitalized.

Name	Always	Not Always
49. Streptococcus		
50. Tylenol		
51. Benadryl		
52. Diagnosis		
53. Analgesic		
54. Merck		
55. Antihistamine		
56. Tampax		

COG PSY ACTIVE LEARNING

Grade: _____

57. Dr. Bruce Mosley asks you to prepare a memorandum for distribution to the entire office. He hands you a note to use as the body of the memo. It reads as follows:
On May 9, Jerry Henderson, a representative of Conrad Insurance, will be visiting the office during the morning. Please extend him the utmost courtesy and introduce yourself if you have not yet met him. Jerry is a wonderful man who has been very helpful to our practice. I will be unavailable during the morning as a result of his visit. Please direct questions to Shelly or Dr. Garcia. Of course, I may be contacted in case of an emergency. Using the sample memorandum format in **Figure 7-5** of your text, construct the memo.

COG IDENTIFICATION

Grade: _____

58. You have been asked to send a summary of a patient's recent visit to a specialist. Review the list of forms of written communication below and place a check mark to indicate whether it is an appropriate means of written communication.

Form	Appropriate	Not Appropriate
a. A formal letter labeled confidential		
b. An e-mail marked urgent		
c. A memorandum		
d. A fax with a confidentiality statement		
e. A memorandum labeled urgent		

59. You always take the minutes at the staff meeting, but you will be on vacation during the next meeting. Identify and list for your coworker what information belongs in the minutes.

_____

_____

_____

60. Dr. Shadrick is at a week-long conference in another state. She needs a patient's complete history to present to the conference one day from now, but has forgotten it at the office. Name three suitable delivery options.

a. _____

b. _____

c. _____

61. Which of the following is/are good practice(s) with regard to handling mail? Place a check mark in the correct box below to answer "Yes" or "No."

Practice	Yes	No
a. Handling promotional materials last		
b. Opening mail marked "confidential" addressed to a physician		
c. Asking a physician or office manager about a piece of mail you are unsure about		
d. Leaving patient correspondence in an external mailbox		
e. Disposing of a physician's personal mail if they are away		
f. Informing a covering physician about mail requiring urgent attention		
g. Prioritizing patient care-related mail over pharmaceutical samples		

AFF PSY WHAT WOULD YOU DO?

Grade: _____

62. You are asked to open the mail today. There is a variety of material including several letters addressed to the physician marked "Urgent," "Confidential," and "Personal." Some of the other mail is from patients, but it is not marked in any unusual fashion. Other letters are from insurance companies with which your office is associated. There are also several advertisements and promotional mailings from medical supply companies, pharmaceutical companies, and insurance companies. In addition, there are pieces of mail that do not include a return address. Explain the procedure you would follow in dealing with this mail.

_____

_____

_____

_____

PSY PATIENT EDUCATION

Grade: _____

63. The office's policy is to mail a welcome letter to new patients. Make a list of information that should be included in this letter so the patient is prepared for her first visit.

_____

_____

_____

_____

AFF **CASE STUDIES FOR CRITICAL THINKING**

Grade: _____

The office manager has asked you to compose a letter to every patient in the practice explaining why their physician will be out of the office for 10 months. The physician is having extensive cosmetic surgery and is taking a medical leave of absence.

64. Your letter should _____ should not _____ include the reason for the absence.

65. Circle the more appropriate sentence for your letter from the two choices below:
   a. This letter is to tell you that Dr. Smith will not be here for the next 10 months, effective October 1, 2025.
   b. This letter is to inform you that Dr. William Smith will be taking a 10-month leave of absence beginning October 1, 2025.

66. Circle the more appropriate sentence for your letter from the two choices below:
   a. We hope you will continue to receive medical care from our office. We have 12 other providers who will be available to handle your healthcare needs.
   b. Dr. Smith wants you to see one of our other many excellent providers in the interim.

PSY PROCEDURE 7-1 **Composing a Business Letter**

Name: _____ **Date:** _____ **Time:** _____ **Grade:** _____

EQUIPMENT/SUPPLIES: Computer with word processing software, 8 1/2 × 11 white paper, #10 sized envelope

STANDARDS: Given the needed equipment and a place to work, the student will perform this skill with _____ % accuracy in a total of _____ minutes. *(Your instructor will tell you what the percentage and time limits will be before you begin.)*

KEY: 4 = Satisfactory 0 = Unsatisfactory NA = This step is not counted

PROCEDURE STEPS	SELF	PARTNER	INSTRUCTOR
1. Move cursor down two lines below the letterhead and enter today's date, flush left.	❏	❏	❏
2. Flush left, move cursor down two lines and enter the inside address using the name and address of the person to whom you are writing.	❏	❏	❏
3. Enter a reference line.	❏	❏	❏
4. Double-space and type the salutation followed by a colon.	❏	❏	❏
5. Double-space between paragraphs.	❏	❏	❏
6. Double-space and flush left, enter the complimentary close.	❏	❏	❏
7. Move cursor down four spaces and enter the sender's name.	❏	❏	❏
8. Double-space and enter initials of the sender in all caps.	❏	❏	❏
9. Enter a slash and your initials in lower case letters.	❏	❏	❏
10. Enter c: and names of those who get copies of the letter.	❏	❏	❏
11. Enter Enc: and the number and description of each enclosed sheet.	❏	❏	❏
12. Print on letterhead.	❏	❏	❏
13. Proofread the letter.	❏	❏	❏
14. Attach the letter to the patient's chart.	❏	❏	❏
15. Submit to the sender of the letter for review and signature.	❏	❏	❏
16. Make a copy of the letter for the patient's chart.	❏	❏	❏
17. Address envelopes using all caps and no punctuation.	❏	❏	❏
18. **AFF** Explain how you would respond in this situation: your physician receives the letter you prepared and asks you to insert a comma where you know a comma is not correct.	❏	❏	❏

(continues)

_____

_____

_____

_____

_____

CALCULATION

Total Possible Points: _____

Total Points Earned: _____ Multiplied by 100 = _____ Divided by Total Possible Points = _____ %

PASS   FAIL   COMMENTS:
❏   ❏

Student's signature _____ Date _____

Partner's signature _____ Date _____

Instructor's signature _____ Date _____

PSY PROCEDURE 7-2 Opening and Sorting Incoming Mail

Name: _____ Date: _____ Time: _____ Grade: _____

EQUIPMENT/SUPPLIES: Letter opener, paper clips, directional tabs, date stamp

STANDARDS: Given the needed equipment and a place to work, the student will perform this skill with _____ % accuracy in a total of _____ minutes. *(Your instructor will tell you what the percentage and time limits will be before you begin.)*

KEY: 4 = Satisfactory   0 = Unsatisfactory   NA = This step is not counted

PROCEDURE STEPS	SELF	PARTNER	INSTRUCTOR
1. Gather the necessary equipment.	❑	❑	❑
2. Open all letters and check for enclosures.	❑	❑	❑
3. Paper clip enclosures to the letter.	❑	❑	❑
4. Date-stamp each item.	❑	❑	❑
5. Sort the mail into categories and deal with it appropriately. Generally, you should handle the following types of mail as noted: • Correspondence regarding a patient: Place on the physician's desk for review. If using a paper medical record, attach letters, test results, etc., to the patient's chart with a paper clip; place the chart in a pile for the physician to review. • Payments and other checks: Record promptly all insurance payments and checks and deposit them according to office policy; account for all drug samples and appropriately log them into the sample book.	❑	❑	❑
6. Dispose of miscellaneous advertisements unless otherwise directed.	❑	❑	❑
7. Distribute the mail to the appropriate staff members (physician, office manager, billing manager, etc.).	❑	❑	❑
8. **AFF** Explain how you would handle a letter marked "Personal and confidential."	❑	❑	❑

_____

_____

_____

_____

(continues)

PSY PROCEDURE 7-2 | **Opening and Sorting Incoming Mail** (continued)

CALCULATION

Total Possible Points: _____

Total Points Earned: _____ Multiplied by 100 = _____ Divided by Total Possible Points = _____ %

PASS   FAIL   COMMENTS:
❑   ❑

Student's signature _____ Date _____

Partner's signature _____ Date _____

Instructor's signature _____ Date _____

CHAPTER 8

Health Information Management and Protection

LEARNING OUTCOMES

COG Cognitive Domain*

1. Spell and define the key terms
2. *Identify components of the Health Insurance Portability and Accountability Act (HIPAA)*
3. Explain the requirements of the Health Insurance Portability and Accountability Act relating to the sharing and saving of personal and protected health information
4. Describe the standard medical record, electronic medical record, and electronic health record systems (EHRs)
5. Explain the process for releasing medical records to third-party payers and individual patients
6. Define and describe types of information contained in the patient's medical record
7. *Identify subjective and objective information*
8. Identify methods of organizing the patient's medical record based on problem-oriented medical record (POMR) and source-oriented medical record (SOMR).
9. Explain how to make an entry in a patient's medical record, using abbreviations when appropriate
10. Explain how to make a correction in a standard and electronic health record

11. Describe filing indexing rules and procedures
12. Identify equipment and supplies needed to create and store medical records
13. Explain the guidelines of sound policies for record retention
14. Describe the proper disposal of paper and electronic protected health information (PHI)
15. Describe the implications of HIPAA for the medical assistant in various medical settings
16. *Identify Health Information Technology for Economic and Clinical Health (HITECH) Act*
17. *Identify the importance of data backup*
18. Explain the HER Incentive Programs as they apply to EMR

PSY Psychomotor Domain*

1. Create and organize a patient's medical record (Procedure 8-1)
2. File patient medical records (Procedure 8-2)
3. Respond to issues of confidentiality (Procedure 8-3)
4. *Apply HIPAA rules with regard to privacy/release of information (Procedure 8-3)*
5. *Document patient care accurately in the medical record (Procedure 8-4)*

AFF Affective Domain*

1. Demonstrate sensitivity to patient rights
2. Demonstrate awareness of the consequences of not working within the legal scope of practice
3. Recognize the importance of local, state, and federal legislation and regulations in the practice setting
4. Protect the integrity of the medical record

*MAERB Standards are italicized.

ABHES Competencies

1. Follow documentation guidelines
2. Institute federal and state guidelines when releasing medical records and entering orders in and utilizing electronic health records
3. Demonstrate compliance with HIPAA guidelines and the Health Information Technology for Economic and Clinical Health (HITECH) Act
4. Follow documentation guidelines
5. Gather and process documents

Name: _____   Date: _____   Grade: _____

COG MULTIPLE CHOICE

1. Who coordinates and oversees the various aspects of HIPAA compliance in a medical office?
   a. Medicaid and Medicare
   b. HIPAA officer
   c. Privacy officer
   d. Office manager
   e. Law enforcement

2. A release of records request must contain the patient's:
   a. next of kin.
   b. home phone number.
   c. original signature.
   d. medical history.
   e. date of birth.

3. Which is an example of protected health information?
   a. Published statistics by a credible source
   b. Insurance company's mailing address
   c. Physician's pager number
   d. First and last name associated with a diagnosis
   e. Poll published in a medical journal

4. If patients believe their rights have been denied or their health information isn't being protected, they can file a complaint with the:
   a. Journal of American Medical Assistants.
   b. American Medical Association.
   c. provider or insurer.
   d. medical assistant.
   e. state's attorney.

5. The only time an original record should be released is when the:
   a. patient asks for the record.
   b. patient is in critical condition.
   c. record is subpoenaed by the court of law.
   d. physician is being sued.
   e. patient terminates the relationship with the physician.

6. Do medical records have the same content if they are on paper or a computer disk?
   a. Yes
   b. No
   c. Sometimes
   d. Most of the time
   e. Never

7. Documentation of each patient encounter is called:
   a. consultation reports.
   b. medication administration.
   c. correspondence.
   d. narrative.
   e. progress notes.

8. Improved medication management is a feature of:
   a. SOAP.
   b. electronic health records.
   c. clearinghouses.
   d. PHI.
   e. workers' compensation.

9. To maintain security, a facility should:
   a. design a written confidentiality policy for employees to sign.
   b. provide public access to medical records.
   c. keep a record of all passwords and give a copy to each employee.
   d. keep doors unlocked during the evening hours only.
   e. have employees hide patient information from other coworkers.

10. Under source-oriented records, the most recent documents are placed on top of previous sheets, which is called:
    a. chronological order.
    b. reverse chronological order.
    c. alphabetical order.
    d. subject order.
    e. numeric order.

11. The acronym "SOAP" stands for:
    a. subjective-objective-adjustment-plan.
    b. subjective-objective-accounting-plan.
    c. subjective-objective-assessment-plan.
    d. subjective-objective-accounting-problem.
    e. subjective-objective-assessment-problem.

12. The acronym "POMR" stands for:
    a. presentation-oriented medical record.
    b. protection-oriented medical record.
    c. performance-oriented medical record.
    d. professional-oriented medical record.
    e. problem-oriented medical record.

13. Which of the following is contained in a POMR database?
a. Marketing tools
b. Field of interest
c. Job description
d. Review of systems
e. Accounting review

14. Which of the following will reflect each encounter with the patient chronologically, whether by phone, by e-mail, or in person?
a. Microfilm
b. Narrative
c. Progress notes
d. Subject filing
e. Flow sheet

15. Shingling is:
a. printing replies to a patient's e-mail.
b. recording laboratory results in the patient's chart.
c. telephone or electronic communications with patients.
d. taping the paper across the top to a regular-size sheet.
e. filing records in chronological order.

16. How long are workers' compensation cases kept open after the last date of treatment for any follow-up care that may be required?
a. 6 months
b. 1 year
c. 2 years
d. 5 years
e. 10 years

17. A cross-reference in numeric filing is called a(n):
a. open file.
b. locked file.
c. straight digit file.
d. master patient index.
e. duplication index.

18. Security experts advise storing backup disks:
a. in the office.
b. offsite.
c. at the physician's home.
d. on every computer.
e. at the library.

19. Drawer files are a type of:
a. filing cabinet.
b. storage container.
c. computer system.
d. shelving unit.
e. subject filing.

20. The statute of limitations is:
a. the end of a provider's ability to legally practice.
b. the record retention system.
c. a miniature photographic system.
d. the legal time limit set for filing a lawsuit against an alleged wrongdoer.
e. the number of records a storage system is able to hold.

COG MATCHING

Grade: _____

Match the following key terms to their definitions.

Key Terms
21. _____ alphabetic filing
22. _____ chief complaint
23. _____ chronological order
24. _____ clearinghouse
25. _____ covered entity
26. _____ cross-reference
27. _____ demographic data
28. _____ electronic health records (EHR)
29. _____ flow sheet
30. _____ medical history forms
31. _____ microfiche
32. _____ microfilm
33. _____ narrative
34. _____ numeric filing

Definitions
a. information about patients that is recorded and stored on a computer
b. photographs of records in a reduced size
c. a paragraph indicating the contact with the patient, what was done for the patient, and the outcome of any action
d. a specific account of the chief complaint, including time frames and characteristics
e. a common method of compiling information that lists each problem of the patient, usually at the beginning of the folder, and references each problem with a number throughout the folder
f. notation in a file indicating that a record is stored elsewhere and giving the reference; verification to another source; checking the tabular list against the alphabetic list in ICD-9 coding
g. entity that takes claims and other electronic data from providers, verifies the information, and forwards the proper forms to the payers for physicians

Key Terms	Definitions
35. _____ protected health information (PHI)	**h.** employer insurance for treatment of an employee's injury or illness related to the job
36. _____ present illness	**i.** any information that can be linked to a specific person
37. _____ problem-oriented medical record (POMR)	**j.** items placed with oldest first
	k. sheets of microfilm
38. _____ reverse chronological order	**l.** arranging files according to their title, grouping similar subjects together
39. _____ SOAP	**m.** a style of charting that includes subjective, objective, assessment, and planning notes
40. _____ subject filing	
41. _____ workers' compensation	**n.** arranging of names or titles according to the sequence of letters in the alphabet
	o. health plan; healthcare clearinghouse; or healthcare provider who transmits any health information in electronic form in connection with a transaction covered under HIPAA
	p. placing in order of time; usually the most recent is placed foremost
	q. information relating to the statistical characteristics of populations
	r. color-coded sheets that allow information to be recorded in graphic or tabular form for easy retrieval
	s. arranging files by a numbered order
	t. main reason for the visit to the medical office
	u. record containing information about a patient's past and present health status

SHORT ANSWER

Grade: _____

42. List the four steps you should take to ensure that files are stored and retrieved quickly and efficiently.

_____

_____

_____

_____

43. Describe the difference between standard and EHRs.

_____

_____

_____

_____

44. When documenting in a medical record or file, why should you use caution when using abbreviations?

_____

_____

_____

_____

45. How does a numeric filing system help a medical office meet HIPAA's privacy requirements?

_____

_____

_____

_____

46. Documentation is a large part of your job as a medical assistant. Legible, correct, and thorough documentation is necessary. List three instances, other than patient visits, when documentation is required.

_____

_____

_____

_____

47. When a healthcare provider's practice ends, either from retirement or death, what happens to the records?

_____

_____

_____

_____

48. Those who must abide by HIPAA are called "covered entities." List the three groups that are considered covered entities.

_____

_____

_____

_____

COG PSY ACTIVE LEARNING
Grade: _____

49. If you were opening a new medical facility, consider whether you would want staff members using abbreviations in patient records. Then create a list of 20 acceptable abbreviations that may be used in your new facility. Next, create a "Do Not Use" list for abbreviations that may be confusing and should not be included in records. Visit the website for the Joint Commission at www.jointcommission.org and include all of those abbreviations in addition to five other abbreviations of your own choice.

50. Interview a fellow student with a hypothetical illness. Document the visit with the chief complaint and history of present illness.

51. The office in which you work receives lab results on a printer throughout the day. Write an office policy for maintaining confidentiality with the PHI being transmitted electronically.

52. Your medical office uses an alphabetic filing system. Place the following names in the correct order to show how you would place each record in a filing system.

Brandon P. Snow	Kristen F. Darian-Lewes	Shante L. Dawes	Emil S. Faqir, Jr.
Shaunice L. DeBlase	Juan R. Ortiz	Kim Soo	Fernando P. Vasquez, DO

a. _____

b. _____

c. _____

d. _____

e. _____

f. _____

g. _____

h. _____

COG IDENTIFICATION

Grade: _____

53. HIPAA has privacy rules that protect your personal health information. Under HIPAA, covered entities must take certain safety measures to protect patients' information. Read the paragraph below. For each blank, there are two choices. Circle the correct word or phrase for each sentence.

Covered entities must designate a (a) (HIPAA officer, privacy officer) to keep track of who has access to health information. They must also adopt written (b) (privacy, healthcare) procedures. Under HIPAA, patients have the right to decide if they provide (c) (permission, marketing) before their health information can be used or shared for certain purposes. They also have the right to get a (d) (narrative, report) on when and why their healthcare information was shared for certain purposes.

COG PSY IDENTIFICATION

Grade: _____

The rules for releasing medical records and authorization are meant to protect patients' privacy rights. Read the questions below regarding the release of medical records and circle "Yes" or "No" for each question.

54. May an 18-year-old patient get copies of their own medical records? Yes No

55. May all minors seek treatment for sexually transmitted diseases and birth control without parental knowledge or consent? Yes No

56. When a patient requests copies of their own records, does the doctor make the decision about what to copy? Yes No

57. Must the authorization form give the patient the opportunity to limit the information released? Yes No

58. When a patient authorizes the release of information, may he request that the physician leave out information pertinent to the situation? Yes No

⬡ FILL IN THE BLANKS

HIPAA requirements provide guidelines and suggestions for safe computer practices when storing or transferring patient information. The following is a list of guidelines that medical facilities are urged to follow. Complete each sentence with the appropriate word from the word bank below.

59. Store _____ in a bank safe deposit box.

60. Change log-in _____ and passwords every 30 days.

61. Turn _____ away from areas where information may be seen by patients.

62. Use _____ with _____ other than letters.

63. Prepare a backup _____ for use when the computer system is down.

Word Bank			
characters	plan	disks	information
codes	passwords	template	terminals
Note: Not all words will be used.			

MATCHING

A standard medical record in an outpatient facility, known as a chart or file, contains clinical information as well as billing and insurance information. In the clinical section of the file, you will often find certain types of information. In the columns below, draw a diagonal line to match the clinical type of information with its correct description.

Name of Clinical Information
64. Chief complaint
65. Family and personal history
66. Progress notes
67. Diagnosis or medical impression
68. Correspondence pertaining to patient

Description
a. Documentation of each patient encounter
b. Provider's opinion of the patient's problem
c. Symptoms that led the patient to seek the physician's care
d. Letters or memos generated in the facility and sent out
e. Review of major illnesses of family members

TRUE OR FALSE?

69. True or False? Determine whether the following statements are true or false. If false, explain why.

a. HIPAA allows patients to ask to see and get a copy of their health records.

_____

b. To maintain secure files, you should change log-in codes and passwords every 10 days.

_____

c. Medical history forms are commonly used to gather information from the patient before the visit with the physician.

_____

d. Before treating a patient for a possible workers' compensation case, you must first obtain verification from the employer unless the situation is life threatening.

_____

AFF **WHAT WOULD YOU DO?**

70. A mother is accused of physically abusing her 16-year-old daughter, a patient with your facility. A police officer who has been asked to investigate visits to the medical office asks for the patient's medical records. What would you do?

_____

_____

_____

_____

71. You're in the medical office and you suddenly realize that you've forgotten to document a telephone conversation you had with a patient 2 days ago. What would you do?

_____

_____

_____

_____

AFF **CASE STUDIES FOR CRITICAL THINKING A**

You are tasked with creating the office policy for record retention for your facility.

72. Circle any appropriate actions from the list below.
   a. Research federal law that mandates how long you must keep records.
   b. Research the state laws that determine the statute of limitations for your state.
   c. Make sure the time limit for retaining records includes inactive and closed files.
   d. Set the time limits for retaining children's records from their 18th birthday.
   e. Set the time limits for retaining the records of adults and children to be the same for ease of remembering.
   f. Have the policy approved by the physician and/or appropriate employee.

73. This task is not in your job description, and you feel that you are not qualified to set policy for the facility. Circle the appropriate actions from the list below.
   a. Tell your supervisor of your concerns and ask for their guidance.
   b. Consider this a great opportunity to show your employer your skills.
   c. Ask the attorney for the facility to create the policy for you.
   d. Ask the attorney not to tell your supervisor that he helped you.
   e. Do the task, but make sure everyone in the office knows who did it.
   f. Do the task without assistance and ask for a promotion and/or raise when finished.

74. What is the statute of limitations for patients to file malpractice or negligence lawsuits in your state? _____

AFF CASE STUDIES FOR CRITICAL THINKING B

Grade: _____

Your mother's best friend is a patient in the office where you work. You have known her all of your life. She has just been seen for a suspicious lump in her breast. She is very nervous and calls you at home that night to see if you know the results of her test. You saw the stat biopsy report before you left work and you know that the lump is malignant. She was given an appointment in 2 days for the physician to give her the results.

75. Circle all appropriate actions from the list below.
   a. Tell her that it is not in your scope of practice to give patients results without specific instructions from a provider, even if they are friends.
   b. To minimize the time she must anxiously wait, try to move her appointment to tomorrow as soon as you get to work in the morning.
   c. Tell her that the report was not good and to bring someone with her to the visit.
   d. Call the physician at home to ask if you can tell her.
   e. Tell her that you do not know the results of the test, but even if you did you could not tell her.
   f. Call your mother, tell her the situation, and ask for her advice.

76. Let's say you tell the patient that you cannot give test results, and she replies, "I have a right to know what is wrong with me." Circle all of the appropriate responses below.
   a. Only a provider can give test results in my office unless they specifically direct an employee to do so.
   b. I am a professional, and I don't really care about your rights.
   c. I know you are my mother's friend, but I am a CMA, and I follow the rules.
   d. Giving you the results of your biopsy may have caused me to get fired. I'm not getting fired for you or anybody.
   e. You do have that right, but I do not have the right to tell you.
   f. Talk to the physician about it.

77. Why is it important for the physician to give test results such as the one in the case study?

_____

_____

_____

_____

PSY PROCEDURE 8-1 | Establishing, Organizing, and Maintaining a Paper Medical File

Name: _____ Date: _____ Time: _____ Grade: _____

EQUIPMENT/SUPPLIES: File folder; metal fasteners; hole punch; five divider sheets with tabs, title, year, and alphabetic or numeric labels

STANDARDS: Given the needed equipment and a place to work, the student will perform this skill with _____ % accuracy in a total of _____ minutes. *(Your instructor will tell you what the percentage and time limits will be before you begin.)*

KEY: 4 = Satisfactory   0 = Unsatisfactory   NA = This step is not counted

PROCEDURE STEPS	SELF	PARTNER	INSTRUCTOR
1. Place the label along the tabbed edge of the folder so that the title extends out beyond the folder itself. (Tabs can be either the length of the folder or tabbed in various positions, such as left, center, and right.)	❏	❏	❏
2. Place a year label along the top edge of the tab before the label with the title. This will be changed each year the patient has been seen. *Note:* Do not automatically replace these labels at the start of a new year; remove the old year and replace with a new one only when the patient comes in for the first visit of the new year.	❏	❏	❏
3. Place the appropriate alphabetic or numeric labels below the title.	❏	❏	❏
4. Apply any additional labels that your office may decide to use.	❏	❏	❏
5. Punch holes and insert demographic and financial information on the left side of the chart using top fasteners across the top.	❏	❏	❏
6. Make tabs for: Ex. H&P, Progress Notes, Medication Log, Correspondence, and Test Results.	❏	❏	❏
7. Place pages behind appropriate tabs.	❏	❏	❏
8. **AFF** Explain what you would do when you receive a revised copy correcting an error on a document already in a patient's chart.	❏	❏	❏

_____

_____

_____

_____

| PSY | PROCEDURE 8-1 | **Establishing, Organizing, and Maintaining a Paper Medical File** (continued) |

CALCULATION

Total Possible Points: _____

Total Points Earned: _____ Multiplied by 100 = _____ Divided by Total Possible Points = _____ %

PASS   **FAIL**   **COMMENTS:**

❏   ❏

Student's signature _____ Date _____

Partner's signature _____ Date _____

Instructor's signature _____ Date _____

PSY P R O C E D U R E 8 - 2   **Filing Medical Records**

Name: _____ **Date:** _____ **Time:** _____ **Grade:** _____

EQUIPMENT/SUPPLIES: Simulated patient file folder, several single sheets to be filed in the chart, file cabinet with other file

STANDARDS: Given the needed equipment and a place to work, the student will perform this skill with _____ % accuracy in a total of _____ minutes. *(Your instructor will tell you what the percentage and time limits will be before you begin.)*

KEY: 4 = Satisfactory   0 = Unsatisfactory   NA = This step is not counted

PROCEDURE STEPS	SELF	PARTNER	INSTRUCTOR
1. Double check spelling of names on the chart and any single sheets to be placed in the folder.	❑	❑	❑
2. Condition any single sheets, etc.	❑	❑	❑
3. Place sheets behind proper tab in the chart.	❑	❑	❑
4. Remove guide.	❑	❑	❑
5. Place the folder between the two appropriate existing folders, taking care to place the folder between the two charts.	❑	❑	❑
6. Scan color coding to ensure none of the charts in that section are out of order.	❑	❑	❑
7. **AFF** Explain what you would do when you find a chart out of order. Should you bring it to the attention of your supervisor?	❑	❑	❑

_____

_____

_____

_____

_____

CALCULATION

Total Possible Points: _____

Total Points Earned: _____ Multiplied by 100 = _____ Divided by Total Possible Points = _____ %

PASS   FAIL   COMMENTS:
❑   ❑

Student's signature _____ Date _____

Partner's signature _____ Date _____

Instructor's signature _____ Date _____

PSY PROCEDURE 8-3 | Releasing Medical Records

Name: _____ Date: _____ Time: _____ Grade: _____

EQUIPMENT/SUPPLIES: Simulated patient medical record (paper or electronic)

STANDARDS: Given the needed equipment and a place to work, the student will perform this skill with _____ % accuracy in a total of _____ minutes. *(Your instructor will tell you what the percentage and time limits will be before you begin.)*

KEY: 4 = Satisfactory   0 = Unsatisfactory   NA = This step is not counted

PROCEDURE STEPS	SELF	PARTNER	INSTRUCTOR
1. Verify the patient's name and another piece of identifying information in order to pull the correct medical record.	❏	❏	❏
2. Determine if a release of medical record must be signed before the records can be released.	❏	❏	❏
3. Choose the correct document(s) to be released and provide a copy of the documentation if it is not sent electronically.	❏	❏	❏
4. Determine whether a fee should be assessed for copies of the medical record.	❏	❏	❏
5. **AFF** Explain how you would handle copying the requested medical documentation when using a copier.	❏	❏	❏

_____

_____

_____

_____

_____

CALCULATION

Total Possible Points: _____

Total Points Earned: _____ Multiplied by 100 = _____ Divided by Total Possible Points = _____ %

PASS   FAIL   COMMENTS:
❏   ❏

Student's signature _____ Date _____

Partner's signature _____ Date _____

Instructor's signature _____ Date _____

PSY PROCEDURE 8-4   **Document Patient Care Accurately in the Medical Record**

Name: _____   Date: _____   Time: _____   Grade: _____

EQUIPMENT/SUPPLIES: Simulated patient medical record (paper or electronic) and progress note

STANDARDS: Given the needed equipment and a place to work, the student will perform this skill with _____ % accuracy in a total of _____ minutes. *(Your instructor will tell you what the percentage and time limits will be before you begin.)*

KEY: 4 = Satisfactory   0 = Unsatisfactory   NA = This step is not counted

PROCEDURE STEPS	SELF	PARTNER	INSTRUCTOR
1. Go to a private room with limited background noise and a telephone.	❏	❏	❏
2. Verify the patient's name and another piece of identifying information such as a date of birth.	❏	❏	❏
3. Confirm the date and time of the phone conversation in the EHR or enter it with the patient's name and date of birth in the medical record.	❏	❏	❏
4. Ask appropriate, open-ended questions to gather information about the patient's current health status, seeking clarification when necessary.	❏	❏	❏
5. Accurately and concisely document the patient's responses during the phone conversation in the patient's medical record.	❏	❏	❏
6. Authenticate the medical record by signing or initialing your name.	❏	❏	❏
7. **AFF** Explain how you would respond if the patient's symptoms had worsened since the last visit with the physician.	❏	❏	❏

_____

_____

_____

_____

CALCULATION

Total Possible Points: _____

Total Points Earned: _____ Multiplied by 100 = _____ Divided by Total Possible Points = _____ %

PASS   **FAIL**   **COMMENTS:**
❏   ❏

Student's signature _____ Date _____

Partner's signature _____ Date _____

Instructor's signature _____ Date _____

CHAPTER 9

Electronic Applications in the Medical Office

LEARNING OUTCOMES

OOG Cognitive Domain*

1. Spell and define the key words
2. Identify the basic computer components
3. *Recognize the purpose of routine maintenance of equipment*
4. Explain the basics of connecting to the Internet
5. Discuss the safety concerns for online searching
6. Describe how to use a search engine
7. Describe the benefits of an Intranet and explain how it differs from the Internet
8. Describe the various types of clinical software that might be used in a physician's office
9. Describe the various types of administrative software that might be used in a physician's office
10. *Identify the components of an Electronic Medical Record, Electronic Health Record, and Practice Management System*
11. Describe the considerations for purchasing a computer
12. Describe the steps in making the transition from paper to electronic records
13. Discuss the ethics related to computer access
14. *Identify the importance of backup*
15. *Identify the medical assistant's role in telehealth*

AFF Affective Domain*

1. *Reassure patients of the integrity of the information in the medical record when there is a loss of access to the EMR and PMS*
2. *Demonstrate tactfulness when participating in a telehealth interaction*

PSY Psychomotor Domain*

1. Perform routine maintenance of administrative or clinical equipment (Procedure 9-1)
2. Use the Internet to access information related to the medical office (Procedure 9-2)
3. *Input patient data utilizing an electronic system* (Procedure 9-3 and Procedure 9-4)
4. *Participate in a telehealth interaction with a patient* (Procedure 9-4)
5. Develop a plan in the event of loss of access for more than 24 hours to the EMR and PMS to ensure information integrity and patient care (Procedure 9-5)

MAERB Standards are italicized

ABHES Competencies

1. Display effective interpersonal skills with patients and healthcare team
2. Gather and process documents
3. Navigate electronic health records systems and practice management software
4. Display professionalism through written and verbal communications
5. Perform basic computer skills

Name: _____   Date: _____   Grade: _____

OOG MULTIPLE CHOICE

1. Another name for a central processing unit is a:
   a. silicon chip.
   b. USB port.
   c. modem.
   d. microprocessor.
   e. handheld computer.

2. The purpose of a zip drive in a computer is to:
   a. scan information.
   b. delete information.
   c. store information.
   d. research information.
   e. translate information.

3. The acronym *DSL* stands for:
   a. data storage location.
   b. digital subscriber line.
   c. digital storage link.
   d. data saved/lost.
   e. digital software link.

4. In a physician's practice, the HIPAA officer:
   a. checks for security threats or gaps in electronic information.
   b. purchases new technological equipment.
   c. maintains computer equipment and fixes problems.
   d. trains staff in how to use computer equipment.
   e. monitors staff who may be misusing computer equipment.

Scenario for questions 5 and 6: A parent approaches you and asks how he can keep his 9-year-old daughter safe on the Internet.

5. Which of these actions would you recommend to the parent?
   a. Don't allow the daughter on the Internet after 7 PM.
   b. Stand behind the daughter the entire time she is using the Internet.
   c. Don't permit the daughter to use the Internet until she is 10 years old.
   d. Add a filter to the daughter's computer to only allow safe sites as decided by the parent.
   e. Ask other parents for advice.

6. Which of these websites might be helpful to the parent?
   a. www.skyscape.com
   b. www.google.com
   c. www.ezclaim.com
   d. www.netnanny.com
   e. www.nextgen.com

7. To protect your computer from a virus, you should:
   a. make sure that your computer is correctly shut down every time you use it.
   b. avoid opening any attachments from unknown websites.
   c. only download material from government websites.
   d. consult a computer technician before you use new software.
   e. only open one website at a time.

8. What is the advantage of encrypting an e-mail?
   a. It makes the e-mail arrive at its intended destination faster
   b. It marks the e-mail as *urgent*
   c. It scrambles the e-mail so that it cannot be read until it reaches the recipient
   d. It translates the e-mail into another language
   e. It informs the sender when the e-mail has been read by the recipient

9. Which of these is an example of an inappropriate e-mail?
   a. "There will be a staff meeting on Wednesday at 9 AM."
   b. "Please return Mrs. Jay's call: Her number is 608-223-3444."
   c. "If anyone has seen a lost pair of sunglasses, please return them to reception."
   d. "Mr. Orkley thinks he is having a stroke. Please advise."
   e. "Mrs. Jones called to confirm her appointment."

10. Which of the following is not a peripheral?
    a. Router
    b. Monitor
    c. Keyboard
    d. Modem
    e. Hard drive

11. Which of these would you most likely find on an Intranet?
    a. Advice about health insurance
    b. Minutes from staff meetings
    c. Information about Medicare
    d. Descriptions of alternative treatments
    e. National guidelines on medical ethics

12. What is the difference between clinical and administrative software packages?
    a. Clinical software helps provide good medical care, whereas administrative software keeps the office efficient
    b. Administrative software is designed to be used by medical assistants, whereas clinical software is used by physicians
    c. Clinical software is cheaper than administrative software because it offers fewer technical features
    d. Administrative software lasts longer than clinical software because it is of higher quality
    e. Clinical software does not allow users to access it without a password, whereas anyone can use administrative software

13. Which of these should you remember to do when paging a physician?
    a. Follow up the page with a phone call to make sure the physician got the message
    b. Keep track of what time the message is sent and repage if there is no response
    c. Document the fact that you sent a page to the physician
    d. Contact the person who left the message to let them know you have paged the physician
    e. E-mail the physician with a copy of the paged message

14. You can use the Microsoft Outlook program to:
    a. contact patients about appointment changes.
    b. coordinate internal meetings and calendars.
    c. print patient reminders for annual checkups.
    d. create slideshow presentations for meetings.
    e. page office staff when a meeting is about to start.

15. Which of these is an important consideration when purchasing a new computer for the office?
    a. Whether the computer's programs are HIPAA compliant
    b. Whether the computer will be delivered to the office
    c. The number of people who will be using the computer
    d. The amount of space the computer will take up in the office
    e. Which is the best-selling computer on the market?

16. When assigning computer login passwords to staff, a physician should:
    a. make sure that everyone has the code for the hospital computers.
    b. give staff two log-in passwords: one for professional use and one for personal use.
    c. issue all new employees their own passwords.
    d. make sure that everyone has access to their e-mails, in case they are out of the office.
    e. use a standard login password for all of the office computers.

17. It is a good idea to lock the hard drive when you are moving a computer to:
    a. prevent the zip drive from falling out.
    b. make sure that no information is erased.
    c. stop viruses from attacking the computer.
    d. protect the CPU and disk drives.
    e. avoid damaging the keyboard.

18. A modem is a:
    a. communication device that connects a computer to other computers, including the Internet.
    b. piece of software that enables the user to perform advanced administrative functions.
    c. name for the Internet.
    d. method of storing data on the computer.
    e. type of networking technology for local area networks.

19. Which of the following is true of an abstract found during a literary search?
    a. Abstracts are only found on government websites
    b. Only physicians can access an abstract during a literary search
    c. An abstract is a summary of a journal article
    d. Most medical offices cannot afford to download an abstract
    e. Abstracts can only be printed at a hospital library

20. If a computer is exposed to static electricity, there is the potential risk of:
    a. electrical fire.
    b. memory loss.
    c. dust accumulation.
    d. slow Internet connection.
    e. viruses.

21. You have been asked to train new employees on how to use an administrative application. However, you do not have a lot of time or extra funding to spend on training. Circle the best option for training the new employees.

 a. Have them read the user manual.
 b. Have them call the help desk.
 c. Have them ask another colleague.
 d. Have them take a tutorial on the program.
 e. Hire experts from the software company.

22. When shopping for prescription management software, what is the minimum that a physician should be able to do with the program? Circle the correct answer.

 a. Find a patient name in a database, write the prescription, and download it to the pharmacy.
 b. Find a patient name in a database, check the prescription for contraindication, and download it to the pharmacy.
 c. Find a patient name in a database, write the prescription, and print it out for the patient.
 d. Find a medication in a database, write the prescription, and download the data to a handheld computer.
 e. Find a patient name in a database, write the prescription, download it to the pharmacy, and check that the medication is covered by insurance.

COG MATCHING
Grade: _____

Match the following key terms to their definitions.

Key Terms

23. _____ cookies
24. _____ downloading
25. _____ encryption
26. _____ Ethernet
27. _____ Internet
28. _____ Intranet
29. _____ literary search
30. _____ search engine
31. _____ surfing
32. _____ virus
33. _____ virtual
34. _____ PMS
35. _____ EHR

Definitions

a. a system that allows the computer to be connected to a cable or DSL system
b. a private network of computers that share data
c. a global system used to connect one computer to another
d. tiny files left on your computer's hard drive by a website without your permission
e. a dangerous invader that enters your computer through a source and can destroy your files, software programs, and possibly even the hard drive
f. transferring information from an outside location to your computer's hard drive
g. the process of scrambling e-mail messages so that they cannot be read until they reach the recipient
h. the process of navigating websites
i. a program that allows you to find information on the Web related to specific terms
j. a search that involves finding journal articles that present new facts or data about a given topic
k. simulated by your computer
l. clinical information about patients stored in a digital format
m. software application that handles the business of the practice

COG SHORT ANSWER
Grade: _____

36. List three benefits of having appointment scheduling software in the office.

_____

_____

_____

_____

37. You receive an e-mail from a patient saying that his medication is working out well and is not causing any side effects. He will be in for his appointment next Tuesday. How do you document this information in the patient's medical record?

_____

_____

_____

_____

38. What are three benefits of using electronic medical records instead of paper charts?

_____

_____

_____

_____

39. Mr. Jones requires special treatment that uses a laser machine. He makes an appointment for Thursday morning and takes time off from work to attend. When he arrives at the facility, he is told that the machine is only available on Mondays and that the new receptionist was unaware of this fact when she made his appointment. How could an administrative software program have helped to prevent this situation?

_____

_____

_____

_____

COG PSY PATIENT EDUCATION
Grade: _____

40. A patient has told you of his decision to start buying prescription medication on the Internet. What warnings/information should you give to him?

_____

_____

_____

_____

COG PSY ACTIVE LEARNING
Grade: _____

41. Perform research using the Internet to find information about a disease and possible treatments. Try using different key words to see which ones produce the most useful results. Make a list of the websites you have used and observe whether each one has the logo of a verification program such as the HON (Health on the Net) seal.

42. Use the PowerPoint program on the computer to turn your Internet research about a common disease into a presentation. Use the program to make handouts of your presentation for quick office reference. You can use the tutorial feature on the software if you are unsure about how to perform certain functions.

43. Visit the Medicare website at www.medicare.gov. Find the part of the website that addresses FAQs, or frequently asked questions. Choose five of these questions that might be relevant to your patients and print the questions and answers. Then use presentation software to highlight these five questions in a presentation that you will give to your class.

COG IDENTIFICATION

Grade: _____

44. Your office has started converting many of your paper files into digital online files to save time. Recently, you have realized that accessing these records through your Internet service provider (ISP) is taking a very long time. Circle the solutions to this problem.
   a. Upgrade your office's ISP to cable.Q2
   b. Switch your Web browser
   c. Switch your search engine
   d. Upgrade your printer
   e. Eliminate viruses with a virus scan
   f. Upgrade your monitor
   g. Upgrade your office's ISP to DSL

45. A patient has asked you for information on how she can lower her cholesterol. You have decided to surf the Internet to find the latest information. Place a check in the "Yes" column for those keywords that would lead to a faster, more efficient search. Place a check in the "No" column for those keywords that would lead to a slower, less-efficient search.

Key Words	Yes	No
a. Cholesterol		
b. Lowering cholesterol		
c. Cholesterol diet		
d. How do people lower their cholesterol?		
e. Cholesterol reduction		

46. A diabetic patient has been researching information on the disease. He has asked you to review a list of websites he has been reading. Place a check in the "Patient" box for sites that are more useful for patients. Place a check in the "Professional" box for sites that are more useful to physicians and medical assistants.

Websites	Patient	Professional
a. www.mywebmd.com		
b. www.lancet.org		
c. www.jama.com		
d. www.healthfinder.gov		
e. www.tifaq.com		

COG PSY PATIENT EDUCATION

Grade: _____

47. A patient has expressed an interest in learning more about her food allergies on the Internet. You decide to give her advice on what to look out for when surfing. Place a check in the "Yes" column indicating that the statement is good advice. Place a check in the "No" column indicating that the statement is bad advice.

Keywords	Yes	No
a. Almost all testimonials can be trusted.		
b. Don't trust sites that claim to have secret formulas, medical miracles, or breakthroughs.		
c. Some treatments found online are best to not tell your physician about.		
d. No matter how professional the website, you cannot learn lifesaving skills on the Internet.		

TRUE OR FALSE?

Grade: _____

48. Determine whether the following statements are true or false. If false, explain why.

a. The advanced search feature of a search engine should return more results.

_____

b. Internal job postings are often found on the Internet.

_____

c. The most popular program used to write presentations is PowerPoint.

_____

d. A computer system is divided into three areas: hardware, peripherals, and software.

_____

AFF PSY WHAT WOULD YOU DO?

Grade: _____

49. You perform most of the administrative tasks in a physician's office and have been asked for your input concerning a new office computer. The physician asks you which administrative features you would find helpful in a new computer. List three administrative software programs that you would find useful and explain what functions they perform.

_____

_____

_____

_____

50. A patient tells you that her medicine has not been working properly and that she is thinking of researching alternative treatments on the Internet. What is the best advice you can give her?

_____

_____

_____

_____

51. One of your coworkers has a habit of getting up from her computer and leaving confidential patient information visible on the screen. She says that she sits too far away from patients for them to read anything on the screen, but you have seen several patients near the computer while your coworker is away from her desk. What do you say to her?

_____

_____

_____

_____

52. It is your first week working at a physician's office. You notice that the computer is dusty in the morning sunlight. Disks are in a neat pile next to the uncovered computer. What steps would you take to maintain this computer?

_____

_____

_____

_____

AFF CASE STUDIES FOR CRITICAL THINKING

Grade: _____

You are teaching Ginger, a new employee, to use the computer system in the office where you work. She is excited and enthusiastic about her new job. At every possible opportunity, Ginger checks her Facebook and Twitter pages. You know that this is against the office policy regarding accepted use of office computers.

53. Circle all appropriate actions from the list below.
   a. Beg the office manager to get someone else to train Ginger
   b. Show her the policy in the office _Policies and Procedures Manual_
   c. Tell her if she continues this practice she will get fired
   d. Tell her that the IT department can and will track her use of the office computer
   e. Suggest that she wait until she gets off work for personal computer use
   f. Suggest that people should talk to each other the way they used to, face to face

54. Circle the accurate statements from the list below. Businesses control personal use of their computers because:
   a. it reduces wear and tear on the computers.
   b. it is inefficient for employees to be doing personal things while at work.
   c. it is dishonest to use someone else's computer.
   d. it is unprofessional and unethical.
   e. you should never disobey the office rules, no matter what.
   f. they are not paying you to be on Facebook and Twitter.
   g. it is illegal.

55. You are teaching Ginger how to care for her computer. Why is it important to perform routine maintenance on the office computer? Circle all appropriate answers from the list below.

  a. It enhances the performance and prolongs the life of the equipment
  b. It is a rule and you *always* follow the rules, no matter what
  c. It shows that you are a clean person
  d. It looks bad for the patients to see dust
  e. It is in the office *Policy and Procedure Manual*

PSY PROCEDURE 9-1 Care for and Maintain Computer Hardware

Name: _____ **Date:** _____ **Time:** _____ **Grade:** _____

EQUIPMENT/SUPPLIES: Computer CPU, monitor, keyboard, mouse, printer, duster, simulated warranties

STANDARDS: Given the needed equipment and a place to work, the student will perform this skill with _____ % accuracy in a total of _____ minutes. *(Your instructor will tell you what the percentage and time limits will be before you begin.)*

KEY: 4 = Satisfactory 0 = Unsatisfactory NA = This step is not counted

PROCEDURE STEPS	SELF	PARTNER	INSTRUCTOR
1. Place the monitor, keyboard, and printer in a cool, dry area out of direct sunlight.	❏	❏	❏
2. Place the computer desk on an antistatic floor mat or carpet.	❏	❏	❏
3. Clean the monitor screen with antistatic wipes.	❏	❏	❏
4. Use dust covers for the keyboard and the monitor when they are not in use.	❏	❏	❏
5. Lock the hard drive when moving the computer.	❏	❏	❏
6. Keep keyboard and mouse free of debris and liquids; dust and/or vacuum the keyboard.	❏	❏	❏
7. Create a file for maintenance and warranty contracts for the computer system.	❏	❏	❏
8. Handle data storage disks with special care.	❏	❏	❏
9. **AFF** If you were the office manager, explain how you would respond to an employee who continued to spill soft drinks on her keyboard.	❏	❏	❏

_____

_____

_____

_____

_____

CALCULATION

Total Possible Points: _____

Total Points Earned: _____ Multiplied by 100 = _____ Divided by Total Possible Points = _____ %

PASS **FAIL** **COMMENTS:**
❏ ❏

Student's signature _____ Date _____

Partner's signature _____ Date _____

Instructor's signature _____ Date _____

PSY PROCEDURE 9-2 **Searching on the Internet**

Name: _____ **Date:** _____ **Time:** _____ **Grade:** _____

EQUIPMENT/SUPPLIES: Computer with Web browser software, modem, active Internet connection account

STANDARDS: Given the needed equipment and a place to work, the student will perform this skill with _____ % accuracy in a total of _____ minutes. *(Your instructor will tell you what the percentage and time limits will be before you begin.)*

KEY: 4 = Satisfactory 0 = Unsatisfactory NA = This step is not counted

PROCEDURE STEPS	SELF	PARTNER	INSTRUCTOR
1. Connect computer to the Internet.	❏	❏	❏
2. Locate a search engine.	❏	❏	❏
3. Select two or three key words and type them in the appropriate place on the web page.	❏	❏	❏
4. View the number of search results. If no sites are found, check spelling and retype or choose new key words.	❏	❏	❏
5. If the search produces a long list, do an advanced search and refine keywords.	❏	❏	❏
6. Select an appropriate site and open its home page.	❏	❏	❏
7. If satisfied with the site's information, either download the material or bookmark the page. If unsatisfied with its information, either visit a site listed on the results page or return to the search engine.	❏	❏	❏
8. **AFF** You sit down to use your office computer to search for information with a patient when a coworker's Facebook page pops up. You are embarrassed at the lack of professionalism this displays in front of the patient. Explain how you would respond in this situation.	❏	❏	❏

_____

_____

_____

_____

_____

CALCULATION

Total Possible Points: _____

Total Points Earned: _____ Multiplied by 100 = _____ Divided by Total Possible Points = _____ %

PASS   FAIL   COMMENTS:
❏   ❏

Student's signature _____ Date _____

Partner's signature _____ Date _____

Instructor's signature _____ Date _____

PSY PROCEDURE 9-3 **Entering Patient Demographics into a Practice Management System**

Name: _____ Date: _____ Time: _____ Grade: _____

EQUIPMENT/SUPPLIES: Computer, completed patient demographics form, and a practice management system

STANDARDS: Given the needed equipment and a place to work, the student will perform this skill with _____ % accuracy in a total of _____ minutes. *(Your instructor will tell you what the percentage and time limits will be before you begin.)*

KEY: 4 = Satisfactory   0 = Unsatisfactory   NA = This step is not counted

PROCEDURE STEPS	SELF	PARTNER	INSTRUCTOR
1. Open the practice management application and verify that the patient is not already in the system.	❏	❏	❏
2. Open the patient module, enter all of the patient's personal information on the demographics tab, and save.	❏	❏	❏
3. Enter the insurance/subscriber information for the primary insurance and save.	❏	❏	❏
4. Verify that correct information has been entered from the patient information form.	❏	❏	❏
5. **AFF** While entering the patient's demographic information, you are interrupted by the physician and walk away from your computer. What choices could you have made to protect the patient's private information?	❏	❏	❏

_____

_____

_____

_____

CALCULATION

Total Possible Points: _____

Total Points Earned: _____ Multiplied by 100 = _____ Divided by Total Possible Points = _____ %

PASS   **FAIL**   **COMMENTS:**
 ❏   ❏

Student's signature _____ Date _____

Partner's signature _____ Date _____

Instructor's signature _____ Date _____

PSY PROCEDURE 9-4 **Utilizing Telecommunications for a Healthcare Encounter**

Name: _____ Date: _____ Time: _____ Grade: _____

EQUIPMENT/SUPPLIES: Computer with audio and video capabilities and an electronic medical record.

STANDARDS: Given the needed equipment and a place to work, the student will perform this skill with _____ % accuracy in a total of _____ minutes. *(Your instructor will tell you what the percentage and time limits will be before you begin.)*

KEY: 4 = Satisfactory 0 = Unsatisfactory NA = This step is not counted

PROCEDURE STEPS	SELF	PARTNER	INSTRUCTOR
1. Prior to the visit, verify that the patient has been given information needed for accessing the telehealth visit (via smartphone, computer, or tablet), including the telecommunications platform that will be used with login information (the patient EHR portal, Zoom, Webex, etc.).	❏	❏	❏
2. Go to a private room with limited background noise, adequate lighting, Internet capabilities, and a computer with audio and video.	❏	❏	❏
3. Determine if patient consent is needed for the visit based on state informed consent laws.	❏	❏	❏
4. Enter the telecommunications platform to be used for the visit and greet the patient.	❏	❏	❏
5. Verify the patient's name and another piece of identifying information and access the correct medical record.	❏	❏	❏
6. Document the patient's chief complaint in the electronic medical record.	❏	❏	❏
7. Explain how you would respond if a patient had a family member present during the telehealth visit.	❏	❏	❏

PSY PROCEDURE 9-5 **Contingency Plan for Loss of Information Technology**

Name: _____ **Date:** _____ **Time:** _____ **Grade:** _____

EQUIPMENT/SUPPLIES: Computer with word processing software, 8-1/2 X 11 white paper

STANDARDS: Given the needed equipment and a place to work, the student will perform this skill with _____ % accuracy in a total of _____ minutes. *(Your instructor will tell you what the percentage and time limits will be before you begin.)*

KEY: 4 = Satisfactory 0 = Unsatisfactory NA = This step is not counted

PROCEDURE STEPS	SELF	PARTNER	INSTRUCTOR
1. Identify who is responsible for backing up the EMR and PMS data on the network servers on a regular basis and where the information will be stored.	❏	❏	❏
2. Print a copy of the schedule at the beginning of every day.	❏	❏	❏
3. Identify the person responsible for immediately communicating: • The downtime to the staff and keeping everyone advised of connectivity status • Notification of the problem with the EHR and/or PMS vendor • Notification to the network provider if the Internet service is also disrupted	❏	❏	❏
4. Maintain a supply of printed copies of paper documentation tools such as patient demographic sheets, medical history forms, progress notes, and paper medical charts.	❏	❏	❏
5. Identify a private, secure area to store the paper medical records until the EMR and PMS systems are functioning again.	❏	❏	❏
6. Identify the person responsible for entering patient information into the PMS and EHR and, if necessary, recovering data that has been backed up as soon as access to the computers and/or Internet become available.	❏	❏	❏
7. Schedule and participate in a debriefing with all staff to reflect and discuss how the IT Emergency Action Plan worked and make revisions, if necessary.	❏	❏	❏
8. Require all staff to review upon hire and participate at least annually in the IT Emergency Action Plan training and drills.	❏	❏	❏
9. Explain how you would reassure a patient that the PHI in the EHR is secure even though you cannot access it during an office IT emergency.	❏	❏	❏

CHAPTER 10

Managing the Medical Office

LEARNING OUTCOMES

COG Cognitive Domain*

1. Spell and define the key terms
2. Describe what is meant by organizational structure
3. List seven responsibilities of the medical office manager
4. Explain the five staffing issues that a medical office manager will be responsible for handling
5. *Identify legal and illegal interview questions*
6. List the types of policies and procedures that should be included in a medical office's policy and procedures manual
7. List five types of promotional materials that a medical office may distribute
8. Describe three purposes of a budget
9. *Identify steps involved in completing an inventory*
10. Define risk management
11. List three services provided by most medical malpractice companies
12. List six guidelines for completing incident reports
13. *Identify the process in compliance reporting:*
    a. *Unsafe activities*
    b. *Errors in patient care*
    c. *Conflicts of interest*
    d. *Incident reports*
14. List four regulatory agencies that require medical offices to have quality improvement programs

15. Explain the purpose of participating in the Joint Commission
16. Describe the steps to developing a quality improvement program
17. *Identify workplace safeguards*
18. *Identify the purpose of Safety Data Sheets (SDS) in a healthcare setting*
19. *Identify fire safety issues in an ambulatory healthcare environment*
20. *Identify the processes for disposal of:*
    a. *biohazardous waste*
    b. *chemicals*
21. *Identify principles of*
    a. *Body mechanics*
    b. *Ergonomics*
22. *Identify safety techniques that can be used in responding to accidental exposure to:*
    a. *Blood*
    b. *Other body fluids*
    c. *Needle sticks*
    d. *Chemicals*
23. *Identify emergency practices for evacuation of a healthcare setting*
24. *Identify critical elements of an emergency plan for response to a natural disaster or other emergency*
25. *Identify physical manifestations and emotional behaviors on persons involved in an emergency*

PSY Psychomotor Domain*

1. Create a policy and procedures manual (Procedure 10-1)

2. *Perform an inventory of supplies (Procedure 10-2)*
3. *Evaluate an environment to identify unsafe conditions (Procedure 10-3)*
4. *Complete an incident report related to an error in patient care (Procedure 10-4)*
5. Apply local, state, and federal healthcare legislation and regulation appropriate to the medical assisting practice setting (Procedure 10-3)
6. *Comply with safety practices (Procedure 10-5)*

AFF Affective Domain*

1. *Recognize the physical and emotional effects on persons involved in an emergency situation*
2. *Demonstrate self-awareness in responding to emergency situations*
3. Recognize the importance of local, state, and federal legislation and regulation in the practice setting

*MAERB Standards are italicized.

ABHES Competencies

1. Maintain inventory, equipment, and supplies
2. Perform risk management procedures
3. Comply with federal, state, and local health laws and regulations

Name: _____   Date: _____   Grade: _____

COG MULTIPLE CHOICE

Scenario for questions 1 and 2: It's your first day on the job as the medical office manager, so there is a lot you don't know yet about this office.

1. You want to know who is responsible for what in the office. Where is the best place to find that information?
   a. Payroll records
   b. The work schedule
   c. The chain-of-command chart
   d. The recent employee evaluations
   e. The bulletin board

2. You know the office is running low on paper and syringes. You're most likely to find out how to order supplies in:
   a. the QI plan.
   b. the service contracts folder.
   c. the operating budget.
   d. the policy and procedures manual.
   e. the communication notebook.

3. An SDS is required to contain:
   a. general information about safety.
   b. a written hazard communication plan.
   c. information regarding hazardous chemicals found in a facility.
   d. the appropriate amount of bleach that can be stored in a medical office.
   e. a complete list of the hazardous materials in a facility.

4. The office keeps running out of tongue depressors. Which action should you take first?
   a. Establish a recycling program
   b. Determine whether someone is stealing supplies
   c. Review the system for keeping track of supplies
   d. Tell the physicians not to use so many tongue depressors
   e. Borrow some tongue depressors from the nearest medical office

5. Which item should be in any job description?
   a. Age requirements
   b. Salary or hourly pay
   c. Physical requirements
   d. The preferred gender of the applicant
   e. Medical and dental benefits

6. Which task should you be expected to perform as medical office manager?
   a. Clean the waiting room
   b. Assign someone to make coffee
   c. Develop promotional pamphlets
   d. Assist with simple medical procedures
   e. Sign prescription refills

7. Which of the following is a medical office manager's responsibility?
   a. Completing all incident reports
   b. Teaching CPR
   c. Evaluating the physicians
   d. Hiring and firing employees
   e. Teaching employees about malpractice insurance

8. Which statement is true of an incident report about a patient?
   a. It should be mailed to the attorney of your choice
   b. It should be written by a physician
   c. It should be written within 24 hours of the incident
   d. It should be written from the patient's point of view
   e. It should be kept in the medical office

9. Which action should be taken if an employee is stuck by a patient's needle?
   a. The patient should be informed
   b. The physician should take disciplinary action against the employee
   c. The employee should write an incident report
   d. The employee should be kept away from patients
   e. The employee should sign a form admitting liability

10. Which of the following categories is part of a capital budget?
    a. Payroll
    b. Medical supplies
    c. Building maintenance
    d. Heating and air conditioning
    e. Electricity

11. Which item should be part of any medical office budget?
    a. Merit bonuses
    b. Billing service
    c. Continuing education
    d. Magazine subscriptions
    e. Children's play facility

12. Which agency licenses and monitors healthcare organizations and enforces regulations?
    a. CMS
    b. State health department
    c. The Joint Commission
    d. OSHA
    e. HCFA

13. General liability and medical malpractice insurance is for:
    a. all medical professionals.
    b. all physicians.
    c. physicians who perform risky procedures.
    d. medical professionals with high-risk profiles.
    e. physicians and nurses.

14. The first step in creating a quality improvement plan is to:
    a. form a task force.
    b. identify the problem.
    c. establish a monitoring plan.
    d. assign an expected threshold.
    e. explore the problem.

15. Which of the following items should be included in an emergency kit?
    a. Alcohol wipes
    b. Syringe
    c. Penicillin
    d. Oscilloscope
    e. Sample containers

16. If you fill out an incident report, you should:
    a. keep a copy of the report.
    b. have a supervisor review it.
    c. give your title but not your name.
    d. fill out only the sections that apply.
    e. summarize what happened in the report.

17. Which of the following is used to estimate expenditures and revenues?
    a. Budget
    b. Tracking file
    c. Expected threshold
    d. Financial statement
    e. Inventory log

18. Risk management is a(n):
    a. process begun only after a sentinel event.
    b. process intended to identify potential problems.
    c. external process that deals with OSHA violations.
    d. internal process that deals with recurring problems.
    e. process undertaken by managers to reduce annual expenditure.

19. Which of the following is true of an expected threshold for a quality improvement program?
    a. It is the expected percentage reduction in risk
    b. It is a way to measure the success of the program
    c. It should be set higher for more dangerous problems
    d. It should be set lower than you think you can achieve
    e. It should only be used for particularly severe problems

20. General liability and medical malpractice insurance is needed:
    a. only by employees in offices that use new medical procedures.
    b. by physicians sued for malpractice, but not by nurses or office personnel.
    c. to protect medical professionals from financial loss due to lawsuits or settlements.
    d. because visitors who are hurt in the waiting room can sue unless an incident report is completed.

COG MATCHING

Grade: _____

Match the following key terms to their definitions.

Key Terms
21. _____ bioterrorism
22. _____ body mechanics
23. _____ budget
24. _____ compliance officer
25. _____ epidemic
26. _____ ergonomics
27. _____ expected threshold
28. _____ incident report
29. _____ job description

Definitions
a. numerical goal for a given problem
b. statement of work-related responsibilities
c. series of steps required to perform a given task
d. written account of untoward patient, visitor, or staff event
e. description of the goals of the practice and whom it serves
f. statement regarding the organization's rules on a given topic
g. purposeful infliction of a dangerous agent into a populated area with intent to harm
h. financial planning tool used to estimate anticipated expenditures and revenues

Key Terms

30. _____ mission statement
31. _____ organizational chart
32. _____ pandemic
33. _____ policy
34. _____ procedure
35. _____ quality improvement
36. _____ task force

Definitions

i. staff member who ensures compliance with the rules and regulations of the office

j. implementation of practices that will help ensure high-quality patient care and service

k. flow sheet that allows staff to identify team members and see where they fit into the team

l. group of employees with different roles brought together to solve a problem

m. using the correct muscles and posture to complete a task safely and efficiently

n. the study of the fit between a worker and their physical work environment

o. a disease affecting many people in a specific geographic area

p. a disease infecting numerous people in many areas of the world at the same time

SHORT ANSWER

Grade: _____

37. List three responsibilities of the office manager regarding service contractors.

_____

_____

_____

_____

_____

38. List five types of promotional materials that a medical office might use.

_____

_____

_____

_____

39. List six items that should be included in employee fire safety training.

_____

_____

_____

_____

40. List the four basic principles of proper body mechanics.

_____

_____

_____

_____

41. List five techniques used to reduce fatigue as you work.

_____

_____

_____

_____

_____

COG IDENTIFICATION

Grade: _____

42. Below is a list of the steps for creating a quality improvement plan. Put the steps in logical order. Then explain the reason for each step.

Steps

Assign an expected threshold.
Document the entire process.
Establish a monitoring plan.
Explore the problem and propose solutions.
Form a task force.
Identify the problem.
Implement the solution.
Obtain feedback.

Step	Reason
1.	
2.	
3.	
4.	
5.	
6.	
7.	
8.	

⬛ YES OR NO?

Grade: _____

Answer "Yes," "No," or "Yes But" to the following questions about evaluating employees. If you answer "No" or "Yes But," be able to explain why.

	Yes	No	Yes But ...
43. Are employee evaluations your responsibility as a medical office manager?			
44. Should new employees be evaluated annually?			
45. Should you coach new employees about how to do their jobs well?			
46. Can annual performance appraisals be done orally?			
47. Should you communicate with employees about performance problems when one of the physicians asks you to?			
48. Should you inform a good employee yearly that they are doing a good job?			

⬛ IDENTIFICATION

Grade: _____

49. Medical offices usually have an operating budget and a capital budget. Separate the following items into the two categories by checking the column for operating budget or capital budget.

Budget Item	Operating Budget	Capital Budget
a. Payroll		
b. Medical equipment		
c. Office supplies		
d. Internet service		
e. Medical supplies		
f. Building maintenance		
g. Telephone service		
h. Electricity		
i. Expensive furniture		
j. Patient materials		
k. Continuing education		

COG **PSY** **ACTIVE LEARNING**

Grade: _____

50. When you complete your study program, you would like to find a job as a medical office manager. Write the job description for your ideal job. Be sure to include all of the essential elements, including a position summary, hours, location, and duties.

51. Your office manager has assigned you to a task force that will write a plan for fire prevention in your office. Your role in the group is to establish the headings for the plan. List five items that should be included.

_____

_____

_____

_____

_____

_____

_____

_____

52. Working together with a partner, search the local classified ads for an open job as a medical office manager. Then prepare to role-play the interview process with your partner, taking turns acting as the interviewer and the interviewee. Make a list of questions that you would ask as both the interviewer and the interviewee. Switch places so you both get to experience the job interview process from each perspective.

_____

_____

_____

_____

COG **IDENTIFICATION**

Grade: _____

53. Circle all of the following tasks that are the responsibility of the medical office manager.

a. Scheduling staff

b. Ordering supplies

c. Writing the budget

d. Keeping up to date on legal issues

e. Assisting with medical procedures

f. Cleaning the office and waiting room

g. Revising policy and procedures manuals

h. Presenting continuing education seminars

i. Developing HIPAA and OSHA regulations

j. Developing promotional pamphlets or newsletters

54. Inventory control is the responsibility of the office manager. On the checklist below, put an **M** beside the inventory tasks the manager should do and an **A** beside the things an assistant or other office staff member can do.

_____ Receive supplies

_____ Initial the packing slip

_____ Develop a system to keep track of supplies

_____ Determine the procedures for ordering supplies

_____ Transfer supplies from packing boxes to supply shelves

_____ Check the packing slip against the actual supply contents

_____ Keep receipts or packing slips in a bills-pending file for payment

_____ Develop a process to check that deliveries of supplies are complete and accurate

COG YES OR NO?

Grade: _____

55. Indicate by a check mark in the "Yes" or "No" column whether an item should be included in a medical office's policy and procedures manual.

Policy	Yes	No
a. A chain-of-command chart		
b. A list of employee benefits		
c. Infection control guidelines		
d. The office operating budget		
e. Annual employee evaluations		
f. Procedures for bill collections		
g. Copies of completed incident reports		
h. A description of the goals of the practice		
i. Responsibilities and procedures for ordering supplies		
j. A list of responsibilities for the last employee to leave the office each day		

COG LISTING

Grade: _____

56. List six of the elements that should be included in any job description.

a. _____

b. _____

c. _____

d. _____

e. _____

f. _____

57. In addition to writing job descriptions and managing employee evaluations, list the three other staffing issues that are the medical office manager's responsibility.

a. _____

b. _____

c. _____

58. List three services provided by most medical malpractice companies.

a. _____

b. _____

c. _____

COG FALSE THEN TRUE

Grade: _____

59. Each of the following statements about incident reports is false or incomplete. Rewrite each statement to make it true and complete.

a. You should write up an incident report as the event was reported to you.

_____

b. The witness should summarize and explain the event.

_____

c. You should remain anonymous when you fill out a report.

_____

d. The form should be completed within 48 hours of the event.

_____

e. If a particular section of the report does not apply, it should be left blank.

_____

f. Keep a copy of the incident report for your own personal record.

_____

g. If the incident happened to a patient, put a copy of the report in the patient's chart.

_____

h. The report should be reviewed by a supervisor to make sure the office is not liable.

_____

i. Incident reports are written when negative events happen to patients or visitors.

_____

COG MATCHING

Grade: _____

60. Below is a list of four regulatory agencies that require medical offices to have quality improvement programs. Draw a line between the two columns to match the regulatory agency with its description.

Agencies	Descriptions
1. CMS	**a.** Federal agency that regulates and runs Medicare and Medicaid
2. OSHA	**b.** Nonfederal agency to license and monitor healthcare organizations and enforce regulations
3. The Joint Commission	**c.** Federal agency that enforces regulations to protect the health and welfare of patients and employees
4. State health department	**d.** Agency that sets voluntary healthcare standards and evaluates a healthcare organization's implementation of those standards

COG WHICH IS WHICH?

Grade: _____

61. Explain how quality improvement programs and risk management work together in a medical office.

_____

_____

_____

_____

COG TRUE OR FALSE?

Grade: _____

62. Determine whether the following statements are true or false. If false, explain why.

a. Healthcare organizations are required to follow the regulations of the Joint Commission.

_____

b. Accreditation by The Joint Commission is valid for 5 years.

_____

c. If The Joint Commission's initial site review identifies unsatisfactory areas, the healthcare organization may later prove that corrections have been made by passing a focus survey.

_____

d. The healthcare organization should prepare for the Joint Commission survey by assessing its compliance with OSHA standards.

_____

AFF WHAT WOULD YOU DO?

Grade: _____

63. As you enter the office on the first day of your new job as the medical office manager, you notice a thick layer of dust on the plastic plants in the waiting room and see that the magazines are old and tattered. The staff greets you with enthusiasm, saying you are just what they need to deal with the patients' complaints about spending too much time waiting to be seen. Someone has left an incident report file on your desk. You look through it right away and learn that a needlestick has been reported almost every Wednesday evening for a month. What would you do first, and why?

_____

_____

_____

_____

64. You have a patient who lost her home and several pets to a recent tornado in your city. You know she is at risk for the development of a major psychiatric disorder. What are five ways to help this patient who has been exposed to trauma from natural or manmade disasters?

_____

_____

_____

_____

65. Mrs. Hadley, who is blind and walks with a cane, slipped on the wet floor near a leaky water cooler and fell, cutting her forearm. One of the nurses examined and treated her wound and apologized. Mrs. Hadley said it was no problem and left the office. The nurse told you she wasn't going to file an incident report because the wound was minor and Mrs. Hadley had accepted her apology. As the medical office manager, what should you do?

_____

_____

_____

_____

AFF **CASE STUDIES FOR CRITICAL THINKING**

Grade: _____

You have been asked by your physician employer to inspect the office for possible safety hazards. He wants a report of any negative findings by the end of the week.

66. Circle the most appropriate first step.

    a. Ask if you can assign a task force to help you

    b. Design a form for checking off items as you inspect them

    c. Tell him you are too busy with patients to take on such a large task

    d. Call the local fire department to perform the inspection

    e. Call the local OSHA representative to perform the inspection

67. From the following list of actions, circle all that are appropriate.

    a. Check closets for the storage of flammable liquids

    b. Check areas where oxygen is in use

    c. Check to be sure all cylinders and tanks that contain flammable gases or liquids are uncapped and ready for use

    d. Check to see that equipment and carts are on the right side of each hallway

    e. Check the CMA schedule to be sure there is enough coverage to keep everyone safe

PSY PROCEDURE 10-1 **Create a Procedures Manual**

Name: _____ Date: _____ Time: _____ Grade: _____

EQUIPMENT/SUPPLIES: Word processor, three-ring binder, paper, choose any procedure approved by your instructor

STANDARDS: Given the needed equipment and a place to work, the student will perform this skill with _____ % accuracy in a total of _____ minutes. *(Your instructor will tell you what the percentage and time limits will be before you begin.)*

KEY: 4 = Satisfactory 0 = Unsatisfactory NA = This step is not counted

PROCEDURE STEPS	SELF	PARTNER	INSTRUCTOR
1. Check the latest information from key governmental agencies, local, and state health departments, and healthcare organizations, such as OSHA and the CDC to make sure that the policies and procedures being written comply with federal and state legislation and regulations.	❏	❏	❏
2. Gather product information; consult government agencies, if needed. Secure educational pamphlets.	❏	❏	❏
3. Title the procedure properly.	❏	❏	❏
4. Number the procedure appropriately.	❏	❏	❏
5. Define the overall purpose of the procedure in a sentence or two explaining the intent of the procedure.	❏	❏	❏
6. List all necessary equipment and forms. Include everything needed to complete the task.	❏	❏	❏
7. List each step with its rationale.	❏	❏	❏
8. Provide spaces for signatures.	❏	❏	❏
9. Record the date the procedure was written.	❏	❏	❏
10. Describe how you would explain to employees why they were asked to work in a group to create a procedure manual.	❏	❏	❏

_____

_____

_____

_____

CALCULATION

Total Possible Points: _____

Total Points Earned: _____ Multiplied by 100 = _____ Divided by Total Possible Points = _____ %

(continues)

PSY   P R O C E D U R E   1 0 - 1   **Create a Procedures Manual** (continued)

PASS   FAIL   COMMENTS:
❑   ❑

Student's signature _____   Date _____

Partner's signature _____   Date _____

Instructor's signature _____   Date _____

PSY   PROCEDURE 10-2   **Perform an Office Inventory**

Name: _____   Date: _____   Time: _____   Grade: _____

EQUIPMENT: Inventory form, reorder form

STANDARDS: Given the needed equipment and a place to work, the student will perform this skill with _____ % accuracy in a total of _____ minutes. *(Your instructor will tell you what the percentage and time limits will be before you begin.)*

KEY: 4 = Satisfactory   0 = Unsatisfactory   NA = This step is not counted

PROCEDURE STEPS	SELF	PARTNER	INSTRUCTOR
1. Using forms supplied by your instructor, count and record the amounts of specified supplies	❏	❏	❏
2. Record amount of each item	❏	❏	❏
3. Compare amount on hand with amount needed	❏	❏	❏
4. Complete reorder form based on these numbers	❏	❏	❏
5. Submit reorder forms to office manager	❏	❏	❏
6. Document your actions according to the ordering procedure	❏	❏	❏
7. Explain how you would respond to an employee who continually takes a vacation day when the office plans to take inventory	❏	❏	❏

_____

_____

_____

_____

CALCULATION

Total Possible Points: _____

Total Points Earned: _____ Multiplied by 100 = _____ Divided by Total Possible Points = _____ %

PASS   FAIL   COMMENTS:
  ❏   ❏

Student's signature _____   Date _____

Partner's signature _____   Date _____

Instructor's signature _____   Date _____

PSY PROCEDURE 10-3   **Perform Medical Office Safety Checklist**

Name: _____ Date: _____ Time: _____ Grade: _____

EQUIPMENT: Office Safety Checklist, pen

STANDARDS: Given the needed equipment and a place to work, the student will perform this skill with _____ % accuracy in a total of _____ minutes. *(Your instructor will tell you what the percentage and time limits will be before you begin.)*

KEY: 4 = Satisfactory   0 = Unsatisfactory   NA = This step is not counted

PROCEDURE STEPS	SELF	PARTNER	INSTRUCTOR
1. After obtaining a floor plan of the medical office, perform a general visual inspection of every room/area for potential hazards	❏	❏	❏
2. Inspect office equipment for potential hazards	❏	❏	❏
3. Examine all fire extinguishers and determine that they are in their appropriate places, fully charged, and operating properly	❏	❏	❏
4. Verify that the following items are properly displayed: evacuation routes in every room; and an OSHA poster (publication 3165) in a prominent location in the office. Also, verify that lighted exit signs are working	❏	❏	❏
5. Verify that the SDS are accessible to all employees in a prominent location in the office	❏	❏	❏
6. Advise the physician of any hazardous situations that you may find that need corrective action	❏	❏	❏

_____

_____

_____

_____

CALCULATION

Total Possible Points: _____

Total Points Earned: _____ Multiplied by 100 = _____ Divided by Total Possible Points = _____ %

PASS   FAIL   COMMENTS:
❏   ❏

Student's signature _____ Date _____

Partner's signature _____ Date _____

Instructor's signature _____ Date _____

Great Falls Health System Physician Offices
WORKPLACE SAFETY CHECKLIST

Name of person conducting the inspection:	Inspection Date:

GENERAL VISUAL INSPECTION:

Reception Area	Yes	No	Comments
1. Is this area clean and uncluttered?			
2. Is there a posted office diagram showing evacuation routes in the event of an emergency?			
3. Are the exits unobstructed?			
4. Are the emergency exit lights working properly?			
5. Is there anything stacked up that could fall?			
6. Are all electrical cables in good condition (not frayed or damaged) and neatly tied up?			
7. Is electrical equipment working properly with adequate ventilation?			
8. Is there adequate clearance for electrical equipment from combustible material?			
Exam Room 1	**Yes**	**No**	**Comments**
1. Is this area clean and uncluttered?			
2. Is there a posted office diagram showing evacuation routes in the event of an emergency?			
3. Are the exits unobstructed?			
4. Are the emergency exit lights working properly?			
5. Is there anything stacked up that could fall?			
6. Are all electrical cables in good condition (not frayed or damaged) and neatly tied up?			
7. Is electrical equipment working properly with adequate ventilation?			
8. Is there adequate clearance for electrical equipment from combustible material?			
Exam Room 2	**Yes**	**No**	**Comments**
1. Is this area clean and uncluttered?			
2. Is there a posted office diagram showing evacuation routes in the event of an emergency?			
3. Are the exits unobstructed?			

	Yes	No	Comments
4. Are the emergency exit lights working properly?			
5. Is there anything stacked up that could fall?			
6. Are all electrical cables in good condition (not frayed or damaged) and neatly tied up?			
7. Is electrical equipment working properly with adequate ventilation?			
8. Is there adequate clearance for electrical equipment from combustible material?			
Lunch Room/Break Area	**Yes**	**No**	**Comments**
1. Is this area clean and uncluttered?			
2. Is there a posted office diagram showing evacuation routes in the event of an emergency?			
3. Are the exits unobstructed?			
4. Are the emergency exit lights working properly?			
5. Is there anything stacked up that could fall?			
6. Are all electrical cables in good condition (not frayed or damaged) and neatly tied up?			
7. Is electrical equipment working properly with adequate ventilation?			
8. Is there adequate clearance for electrical equipment from combustible material?			
9. Is the OSHA poster "Job Safety and Health" prominently displayed?			
Fire Emergencies	**Yes**	**No**	
1. Are fire extinguishers visible and current throughout the office?			
2. Have all fire extinguishers been checked within the last 6 months?			

CLINICAL AREA INSPECTIONS:

All Exam Rooms:	**Yes**	**No**	**Comments**
1. Are medical records inaccessible and PHI protected while in the exam rooms?			
2. Are there any syringes or needles accessible in the exam rooms?			
3. Are medications accessible in the exam rooms?			
4. Are there Sharps containers in each exam room for disposal of needles and biohazard material?			

Lab Area:			
1. Is food kept in the lab refrigerator?			
2. Is there food or drink consumed in the lab area?			
3. Do specimen containers have biohazard labels?			
4. Are chemicals stored in an unlabeled container?			
5. Is there a biohazard container in the lab?			
Personal Protective Equipment Inspection:	Yes	No	
1. Are employees provided with and using proper PPE for procedures in which there is a potential for contamination with bloodborne pathogens?			
2. Are the Safety Data Sheets current and accessible to all employees			

EMPLOYEE TRAINING:

Required Training Inservices	Yes	No	Last Training Date:
1. Training for proper selection and use of PPE			
2. Bloodborne Pathogens Training			
3. Emergency Preparedness Training			
4. Fire Safety Training including use of fire extinguishers			
5. HIPAA Privacy Training			

PSY PROCEDURE 10-4 **Complete an Incident Report**

Name: _____ **Date:** _____ **Time:** _____ **Grade:** _____

EQUIPMENT: Incident Form, pen

STANDARDS: Given the needed equipment and a place to work, the student will perform this skill with _____ % accuracy in a total of _____ minutes. *(Your instructor will tell you what the percentage and time limits will be before you begin.)*

KEY: 4 = Satisfactory 0 = Unsatisfactory NA = This step is not counted

PROCEDURE STEPS	SELF	PARTNER	INSTRUCTOR
1. Recognize the error in patient care or accident occurring in the office	❑	❑	❑
2. Complete the incident report as per office policies and procedures	❑	❑	❑
3. Sign and date the incident report form and file with the office or practice manager	❑	❑	❑
4. Explain what steps can be taken to ensure that this accident does not occur in the future	❑	❑	❑

_____

_____

_____

_____

CALCULATION

Total Possible Points: _____

Total Points Earned: _____ Multiplied by 100 = _____ Divided by Total Possible Points = _____ %

PASS **FAIL** **COMMENTS:**
❑ ❑

Student's signature _____ Date _____

Partner's signature _____ Date _____

Instructor's signature _____ Date _____

WORK PRODUCT 1

Grade: _____

PERFORM AN INVENTORY OF SUPPLIES

When you are working in a medical office, you may need to keep an inventory of all supplies. The inventory will help you decide when to order new supplies. It will also help you calculate how much money you will need to spend on supplies. Supplies are those items that are consumed quickly and need to be reordered on a regular basis.

If you are currently working in a medical office, use the form below to take an inventory of the supplies in the office. If you do not have access to a medical office, complete an inventory of the supplies in your kitchen or bathroom at home.

**Third Street
Physician's Office, Inc.**
123 Main Street
Baltimore, MD 21201
410-895-6214

Supply Inventory

Item Description	Item Number or Code	Number Needed in Stock	Number Currently in Stock	Date Ordered	Number Ordered	Unit Price	Total	Actual Delivery Date

WORK PRODUCT 2

Grade: _____

PERFORM AN INVENTORY OF EQUIPMENT

When you are working in a medical office, you may need to keep an inventory of all equipment. The inventory will help you decide when to order new equipment. It will also help you calculate how much money you will need to spend on new equipment. Equipment includes items that can be used over and over and generally last many years.

If you are currently working in a medical office, use the form below to take an inventory of the equipment in the office. If you do not have access to a medical office, complete an inventory of the equipment in your kitchen or bathroom at home.

Third Street
Physician's Office, Inc.
123 Main Street
Baltimore, MD 21201
410-895-6214

Equipment Inventory

Item Description	Item Number or Code	Purchase Date	Condition	Comments	Expected New Purchase Date	Cost if Purchased This Year

WORK PRODUCT 3

Grade: _____

USE METHODS OF QUALITY CONTROL

Louise Baggins, a 55-year-old patient, was visiting the physician for a physical exam. While waiting for her appointment, she asked you to direct her to the restroom. On her way into the restroom, she slipped and fell on a magazine that had fallen on the floor in the reception area. You did not see her fall, but she yelled out in pain after she fell. She was able to get up on her own but injured her wrist. Her wrist was immediately red, swollen, and painful to touch. Dr. Mikuski looked at her wrist and suggested she go to the hospital emergency room to have x-rays. You called an ambulance to transfer Mrs. Baggins to the hospital.

Fill in the incident report below to document this event.

Great Falls Health System Physician Offices

Employee Incident/Injury Report Form

Please complete this form as soon as possible when an accident, injury, or illness occurs in the workplace.

Employee Name:	Title:
Location:	Date and Time of Injury/Illness:
Person or Employee the Injury/Illness Reported to:	Title of Person or Employee Injury or Illness Reported to:

Describe the details of your accident, injury, or illness. Be as specific as possible:

_____

_____

_____

_____

Explain what you were doing at the time of your accident, injury, or illness:

_____

_____

_____

For injuries, list the part or parts of your body that were injured. Be specific (i.e., right index finger, left ankle, etc…):

_____

_____

_____

If there was a delay in reporting the injury or illness, explain the reason for this delay:

_____

_____

_____

_____

(continues)

Names and Titles of Any Witnesses to your Injury or Illness:

_____

_____

_____

_____

Employee Signature: **Date:**

WORK PRODUCT 4

Grade: _____

USE METHODS OF QUALITY CONTROL

After Mrs. Baggins fell in the reception area (see Work Product 3), your supervisor asks you to review any other injuries in the reception area in the past 6 months. There are seven incident reports involving patient falls, and all of those occurred in some part of the reception area. Three patients slipped by the doorway on rainy days. Two more tripped on the corner of the doormat. The last two patients fell in the main lobby—one tripped over a children's toy, and the other slipped on a magazine, just like Mrs. Baggins did.

You are named to represent the medical assistants on a task force addressing these complaints. Assign an expected threshold using measurable, realistic goals. Explore the problem and propose solutions. Establish a QI monitoring plan explaining how data will be collected. Document the entire process and print the information to attach to this sheet. Using the blank memorandum below, write a memo to the staff with instructions to implement the solutions.

Memo

To:

From:

Date:

Re:

Managing the Finances in the Practice

CHAPTER 11

Diagnostic Coding

LEARNING OUTCOMES

COG Cognitive Domain*

1. Spell and define the key terms
2. Describe the relationship between coding and reimbursement
3. *Identify the current diagnostic coding system*
4. Explain the format of the ICD-10-CM
5. Describe the types of conventions used in ICD-10-CM
6. Explain the types and uses of abbreviations and symbols used in ICD-10-CM
7. Describe how to use the most current diagnostic coding classification system
8. Describe the process of locating a diagnosis code using ICD-10-CM
9. *Define medical necessity*

PSY Psychomotor Domain*

1. *Perform diagnostic coding (Procedure 11-1)*

AFF Affective Domain*

1. Work with a physician to achieve the maximum reimbursement
2. *Utilize tactful communication skills with medical providers to ensure accurate code selection*

MAERB Standards are italicized.

ABHES Competencies

1. Follow documentation guidelines
2. Perform billing and collection procedures and diagnostic and procedural coding
3. Comply with federal, state, and local health laws and regulations as they relate to health care

Name: _____   Date: _____   Grade: _____

COG MULTIPLE CHOICE

1. Which most accurately states the purpose of coding?
 a. Coding assists patients in accessing insurance databases
 b. Coding determines the reimbursement of medical fees
 c. Coding is used to track a physician's payments
 d. Coding is used to index patients' claim forms
 e. Coding identifies patients in a database

2. A patient signs an advance beneficiary notice (ABN) to:
 a. consent to medically necessary procedures.
 b. assign payment to Medicare.
 c. accept responsibility for payment.
 d. assign responsibility for payment to a beneficiary.
 e. consent to a medically unnecessary procedure.

3. The content of ICD-10-CM is a(n):
 a. classification of diseases and list of procedures.
 b. statistical grouping of trends in diseases.
 c. clinical modification of codes used by hospitals.
 d. index of diseases.
 e. international document for monitoring coding.

4. Which is true of ICD-10-PCS?
 a. It is organized by location on the patient's body
 b. It is used to code mostly outpatient procedures
 c. It is an alphabetical listing of diseases
 d. It is used by hospitals to report procedures and services
 e. It is an index of Volumes 1 and 2

5. Physicians' services are reported:
 a. on the UB-04.
 b. on the CMS-1500.
 c. on the uniform bill.
 d. on the advance beneficiary notice.
 e. on bills from health institutions.

6. Which of these would not be considered outpatient coding?
 a. Hospital same-day surgery
 b. Hour-long testing in a hospital CAT scan
 c. Treatment in the emergency room
 d. Observation status in a hospital
 e. Meals and testing during a hospital stay

7. In ICD-10-CM chapters are grouped:
 a. by alphabetic ordering of diseases and injuries.
 b. alphabetically by eponym.
 c. by location in the body.
 d. by etiology and anatomic system.
 e. by surgical specialty.

8. The fourth and fifth digits in an ICD-10-CM code indicate the:
 a. anatomical location where a procedure was performed.
 b. number of times a test was executed.
 c. more details about the disease or condition.
 d. code for the patient's general disease.
 e. traumatic origins of a disease (i.e., injury, deliberate violence).

9. A code from Chapter 21 in ICD-10-CM might indicate a(n):
 a. immunization.
 b. poisoning.
 c. external cause of injury
 d. diagnosis.
 e. treatment.

10. Codes Chapter 21 in ICD-10-CM are used:
 a. for inpatient coding only.
 b. when reimbursement is not needed.
 c. when a patient is not sick.
 d. to code poisonings and adverse effects.
 e. for infectious diseases.

11. What is the purpose of ICD-10-CM Chapter 20 codes?
 a. They code for immunizations and other preventive procedures
 b. They are used to code medical testing before a diagnosis
 c. They assist insurance companies in making reimbursements
 d. They indicate how an injury or poisoning occurred
 e. They indicate if a procedure was inpatient or outpatient

12. Certain ICD-10-CM Chapter 21 codes may be listed as primary on the CMS-1500 claim form:
  a. depending on the reason for the encounter.
  b. in most diagnostic coding situations.
  c. only for inpatient coding.
  d. only for outpatient coding.
  e. when the medical record is not specific enough to code from another chapter.

13. After finding a code in Volume 2 in ICD-10-CM, you should:
  a. record the code on the CMS-1500.
  b. consult Volume 3 for subordinate terms.
  c. cross-reference the code with Volume 1.
  d. indicate if the code is inpatient or outpatient.
  e. record the code on the UB-04.

14. If no diagnosis is documented in the medical record, coders must use:
  a. the disease that the provider believes the patient may have.
  b. the patient's signs and symptoms.
  c. a diagnosis from ICD-10-CM Chapter 21.
  d. a code that will support reimbursement.
  e. the coder's best judgment.

15. One example of an eponym is:
  a. Crohn's disease.
  b. bacterial meningitis.
  c. influenza virus.
  d. pruritus.
  e. pneumonia.

16. What is the first step to locating a diagnostic code?
  a. Determine where the diagnosis occurs in the body
  b. Choose the main term within the diagnostic statement
  c. Begin looking up the diagnosis in the tabular index
  d. Consult the CMS-1500 for reimbursement codes
  e. Use Volume 1 of the ICD-10-CM to find the disease

17. Which code is listed first on a CMS-1500?
  a. A reasonable second opinion
  b. Relevant laboratory work
  c. Diagnostic tests
  d. The symptoms of an illness
  e. The primary diagnosis

18. How do you code for late effects?
  a. Code for the treatment of the disease that causes late effects
  b. Code for the disease that is causing the current condition
  c. First code for the current condition, and then list the cause
  d. Only code for the current condition
  e. Only code for the cause of the current condition

19. You should not code for a brain tumor:
  a. when the patient comes in for an MRI.
  b. after the tumor is confirmed on an MRI.
  c. when the diagnosed patient comes in for treatment.
  d. any time after the patient has been diagnosed.
  e. when the patient seeks specialist care.

COG MATCHING

Grade: _____

Match the following key terms to their definitions.

Key Terms

20. _____ advance beneficiary notice
21. _____ audits
22. _____ conventions
23. _____ cross-reference
24. _____ chapter 20
25. _____ eponym
26. _____ etiology
27. _____ inpatient
28. _____ International Classification of Diseases, Clinical Modification
29. _____ late effects
30. _____ main terms
31. _____ medical necessity
32. _____ outpatient
33. _____ primary diagnosis
34. _____ service
35. _____ specificity
36. _____ chapter 21

Definitions

a. ICD-10-CM codes indicating the external causes of injuries and poisoning
b. conditions that result from another condition
c. general notes, symbols, typeface, format, and punctuation that direct and guide a coder to the most accurate diagnosis code
d. the condition or chief complaint that brings a person to a medical facility for treatment
e. a procedure or service that would have been performed by any reasonable physician under the same or similar circumstances
f. a document that informs covered patients that Medicare may not cover a certain service and the patient will be responsible for the bill
g. a word based on or derived from a person's name
h. ICD-10-CM codes assigned to patients who receive service but have no illness, injury, or disorder
i. the billable tasks performed by a physician
j. refers to a medical setting in which patients are admitted for diagnostic, radiographic, or treatment purposes
k. an investigation performed by government, managed healthcare companies, and healthcare organizations to determine compliance and to detect fraud
l. a system for transforming verbal descriptions of disease, injuries, conditions, and procedures to numeric codes
m. refers to the cause of disease
n. refers to a medical setting in which patients receive care but are not admitted
o. verification against another source
p. relating to a definite result
q. words in a multiple-word diagnosis that a coder should locate in the alphabetic listing

COG SHORT ANSWER

Grade: _____

37. Why is the ICD-10-PCS not used at a hospital's emergency department?

_____

_____

_____

_____

38. What is the title of the new edition of the ICD manuals?

_____

_____

_____

_____

39. You are reading a patient's chart and notice that it is marked with a code from ICD-10-CM Chapter 21. However, the patient has experienced no physical injuries. Why might a code from this chapter be used in this situation?

_____

_____

_____

_____

40. You ask a veteran medical assistant for advice on coding, especially how to go about finding a diagnosis with more than one word. Her response is, "Find the condition, not the location." What does she mean by this?

_____

_____

_____

_____

41. What is listed first in the diagnosis section of the CMS-1500? What does it represent?

_____

_____

_____

_____

42. If a construction worker falls from a ladder and suffers an ankle fracture, what supplemental code is used for ICD10-CM?

_____

_____

_____

_____

43. When would you use an ICD-10-CM Z-code for laboratory examination?

_____

_____

_____

_____

44. What should you do after finding a seemingly appropriate code in the alphabetic listing of ICD-10-CM?

_____

_____

_____

_____

45. If you do not know the medical terminology for a diagnosis for a common problem, what would be a good first plan of action?

_____

_____

_____

_____

46. What is the purpose of additional digits often appended to categories?

_____

_____

_____

_____

COG PSY ACTIVE LEARNING

Grade: _____

47. A reasonable and capable physician believes that a patient needs a chest x-ray to rule out pneumonia. Does the procedure meet the grounds for medical necessity? Why? Why not?

_____

_____

_____

_____

48. A patient comes in complaining of chest pain, and tests are ordered to rule out myocardial infarction. When you enter the codes for this patient encounter, you code that the patient has "acute myocardial infarction." Why would it be better to code this encounter "chest pain"?

_____

_____

_____

_____

49. George Cregan has been seen by the physician for controlled non-insulin-dependent type 2 diabetes mellitus for about 10 years. While being seen for a routine check of his blood sugar, he complains of numbness and tingling in his left lower leg and foot. An x-ray of both legs is performed because poor circulation in the extremities can be a complication of diabetes. The x-ray confirms the diagnosis of peripheral neuropathy. Which diagnosis code should be listed with the office visit? Which code indicates the reason for the x-ray? Which code should be placed on the CMS-1500 first as the primary diagnosis or reason for the visit?

_____

_____

_____

_____

Determine the main term for the following multiple-word diagnoses.

Diagnosis	Main Term
50. Chronic fatigue syndrome	
51. Severe acute respiratory syndrome	
52. Hemorrhagic encephalitis	
53. Acute fulminating multiple sclerosis	
54. Fractured left tibia	
55. Breast cyst	

IDENTIFICATION

Grade: _____

56. Review the list of circumstances below and place a check mark to indicate whether a patient would be forced, given the circumstance, to sign an ABN. All of the patients below are covered by Medicare.

Circumstance	ABN	No ABN
a. The patient wishes to receive a service or procedure that is not covered by Medicare		
b. The patient is undergoing a regularly scheduled checkup		
c. The patient demands to be tested for an illness that the physician considers an impossibility		
d. The patient has a badly sprained ankle and wishes to be treated		
e. The patient is undergoing x-ray imaging per order of a physician		

57. When it comes to coding, it makes a difference if the patient is seen in an inpatient or outpatient facility. Review the list of places below. Place an *I* next to those places that are considered "Inpatient" and an *O* next to those places that are considered "Outpatient."

a. _____ Hospital clinic

b. _____ Healthcare provider's office

c. _____ Hospital for less than 24 hours

d. _____ Hospital for 24 hours or more

e. _____ Hospital emergency room

58. Circle the main terms where you will find obstetric conditions.

delivery	fetus	pregnancy	labor
baby	obstetrics	puerperal	gestational

COG TRUE OR FALSE?

_____ Grade: _____

True or False? Determine whether the following statements are true or false. If false, explain why.

59. Only the first three digits of a code are necessary.

_____

_____

60. One should never code directly from the alphabetic index.

_____

_____

61. The main term describes a condition, not an aspect of anatomy.

_____

_____

62. In the outpatient setting, coders list conditions after the patient's testing is complete.

_____

_____

AFF WHAT WOULD YOU DO?

_____ Grade: _____

63. A patient calls complaining of pain and swelling in the right hand since awakening this morning. The patient comes in, sees the doctor, and returns to the front desk with an encounter form that states his diagnosis is "gout." In order to make this diagnosis, the physician would need to know the patient's uric acid level. You know that the patient just had blood drawn for the test. It is a test that must be sent to an outside lab. Do you still code today's visit as "gout"? What would you do?

_____

_____

_____

_____

64. A patient is concerned that her insurance provider will not cover her visit because the diagnosis is for a very minor ailment. She requests that you mark her CMS-1500 with a more severe disorder that demands similar treatment. How would you deal with this situation? What would you tell the patient? How might you involve the physician?

_____

_____

_____

_____

65. A patient entered the office complaining of abdominal pain that radiates into the right lower quadrant. After examination, the physician decided to order laboratory tests in order to rule out the possibility of appendicitis. Which code should be placed on the CMS-1500 first as the primary diagnosis or reason for the visit? Why?

_____

_____

_____

_____

AFF CASE STUDIES FOR CRITICAL THINKING

Grade: _____

Your physician employer works with you closely to choose the most appropriate codes. He tells you that he would like for you to code patients who have B_{12} injections with "pernicious anemia." You ask if these patients should have a lab work to substantiate that diagnosis, and he says, "don't worry about that."

66. What would you say to him?

_____

_____

_____

_____

67. What would be the possible consequences of such an action?

_____

_____

_____

_____

68. Which of these is an unethical act? Explain why.

a. Coding multiple conditions on the same CMS-1500

_____

_____

_____

b. Coding an unsupported diagnosis in order to make a service appear medically necessary

_____

_____

_____

c. Using a code from Chapter 20 in ICD-10-CM to better explain the reason for a patient's visit

_____

_____

_____

d. Using diagnosis coding search software to more easily access the codes contained in the ICD-10-CM

_____

_____

_____

PSY PROCEDURE 11-1 Locating A Diagnostic Code

Name: _____ **Date:** _____ **Time:** _____ **Grade:** _____

EQUIPMENT: Diagnosis, current volume of ICD-10-CM codebook, medical dictionary.

STANDARDS: Given the needed equipment and a place to work, the student will perform this skill with _____ % accuracy in a total of _____ minutes. *(Your instructor will tell you what the percentage and time limits will be before you begin.)*

KEY: 4 = Satisfactory 0 = Unsatisfactory NA = This step is not counted

PROCEDURE STEPS	SELF	PARTNER	INSTRUCTOR
1. Using the diagnosis "chronic rheumatoid arthritis," choose the main term within the diagnostic statement. If necessary, look up the word(s) in your dictionary	❏	❏	❏
2. Locate the main term in the alphabetic index	❏	❏	❏
3. Refer to all notes and conventions under the main term	❏	❏	❏
4. Find the appropriate indented subordinate term	❏	❏	❏
5. Follow any relevant instructions, such as "see also"	❏	❏	❏
6. Confirm the selected code by cross-referencing to the tabular index. Make sure you have added any fourth or fifth digits necessary	❏	❏	❏
7. Assign the code	❏	❏	❏
8. **AFF** Your office manager instructs you to assign a diagnosis code to a claim for a patient whom you know does not have the diagnosis. Explain how you would respond	❏	❏	❏

_____

_____

_____

_____

CALCULATION

Total Possible Points: _____

Total Points Earned: _____ Multiplied by 100 = _____ Divided by Total Possible Points = _____ %

PASS FAIL COMMENTS:
❏ ❏

Student's signature _____ Date _____

Partner's signature _____ Date _____

Instructor's signature _____ Date _____

WORK PRODUCT 1

Grade: _____

Underline the main term in these diagnoses with more than one word. Using a current diagnosis coding book, code the diagnoses:

1. Sick sinus syndrome
2. Congestive heart failure with malignant hypertension
3. Bilateral stenosis of carotid artery
4. Aspiration pneumonia
5. Massive blood transfusion thrombocytopenia
6. Acute rheumatic endocarditis
7. Acute viral conjunctivitis with hemorrhage
8. *Escherichia coli* intestinal infection
9. Postgastrectomy diarrhea
10. Congenital syphilitic osteomyelitis

WORK PRODUCT 2

Grade: _____

Determine the diseases associated with the following ICD-10-CM codes:

1. K50.10

   _____

2. O92.5

   _____

3. F90.9

   _____

4. M76.60

   _____

5. M54.31

   _____

WORK PRODUCT 3

Grade: _____

Determine the supplemental *External Causes of Injury (or Morbidity)* for the following:

Description	ICD-10-CM Code
Injured when hot air balloon crashed	
Skin frozen, contact with dry ice	
Bicyclist injured by train in a traffic accident	
Injured by fireworks	
Hand slashed by circular saw	

WORK PRODUCT 4

Grade: _____

CODE SEQUENCING

Kayla Moore, age 38 years, is seen in the clinic today. She has a few chronic conditions but is seen today for fluttering in her chest. Because she is here, and it is time for her regular diabetes checkup; the doctor orders a test to check on her blood sugar. Because Ms. Moore is a breast cancer survivor, in addition, she was given a mammogram. Her physician also prescribed a tetanus booster, because she has been renovating an old stable and has suffered several small skin punctures over the past few weeks. Her encounter form indicates the following charges:

- An EKG to monitor a previously diagnosed arrhythmia

- Fasting blood sugar for known diabetes

- Mammogram

- Tetanus booster

- List the diagnoses in the proper order to be placed on line #21 of the CMS-1500 form

1. _____   3. _____

2. _____   4. _____

CHAPTER 12

Outpatient Procedural Coding

LEARNING OUTCOMES

COG Cognitive Domain*

1. Spell and define the key terms
2. *Identify the current procedural coding systems, including Healthcare Common Procedure Coding Systems II (HCPCS Level II)*
3. Explain the format of level I, Current Procedural Terminology (CPT-4), and its use
4. Describe the relationship between coding and reimbursement
5. Describe how to use the most current procedure coding system
6. *Identify the effects of upcoding and downcoding*
7. Describe how to use the most current HCPCS coding
8. Describe the concept of RBRVS
9. Define both medical terms and abbreviations related to all body systems
10. Describe medical necessity as it applies to procedural coding

PSY Psychomotor Domain*

1. *Perform procedural coding (Procedure 12-1)*

AFF Affective Domain*

1. Work with physician to achieve the maximum reimbursement
2. *Demonstrate tactfulness when communicating with medical providers to ensure accurate code selection*

3. Apply ethical behaviors, including honesty/integrity in performance of medical assisting practice

MAERB Standards are italicized.

ABHES Competencies

1. Follow documentation guidelines
2. Perform billing and collection procedures
3. Comply with federal, state, and local health laws and regulations as they relate to healthcare

Name: _____ Date: _____ Grade: _____

⬤⬤⬤ MULTIPLE CHOICE

1. In the case of an unlisted code, the medical assistant should:
   a. notify the American Medical Association (AMA) so that a new code is issued.
   b. submit a copy of the procedure report with the claim.
   c. obtain authorization from the AMA to proceed with the procedure.
   d. include the code that fits the best and add a note to explain the differences.
   e. not charge the patient for the procedure.

2. Which kind of information appears in a special report?
   a. Type of medicine prescribed
   b. Patient history
   c. Allergic reactions
   d. Possible procedural risks
   e. Equipment necessary for the treatment

3. On a medical record, the key components contained in E/M codes indicate:
   a. the scope and result of a medical visit.
   b. the duties of a physician toward his patients.
   c. the definition and description of a performed procedure.
   d. the services that a medical assistant may perform.
   e. the charges that are owed to the insurance company.

4. Time becomes a key component in a medical record when:
   a. the visit lasts more than 1 hour.
   b. more than half of the visit is spent counseling.
   c. the physician decides on a series of regular visits.
   d. the visit lasts longer than it was initially established.
   e. the patient is constantly late for their appointments.

5. When assigning a level of medical decision making, you should consider the:
   a. medication the patient is on.
   b. available coding for the procedure.
   c. the number of diagnoses given to a patient
   d. insurance coverage allowed to the patient.
   e. patient's medical history.

6. In the anesthesia section, the physical status modifier indicates the patient's:
   a. medical history.
   b. condition after surgery.
   c. good health before surgery.
   d. reactions to past anesthesia.
   e. condition prior to the administration of anesthesia.

7. Which of the following is included in a surgical package?
   a. General anesthesia
   b. Hospitalization time
   c. Complications related to the surgery
   d. Prescriptions given after the operation
   e. Uncomplicated follow-up care

8. How are procedures organized in the subsections of the surgery section of the CPT-4?
   a. By invasiveness
   b. By location and type
   c. In alphabetical order
   d. In order of difficulty of procedure
   e. By average recurrence of procedure

9. Which is the first digit that appears on radiology codes?
   a. 1
   b. 6
   c. 7
   d. 8
   e. 9

10. Diagnostic-related groups (DRGs) are a group of:
    a. codes pertaining to one particular treatment.
    b. inpatients sharing a similar medical history.
    c. modifiers attached to a single procedural form.
    d. physicians agreeing on a procedure for a particular medical condition.
    e. inpatients sharing similar diagnoses, treatment, and length of hospital stay.

11. The resource-based relative value scale (RBRVS) gives information on the:
    a. difficulty level of a particular surgical operation.
    b. maximum fee that physicians can charge for a procedure.
    c. reimbursement given to physicians for Medicare services.
    d. average fee asked by physicians for emergency procedures.
    e. minimum amount of time the physician should spend with a patient.

12. The Medicare allowed charge is calculated by:
    a. adding the RVU and the national conversion factor.
    b. dividing the RVU by the national conversion factor.
    c. multiplying the RVU by the national conversion factor.
    d. subtracting the RVU from the national conversion factor.
    e. finding the average between the RVU and the national conversion factor.

13. Upcoding is:
    a. billing more than the proper fee for a service.
    b. correcting an erroneous code in medical records.
    c. auditing claims retroactively for suspected fraud.
    d. comparing the documentation in the record with the codes received.
    e. researching new codes online.

14. Who has jurisdiction over a fraudulent medical practice?
    a. CMS
    b. AMA
    c. Medicare
    d. U.S. Attorney General
    e. State's supreme court

15. The purpose of the Level II HCPCS codes is to:
    a. decode different types of code modifiers.
    b. attribute a code to every step of a medical procedure.
    c. list the practices eligible for reimbursement by Medicare.
    d. identify services, supplies, and equipment not identified by CPT codes.
    e. provide coding information for various types of anesthesia.

16. Which of these sections is included in the HCPCS Level I code listing?
    a. Orthotics
    b. Injectable drugs
    c. Vision care
    d. Dental services
    e. Pathology and laboratory

17. How is a consultation different from a referral?
    a. A consultation is needed when the patient wants to change physicians
    b. A consultation is needed when the physician asks for the opinion of another provider
    c. A consultation is needed when the patient is transferred to another physician for treatment
    d. A consultation is needed when the physician needs a team of doctors to perform a procedure
    e. A consultation is needed before the physician can submit insurance claims

18. Which of the following is contained in Appendix B in the CPT-4?
    a. Legislation against medical fraud
    b. Detailed explanation of the modifiers
    c. Revisions made since the last editions
    d. Explanation on how to file for reimbursement
    e. Examples concerning the Evaluation and Management sections

19. Drug screening is considered *quantitative* when checking:
    a. for the amount of illegal drugs in the blood.
    b. for the presence of illegal drugs in the blood.
    c. for the proper level of therapeutic drugs in the blood.
    d. that the therapeutic drug is not interacting with other medications.
    e. that the drug is not causing an allergic reaction.

20. How many numbers do E/M codes have?
    a. Two
    b. Five
    c. Six
    d. Seven
    e. Ten

COG MATCHING

Match the following key terms to their definitions.

Key Terms

21. _____ Current Procedural Terminology
22. _____ descriptor
23. _____ diagnostic-related group
24. _____ Health Care Common Procedure Coding System
25. _____ key component
26. _____ modifiers
27. _____ outlier
28. _____ procedure
29. _____ resource-based relative value scale
30. _____ upcoding

Definitions

a. a patient whose hospital stay is longer than the amount allowed by the DRG
b. categories used to determine hospital and physician reimbursement for Medicare patients' inpatient services
c. a value scale designed to decrease Medicare Part B costs and establish national standards for coding and payment
d. billing more than the proper fee for a service by selecting a code that is higher on the coding scale
e. description of a service listed with its code number
f. numbers or letters added to a code to clarify the service or procedure provided
g. a comprehensive listing of medical terms and codes for the uniform coding of procedures and services that are provided by physicians
h. a medical service or test that is coded for reimbursement
i. a standardized coding system that is used primarily to identify products, supplies, and services
j. the criteria or factors on which the selection of CPT-4 evaluation and management is based

COG SHORT ANSWER

31. What role do modifiers play in coding?

_____

_____

_____

_____

32. When would you use 99 as the first numbers in your modifier?

_____

_____

_____

_____

33. What is the goal of the RBRVS?

_____

_____

_____

_____

34. How does coding play a part in reimbursement?

_____

_____

_____

_____

35. What are DRGs, and how are they used to determine Medicare payments?

_____

_____

_____

_____

36. List three ways to reduce the likelihood of a Medicare audit of your office.

_____

_____

_____

_____

37. Name four factors that go into radiology coding.

_____

_____

_____

_____

38. Why is it important to check the components of a surgery package with a third-party payer?

_____

_____

_____

_____

39. A patient experiences complications after an appendectomy and has to be hospitalized for several days. Will the time spent in the hospital be coded as part of a surgery package or separately?

_____

_____

_____

_____

COG PSY ACTIVE LEARNING

Grade: _____

Using a current CPT book, assign the appropriate CPT code for the following:

40. occult blood in stool, two simultaneous guaiac tests

_____

41. blood ethanol levels

_____

42. transurethral resection of prostate

_____

43. flexible sigmoidoscopy for biopsy

_____

44. radiation therapy requiring general anesthesia

_____

45. hair transplant, 21 punch grafts

_____

46. breast reduction, left

_____

47. open repair of left Dupuytren contracture

_____

48. partial removal left turbinate

_____

49. newborn clamp circumcision

_____

COG PSY IDENTIFICATION

Grade: _____

What would be the first digit of the following codes?

50. routine prothrombin time

_____

51. ultrasound guidance for amniocentesis

_____

52. well-child check

_____

53. EKG

_____

54. removal of skin tags

_____

COG TRUE OR FALSE?

Grade: _____

Determine whether the following statements are true or false. If false, explain why.

55. It is permissible to leave out modifiers if a note is made on the patient's sheet.

_____

56. When time spent with a patient is more than 50% of the typical time for the visit, time becomes the deciding factor in choosing a code.

_____

57. The number of tests you perform is the final number in the coding.

_____

58. The amount of time a physician spends with a patient has no effect on the coding for that exam.

_____

OOG IDENTIFICATION

Grade: _____

59. Fill in the chart below to show the difference between Level I HPCS and Level II.

Level I	Level II

60. What are the six major sections of the CPT-4?

a. _____

b. _____

c. _____

d. _____

e. _____

f. _____

61. Define the seven components of the E/M codes.

Component	Definition
a. History	
b. Physician examination	
c. Medical decision making	
d. Counseling	
e. Coordination of care	
f. Nature of presenting problem	
g. Time	

⚏ WHAT WOULD YOU DO?

Grade: _____

62. Read the scenario below. Then highlight or underline the medical decision-making section.
Anikka was seen today for a follow-up on her broken wrist. The cast was removed 2 weeks ago, and she said she is still unable to achieve full range of movement in her wrist without pain. On exam, her wrist appeared swollen, and she mentioned tenderness. The x-ray revealed a slight fracture in the carpals. Dr. Levy splinted the wrist and referred her to an orthopedic surgeon for possible surgery. I spoke with Anikka, instructing her to avoid exerting her wrist and to keep it splinted until she has seen the surgeon. Dr. Levy suggested ibuprofen for pain.

63. Now, read the same scenario again. Circle the history section.
Anikka was seen today for a follow-up on her broken wrist. The cast was removed 2 weeks ago, and she said she is still unable to achieve full range of movement in her wrist without pain. On exam, her wrist appeared swollen, and she mentioned tenderness. The x-ray revealed a slight fracture in the carpals. Dr. Levy splinted the wrist and referred her to an orthopedic surgeon for possible surgery. I spoke with Anikka, instructing her to avoid exerting her wrist and to keep it splinted until she has seen the surgeon. Dr. Levy suggested ibuprofen for pain.

64. Read the scenario below.
Mr. Ekko presents today for removal of stitches from a calf wound. Upon inspection, the wound seems to have healed well, but the scar tissue is still slightly inflamed. I prescribed antibacterial cream for him to apply twice a day and instructed him to still keep the area bandaged. I told him to let us know if the swelling has not gone down within a week and to come in if it gets any worse.

Circle the correct level of medical decision making involved.

Straightforward   Low complexity

Moderate complexity   High complexity

⚏ IDENTIFICATION

Grade: _____

Fill in the medical terminology chart below about the CPT subcategory on repair, revision, or reconstruction.

Suffix	Meaning
65. -pexy	
	66. surgical repair
67. -rrhaphy	

AFF **CASE STUDIES FOR CRITICAL THINKING**

Grade: _____

68. A patient will be undergoing surgery to remove her gallbladder. Her insurance company labels this sort of operation as an outpatient surgery. She lives alone and will have no assistance after surgery. She wants to stay in the hospital overnight. The patient asks if you can do anything in the coding of the procedure to make her insurance company pay for a night in the hospital. What do you say to her? Can you do anything to code this information on the claim form for more reimbursement?

_____

_____

_____

_____

PSY PROCEDURE 12-1 **Locating a CPT Code**

Name: _____ **Date:** _____ **Time:** _____ **Grade:** _____

EQUIPMENT: CPT-4 codebook, patient chart, scenario (Work Product 1)

STANDARDS: Given the needed equipment and a place to work, the student will perform this skill with _____ % accuracy in a total of _____ minutes. *(Your instructor will tell you what the percentage and time limits will be before you begin.)*

KEY: 4 = Satisfactory 0 = Unsatisfactory NA = This step is not counted

PROCEDURE STEPS	SELF	PARTNER	INSTRUCTOR
1. Identify the exact procedure performed	❑	❑	❑
2. Obtain the documentation of the procedure in the patient's chart	❑	❑	❑
3. Choose the proper codebook	❑	❑	❑
4. Using the alphabetic index, locate the procedure	❑	❑	❑
5. Locate the code or range of codes given in the tabular section	❑	❑	❑
6. Read the descriptors to find the one that most closely describes the procedure	❑	❑	❑
7. Check the section guidelines for any special circumstances	❑	❑	❑
8. Review the documentation to be sure it justifies the code	❑	❑	❑
9. Determine if any modifiers are needed	❑	❑	❑
10. Select the code and place it in the appropriate field of the CMS-1500 form	❑	❑	❑
11. **AFF** Your physician is helping you find a code in the CPT-4 codebook and chooses a code based on what the surgery entailed. The operative report does not support what the physician said. Explain how you would advise the physician to correct the problem and proceed	❑	❑	❑

_____

_____

_____

_____

PSY PROCEDURE 12-1 **Locating a CPT Code** (continued)

CALCULATION

Total Possible Points: _____

Total Points Earned: _____ Multiplied by 100 = _____ Divided by Total Possible Points = _____ %

PASS   FAIL   COMMENTS:
❏   ❏

Student's signature _____   Date _____

Partner's signature _____   Date _____

Instructor's signature _____   Date _____

WORK PRODUCT 1

Grade: _____

PERFORM PROCEDURAL CODING

Kayla Moore has just completed a general physical. Her examination consisted of the following:

- A 12-lead EKG to monitor a previously diagnosed arrhythmia

- Urine collection to test for diabetes

- Blood sampling to test cholesterol levels

Because Ms. Moore is a breast cancer survivor, in addition to the routine examination, she was given an order for a mammogram. Her physician prescribed a tetanus booster (Td) as well, because she has been renovating an old stable and has suffered several small skin punctures over the past few weeks.

List the procedure codes that may be used for Kayla's visit today.

HEALTH INSURANCE CLAIM FORM

APPROVED BY NATIONAL UNIFORM CLAIM COMMITTEE (NUCC) 02/12

☐☐☐ PICA | | PICA ☐☐☐

| 1. MEDICARE ☐ (Medicare#)   MEDICAID ☐ (Medicaid#)   TRICARE ☐ (ID#/DoD#)   CHAMPVA ☐ (Member ID#)   GROUP HEALTH PLAN ☐ (ID#)   FECA BLK LUNG ☐ (ID#)   OTHER ☐ (ID#) | 1a. INSURED'S I.D. NUMBER (For Program in Item 1) |

2. PATIENT'S NAME (Last Name, First Name, Middle Initial)

3. PATIENT'S BIRTH DATE MM | DD | YY   SEX M ☐ F ☐

4. INSURED'S NAME (Last Name, First Name, Middle Initial)

5. PATIENT'S ADDRESS (No., Street)

6. PATIENT RELATIONSHIP TO INSURED   Self ☐ Spouse ☐ Child ☐ Other ☐

7. INSURED'S ADDRESS (No., Street)

CITY   STATE

8. RESERVED FOR NUCC USE

CITY   STATE

ZIP CODE   TELEPHONE (Include Area Code) (   )

ZIP CODE   TELEPHONE (Include Area Code) (   )

9. OTHER INSURED'S NAME (Last Name, First Name, Middle Initial)

10. IS PATIENT'S CONDITION RELATED TO:

11. INSURED'S POLICY GROUP OR FECA NUMBER

a. OTHER INSURED'S POLICY OR GROUP NUMBER

a. EMPLOYMENT? (Current or Previous) ☐ YES ☐ NO

a. INSURED'S DATE OF BIRTH MM | DD | YY   SEX M ☐ F ☐

b. RESERVED FOR NUCC USE

b. AUTO ACCIDENT? ☐ YES ☐ NO   PLACE (State)

b. OTHER CLAIM ID (Designated by NUCC)

c. RESERVED FOR NUCC USE

c. OTHER ACCIDENT? ☐ YES ☐ NO

c. INSURANCE PLAN NAME OR PROGRAM NAME

d. INSURANCE PLAN NAME OR PROGRAM NAME

10d. CLAIM CODES (Designated by NUCC)

d. IS THERE ANOTHER HEALTH BENEFIT PLAN? ☐ YES ☐ NO   **If yes**, complete items 9, 9a, and 9d.

READ BACK OF FORM BEFORE COMPLETING & SIGNING THIS FORM.
12. PATIENT'S OR AUTHORIZED PERSON'S SIGNATURE I authorize the release of any medical or other information necessary to process this claim. I also request payment of government benefits either to myself or to the party who accepts assignment below.

SIGNED _____ DATE _____

13. INSURED'S OR AUTHORIZED PERSON'S SIGNATURE I authorize payment of medical benefits to the undersigned physician or supplier for services described below.

SIGNED _____

14. DATE OF CURRENT ILLNESS, INJURY, or PREGNANCY (LMP) MM | DD | YY   QUAL.

15. OTHER DATE QUAL. | MM | DD | YY

16. DATES PATIENT UNABLE TO WORK IN CURRENT OCCUPATION MM | DD | YY   FROM   TO   MM | DD | YY

17. NAME OF REFERRING PROVIDER OR OTHER SOURCE

17a.
17b. NPI

18. HOSPITALIZATION DATES RELATED TO CURRENT SERVICES MM | DD | YY   FROM   TO   MM | DD | YY

19. ADDITIONAL CLAIM INFORMATION (Designated by NUCC)

20. OUTSIDE LAB? ☐ YES ☐ NO $ CHARGES

21. DIAGNOSIS OR NATURE OF ILLNESS OR INJURY Relate A-L to service line below (24E)   ICD Ind. |
A. |___   B. |___   C. |___   D. |___
E. |___   F. |___   G. |___   H. |___
I. |___   J. |___   K. |___   L. |___

22. RESUBMISSION CODE   ORIGINAL REF. NO.

23. PRIOR AUTHORIZATION NUMBER

24. A. DATE(S) OF SERVICE From MM DD YY To MM DD YY	B. PLACE OF SERVICE	C. EMG	D. PROCEDURES, SERVICES, OR SUPPLIES (Explain Unusual Circumstances) CPT/HCPCS MODIFIER	E. DIAGNOSIS POINTER	F. $ CHARGES	G. DAYS OR UNITS	H. EPSDT Family Plan	I. ID. QUAL.	J. RENDERING PROVIDER ID. #
1									NPI
2									NPI
3									NPI
4									NPI
5									NPI
6									NPI

25. FEDERAL TAX I.D. NUMBER ☐ SSN ☐ EIN

26. PATIENT'S ACCOUNT NO.

27. ACCEPT ASSIGNMENT? (For govt. claims, see back) ☐ YES ☐ NO

28. TOTAL CHARGE $

29. AMOUNT PAID $

30. Rsvd for NUCC Use

31. SIGNATURE OF PHYSICIAN OR SUPPLIER INCLUDING DEGREES OR CREDENTIALS (I certify that the statements on the reverse apply to this bill and are made a part thereof.)

SIGNED _____ DATE _____

32. SERVICE FACILITY LOCATION INFORMATION
a. NPI   b.

33. BILLING PROVIDER INFO & PH # (   )
a. NPI   b.

CHAPTER 13

Health Insurance and Reimbursement

LEARNING OUTCOMES

COG Cognitive Domain*

1. Spell and define the key terms
2. *Identify types of:*
   a. *third-party plans*
   b. *the steps for filing a third-party claim*
3. Discuss utilization review principles
4. *Identify managed care requirements for patient referral*
5. Compare processes for filing insurance claims both manually and electronically
6. Describe the concept of resource-based relative value scale (RBRVS)
7. Explain the concept of diagnosis-related groups (DRGs)
8. *Identify* processes for:
   a. *Verification of eligibility for services*
   b. *Precertification/ preauthorization*
   c. *Claim tracking*
9. *Identify fraud and abuse as they relate to third-party reimbursement*

10. *Define the following:*
    a. *Advanced beneficiary notice (ABN)*
    b. *Deductible*
    c. *Co-insurance*
    d. *Co-pay*
11. *Identify the purpose and components of the Explanation of Benefits and Remittance Advice*

PSY Psychomotor Domain*

1. *Complete an insurance claim form (Procedure 13-1)*
2. Apply third-party guidelines
3. *Interpret information on an insurance card (Procedure 13-2)*
4. *Obtain precertification or preauthorization, with documentation (Procedure 13-2)*
5. *Verify eligibility for services (Procedure 13-2)*
6. *Input accurate billing information in an electronic system (Procedure 13-2)*
7. *Assist a patient in understanding an Explanation of Benefits (EOB) (Procedure 13-3)*

8. *Utilize medical necessity guidelines (Procedure 13-2)*

AFF Affective Domain*

1. *Demonstrate critical thinking skills to complete an accurate insurance claim form*
2. *Demonstrate empathy when communicating with patient's third-party requirements*
3. Communicate in language the patient can understand regarding managed care and insurance plans
4. Apply ethical behaviors, including honesty/integrity in performance of medical assisting practice

*MAERB Standards are italicized.

ABHES Competencies

1. Process insurance claims
2. Demonstrate professional behaviors

Name: _____ Date: _____ Grade: _____

⬛ MULTIPLE CHOICE

1. Which of the following is frequently not covered in group health benefits packages?
   a. Vision Benefits
   b. Childhood immunizations
   c. Routine diagnostic care
   d. Treatment for substance abuse
   e. Regular physical examinations

2. Any payment for medical services that is not paid by the patient is said to be paid by a(n):
   a. second-party payer.
   b. first-party payer.
   c. insurance party payer.
   d. third-party payer.
   e. healthcare party payer.

3. The criteria a patient must meet for a group benefit plan to provide coverage are called:
   a. eligibility requirements.
   b. patient requirements.
   c. benefit plan requirements.
   d. physical requirements.
   e. insurance requirements.

4. Eligibility for a dependent requires that they are:
   a. unmarried.
   b. employed.
   c. living with the employee.
   d. younger than 18.
   e. an excellent student.

5. Whom should you contact about the eligibility of a patient for the health benefits plan?
   a. Claims administrator
   b. Claims investigator
   c. Insurance salesperson
   d. Insurance reviewer
   e. Claims insurer

Scenario for questions 6 and 7: Aziz pays premiums directly to the insurance company, and the insurance company reimburses him for eligible medical expenses.

6. What type of insurance does Aziz have?
   a. Individual health benefits
   b. Public health benefits
   c. Managed care
   d. PPO
   e. HMO

7. Which of the following is likely true of Aziz's insurance?
   a. The insurance is provided by his employer
   b. Money can be put aside into accounts used for medical expenses
   c. He has a deductible that must be paid before insurance benefits will be reimbursed
   d. All providers are under contract with the insurer
   e. There are two levels of benefits in the health plan

8. An optional health benefits program offered to persons signing up for Social Security benefits is:
   a. Medicare Part A.
   b. Medicare Part B.
   c. Medicaid.
   d. TRICARE/CHAMPVA.
   e. HMO.

9. After the deductible has been met, what percentage of the approved charges does Medicare reimburse to the physician?
   a. 0
   b. 20
   c. 75
   d. 80
   e. 100

10. Which benefits program bases eligibility on a patient's eligibility for other state programs such as welfare assistance?
    a. Workers' Compensation
    b. Medicare
    c. Medicaid
    d. TRICARE/CHAMPVA
    e. Social Security

11. The term Medi-Medi refers to:
    a. Medicare as the primary and Medicaid as the secondary payer
    b. Medicaid as the primary payer
    c. Medicare as the secondary payer
    d. Claim submitted to CMS
    e. Medicare claims filed electronically

12. In a traditional insurance plan:
    a. the covered patient may seek care from any provider.
    b. the insurer has no relationship with the provider.
    c. a patient can be admitted to a hospital only if that admission has been certified by the insurer.
    d. there is no third-party payer.
    e. the patient cannot be billed for the deductible.

13. Which of the following is a plan typically developed by hospitals and physicians to attract patients?
    a. HMO
    b. PPO
    c. HSA
    d. TPA
    e. UCR

14. Which of the following is true about both HMOs and PPOs?
    a. Both allow patients to see any physician of their choice and receive benefits
    b. Both contract directly with participating providers, hospitals, and physicians
    c. Both offer benefits at two levels, commonly referred to as *in-network* and *out-of-network*
    d. Both are not risk-bearing and do not have any financial involvement in the health plan
    e. Both incorporate independent practice associations

15. Which of the following is a government-sponsored health benefits plan?
    a. TRICARE/CHAMPVA
    b. HMO
    c. HSA
    d. PPO
    e. PHO

16. If a provider is unethical, you should:
    a. correct the issue yourself.
    b. immediately stop working for the provider.
    c. comply with all requests to misrepresent medical records but report the physician.
    d. do whatever the physician asks to avoid confrontation.
    e. explain that you are legally bound to truthful billing and report the physician.

17. A patient's ID card:
    a. contains the information needed to file a claim on it.
    b. should be updated at least once every 2 years.
    c. must be cleared before an emergency can be treated.
    d. is updated and sent to Medicaid patients bimonthly.
    e. is not useful for determining if the patient is a dependent.

18. What information is needed to fill out a CMS-1500 claim form?
    a. A copy of the patient's chart
    b. Location where patient will be recovering
    c. Diagnostic codes from encounter form
    d. Copies of hospitalization paperwork
    e. Physician's record and degree

19. Claims that are submitted electronically:
    a. violate HIPAA standards.
    b. contain fewer errors than those that are mailed.
    c. require approval from the patient.
    d. increase costs for Medicare patients.
    e. reduce the reimbursement cycle.

20. Many insurance plans have an amount that must be paid before insurance benefits will be reimbursed. This is referred to as the:
    a. deductible.
    b. coinsurance.
    c. balance billing.
    d. benefits.
    e. claim.

21. Which is true about how a managed care system is different from a traditional insurance coverage system?
    a. They usually are less costly.
    b. They cost more but have more benefits.
    c. They cost the same but have more benefits.
    d. You can only use network physicians.
    e. They do not have preauthorization requirements

COG MATCHING

Match the following key terms to their definitions.

Key Terms

22. _____ assignment of benefits
23. _____ balance billing
24. _____ capitation
25. _____ carrier
26. _____ claims administrator
27. _____ coinsurance
28. _____ coordination of benefits
29. _____ copayments
30. _____ crossover claim
31. _____ deductible
32. _____ dependent
33. _____ eligibility
34. _____ explanation of benefits (EOB)
35. _____ fee-for-service
36. _____ fee schedule
37. _____ group member
38. _____ healthcare savings account (HSA)
39. _____ health maintenance organization (HMO)
40. _____ independent practice association (IPA)
41. _____ managed care
42. _____ Medicare
43. _____ peer-review organization
44. _____ physician hospital organization
45. _____ preferred provider organization (PPO)
46. _____ usual, customary, and reasonable (UCR)
47. _____ utilization review

Definitions

a. an individual who manages the third-party reimbursement policies for a medical practice

b. the part of the payment for a service that a patient must pay

c. the determination of an insured's right to receive benefits from a third-party payer based on criteria such as payment of premiums

d. spouse, children, and sometimes other individuals designated by the insured who are covered under a healthcare plan

e. the transfer of the patient's legal right to collect third-party benefits to the provider of the services

f. a company that assumes the risk of an insurance company

g. a group of physicians and specialists that conducts a review of a disputed case and makes a final recommendation

h. an organization that provides a wide range of services through a contract with a specified group at a predetermined payment

i. billing the patients for the difference between the physician's charges and the Medicare-approved charges

j. an organization of nongroup physicians developed to allow independent physicians to compete with prepaid group practices

k. a coalition of physicians and a hospital contracting with large employers, insurance carriers, and other benefits groups to provide discounted health services

l. an established set of fees charged for specific services and paid by the patient or insurance carrier

m. the practice of third-party payers to control costs by requiring physicians to adhere to specific rules as a condition of payment

n. the method of designating the order in which multiple-carriers pay benefits to avoid duplication of payment

o. a statement from an insurance carrier that outlines which services are being paid

p. a government-sponsored health benefits package that provides insurance for the elderly

q. a claim that moves over automatically from one coverage to another for payment

r. a policyholder who is covered by a group insurance carrier

s. a type of health benefit program whose purpose is to contract with providers, then lease this network of contracted providers to healthcare plans

t. an employee benefit that allows individuals to save money through payroll deduction to accounts that can be used only for medical care

u. a list of pre-established fee allowances set for specific services performed by a provider

v. a managed care plan that pays a certain amount to a provider over a specific time for caring for the patients in the plan, regardless of what or how many services are performed

w. the basis of a physician's fee schedule for the normal cost of the same service or procedure in a similar geographic area and under the same or similar circumstances

x. the agreed-upon amount paid to the provider by a policyholder

y. an analysis of individual cases by a committee to make sure services and procedures being billed to a third-party payer are medically necessary

z. the amount paid by the patient before the carrier begins paying

COG SHORT ANSWER

Grade: _____

48. What does the acronym DRG represent? How are DRGs used?

_____

_____

_____

49. What does the acronym RBRVS represent? Briefly explain RBRVS.

_____

_____

_____

50. What is a third-party payer?

_____

_____

_____

51. Elaine is 22 years old and is still eligible as a dependent. What could be a possible reason for this?

_____

_____

_____

52. Why do managed care programs require approved referrals?

_____

_____

_____

53. What does a gatekeeper physician do?

_____

_____

_____

54. A new patient comes to your office, and he hands you his insurance card. What information can you find on the back of his identification card?

_____

_____

_____

55. What form do you fill out to submit an insurance claim?

_____

_____

_____

56. When is a physician required to file a patient's claim?

_____

_____

_____

57. Why is it important to check the Explanation of Benefits?

_____

_____

_____

58. What is a preexisting condition?

_____

_____

_____

COG PSY ACTIVE LEARNING

Grade: _____

59. Interview three people about their health insurance. Ask them what they like about their service. What do they dislike? Compile a list of their comments to discuss with the class.

60. Visit the website for Medicare at http://www.medicare.gov. Locate their Frequently Asked Questions page. Read over the questions, and choose five that you believe are the most likely to be asked in a medical office. Design a pamphlet for your office that addresses these five questions.

COG IDENTIFICATION

Grade: _____

61. Jim works for a company that offers an employee benefit whereby money is taken out of his paycheck and put toward medical care expenses. What is the name of this practice?

_____

_____

62. Determine which of the following are characteristics of Medicare or Medicaid. Place a check mark in the appropriate column below.

	Medicare	Medicaid
a. Provides coverage for low-income or indigent persons of all ages		
b. In a crossover claim, this is the primary coverage		
c. Implemented on a state or local level		
d. Physician reimbursement is considerably less than other insurances		
e. Patients receive a new ID card each month		
f. Program is broken down into part A and part B		
g. Provides coverage for persons suffering from end-stage renal disease		

63. Read each person's health insurance scenario and then match it with the correct type of health insurance plan.

Scenario		Health Insurance Plan	
a.	Sandra was recently let go from her job and is unemployed.	**1.**	group
b.	Thomas has a plan that has less generous coverage and may limit or eliminate benefits for certain illnesses or injuries.	**2.**	individual health
c.	Mario just started a new job and signed up for health insurance at work.	**3.**	government

AFF WHAT WOULD YOU DO?   Grade: _____

64. Claims are sometimes denied, and it is your responsibility to take corrective actions. Read the scenarios below, and briefly state what action you should take.

    a. Services are not covered by the plan. _____

    b. Coding is deemed inappropriate for services provided. _____

    c. Data are incomplete. _____

    d. The patient cannot be identified as a covered person. _____

    e. The patient is no longer covered by the plan. _____

65. Kairi is a dependent, and both of her parents have healthcare plans. There are no specific instructions about which plan is primary, so how do you choose which plan to use?

_____

_____

_____

_____

66. Describe the two main characteristics of primary and secondary insurance below.

Primary Insurance	Secondary Insurance

COG TRUE OR FALSE?   Grade: _____

67. Determine if the statements below are true or false. If false, explain why.

    a. Approximately 80% of Americans are enrolled in health benefits plans of one sort or another.

_____

    b. A network of providers that make up the PHO may have no financial obligation to subscribers.

_____

    c. In managed care, a patient is not usually required to use network providers to receive full coverage.

_____

    d. An HMO requires the patient to pay the provider directly, then reimburses the patient.

_____

PSY WHAT WOULD YOU DO?

_____ Grade: _____

68. Mrs. Smith is moving out of the area and is seeing Dr. Jones, her primary care physician, for the last time. After the move, Mrs. Smith will have to choose a new physician. Mrs. Smith has the choice of an HMO or a PPO. Mrs. Smith asks you to explain the difference. How would you teach Mrs. Smith about the differences between an HMO and a PPO?

_____

_____

_____

_____

69. Mandy's primary care physician is included under her health plan. However, she has recently been experiencing chest pains, and her physician refers her to a cardiologist. What would you to do to help make sure the specialist's visit is covered?

_____

_____

_____

_____

AFF CASE STUDIES FOR CRITICAL THINKING

_____ Grade: _____

You are tasked with arranging a referral for Mrs. Williams. She has Blue Cross Blue Shield of VA. She needs a carpal tunnel release. She insists that her insurance will pay, but when you call for preauthorization, you are told her policy is no longer in effect. She did not pay her premium last month, and the policy was cancelled. Apparently, she has not been notified.

70. Word for word, what would you say to her?

_____

_____

_____

_____

71. Circle all appropriate contacts below that you could suggest to Mrs. Williams.

    a. The Yellow Pages

    b. The local Department of Social Services

    c. An attorney

    d. Another physician. She probably will not be able to pay

    e. A free clinic

    f. Her employer

    g. The phone number on the back of her insurance card

PSY PROCEDURE 13-1 **Completing a CMS-1500 Claim Form**

Name: _____ **Date:** _____ **Time:** _____ **Grade:** _____

EQUIPMENT: Case scenario (see work product), completed encounter form, blank CMS-1500 Claim Form, pen

STANDARDS: Given the needed equipment and a place to work, the student will perform this skill with _____ % accuracy in a total of _____ minutes. *(Your instructor will tell you what the percentage and time limits will be before you begin.)*

KEY: 4 = Satisfactory   0 = Unsatisfactory   NA = This step is not counted

PROCEDURE STEPS	SELF	PARTNER	INSTRUCTOR
1. Using the information provided in the case scenario, complete the demographic information in lines 1 through 11d	❏	❏	❏
2. Insert "SOF" (signature on file) on lines 12 and 13. Check to be sure there is a current signature on file in the chart and that it is specifically for the third-party payer being filed	❏	❏	❏
3. If the services being filed are for a hospital stay, insert information in lines 16, 18, and 32	❏	❏	❏
4. If the services are related to an injury, insert the date of the accident in line 14	❏	❏	❏
5. Enter the name of the referring provider and NPI with the appropriate qualifier in lines 17 and 17b.	❏	❏	❏
6. List the ICD-10-CM codes with the primary reason for the encounter as well as other diagnoses as documented by the physician on line 21, A through L	❏	❏	❏
7. Insert dates of service in the unshaded portion of lines 24A, rows 1 through 6, in both "from" and "to" for each service or procedure)	❏	❏	❏
8. Reference the code where the service was rendered on line 24, column B	❏	❏	❏
9. Complete lines 24D through 24J for each service and procedure including the diagnosis pointer(s), charges, number of units, and rendering provider NPI	❏	❏	❏
10. Enter the federal tax ID number on line 25 and accept assignment on line 27	❏	❏	❏
11. Complete the total charges on line 28	❏	❏	❏
12. Complete blocks 31, 32, and 33	❏	❏	❏
13. Add claim to the pending claims tracking list	❏	❏	❏
14. **AFF** You notice that Mr. Dishman has no signature on file, but the box on line 12 of his claim form says he does. Explain how you would respond	❏	❏	❏

(continues)

PSY PROCEDURE 13-1 **Completing a CMS-1500 Claim Form** (continued)

_____

_____

_____

_____

CALCULATION

Total Possible Points: _____

Total Points Earned: _____ Multiplied by 100 = _____ Divided by Total Possible Points = _____ %

PASS   FAIL   COMMENTS:
❏   ❏

Student's signature _____ Date _____

Partner's signature _____ Date _____

Instructor's signature _____ Date _____

PROCEDURE 13-2 **Obtain Preauthorization for Services**

Name: _____ Date: _____ Time: _____ Grade: _____

EQUIPMENT: Case scenario (see work product 2), patient's demographic information including insurance card information, a physician's order for treatment, preauthorization form, pen

STANDARDS: Given the needed equipment and a place to work, the student will perform this skill with _____ % accuracy in a total of _____ minutes. *(Your instructor will tell you what the percentage and time limits will be before you begin.)*

KEY: 4 = Satisfactory 0 = Unsatisfactory NA = This step is not counted

PROCEDURE STEPS	SELF	PARTNER	INSTRUCTOR
1. Using the information provided in the case scenario, verify the physician's order with the patient's demographic/insurance information	❑	❑	❑
2. Complete the preauthorization form (preauthorization form) as provided by the insurance company or the practice's form with details involving the requested services including the date the preauthorization is being requested	❑	❑	❑
3. Contact the insurance company's preauthorization department by calling the number listed on the back of the patient's insurance card to verify the patient's eligibility for the services and document on the preauthorization form	❑	❑	❑
4. Determine if the patient's insurance benefits require preauthorization or precertification from the insurance company for the requested service	❑	❑	❑
5. Note the name or identification of the insurance preauthorization representative on the preauthorization form	❑	❑	❑
6. Provide details noted on the completed preauthorization form for the requested services and/or treatment to the insurance preauthorization representative	❑	❑	❑
7. Accurately document the preauthorization number given for the service or treatment on the preauthorization form. This information must be given to the provider performing the authorized services	❑	❑	❑
8. Sign the preauthorization form as the person who got the authorization, and file it in the patient's medical record	❑	❑	❑
9. **AFF** Describe how you would handle advising a patient that their insurance benefits did not cover the ordered service or treatment	❑	❑	❑

_____

_____

_____

_____

(continues)

PSY   PROCEDURE 13-2   **Obtain Preauthorization for Services** (continued)

CALCULATION

Total Possible Points: _____

Total Points Earned: _____ Multiplied by 100 = _____ Divided by Total Possible Points = _____ %

PASS   FAIL   COMMENTS:
❏   ❏

Student's signature _____   Date _____

Partner's signature _____   Date _____

Instructor's signature _____   Date _____

PSY PROCEDURE 13-3 | **Accurately Describe Information on an Explanation of Benefits**

Name: _____ Date: _____ Time: _____ Grade: _____

EQUIPMENT: Case scenario (see work product 3), insurance explanation of benefits

STANDARDS: Given the needed equipment and a place to work, the student will perform this skill with _____ % accuracy in a total of _____ minutes. *(Your instructor will tell you what the percentage and time limits will be before you begin.)*

KEY: 4 = Satisfactory   0 = Unsatisfactory   NA = This step is not counted

PROCEDURE STEPS	SELF	PARTNER	INSTRUCTOR
1. Review the Explanation of Benefits (EOB) to determine what was billed and what was paid for the correct date of service	❏	❏	❏
2. Determine the insurance allowed amount(s) for the services and procedures for the correct date of service	❏	❏	❏
3. Calculate the patient's financial responsibility for the services if the physician has a contracted fee schedule and accepts the EOB allowed amount	❏	❏	❏
4. Determine the patient's financial responsibility of the services if the physician does not have a contracted fee schedule with the insurance company	❏	❏	❏
5. **AFF** Explain how you would respond to a patient who becomes angry because it looks like the practice charges too much based on how much the insurance "allowed"	❏	❏	❏

WORK PRODUCT 1

Grade: _____

COMPLETE INSURANCE CLAIM FORMS

Jackson Dishman is seen in the office for acute abdominal pain. Complete the CMS-1500 form using the information provided below:

297-01-2222
Jackson W. Dishman   Group #68735
123 Smith Avenue
Winston-Salem NC 27103   Date of Birth: 06-01-53

He is charged for an office visit, which carries the CPT code 99213 and costs $150.00. The doctor orders a complete blood count and has the RMA do a venipuncture (the CPT code 36415); and the charge is $50.00. The patient pays nothing today. The physician sends Mr. Dishman home with a diagnosis of acute right lower abdominal pain (IDC-10-CM code is R10.31). He is to return in 2 days unless the pain becomes unbearable.

HEALTH INSURANCE CLAIM FORM

APPROVED BY NATIONAL UNIFORM CLAIM COMMITTEE (NUCC) 02/12

| | PICA | | | | | | PICA | |

CARRIER

□□ PICA

| 1. MEDICARE | MEDICAID | TRICARE | CHAMPVA | GROUP HEALTH PLAN | FECA BLK LUNG | OTHER | 1a. INSURED'S I.D. NUMBER (For Program in Item 1) |
| □ (Medicare#) | □ (Medicaid#) | □ (ID#/DoD#) | □ (Member ID#) | □ (ID#) | □ (ID#) | □ (ID#) | |

2. PATIENT'S NAME (Last Name, First Name, Middle Initial)

3. PATIENT'S BIRTH DATE MM DD YY   SEX   M □   F □

4. INSURED'S NAME (Last Name, First Name, Middle Initial)

5. PATIENT'S ADDRESS (No., Street)

6. PATIENT RELATIONSHIP TO INSURED   Self □ Spouse □ Child □ Other □

7. INSURED'S ADDRESS (No., Street)

CITY   STATE

8. RESERVED FOR NUCC USE

CITY   STATE

ZIP CODE   TELEPHONE (Include Area Code) ( )

ZIP CODE   TELEPHONE (Include Area Code) ( )

9. OTHER INSURED'S NAME (Last Name, First Name, Middle Initial)

10. IS PATIENT'S CONDITION RELATED TO:

11. INSURED'S POLICY GROUP OR FECA NUMBER

a. OTHER INSURED'S POLICY OR GROUP NUMBER

a. EMPLOYMENT? (Current or Previous)   □ YES   □ NO

a. INSURED'S DATE OF BIRTH MM DD YY   SEX   M □   F □

b. RESERVED FOR NUCC USE

b. AUTO ACCIDENT?   □ YES   □ NO   PLACE (State) ⌴

b. OTHER CLAIM ID (Designated by NUCC)

c. RESERVED FOR NUCC USE

c. OTHER ACCIDENT?   □ YES   □ NO

c. INSURANCE PLAN NAME OR PROGRAM NAME

d. INSURANCE PLAN NAME OR PROGRAM NAME

10d. CLAIM CODES (Designated by NUCC)

d. IS THERE ANOTHER HEALTH BENEFIT PLAN?   □ YES   □ NO   *If yes*, complete items 9, 9a, and 9d.

READ BACK OF FORM BEFORE COMPLETING & SIGNING THIS FORM.
12. PATIENT'S OR AUTHORIZED PERSON'S SIGNATURE I authorize the release of any medical or other information necessary to process this claim. I also request payment of government benefits either to myself or to the party who accepts assignment below.

SIGNED _____   DATE _____

13. INSURED'S OR AUTHORIZED PERSON'S SIGNATURE I authorize payment of medical benefits to the undersigned physician or supplier for services described below.

SIGNED _____

PATIENT AND INSURED INFORMATION

14. DATE OF CURRENT ILLNESS, INJURY, or PREGNANCY (LMP) MM DD YY   QUAL.

15. OTHER DATE QUAL.   MM DD YY

16. DATES PATIENT UNABLE TO WORK IN CURRENT OCCUPATION MM DD YY   FROM   TO   MM DD YY

17. NAME OF REFERRING PROVIDER OR OTHER SOURCE   17a.   17b. NPI

18. HOSPITALIZATION DATES RELATED TO CURRENT SERVICES MM DD YY   FROM   TO   MM DD YY

19. ADDITIONAL CLAIM INFORMATION (Designated by NUCC)

20. OUTSIDE LAB?   □ YES   □ NO $ CHARGES

21. DIAGNOSIS OR NATURE OF ILLNESS OR INJURY Relate A-L to service line below (24E)   ICD Ind. ⌴

A. |_____   B. |_____   C. |_____   D. |_____
E. |_____   F. |_____   G. |_____   H. |_____
I. |_____   J. |_____   K. |_____   L. |_____

22. RESUBMISSION CODE   ORIGINAL REF. NO.

23. PRIOR AUTHORIZATION NUMBER

24. A. DATE(S) OF SERVICE						B. PLACE OF SERVICE	C. EMG	D. PROCEDURES, SERVICES, OR SUPPLIES (Explain Unusual Circumstances)		E. DIAGNOSIS POINTER	F. $ CHARGES	G. DAYS OR UNITS	H. EPSDT Family Plan	I. ID. QUAL.	J. RENDERING PROVIDER ID. #
From			To					CPT/HCPCS	MODIFIER						
MM	DD	YY	MM	DD	YY										
1															NPI
2															NPI
3															NPI
4															NPI
5															NPI
6															NPI

PHYSICIAN OR SUPPLIER INFORMATION

25. FEDERAL TAX I.D. NUMBER   □ SSN □ EIN

26. PATIENT'S ACCOUNT NO.

27. ACCEPT ASSIGNMENT? (For govt. claims, see back)   □ YES   □ NO

28. TOTAL CHARGE $

29. AMOUNT PAID $

30. Rsvd for NUCC Use

31. SIGNATURE OF PHYSICIAN OR SUPPLIER INCLUDING DEGREES OR CREDENTIALS (I certify that the statements on the reverse apply to this bill and are made a part thereof.)

SIGNED _____   DATE _____

32. SERVICE FACILITY LOCATION INFORMATION

a.   b.

33. BILLING PROVIDER INFO & PH # ( )

a.   b.

NUCC Instruction Manual available at: www.nucc.org   *PLEASE PRINT OR TYPE*   APPROVED OMB-0938-1197 FORM 1500 (02-12)

WORK PRODUCT 2

COMPLETE PREAUTHORIZATION FOR SERVICES

Charlene Adams has been having right shoulder pain for the last 3 months that is causing her to wake several times during the night because of the severe pain. Dr. Kyle Dunn has requested an MRI of her right shoulder with contrast, and her insurance requires preauthorization. Complete a preauthorization form using the information provided below for Charlene Adams, Date of Birth 03/22/1984, SSN#XXX-XX-9770, 167 Maple Ave., Winston-Salem, NC 27103.

PRIMARY INSURANCE INFORMATION:

Southeast Insurance HMO	Southeast Insurance	
GRP: R845B		
ID: 301993KR	Providers: Please file the medical claims with Southeast at: P.O. Box 4445668 Atlanta, GA 30101-5668	Preauthorization: 1-888-708-3562
PCP: Kyle Dunn, M.D.		Deductibles/Coinsurance Applies: $2,500 deductible
Subscriber: Charlene Adams		Co-pay: PCP $ 30.00
MEMBERS SERVICES 1-800-123-9876		Co-pay: SPC $ 50.00
PROVIDER SERVICES/PREAUTHORIZATIONS: 1-888-123-54321		ER $ 250.00
		www.southeastmemberservices.com
	www.southeasthmoplans.com	

The diagnosis is right shoulder pain, ICD-10-CM M25.511, and preauthorization is necessary for CPT 73222. The patient recently finished 10 physical therapy sessions for her right shoulder without relief. Ms. Adams is also an insulin-dependent diabetic.

Great Falls Health System Physician Offices

Insurance Preauthorization/Precertification Form

Please complete this form as accurately and with as many details as possible when preauthorizing or precertifying services or treatments with insurance companies. The completed form is filed in the patient's medical record for future reference.

Employee Name and Title:	Date of Completion:
Ordering Physician:	
Patient's Name:	
Patient's DOB:	Insurance ID:
Insurance Company:	
Description of service or treatment requested with CPT Code(s):	
Diagnoses codes supporting medical necessity for the service or treatment requested:	
Comorbid conditions and diseases (Diagnoses Codes):	
Other information to support medical necessity (i.e., physical therapy, medication regimen, etc.):	
Name or ID number of Insurance Representative:	
AUTHORIZATION NUMBER:	AUTHORIZED FROM: TO:
Employee Signature:	Date Authorization Obtained:

WORK PRODUCT 3

Grade: _____

INTERPRET INSURANCE EXPLANATION OF BENEFITS

Southeast Insurance					
Explanation of Benefits					
Employee Name: Charlene Adams				Date of Service: 10/15/2025	
SSN: XXX-XX-9770				Provider: Dr. Dunn	
Subscriber No. 301993KR				Provider TIN: 31-7766554	
Group No. R845B					
Date of Service	Comment Code	Amount of Charge	Amount Allowed	Co-Insurance	Amount Paid
10/15/2025	57	$150.00	$ 116.00	80%	$ 92.80
Comment Code: 57 – Amount charged exceeds Usual and Customary				Total Paid	$ 92.80

CHAPTER 14

Accounting Responsibilities

LEARNING OUTCOMES

COG Cognitive Domain*

1. Spell and define the key terms
2. *Define the following bookkeeping terms:*
   a. *Charges*
   b. *Payments*
   c. *Accounts receivable*
   d. *Accounts payable*
   e. *Adjustments*
   f. *end-of-day reconciliation*
3. Explain the concept of the pegboard bookkeeping system
4. Describe the functions of a computer accounting system
5. Explain banking services, including types of accounts and fees
6. Describe the accounting equation
7. Explain the process of ordering supplies and paying invoices
8. Explain basic booking computations
9. Differentiate between bookkeeping and accounting
10. Describe banking procedures as related to the ambulatory care setting
11. Compare types of endorsement
12. Differentiate between accounts payable and accounts receivable
13. Describe common periodic financial reports
14. *Define the following: allowed amount*
15. *Identify types of adjustments made to patient accounts including:*
    a. *Non-sufficient funds (NSF) check*
    b. *Collection agency transaction*
    c. *Credit balance*
    d. *Third party*

PSY Psychomotor Domain*

1. Prepare a bank deposit (Procedure 14-9)
2. *Perform accounts receivable procedures to patient accounts, including posting:*
   a. *Charges (Procedure 14-1)*
   b. *Payments (Procedure 14-2)*
   c. *Adjustments (Procedures 14-4, 14-5, 14-6)*
   d. Process a credit balance (Procedure 14-3)
   e. Process refunds (Procedure 14-4)
   f. Post NSF checks (Procedure 14-7)
   g. Post collection agency payments (Procedure 14-6)
3. Perform end-of-day reconciliation (Procedure 14-8)
4. Reconcile a bank statement (Procedure 14-10)
5. Maintain a petty cash account (Procedure 14-11)
6. Write a check (Procedure 14-12)

AFF Affective Domain*

1. *Demonstrate critical thinking skills in end-of-day reconciliation*
2. *Recognize personal boundaries with confidential patient financial information*

MAERB Standards are italicized.

ABHES Competencies

1. Perform billing and collection procedures
2. Perform accounts receivable procedures
3. Use manual or computerized bookkeeping systems

Name: _____   Date: _____   Grade: _____

⬛︎ MULTIPLE CHOICE

1. The best place to put petty cash is:
   a. in the same drawer as the other cash and checks.
   b. in a separate, secured drawer.
   c. in an envelope stored in the staff room.
   d. in the physician's office.
   e. in a locked supply cabinet.

2. Which of the following information is found on a patient's ledger card?
   a. Date of birth
   b. Social Security number
   c. Blood type
   d. Insurance information
   e. Marital status

3. The purpose of the posting proofs section is to:
   a. enter the day's totals and balance the daysheet.
   b. update and maintain a patient's financial record.
   c. make note of any credit the patient has on file.
   d. make note of any debit the patient has on file.
   e. allow for any adjustments that need to be made.

4. Which of the following might you purchase using petty cash?
   a. Cotton swabs
   b. Thermometer covers
   c. Office supplies
   d. Nonlatex gloves
   e. New x-ray machine

Scenario for questions 5 and 6: A new patient comes in and gives you his insurance card. The patient's insurance allows $160.00 for a routine checkup. Of this, insurance will pay 75% of his bill.

5. How much will the patient need to pay?
   a. $0
   b. $40.00
   c. $120.00
   d. $75.00
   e. $160.00

6. How much will the insurance company pay?
   a. $120.00
   b. $40.00
   c. $160.00
   d. $32.00
   e. $0

7. A check register is used to:
   a. hold checks until they are ready for deposit.
   b. create a checklist of daily office duties.
   c. make a list of payments the office is still owed.
   d. record all checks that go in and out of the office.
   e. remind patients when their payments are due.

8. Ideally, if you are using a pegboard accounting system, what is the best way to organize your ledgers?
   a. File all ledgers alphabetically in a single tray
   b. Alphabetically file paid ledgers in one tray and ledgers with outstanding balances in another
   c. Numerically file paid ledgers in the front of the tray and ledgers with outstanding balances in the back
   d. Alphabetically file paid ledgers into the patient's folders and ledgers with outstanding balances in a tray
   e. File all ledgers into the patient's files

9. Accounts receivable is:
   a. a record of all monies owed to the practice.
   b. the people the practice owes money to.
   c. the transactions transferred from a different office.
   d. any outstanding inventory bills.
   e. a list of patients who have paid in the last month.

10. It is unsafe to use credit card account numbers on purchases made:
   a. over the phone.
   b. by fax.
   c. through e-mail.
   d. from a catalog.
   e. in person.

11. When you have a deposit that includes cash, what is the only way you should get it to the bank?
   a. Deliver it by hand
   b. Deliver it into a depository
   c. Send it by mail with enough postage
   d. Deliver checks by mail and cash by hand
   e. Do not accept cash as payment

12. Which of the following is a benefit of paying bills by computer?
    a. You do not need to keep a record of paying your bills
    b. Entering data into the computer is quick and easy
    c. Information can be "memorized" and stored
    d. You can divide columns into groups of expenses (rent, paychecks, etc.)
    e. You can easily correct any errors

13. Most medical offices generally use:
    a. standard business checks.
    b. certified checks.
    c. traveler's checks.
    d. money orders.
    e. cash deposits.

14. What is a quick way to find order numbers when making a purchase?
    a. Check the packing slip of a previous order
    b. Find a previous bill for any item numbers
    c. Check past purchase orders for their order numbers
    d. Call the supplier for a list of item numbers
    e. Look at the supplier's website

15. Summation reports are:
    a. lists of all the clients who entered the office.
    b. reports that track all expenses and income.
    c. computer reports that compile all daily totals.
    d. lists that analyze an office's activities.
    e. reports the IRS sends an office being audited.

16. Why is the adjustment column so important?
    a. It assists you in deciding the discount percentage
    b. It records all transactions a patient has made in your office
    c. It allows you to adjust the account balance for discounts
    d. It keeps track of any changes a patient has in health care
    e. It keeps track of bounced checks

17. Which of the following is NOT an important reason for performing an office inventory of equipment and supplies?
    a. It will help you know when to order new supplies and/or equipment
    b. It will help you calculate how much money you will need to spend on new equipment
    c. It will alert you of any misuse/theft of supplies or equipment
    d. The information will be needed for tax purposes
    e. It will help you see if you will have excess supplies to share with employees

18. In a bookkeeping system, things of value relating to the practice are called:
    a. assets.
    b. liabilities.
    c. debits.
    d. credits.
    e. audits.

19. The amount of capital the physician has invested in the practice is referred to as:
    a. assets.
    b. credits.
    c. equity.
    d. liabilities.
    e. invoices.

20. Overpayments under $5 are generally:
    a. sent back to the patient.
    b. placed in petty cash.
    c. left on the account as a credit.
    d. deposited in a special overpayment account.
    e. mailed to the insurance company.

⬢ MATCHING

Grade: _____

Match the following key terms to their definitions.

Key Terms

21. _____ accounting cycle
22. _____ accounts payable
23. _____ adjustment
24. _____ audit
25. _____ balance
26. _____ bookkeeping
27. _____ charge slip
28. _____ check register
29. _____ check stub
30. _____ credit
31. _____ day sheet
32. _____ debit
33. _____ encounter form
34. _____ Internal Revenue Service (IRS)
35. _____ invoice
36. _____ accounts receivable
37. _____ ledger card
38. _____ packing slip
39. _____ posting
40. _____ profit-and-loss statement
41. _____ purchase order
42. _____ returned check fee
43. _____ service charge
44. _____ summation report

Definitions

a. a preprinted three-part form that can be placed on a day sheet to record the patient's charges and payments along with other information in an encounter form
b. a charge or money owed to an account
c. a record of all money owed to the business
d. a document that accompanies a supply order and lists the enclosed items
e. any report that provides a summary of activities, such as a payroll report or profit-and-loss statement
f. a daily business record of charges and payments
g. a statement of income and expenditures; shows whether in a given period a business made or lost money and how much
h. statement of debt owed; a bill
i. a review of an account
j. a consecutive 12-month period for financial recordkeeping following either a fiscal year or the calendar year
k. a balance in one's favor on an account; a promise to pay a bill at a later date; record of payment received
l. listing financial transactions in a ledger
m. a continuous record of business transactions with debits and credits
n. change in a posted account
o. a federal agency that regulates and enforces various taxes
p. amount of money a bank or business charges for a check written on an account with insufficient funds
q. amounts of money the practice owes
r. organized and accurate recordkeeping system of financial transactions
s. a document that lists required items to be purchased
t. preprinted patient statement that lists codes for basic office charges and has sections to record charges incurred in an office visit, the patient's current balance, and next appointment
u. that which is left over after the additions and subtractions have been made to an account
v. piece of paper that indicates to whom a check was issued, in what amount, and on what date
w. a document used to record the checks that have been written
x. a charge by a bank for various services

⬢ SHORT ANSWER

Grade: _____

45. What are banking services?

_____
_____
_____
_____

46. Why is correction fluid not used in a medical office, and what is the proper procedure to correct a mistake?

_____

_____

_____

_____

47. What are four steps you can take if an item you ordered was not delivered?

_____

_____

_____

_____

48. List four items that should be readily available in case your office is audited.

_____

_____

_____

_____

49. What is a returned check fee?

_____

_____

_____

_____

50. Why might you run a trial daily report before you run a final daily report?

_____

_____

_____

_____

51. The office you are working in has recently updated its bookkeeping system from pegboard to computer. Now, the physician wants to utilize all the capabilities the new system offers. One function that interests her is the computer accounting reports. List the different types of reports and briefly describe their uses.

_____

_____

_____

_____

COG PSY ACTIVE LEARNING

Grade: _____

52. During a staff meeting, the issue of ordering supplies comes up. The office has been buying small quantities of all supplies, causing some items to quickly run out, while others are stockpiled in disuse. The physician wants to figure out a way to spend the budget more efficiently and asks you to be in charge of the next order. What steps can you take to determine which items you will order in the office's next purchase? How can you further improve the office's expenditure?

_____

_____

_____

_____

53. Your office currently is using a checking account at a local bank. However, the physician you work for is thinking about changing over to a money market account because he has heard the interest is much better in a money market account. He knows about an offer through another bank that will waive the minimum balance of $500 for 3 months. What important information should you research before you give him your opinion? Discuss the differences between a checking account and a money market account and include the advantages and disadvantages of switching accounts.

_____

_____

_____

_____

COG IDENTIFICATION

Grade: _____

54. There are several advantages of a computerized system over a manual system. Read the selection below and circle the functions that are computerized accounting functions only.

a. Entries are recorded in a patient's file

b. Quickly create invoices and receipts

c. Calculation of each transaction is made, as well as a total at the end of the day

d. Performs bookkeeping, making appointments, and generating office reports

e. Daily activities are recorded

f. Bill reminders are placed to keep track of expenses

55. A medical office is just starting up, and one of the first things the bookkeeper needs to do is find a bank. Fill in the chart below with descriptions of checking, savings, and money market accounts.

Checking Account	Savings Account	Money Market Account

56. The office you are working in has an accounting cycle that begins in June. Describe what the accounting cycle is, and what kind of year your office follows.

_____

_____

_____

_____

57. The office manager ordered a new endorsement stamp from the bank. In the meantime, you need to deposit a check for Rinku Banjere, MD, into account number 123-4567-890. Endorse the check below for deposit.

ENDORSE HERE
DO NOT SIGN/WRITE/STAMP BELOW THIS LINE
FOR FINANCIAL INSTITUTION USE ONLY

PSY WHAT WOULD YOU DO?

Grade: _____

58. A patient's check has been returned for insufficient funds. The patient asks you to send it back through the bank. What would you do?

_____

_____

_____

_____

59. Explain the process of ordering supplies and paying invoices.

_____

_____

_____

_____

COG TRUE OR FALSE?

Grade: _____

Determine whether the following statements are true or false. If false, explain why.

60. Once you have entered a patient transaction on the day sheet, you give the ledger to the patient as a receipt.

_____

61. As long as your bookkeeping records are accurate and the figures balance, you do not need to save receipts.

_____

62. You should always compare the prices and quality of office supplies when you are placing an order.

_____

63. Audits are performed in the office yearly by the IRS.

_____

64. Packing slips are used by the manufacturer and can be destroyed upon opening a package of supplies.

_____

COG PATIENT EDUCATION

Grade: _____

65. Your patient is a young woman who does not understand what happens to the difference between what a physician charges and what her insurance company will pay. In her case, the physician's charge is $100, but insurance only allows for $80. The insurance company will pay for 75% of the cost. How much will the patient pay? Explain to her how this works, and how the charge is determined.

_____

_____

_____

_____

AFF CASE STUDIES FOR CRITICAL THINKING

Grade: _____

You have been working at a small, one-physician practice for about 2 weeks. You share the front office with the office manager, who has been working there for 20 years. She goes on vacation and in the course of covering some of her duties, you discover suspicious entries in the accounts payable records. You wonder if she is paying her own bills out of the office account.

66. What should you do? Choose all appropriate actions from the list below.

    a. Nothing, she is your boss and you are new here.

    b. Ask your coworkers for advice.

    c. Question her about what you found when she returns.

    d. Tell the physician immediately.

    e. Tell the physician's wife of your suspicions.

    f. Keep it to yourself; it is none of your business.

    g. Post the situation on Facebook and ask for advice.

    h. Investigate further while she is away by going over all of the check entries.

PSY PROCEDURE 14-1 Post Charges on a Day Sheet

Name: _____ **Date:** _____ **Time:** _____ **Grade:** _____

EQUIPMENT/SUPPLIES: Pen, pegboard, calculator, day sheet, encounter forms, ledger cards, previous day's balance, list of patients and charges, fee schedule

STANDARDS: Given the needed equipment and a place to work, the student will perform this skill with _____ % accuracy in a total of _____ minutes. *(Your instructor will tell you what the percentage and time limits will be before you begin.)*

KEY: 4 = Satisfactory 0 = Unsatisfactory NA = This step is not counted

PROCEDURE STEPS	SELF	PARTNER	INSTRUCTOR
1. Place a new day sheet on the pegboard and record the totals from the previous day sheet	❏	❏	❏
2. Align the patient's ledger card with the first available line on the day sheet	❏	❏	❏
3. Place the receipt to align with the appropriate line on the ledger card	❏	❏	❏
4. Record the number of the receipt in the appropriate column	❏	❏	❏
5. Write the patient's name on the receipt	❏	❏	❏
6. Record any existing balance the patient owes in the previous balance column of the day sheet	❏	❏	❏
7. Record a brief description of the charge in the description line	❏	❏	❏
8. Record the total charges in the charge column. Press hard so that the marks go through to the ledger card and the day sheet	❏	❏	❏
9. Add the total charges to the previous balance and record in the current balance column	❏	❏	❏
10. Return the ledger card to appropriate storage	❏	❏	❏

_____

_____

_____

_____

PSY PROCEDURE 14-1 **Post Charges on a Day Sheet** (continued)

CALCULATION

Total Possible Points: _____

Total Points Earned: _____ Multiplied by 100 = _____ Divided by Total Possible Points = _____ %

PASS   FAIL   COMMENTS:
❏   ❏

Student's signature _____ Date _____

Partner's signature _____ Date _____

Instructor's signature _____ Date _____

PROCEDURE 14-2 — Post Payments on a Day Sheet

PSY

Name: _____ **Date:** _____ **Time:** _____ **Grade:** _____

EQUIPMENT/SUPPLIES: Pen, pegboard, calculator, daysheet, encounter forms, ledger cards, previous day's balance, list of patients and charges, fee schedule

COMPUTER AND MEDICAL OFFICE SOFTWARE: Follow the software requirements for posting credits to patient accounts.

STANDARDS: Given the needed equipment and a place to work, the student will perform this skill with _____ % accuracy in a total of _____ minutes. *(Your instructor will tell you what the percentage and time limits will be before you begin.)*

KEY: 4 = Satisfactory 0 = Unsatisfactory NA = This step is not counted

PROCEDURE STEPS	SELF	PARTNER	INSTRUCTOR
1. Place a new day sheet on the pegboard and record the totals from the previous day sheet	❏	❏	❏
2. Align the patient's ledger card with the first available line on the day sheet	❏	❏	❏
3. Place receipt to align with the appropriate line on the ledger card	❏	❏	❏
4. Record the number of the receipt in the appropriate column	❏	❏	❏
5. Write the patient's name on the receipt	❏	❏	❏
6. Record any existing balance the patient owes in the previous balance column of the day sheet	❏	❏	❏
7. Record the source and type of the payment in the description line	❏	❏	❏
8. Record appropriate adjustments in the adjustment column	❏	❏	❏
9. Record the total payment in the payment column. Press hard so that marks go through to the ledger card and the day sheet	❏	❏	❏
10. Subtract the payment and adjustments from the outstanding/ previous balance, and record the current balance	❏	❏	❏
11. Return the ledger card to appropriate storage	❏	❏	❏

_____

_____

_____

_____

PSY PROCEDURE 14-2 **Post Payments on a Day Sheet** (continued)

CALCULATION

Total Possible Points: _____

Total Points Earned: _____ Multiplied by 100 = _____ Divided by Total Possible Points = _____ %

PASS   FAIL   COMMENTS:
❏   ❏

Student's signature _____   Date _____

Partner's signature _____   Date _____

Instructor's signature _____   Date _____

PSY PROCEDURE 14-3 — Process a Credit Balance

Name: _____ **Date:** _____ **Time:** _____ **Grade:** _____

EQUIPMENT/SUPPLIES: Pen, pegboard, calculator, day sheet, ledger card

STANDARDS: Given the needed equipment and a place to work, the student will perform this skill with _____ % accuracy in a total of _____ minutes. *(Your instructor will tell you what the percentage and time limits will be before you begin.)*

KEY: 4 = Satisfactory 0 = Unsatisfactory NA = This step is not counted

PROCEDURE STEPS	SELF	PARTNER	INSTRUCTOR
1. Determine the reason for the credit balance	❏	❏	❏
2. Place brackets around the balance, indicating that it is a negative number	❏	❏	❏
3. Write a refund check and follow the steps in Procedure 14-4	❏	❏	❏

_____

_____

_____

_____

CALCULATION

Total Possible Points: _____

Total Points Earned: _____ Multiplied by 100 = _____ Divided by Total Possible Points = _____ %

PASS **FAIL** **COMMENTS:**
❏ ❏

Student's signature _____ Date _____

Partner's signature _____ Date _____

Instructor's signature _____ Date _____

PSY PROCEDURE 14-4 | **Process Refunds**

Name: _____ **Date:** _____ **Time:** _____ **Grade:** _____

EQUIPMENT/SUPPLIES: Pen, pegboard, calculator, day sheet, ledger card, checkbook, check register, word processor letterhead, envelope, postage, copy machine, patient's chart, refund file

STANDARDS: Given the needed equipment and a place to work, the student will perform this skill with _____ % accuracy in a total of _____ minutes. *(Your instructor will tell you what the percentage and time limits will be before you begin.)*

KEY: 4 = Satisfactory 0 = Unsatisfactory NA = This step is not counted

PROCEDURE STEPS	SELF	PARTNER	INSTRUCTOR
1. Determine who gets the refund, the patient or the insurance company	❏	❏	❏
2. Pull patient's ledger card and place on current day sheet aligned with the first available line	❏	❏	❏
3. Post the amount of the refund in the adjustment column in brackets, indicating it is a debit, not a credit, adjustment	❏	❏	❏
4. Add the adjustment to the outstanding/previous balance, and record in the current balance column	❏	❏	❏
5. Write "Refund to Patient" or "Refund to _____" (name of insurance company) in the description column	❏	❏	❏
6. Write a check for the credit amount made out to the appropriate party	❏	❏	❏
7. Record the amount and name of payee in the check register	❏	❏	❏
8. Mail check with letter of explanation to patient or insurance company	❏	❏	❏
9. Place copy of check and copy of letter in the patient's record or in the refund file	❏	❏	❏
10. Return the patient's ledger card to its storage area	❏	❏	❏

_____

_____

_____

_____

(continues)

FSY PROCEDURE 14-4   **Process Refunds** (continued)

CALCULATION

Total Possible Points: _____

Total Points Earned: _____ Multiplied by 100 = _____ Divided by Total Possible Points = _____ %

PASS   FAIL   COMMENTS:
❏   ❏

Student's signature _____ Date _____

Partner's signature _____ Date _____

Instructor's signature _____ Date _____

PSY PROCEDURE 14-5	Post Adjustments to a Day Sheet

Name: _____ **Date:** _____ **Time:** _____ **Grade:** _____

EQUIPMENT/SUPPLIES: Pen, pegboard, calculator, day sheet, encounter forms, ledger cards, previous day's balance, list of patients and charges, fee schedule

COMPUTER AND MEDICAL OFFICE SOFTWARE: Follow the software requirements for posting credits to patient accounts

STANDARDS: Given the needed equipment and a place to work, the student will perform this skill with _____ % accuracy in a total of _____ minutes. *(Your instructor will tell you what the percentage and time limits will be before you begin.)*

KEY: 4 = Satisfactory 0 = Unsatisfactory NA = This step is not counted

PROCEDURE STEPS	SELF	PARTNER	INSTRUCTOR
1. Pull patient's ledger card and place on current day sheet aligned with the first available line	❑	❑	❑
2. Post the amount to be written off in the adjustment column as a credit adjustment	❑	❑	❑
3. Subtract the adjustment from the outstanding/previous balance, and record in the current balance column	❑	❑	❑
4. Return the ledger card to appropriate storage	❑	❑	❑

_____

_____

_____

_____

CALCULATION

Total Possible Points: _____

Total Points Earned: _____ Multiplied by 100 = _____ Divided by Total Possible Points = _____ %

PASS   FAIL   COMMENTS:
❑   ❑

Student's signature _____ Date _____

Partner's signature _____ Date _____

Instructor's signature _____ Date _____

PSY PROCEDURE 14-6   Post Collection Agency Payments

Name: _____ Date: _____ Time: _____ Grade: _____

EQUIPMENT/SUPPLIES: Pen, pegboard, calculator, day sheet, patient's ledger card

STANDARDS: Given the needed equipment and a place to work, the student will perform this skill with _____ % accuracy in a total of _____ minutes. *(Your instructor will tell you what the percentage and time limits will be before you begin.)*

KEY: 4 = Satisfactory   0 = Unsatisfactory   NA = This step is not counted

PROCEDURE STEPS	SELF	PARTNER	INSTRUCTOR
1. Review check stub or report from the collection agency explaining the amounts to be applied to the accounts	❑	❑	❑
2. Pull the patients' ledger cards	❑	❑	❑
3. Post the amount to be applied in the payment column for each patient	❑	❑	❑
4. Adjust off the amount representing the percentage of the payment charged by the collection agency	❑	❑	❑

_____

_____

_____

_____

CALCULATION

Total Possible Points: _____

Total Points Earned: _____ Multiplied by 100 = _____ Divided by Total Possible Points = _____ %

PASS   **FAIL**   **COMMENTS:**
❑   ❑

Student's signature _____ Date _____

Partner's signature _____ Date _____

Instructor's signature _____ Date _____

PSY PROCEDURE 14-7   Process NSF Checks

Name: _____ Date: _____ Time: _____ Grade: _____

EQUIPMENT/SUPPLIES: Pen, pegboard, calculator, day sheet, patient's ledger card

STANDARDS: Given the needed equipment and a place to work, the student will perform this skill with _____ % accuracy in a total of _____ minutes. (Your instructor will tell you what the percentage and time limits will be before you begin.)

KEY: 4 = Satisfactory   0 = Unsatisfactory   NA = This step is not counted

PROCEDURE STEPS	SELF	PARTNER	INSTRUCTOR
1. Pull patient's ledger card and place on current day sheet aligned with the first available line	❏	❏	❏
2. Write the amount of the check in the payment column in brackets indicating it is a debit, not a credit, adjustment	❏	❏	❏
3. Add it to the outstanding/previous balance and record in the current balance column	❏	❏	❏
4. Write "Check Returned For Nonsufficient Funds" in the description column	❏	❏	❏
5. Post a returned check charge with an appropriate explanation in the charge column	❏	❏	❏
6. Write "Bank Fee for Returned Check" in the description column	❏	❏	❏
7. Call the patient to advise him of the returned check and the fee	❏	❏	❏
8. Construct a proper letter of explanation and a copy of the ledger card and mail to the patient	❏	❏	❏
9. Place a copy of the letter and the check in the patient's file	❏	❏	❏
10. Make arrangements for the patient to pay cash	❏	❏	❏
11. Flag the patient's account as a credit risk for future transactions	❏	❏	❏
12. Return the patient's ledger card to its storage area	❏	❏	❏
13. **AFF** You see a patient whose check was returned for nonsufficient funds out at a soccer game. Another parent comments to you about this individual's constant bragging about his new car. Explain how you would respond	❏	❏	❏

_____

_____

_____

_____

(continues)

PSY PROCEDURE 14-7 **Process NSF Checks** (continued)

CALCULATION

Total Possible Points: _____

Total Points Earned: _____ Multiplied by 100 = _____ Divided by Total Possible Points = _____ %

PASS   **FAIL**   **COMMENTS:**

❑   ❑

Student's signature _____   Date _____

Partner's signature _____   Date _____

Instructor's signature _____   Date _____

PSY PROCEDURE 14-8 **Balance a Day Sheet**

Name: _____ Date: _____ Time: _____ Grade: _____

EQUIPMENT/SUPPLIES: Day sheet with totals brought forward, simulated exercise, calculator, pen

STANDARDS: Given the needed equipment and a place to work, the student will perform this skill with _____ % accuracy in a total of _____ minutes. *(Your instructor will tell you what the percentage and time limits will be before you begin.)*

KEY: 4 = Satisfactory 0 = Unsatisfactory NA = This step is not counted

PROCEDURE STEPS	SELF	PARTNER	INSTRUCTOR
1. Be sure the totals from the previous day sheet are recorded in the column for previous totals	❏	❏	❏
2. Total the charge column and place that number in the proper blank	❏	❏	❏
3. Total the payment column and place that number in the proper blank	❏	❏	❏
4. Total the adjustment column and place that number in the proper blank	❏	❏	❏
5. Total the current balance column and place that number in the proper blank	❏	❏	❏
6. Total the previous balance column and place that number in the proper blank	❏	❏	❏
7. Take the grand total of the previous balances, add the grand total of the charges, and subtract the grand total of the payments and adjustments. This number must equal the grand total of the current balance	❏	❏	❏
8. If the numbers do not match, calculate your totals again, and continue looking for errors until the numbers match. This will prove that the day sheet is balanced, and there are no errors	❏	❏	❏
9. Record the totals of the columns in the proper space on the next day sheet. You will be prepared for balancing the new day sheet	❏	❏	❏
10. **ARF** After calculating the end-of-the-day totals on today's day sheet, it does not balance. What should you do?	❏	❏	❏

_____

_____

_____

_____

(continues)

PSY PROCEDURE 14-8 **Balance a Day Sheet** (continued)

CALCULATION

Total Possible Points: _____

Total Points Earned: _____ Multiplied by 100 = _____ Divided by Total Possible Points = _____ %

PASS **FAIL** **COMMENTS:**
❏ ❏

Student's signature _____ Date _____

Partner's signature _____ Date _____

Instructor's signature _____ Date _____

PSY PROCEDURE 14-9 — Complete a Bank Deposit Slip and Make a Deposit

Name: _____ **Date:** _____ **Time:** _____ **Grade:** _____

EQUIPMENT/SUPPLIES: Calculator with tape, currency, coins, checks for deposit, deposit slip, endorsement stamp, deposit envelope

STANDARDS: Given the needed equipment and a place to work, the student will perform this skill with ____ % accuracy in a total of ____ minutes. *(Your instructor will tell you what the percentage and time limits will be before you begin.)*

KEY: 4 = Satisfactory   0 = Unsatisfactory   NA = This step is not counted

PROCEDURE STEPS	SELF	PARTNER	INSTRUCTOR
1. Separate cash from checks	❑	❑	❑
2. Arrange bills face up and sort with the largest denomination on top	❑	❑	❑
3. Record the total in the cash block on the deposit slip	❑	❑	❑
4. Endorse the back of each check with "For Deposit Only"	❑	❑	❑
5. Record the amount of each check beside an identifying number on the deposit slip	❑	❑	❑
6. Total and record the amounts of checks in the total of checks line on the deposit slip	❑	❑	❑
7. Total and record the amount of cash and the amount of checks	❑	❑	❑
8. Record the total amount of the deposit in the office checkbook register	❑	❑	❑
9. Make a copy of both sides of the deposit slip for office records	❑	❑	❑
10. Place the cash, checks, and the completed deposit slip in an envelope or bank bag for transporting to the bank for deposit	❑	❑	❑

_____
_____
_____
_____

(continues)

PSY P R O C E D U R E 1 4 - 9   **Complete a Bank Deposit Slip and Make a Deposit** (continued)

CALCULATION

Total Possible Points: _____

Total Points Earned: _____ Multiplied by 100 = _____ Divided by Total Possible Points = _____ %

PASS   **FAIL**   **COMMENTS:**
  ❑   ❑

Student's signature _____   Date _____

Partner's signature _____   Date _____

Instructor's signature _____   Date _____

FSY PROCEDURE 14-10 **Reconcile a Bank Statement**

Name: _____ Date: _____ Time: _____ Grade: _____

EQUIPMENT/SUPPLIES: Simulated bank statement, reconciliation worksheet, calculator, pen

STANDARDS: Given the needed equipment and a place to work, the student will perform this skill with _____ % accuracy in a total of _____ minutes. *(Your instructor will tell you what the percentage and time limits will be before you begin.)*

KEY: 4 = Satisfactory 0 = Unsatisfactory NA = This step is not counted

PROCEDURE STEPS	SELF	PARTNER	INSTRUCTOR
1. Compare the opening balance on the new statement with the closing balance on the previous statement	❏	❏	❏
2. List the bank balance in the appropriate space on the reconciliation worksheet	❏	❏	❏
3. Compare the check entries on the statement with the entries in the check register	❏	❏	❏
4. List the amounts of checks without check marks (outstanding checks)	❏	❏	❏
5. Total outstanding checks	❏	❏	❏
6. Subtract from the checkbook balance items such as withdrawals, automatic payments, or service charges that appeared on the statement but not in the checkbook	❏	❏	❏
7. Add to the bank statement balance any deposits not shown on the bank statement	❏	❏	❏
8. Make sure the balance in the checkbook and the bank statement agree	❏	❏	❏

_____

_____

_____

_____

CALCULATION

Total Possible Points: _____

Total Points Earned: _____ Multiplied by 100 = _____ Divided by Total Possible Points = _____ %

PASS FAIL COMMENTS:
❏ ❏

Student's signature _____ Date _____

Partner's signature _____ Date _____

Instructor's signature _____ Date _____

PSY PROCEDURE 14-11   **Maintain a Petty Cash Account**

Name: _____ Date: _____ Time: _____ Grade: _____

EQUIPMENT/SUPPLIES: Cash box, play money, checkbook, simulated receipts, and/or vouchers representing expenditures

STANDARDS: Given the needed equipment and a place to work, the student will perform this skill with _____ % accuracy in a total of _____ minutes. *(Your instructor will tell you what the percentage and time limits will be before you begin.)*

KEY: 4 = Satisfactory   0 = Unsatisfactory   NA = This step is not counted

PROCEDURE STEPS	SELF	PARTNER	INSTRUCTOR
1. Count the money remaining in the box	❏	❏	❏
2. Total the amounts of all vouchers in the petty cash box and determine the amount of expenditures	❏	❏	❏
3. Subtract the amount of receipts from the original amount in petty cash, to equal the amount of cash remaining in the box	❏	❏	❏
4. Balance the cash against the receipts	❏	❏	❏
5. Write a check only for the amount that was used	❏	❏	❏
6. Record totals on the memo line of the check stub	❏	❏	❏
7. Sort and record all vouchers to the appropriate accounts	❏	❏	❏
8. File the list of vouchers and attached receipts	❏	❏	❏
9. Place cash in petty cash fund	❏	❏	❏
10. **AFF** A coworker asks to borrow money from petty cash for bus fare home. She promises to pay it back tomorrow. Explain how you would respond	❏	❏	❏

_____

_____

_____

_____

CALCULATION

Total Possible Points: _____

Total Points Earned: _____ Multiplied by 100 = _____ Divided by Total Possible Points = _____ %

PASS   FAIL   COMMENTS:
❏   ❏

Student's signature _____ Date _____

Partner's signature _____ Date _____

Instructor's signature _____ Date _____

PSY PROCEDURE 14-12 | **Write a Check**

Name: _____ **Date:** _____ **Time:** _____ **Grade:** _____

EQUIPMENT/SUPPLIES: Simulated page of checks from checkbook, scenario giving amount of check, check register

STANDARDS: Given the needed equipment and a place to work, the student will perform this skill with _____ % accuracy in a total of _____ minutes. *(Your instructor will tell you what the percentage and time limits will be before you begin.)*

KEY: 4 = Satisfactory   0 = Unsatisfactory   NA = This step is not counted

PROCEDURE STEPS	SELF	PARTNER	INSTRUCTOR
1. Fill out the check register with the following information: **a.** check number **b.** date **c.** payee information **d.** amount **e.** previous balance **f.** new balance	❏	❏	❏
2. Enter date on check	❏	❏	❏
3. Enter payee on check	❏	❏	❏
4. Enter the amount of check using numerals	❏	❏	❏
5. Write out the amount of the check beginning as far left as possible and make a straight line to fill in space between dollars and cents	❏	❏	❏
6. Record cents as a fraction with 100 as the denominator	❏	❏	❏
7. Obtain appropriate signature(s)	❏	❏	❏
8. Proofread for accuracy	❏	❏	❏

_____

_____

_____

_____

_____

CALCULATION

Total Possible Points: _____

Total Points Earned: _____ Multiplied by 100 = _____ Divided by Total Possible Points = _____ %

PASS **FAIL**   **COMMENTS:**
❏   ❏

Student's signature _____ Date _____

Partner's signature _____ Date _____

Instructor's signature _____ Date _____

WORK PRODUCT 1

Grade: _____

PROCESS A CREDIT BALANCE

Mr. Juan Rodriguez has switched to a different medical insurance company. His copay with his old carrier was $35 per visit. His new copay is $20 per visit. However, there was a billing oversight, and Mr. Rodriguez paid his old copay. Process Mr. Rodriguez's credit balance on the day sheet.

CREDITS

Date	Description	Charges	Payments	Adjust ments	Current Balance	Previous Balance	NAME

Totals This Page				
Totals Previous Page				
Month-To-Date Totals				

WORK PRODUCT 2

Grade: _____

PROCESS A REFUND

Mr. Rodriguez has a credit balance of $15 on his account. You need to mail him a refund check. Post this transaction on the day sheet.

Date	Description	Charges	Payments	Adjustments	Current Balance	Previous Balance	NAME

CREDITS (spanning Payments, Adjustments)

	Charges	Payments	Adjustments	Current Balance
Totals This Page				
Totals Previous Page				
Month-To-Date Totals				

WORK PRODUCT 3

Grade: _____

POST ADJUSTMENTS

Mr. Rodriguez visits your office for an x-ray of his knee. Your office normally charges $225 for a knee x-ray. However, your physician is a participating provider in Mr. Rodriguez's insurance carrier. His insurance pays your office only $175 for a knee x-ray. Post the proper adjustment on the day sheet.

CREDITS

Date	Description	Charges	Payments	Adjustments	Current Balance	Previous Balance	NAME

Totals This Page
Totals Previous Page
Month-To-Date Totals

WORK PRODUCT 4

Grade: _____

POST NSF CHECKS

You have just received a check that was returned for nonsufficient funds. The check was written by Martha Montgomery for $750. Post the proper information on the day sheet.

CREDITS

Date	Description	Charges	Payments	Adjust ments	Current Balance	Previous Balance	NAME

	Charges	Payments	Adjustments	Current Balance	Previous Balance
Totals This Page					
Totals Previous Page					
Month-To-Date Totals					

WORK PRODUCT 5

Grade: _____

POST COLLECTION AGENCY PAYMENTS

You receive a check for $787.50 and the following statement from your collection agency.
Jones & Jones Collections
Account:d. Larsen, MD

Debtor	Amount Collected	Fee	Balance
Martha Montgomery	$750.00	$187.50	$562.50
Johan Johansen	$300.00	$75.00	$225.00
		Total	$787.50

Post the payments to the day sheet.

CREDITS

Date	Description	Charges	Payments	Adjust ments	Current Balance	Previous Balance	NAME

Totals This Page				
Totals Previous Page				
Month-To-Date Totals				

WORK PRODUCT 6

Grade: _____

POSTING PAYMENTS FROM MEDICARE

On a blank day sheet provided, post the following Medicare payments. You will need to calculate the adjustments by subtracting the amount allowed from the amount charged. The patient's previous balance will be the amount charged back on the date of service.

Keep in mind that on an actual Medicare EOB, the CPT-4 codes would be used instead of OV, x-ray, etc.

MEDICARE EXPLANATION OF BENEFITS

Name	Charges	Date of Service	Amount Allowed	Amount Paid to Provider	Patient's Responsibility
Smith, John	OV 40.00	3-2-xx	18.00	14.40	3.60
Jones, Anne Total:	OV 100.00 Lab 50.00 150.00	3-2-xx	65.00 50.00 115.00	52.00 40.00 92.00	13.00 10.00 23.00
Stevens, Sally Total:	OV 150.00 X-ray 200.00 350.00	3-2-xx	120.00 160.00 280.00	96.00 128.00 224.00	24.00 32.00 56.00
Reynolds, Susan	Consult 300.00	3-2-xx	250.00	200.00	50.00

CREDITS

Date	Description	Charges	Payments	Adjustments	Current Balance	Previous Balance	NAME

Totals This Page
Totals Previous Page
Month-To-Date Totals

WORK PRODUCT 7

Grade: _____

PUTTING IT ALL TOGETHER

On a blank day sheet provided, complete 1–8.

Post the following transactions on the day sheet provided. Use today's date.

1. Stanley Gleber came in and paid $25.00 in cash on his account. His previous balance is $100.00

2. Lisa Moore sent a check in the mail for $100.00 to be paid on her account, which carries a balance of $500.00

3. Elaine Newman came in and handed you a check she received from Blue Cross Blue Shield for $700.00 to be paid on her account, which has a balance of $900.00. The explanation attached to the check indicates it is for surgery she had on 03/01/09. Your physician does NOT participate with Blue Cross Blue Shield. Post the payment with an appropriate description. Will there be an adjustment?

4. Madeline Bell saw the doctor and brings out an encounter form with a charge for an office visit at $50.00 and lab at $150.00. Post her charges. She does not pay today. Her previous balance was zero

5. Post the collection agency payment for John Simms. His account with a balance of $250.00 was turned over to Equifax on 03/01/12. They collected the entire amount. You receive a check from Equifax. They charge 30% of what they collect, so the check is for 200.00. His balance was not written off when turned over to Equifax, so his previous balance should be 250.00

6. Hazel Wilbourne paid her charges of $200.00 in full at her last visit. Now you receive a check from Aetna for that visit. The check is for $130.00. Your physician participates with this insurance company, which means he agrees to accept what they pay. In other words, you will not bill the patient for the difference. Post the check to Ms. Wilbourne's account

7. Ms. Wilbourne now has a credit balance. You will need to send her a check from the office account as a refund. Post the appropriate entry for this transaction. In accounting, a credit balance is put in angle brackets: <200.00>

8. Calculate and record each column total. Make sure the columns balance by starting with your previous balance, adding the charges, subtracting the payments and adjustments, and this should give you the total of your current balance column. Remember, brackets in accounting mean that you do the opposite when adding your columns, so instead of adding a credit balance when totaling, you will subtract it

CREDITS

Date	Description	Charges	Payments	Adjust ments	Current Balance	Previous Balance	NAME

Totals This Page				
Totals Previous Page				
Month-To-Date Totals				

WORK PRODUCT 8

Grade: _____

PREPARE A BANK DEPOSIT

Prepare a bank deposit for the following:

- Check for $750 from Martin Montgomery.
- Check for $35 from Rita Gonzalez.
- $125 cash

Use fictitious demographic information for the account holder on the deposit slip.

	ITEMS DEPOSITED	DOLLARS	CENTS
Newtown Bank, N.A. **DEPOSIT**	Currency		.
	Coin		.
Name and account number will be verified when presented.	Checks 1		.
Name	Date	2		.
Address	3		.
	4		.
	Sub Total		.
Signature	Sign here only if cash is received from deposit	Less Cash		.
Store Number (Commercial Accounts Only)	Account Number (For CAP Accounts, use 10-digit number.)	Total Deposit	
*	*	$	.

CHAPTER 15

Credit and Collections

LEARNING OUTCOMES

OOG Cognitive Domain*

1. Spell and define the key terms
2. Discuss types of physician's fee schedules
3. *Identify precautions for accepting the following types of payments:*
   a. *Cash*
   b. *Check*
   c. *Credit card*
   d. *Debit card*
4. Identify types of information contained in the patient's billing record
5. Discuss the legal implications of credit collection
6. *Identify patient financial obligations for services rendered*
7. *Identify processes for claim tracking and claim denials*
8. Describe the impact of both the Fair Debt Collection Act and the Federal Truth in Lending Act of 1968 as they apply to collections
9. Describe the concept of RBRVS
10. Describe the implications of HIPAA for the medical assistant in various medical settings
11. Discuss all levels of government legislation and regulation as they apply to medical assisting practice, including FDA and DEA regulations

PSY Psychomotor Domain*

1. Evaluate and manage a patient account (Procedure 15-1)
2. *Inform a patient of financial obligations for services rendered* (Procedure 15-1)
3. Write a collection letter (Procedure 15-2)

AFF Affective Domain*

1. *Demonstrate tactfulness when requesting payment for services rendered*
2. Recognize the importance of local, state, and federal legislation and regulations in the practice setting

MAERB Standards are italicized.

ABHES Competencies

1. Perform billing and collection procedures
2. Assist the physician in navigating issues and concerns that may arise in medical bills
3. Demonstrate professional behavior

Name: _____ Date: _____ Grade: _____

COG MULTIPLE CHOICE

1. The total of all of the charges posted to patients' accounts for the month of May is $16,000. The revenues the practice earned for May total $12,000. What is the collection percentage for May?
   a. 5%
   b. 25%
   c. 75%
   d. 80%
   e. 133%

2. Interest that may be charged to a patient account is determined by:
   a. the physician.
   b. the patient.
   c. the insurance company.
   d. the law.
   e. the state.

3. In the UCR concept, the letters stand for:
   a. user, customer, and regulation.
   b. usual, competitive, and regular.
   c. usage, consumption, and return.
   d. usual, customary, and reasonable.
   e. usage, complaint, and rationale.

4. When credit cards are accepted by a medical practice, the medical practice generally agrees to pay the credit card company:
   a. nothing—it is a benefit of allowing payments to be made using their credit card.
   b. a small percentage of the overall charge amount.
   c. their usual interest rate charged for credit cards.
   d. an amount that is agreed upon between the patient and the credit card company.
   e. 25%.

5. Federal regulations require each medical office to describe its services and procedures and to give the procedure codes and prices by:
   a. giving a list to each patient at check in.
   b. offering the list to each patient at payment.
   c. posting a sign stating that a list is available.
   d. answering a patient's questions about billing.
   e. placing an ad in the newspaper describing the fees.

6. Physicians who chose to become participating providers with third-party payers usually do so in order to:
   a. charge higher fees.
   b. simplify fee schedules.
   c. build a solid patient base.
   d. reduce the time before payment.
   e. share a patient load with another physician.

7. It is a good and ethical business practice to:
   a. take payment in cash only.
   b. accept only patients who have insurance.
   c. refuse patients who have third-party payment plans.
   d. discuss fees with patients before they see a physician.
   e. charge the patient a small fee for paying with a credit card.

8. When dealing with a new patient, you should avoid:
   a. taking cash.
   b. taking a partial payment.
   c. taking a check with two picture IDs.
   d. taking copayment with an insurance card.
   e. taking a payment by credit card.

9. Most fees for medical services:
   a. are paid by insurance companies.
   b. are paid by Medicare and Medicaid.
   c. are paid by patients who are private payers.
   d. are written off on the practice's federal taxes.
   e. are paid to the physician late.

10. When an insurance adjustment is made to a fee:
    a. the patient is charged less than the normal rate.
    b. the medical office receives more than its normal rate.
    c. the insurance carrier pays the adjustment rate.
    d. the insurance carrier's explanation of benefits shows how much the office may collect for the service.
    e. the difference between the physician's normal fee and the insurance carrier's allowed fee is written off.

11. Why would a medical office extend credit to a patient?
    a. To save money
    b. To accommodate the patient
    c. To postpone paying income tax
    d. To charge interest
    e. To make billing more cost-effective

12. Why do many medical offices outsource their credit and billing functions?
    a. They don't want to ask their patients for money directly
    b. They are not licensed to manage credit card transactions
    c. Creating their own installment plans is too complicated legally
    d. Managing patient accounts themselves costs about $5 per month per patient
    e. Billing companies can manage the accounts more cost-effectively

13. It is illegal for a medical office to:
    a. use a collection agency.
    b. disclose fee information to patients who have insurance.
    c. deny credit to patients because they receive public assistance.
    d. charge patients interest, finance charges, or late fees on unpaid balances
    e. change their established billing cycle.

14. If you are attempting to collect a debt from a patient, you must:
    a. use reasonable self-restraint.
    b. call the patient only at home.
    c. hire a licensed bill collection agency.
    d. first take the patient to small claims court.
    e. wait one year before you can ask for payment.

15. When first attempting to collect a debt by telephone, you should:
    a. ask the patient to come in for a checkup.
    b. contact the patient before 8:00 AM or after 9:00 PM.
    c. contact the patient only at his place of employment.
    d. leave a message explaining the situation on the answering machine.
    e. speak only to the patient or leave only your first name and number.

16. When you are collecting a debt from an estate, it is best to:
    a. send a final bill to the estate's executor.
    b. take the matter directly to small claims court.
    c. try to collect within a week of the patient's death.
    d. allow the family a month to mourn before asking for payment.
    e. ask a collection agency to contact the family.

17. If a billing cycle is to be changed, you are legally required to notify patients:
    a. 1 month before their payment is due.
    b. before the next scheduled appointment.
    c. 3 months prior to the billing change.
    d. after you approve the change with the insurance company.
    e. only if they have outstanding payments.

18. When you age an account, you:
    a. write off debts that have been outstanding longer than 120 days.
    b. send bills first to the patients who had the most recent procedures.
    c. organize patient accounts by how long they have been seeing the physician.
    d. calculate the time between the last bill and the date of the last payment.
    e. determine the time between the initial statement and the date of the last payment.

19. A cancellation of an unpaid debt is called a(n):
    a. professional courtesy.
    b. copayment.
    c. write-off.
    d. adjustment.
    e. credit.

20. Which collections method takes the least staff time?
    a. Using a collection agency
    b. Going to small claims court
    c. Billing the patient monthly until paid
    d. Scheduling all payments on the first of the month
    e. Reporting patients to the credit bureaus

⁢OG MATCHING

Grade: _____

Match the following key terms to their definitions.

Key Terms

21. _____ Adjustment
22. _____ Aging schedule
23. _____ Collections
24. _____ Credit
25. _____ Installment
26. _____ Participating provider
27. _____ Patient copayment
28. _____ Professional courtesy
29. _____ Write-off

Definitions

a. Change in a posted account
b. Balance in one's favor on an account
c. Process of seeking payment for overdue bills
d. Arrangement for a patient to pay on an installment plan
e. Charging other healthcare professionals a reduced rate
f. Cancellation of an unpaid debt
g. A certain share of the bill that a managed care company usually requires the patient to pay
h. Physician who agrees to participate with managed care companies and other third-party payers
i. Record of a patient's name, balance, payments made, time of outstanding debt, and relevant comments

⁢OG SHORT ANSWER

Grade: _____

30. Fee setting also considers RBRVS, by which fees are adjusted for geographic differences. What does RBRVS stand for?

_____

_____

_____

_____

31. There should be a sign posted in the office, where patients can see it, giving information about procedure fees. What should be on the sign?

_____

_____

_____

_____

32. Which third-party payers affect fee schedules if the physicians in your office are participating providers, and how many fee schedules might there be?

_____

_____

_____

_____

33. How many times should you contact patients asking them to pay overdue bills? Why?

_____

_____

_____

_____

34. How often should you ask the patient for their insurance card, and what should you do with it when you get it?

_____

_____

_____

_____

35. What are the three most common ways of collecting overdue accounts?

_____

_____

_____

_____

36. What are some of the negative aspects of extending credit to patients? Consider costs, patient attitudes, and legal requirements in your answer.

_____

_____

_____

_____

COG ACTIVE LEARNING
Grade: _____

37. Use the Internet to research the three major credit bureaus and find out how to check a new patient's credit history. Specifically, find out what's available to help you decide how to handle payment from people without traditional credit histories. This group includes college students, young adults, recent immigrants, traditional housewives, and people who choose not to use credit cards.

38. Many people feel uncomfortable asking other people for money. However, you need to feel comfortable discussing finance and account information with patients. Working with a partner, role-play a scenario in which a patient has an overdue account that the medical assistant must address. Take turns playing the parts of the medical assistant and the patient to understand both perspectives.

39. In recent years, the government has called into question the practice of professional courtesy extended to other healthcare professionals. Perform research online or talk to healthcare professionals to find out more about the issues surrounding professional courtesy. Then, write a viewpoint paper arguing for or against the practice of professional courtesy.

COG FALSE THEN TRUE
Grade: _____

40. All the statements below are false or inaccurate. Rewrite each statement so that it accurately reflects the consumer protection laws regarding credit collection.

a. You cannot contact a patient directly about an unpaid bill.

_____

b. You should not try to contact a debtor before 9:00 am or after 5:00 pm.

_____

c. You have every right to call debtors at work.

_____

d. You should keep calling a patient about a debt after turning the case over to a collection agency, in order to increase your chances of recovering the money.

_____

e. It's okay to use abusive language to intimidate a debtor, as long as you don't give false or misleading information.

_____

f. If a patient dies and the estate can't meet all of their debts, the probate court will pay the medical bills first.

_____

COG SHORT ANSWER

Grade: _____

41. List three situations in which calling a patient to collect an overdue payment may be least helpful.

_____

_____

_____

_____

42. What should be in a mailing that asks a patient to settle an overdue account?

_____

_____

_____

_____

43. What is a good way to use a patient's visit as an opportunity to try to collect payment on an overdue bill?

_____

_____

_____

_____

44. What should you say and not say if you call a patient to collect on a bill and you are asked to leave a message?

_____

_____

_____

_____

COG TRUE OR FALSE?

Grade: _____

45. Determine whether the following statements are true or false. If false, explain why.

a. A physician's fee schedule takes into consideration the costs of operating the office, such as rent, utilities, malpractice insurance, and salaries.

_____

b. If a patient has insurance, you must charge him the insurance carrier's allowed fee for a procedure.

_____

c. To maintain good relations with patients, you should be vague and polite when you ask them to pay their bills.

_____

d. You should monitor the activity on a patient's credit account in order to keep the collection ratio low.

_____

PSY AFF WHAT WOULD YOU DO?

Grade: _____

46. You have several patients who have long-standing debts. They don't come into the office anymore, and they don't respond to your telephone calls or letters. You outsourced your overdue billing to a collections agency, but these longtime patients have told you that they have been very upset by the "nastiness" of the collections people who contacted them.

You spoke with a collections agency representative who assured you his employees were doing nothing illegal or inappropriate. You have considered changing collection agencies, but this one's rates are better, and they did collect the debts. What would you do?

_____

_____

_____

_____

47. Mrs. Sanchez is seeing Dr. Roland for the first time and has asked you to explain the physician's fees. How would you explain to Mrs. Sanchez how Dr. Roland establishes the fees he charges his patients?

_____

_____

_____

_____

AFF CASE STUDIES FOR CRITICAL THINKING

Grade: _____

Mr. Green has been a patient with your practice for more than 20 years and has always paid his copayment or bill before he left the office. Recently, however, he has not been paying anything at all, and his outstanding bill is 60 days past due. You have called his home and left several phone messages, but you still haven't heard from him.

48. What should you do? Circle all appropriate actions from the following list.

    a. Send him a letter demanding that he pay his balance immediately

    b. Flag his account for the credit manager to speak with him about his bill when he comes in for a visit

    c. Send a letter asking him to please call the office. State in the letter that you are worried about him

    d. Flag his record to warn anyone making an appointment for him that he is not to be seen until he pays on his bill

    e. Terminate the physician–patient contract in writing

49. A coworker tells you that the patient is very rich. She says that he is just getting old and can't keep up with his bills any longer. Circle all appropriate actions in the list below.

    a. Tell the coworker to mind her own business

    b. Do not consider this gossip in your dealings with the patient

    c. Contact the patient's next of kin and tell them that he needs help

    d. Send the patient a letter telling him you know he has the funds to pay his bill

    e. Do nothing until you reach the patient

    f. Do not mention this new information when you do speak with him

PROCEDURE 15-1 | Evaluate and Manage a Patient's Account

PSY

Name: _____ Date: _____ Time: _____ Grade: _____

EQUIPMENT: Simulation including scenario; sample patient ledger card with transactions; yellow, blue, and red stickers (yellow for accounts 30 days past due; blue for accounts 60 days past due; red for accounts 90 days past due). See Work Product 1.

STANDARDS: Given the needed equipment and a place to work, the student will perform this skill with _____ % accuracy in a total of _____ minutes. *(Your instructor will tell you what the percentage and time limits will be before you begin.)*

KEY: 4 = Satisfactory 0 = Unsatisfactory NA = This step is not counted

PROCEDURE STEPS	SELF	PARTNER	INSTRUCTOR
1. Review the patient's account history to determine the "age" of the account. If payment has not been made between 30 and 59 days from today's date, the account is 40 days past due, and so on	❑	❑	❑
2. Flag the account for appropriate action. Place a yellow flag (sticker) on accounts that are 30 days old. Place a blue flag on accounts that are 60 days old. Place a red flag on accounts that are 90 days old	❑	❑	❑
3. Set aside accounts that have had no payment in 91 days or longer	❑	❑	❑
4. Sort the copies by category: 30, 60, 90 days	❑	❑	❑
5. Write or stamp the copies with the appropriate message	❑	❑	❑
6. Mail the statements to the patients	❑	❑	❑
7. Follow through with the collection process by continually reviewing past due accounts	❑	❑	❑
8. When you call a patient with a seriously past due account, he informs you that he has not paid because his wife passed away and he can hardly get through the day. Explain how you would respond	❑	❑	❑

_____

_____

_____

_____

(continues)

PSY PROCEDURE 15-1 **Evaluate and Manage a Patient's Account** (continued)

CALCULATION

Total Possible Points: _____

Total Points Earned: _____ Multiplied by 100 = _____ Divided by Total Possible Points = _____ %

PASS **FAIL** **COMMENTS:**

❏ ❏

Student's signature _____ Date _____

Partner's signature _____ Date _____

Instructor's signature _____ Date _____

PSY PROCEDURE 15-2 **Composing a Collection Letter**

Name: _____ Date: _____ Time: _____ Grade: _____

EQUIPMENT: Ledger cards generated in Procedure 15-1, word processor, and stationery with letterhead.

STANDARDS: Given the needed equipment and a place to work, the student will perform this skill with _____ % accuracy in a total of _____ minutes. *(Your instructor will tell you what the percentage and time limits will be before you begin.)*

KEY: 4 = Satisfactory 0 = Unsatisfactory NA = This step is not counted

PROCEDURE STEPS	SELF	PARTNER	INSTRUCTOR
1. Review the patients' accounts and sort the accounts by age	❏	❏	❏
2. Design a rough draft of a form letter that can be used for collections	❏	❏	❏
3. In the first paragraph, tell the patient why you are writing	❏	❏	❏
4. Inform the patient of the action you expect. For example: "To avoid further action, please pay $50.00 on this account by Friday, May 1, 20 _____	❏	❏	❏
5. Proofread the rough draft for errors, clarity, accuracy, and retype	❏	❏	❏
6. Take the collection letter to a supervisor or physician for approval	❏	❏	❏
7. Fill in the appropriate amounts and dates on each letter. Ask for at least half of the account balance within a 2-week period	❏	❏	❏
8. Print, sign, and mail the letter	❏	❏	❏
9. You are helping a coworker get her collections letters in the mail. You notice several errors in the letters. Explain how you would respond	❏	❏	❏

_____

_____

_____

_____

_____

CALCULATION

Total Possible Points: _____

Total Points Earned: _____ Multiplied by 100 = _____ Divided by Total Possible Points = _____ %

PASS **FAIL** **COMMENTS:**
❏   ❏

Student's signature _____ Date _____

Partner's signature _____ Date _____

Instructor's signature _____ Date _____

WORK PRODUCT 1

Grade: _____

Perform Accounts Receivable Procedures

Your office's billing cycle posts bills on the first of every month. Review the list of outstanding payments and organize in the Aging of Accounts Receivable Report below.

- Oliver Santino visited the office on April 27 for a physical and blood work. The bill was $250.
- Warren Gates visited the office on May 8. His bill was $55.
- Tamara Jones visited the office on June 18 for a physical examination. The cost for the physical was $125, with an additional $55 for lab work.
- Amir Shell visited the office on June 25 for a physical exam and chest x-rays. The bill was $315.
- Nora Stevenson visited the office on July 9 to have a wound sutured. The bill was $100.

Below is an aging schedule as of August 30, 2012. Fill in the information for these patients. You may enter an account number of 000-00-0000 for all patients.

Aging of Accounts Receivable Report: August 30, 2012

Patient Name	Account Number	Due Date	Amount

Accounts 30 Days Past Due:

Accounts 60 Days Past Due:

Accounts 90 Days Past Due:

Accounts 120 Days or More Past Due:

Total Overdue Accounts Receivable _____

WORK PRODUCT 2

Grade: _____

Perform Billing and Collection Procedures

Caroline Cusick has an outstanding balance of $415 due to the medical office Pediatric Associates, 1415 San Juan Way, Santa Cruz, CA 95060. Write a collection letter to the patient to tell her about her overdue account. Her contact information is as follows: Caroline Cusick, 24 Beach Street, Santa Cruz, CA 95060. Print the letter and attach to this sheet.

PART 3

The Clinical Medical Assistant

UNIT FOUR

Fundamentals of Clinical Medical Assisting

CHAPTER 16

Nutrition and Wellness

LEARNING OUTCOMES

COG Cognitive Domain*

1. Spell and define the key terms
2. *Identify body systems* (Digestive)
3. *Describe the normal function of body organs.*
4. *Identify normal and abnormal results as reported in graphs and/ or tables (BMI)*
5. *Identify dietary nutrients including carbohydrates, fats, proteins, minerals, electrolytes, vitamins, fiber, and water.*
6. *Identify the components of a food label*
7. *Identify the special dietary needs for weight control, cardiovascular disease, hypertension, cancer, lactose sensitivity, gluten free, food allergies, eating disorders*
8. *Identify the function of dietary supplements*
9. List the components of physical fitness
10. Discuss suggestions for a healthy lifestyle
11. Explain the importance of disease prevention
12. List and describe the effects of the substances most commonly abused
13. Recognize the dangers of substance abuse

PSY Psychomotor Domain*

1. Teach a patient how to read food labels (Procedure 16-1)
2. Document patient care accurately in the medical record
3. Develop a meal plan utilizing the basic principles of nutrition (Procedure 16-2)
4. *Instruct a patient according to the patient's special dietary needs (Procedure 16-2)*
5. *Coach patients regarding medical encounters*

AFF Affective Domain*

1. *Demonstrate critical thinking skills*

2. *Protect the integrity of the medical record*
3. *Demonstrate empathy for patient concerns and active listening skills*
4. *Recognize personal boundaries*
5. *Demonstrate respect for individual diversity*
6. *Demonstrate tactfulness and self-awareness*

*MAERB Standards are italicized.

ABHES Competencies

1. Explain the importance of diet and nutrition
2. Educate patients regarding the proper diet and nutrition guidelines
3. Identify categories of patients who require special diets or diet modifications
4. Follow documentation guidelines
5. Partner with healthcare teams to attain optimal patient health outcomes

Name: _____   Date: _____   Grade: _____

COG MULTIPLE CHOICE

Circle the letter preceding the correct answer.

1. The nutrient that cushions and protects body organs and sustains normal body temperature is:
   a. carbohydrate.
   b. fat.
   c. mineral.
   d. protein.
   e. vitamin.

2. The purpose of a therapeutic diet is to:
   a. treat an underlying condition or disease.
   b. enjoy foods that put a person in a good mood.
   c. experiment with foods not normally allowed on other diets.
   d. eat foods the person likes but only in moderation.
   e. replace medications.

3. Which of the following is true about the effects of drugs or alcohol on a developing fetus?
   a. They have no effect on the developing fetus
   b. They could cause the baby to be addicted to the substance after birth
   c. Drugs could cause the brain to stop developing, but alcohol has no effect
   d. They can harm the fetus only if the mother harms herself while using them
   e. They could make the fetus hyper in the womb but cause no long-term effects after birth

4. Which of the following statements about cholesterol are true?
   a. A diet high in fat but low in cholesterol is healthy
   b. Cholesterol is found only in animal products
   c. Cholesterol is found in fresh fruits and vegetables
   d. Since the body cannot produce cholesterol, it must be a part of the diet
   e. Adults should consume at least 350 mg of dietary cholesterol each day

5. Which of the following would leave a person vulnerable to disease?
   a. Keeping your immunizations up-to-date
   b. Washing your hands after using the bathroom
   c. Wearing insect repellent when outside in the summer
   d. Using someone else's antibiotics because they didn't finish them
   e. Washing cutting boards with soap and water after cutting uncooked chicken

6. Although alcohol intoxication may give a person a euphoric feeling, alcohol is a depressant. What does that mean?
   a. It gives the person a sad and gloomy feeling
   b. It causes the person to suffer from depression
   c. It causes increased heart rate and sleeplessness
   d. It speeds up the functioning of the central nervous system
   e. It causes a lack of coordination and impaired brain function

7. The following statement about exercise is true:
   a. It induces stress
   b. It suppresses the production of endorphins
   c. It is effective if done for at least 40 minutes
   d. It reduces the risk of developing certain diseases
   e. Aerobic activities are most effective before the target heart rate is reached

8. Basal metabolic rate is:
   a. the constructive phase of metabolism.
   b. the destructive phase of metabolism.
   c. the baseline metabolic rate that is considered normal for the average adult.
   d. the amount of energy used in a unit of time to maintain vital functions by a fasting, resting person.
   e. the combination of the calories a person can consume and how long it takes to burn those calories.

9. A person who follows a lacto-ovo vegetarian diet eats:
   a. vegetables only.
   b. vegetables and milk and cheese.
   c. vegetables and milk, eggs, and cheese.
   d. vegetables and milk, eggs, and poultry.
   e. vegetables and milk, eggs, and seafood.

10. Which of the following foods is a good source of fiber?
    a. Fish
    b. Milk
    c. Butter
    d. Chicken
    e. Vegetables

11. The five basic food groups include:
    a. dairy, vitamins, produce, meat, and grains.
    b. carbohydrates, fiber, vegetables, fruits, and meat.
    c. oils, lipids, refined sugars, whole grains, and dairy.
    d. grains, vegetables, milk, fruits, and meat and beans.
    e. proteins, carbohydrates, lipids, cholesterol, and minerals.

12. An overweight teenager asks you to suggest a cardiovascular exercise. Which of the following could you suggest?
    a. Yoga
    b. Sit-ups
    c. Stretching
    d. Lifting weights
    e. Jumping rope

13. Which vitamin is important for pregnant women because it reduces the risk of neural tube defects?
    a. Calcium
    b. Folate
    c. Mercury
    d. Potassium
    e. Zinc

14. To determine the correct number of daily servings from each food group, you need to know your:
    a. resting heart rate.
    b. height and weight.
    c. age and gender.
    d. waist measurement and target heart rate.
    e. level of physical activity and blood type.

15. How are refined grains different from whole grains?
    a. Refined grains are full of fiber
    b. Whole grains lack fiber and iron
    c. Whole grains are made with the entire grain kernel
    d. Refined grains contain nutrients like carbohydrates and proteins
    e. Refined grains are darker in color because they have more nutrients

16. Water-soluble vitamins should be consumed:
    a. once a week.
    b. once a month.
    c. twice a week.
    d. daily.
    e. twice a month.

17. Pregnant women are advised to eat no more than one can of tuna per week because of the:
    a. iron content.
    b. lead content.
    c. mercury content.
    d. zinc content.
    e. calcium content.

18. How are substances such as cocaine and marijuana different from alcohol and nicotine?
    a. Alcohol and nicotine are legal; marijuana and cocaine are illegal.
    b. Cocaine and marijuana will not cause sudden death; alcohol and nicotine will cause sudden death.
    c. Alcohol and nicotine do not harm the body; marijuana and cocaine do harm the body.
    d. Cocaine and marijuana are used by people with health problems; alcohol and nicotine are not.
    e. Alcohol and nicotine are not addictive drugs; marijuana and cocaine are addictive drugs.

19. Which of the following drugs damages blood vessels, decreases heart strength, and causes several types of cancer?
    a. Caffeine
    b. Nicotine
    c. Hashish
    d. Mescaline
    e. Phencyclidine

20. Why does inhaling marijuana smoke cause more damage to a person's body than tobacco smoke?
    a. Marijuana smoke is inhaled as unfiltered smoke, so users take in more cancer-causing agents and do more damage to the respiratory system than regular filtered tobacco smoke
    b. Marijuana smoke is thicker and more odorous
    c. Marijuana smoke is inhaled as filtered smoke, so users take in fewer cancer-causing agents and do more damage to the respiratory system than with regular filtered tobacco smoke
    d. Marijuana smoke is inhaled more quickly than tobacco smoke
    e. Marijuana plants are grown in more toxic environments than tobacco plants

COG MATCHING

Grade: _____

Match the essential nutrient with its description by placing the letter preceding the description of its function on the line next to the name of the nutrient.

Nutrients

21. _____ carbohydrates
22. _____ proteins
23. _____ fats
24. _____ vitamins
25. _____ minerals

Definitions

a. cushion and protect body organs and sustain normal body temperature
b. chemical substances that provide the body with energy
c. inorganic substances used in the formation of hard and soft body tissue
d. organic substances that enhance the breakdown of other nutrients in the body
e. substances that contain amino acids and help to build and repair tissue

COG MATCHING

Grade: _____

Match the following terms to the correct definitions. Place the letter preceding the term on the line next to the sentence that best describes its definition.

Key Terms

26. _____ anabolism
27. _____ anencephaly
28. _____ basal metabolic rate
29. _____ body mass index
30. _____ calorie
31. _____ catabolism
32. _____ dental cavities
33. _____ endorphins
34. _____ essential amino acids
35. _____ euphoria
36. _____ homeostasis
37. _____ metabolism
38. _____ minerals
39. _____ spina bifida
40. _____ lipoprotein

Definitions

a. inorganic substances used in the formation of hard and soft body tissue
b. a process in which larger molecules break down into smaller molecules
c. a neural tube defect that causes an incomplete closure of a fetus' spine during early pregnancy
d. a neural tube defect that affects the fetus' brain during early pregnancy
e. a good feeling
f. maintaining a constant internal environment by balancing positive and negative feedback
g. a process in which smaller molecules are converted into larger molecules as food is absorbed into the bloodstream
h. the amount of energy used in a unit of time to maintain vital function by a fasting, resting subject
i. transports cholesterol between the liver and arterial walls
j. the sum of chemical processes that result in growth, energy production, elimination of waste, and body functions performed as digested nutrients are distributed
k. areas of decay in the teeth
l. a pain-relieving substance released naturally from the brain
m. an individual's ratio of fat to lean body mass
n. proteins that come from your diet because the body does not produce them
o. the amount of energy used by the body

COG IDENTIFICATION

Grade: _____

41. Indicate whether the following vitamins are fat-soluble or water-soluble by writing FS (fat-soluble) or WS (water-soluble) on the line preceding the name of the vitamin.

   a. _____ Vitamin A
   b. _____ Vitamin B complex
   c. _____ Vitamin C
   d. _____ Vitamin D
   e. _____ Vitamin E
   f. _____ Vitamin K
   g. _____ Thiamin
   h. _____ Riboflavin
   i. _____ Niacin
   j. _____ Folic acid

cog COMPLETION

Grade: _____

42. Calculate the maximum heart rate and target heart rate for the individuals below based on their ages and desired intensity.

Person	Age	Maximum Heart Rate	Desired Intensity	Target Heart Rate
a. Tara	25		80%	
b. Yolanda	45		65%	
c. Hillel	37		75%	
d. Marco	18		90%	

43. Review the MyPlate diagram in your textbook and answer the following questions:

a. How much food from the grains category should be eaten in a day? _____

b. How many vegetables should be eaten in a day? _____

c. How much fruit should be eaten in a day? _____

d. How much milk should be consumed in a day? _____

e. How much from the meat and beans category should be consumed in a day? _____

44. Answer the following questions based on the food label (Figure 16-4) in your textbook.

a. How many servings are in this can of vegetables? _____

b. What is the serving size? _____

c. How many calories are from fat per serving? _____

d. What is the least amount of sugar you would consume if you ate one cup of this vegetable? _____

e. What is the percentage of sodium in one serving? _____

cog SHORT ANSWER

Grade: _____

45. Explain what BMI stands for and describe how it is calculated.

_____

_____

_____

_____

46. Explain the three basic ways the body expends energy.

a. Basal metabolic rate:

_____

_____

_____

_____

b. Levels of physical activity:

_____

_____

_____

_____

c. Thermic effect of food:

_____

_____

_____

_____

47. What is the best defense against illness?

_____

_____

_____

_____

48. List three techniques that can help lessen stress.

_____

_____

_____

_____

49. Drugs can be classified as stimulants and/or depressants that cause various effects on the body. Read each symptom below and place a check in the appropriate column.

Symptom	Depressant	Stimulant	Both
a. Poor fetal health			
b. Increased heart rate			
c. Psychological and physical dependence			
d. Increased pulse rate			
e. Slow respiratory rate			
f. Sleeplessness and anxiety			
g. Decreased activities of the central nervous system			

50. There are two phases in the process of metabolism: anabolism and catabolism. Indicate on the line provided whether the statement about metabolism describes anabolism (A) or catabolism (C).

a. _____ Constructive phase

b. _____ Amino acids are converted into proteins

c. _____ Destructive phase

d. _____ Smaller molecules are converted into larger molecules

e. _____ Larger molecules are converted into smaller molecules

f. _____ Break down fats to use for energy

g. _____ Complex carbohydrates, such as starch, are converted into simple sugars

51. Look at the list of foods and indicate on the line whether the food contains good fat (G) or bad fat (B). Place the letter G on the line if the item is "good" and B if the item is "bad."

a. _____ Salmon

b. _____ Olive oil

c. _____ Hamburger

d. _____ Margarine

e. _____ Crackers

f. _____ Soybean oil

g. _____ Nuts

h. _____ Cookies

i. _____ Steak

j. _____ Sunflower oil

COG AFF CASE STUDIES FOR CRITICAL THINKING

Grade: _____

52. While conducting a patient interview, your patient, a 20-year-old college student, is concerned about gaining weight. She says she eats the same foods as her roommate, but her roommate does not gain weight, and she has put on 25 pounds since starting school. The roommate has told your patient that she can eat more food because she has a "high" metabolism rate. The patient is not sure what this means. How will you answer your patient? Would you recommend a reduced fat and/or calorie diet? Why or why not?

_____

_____

_____

_____

53. When educating a patient on the difference between whole grains and refined grains, what would you tell your patient?

_____

_____

_____

_____

54. Mr. Consuelo is the president of a large manufacturing company. He is seeing Dr. Smith for frequent headaches. Dr. Smith has diagnosed the headaches as stress-induced and has recommended that Mr. Consuelo develop some coping mechanisms to reduce the stress in his life. As Mr. Consuelo leaves the office, he asks you about ways he can comply with Dr. Smith's recommendation to decrease the stress in his life. What strategies can you offer this patient?

_____

_____

_____

_____

55. Marco is 53 years old and has been smoking since he was 13. He says he would like to try and quit smoking, but he doesn't think it's worth it because the damage is probably already done. What would you say to him?

_____

_____

_____

_____

56. The physician asks you to explain the DASH diet to a patient with high blood pressure. How would you explain this diet including the basic dietary guidelines to a patient who speaks very little English?

_____

_____

_____

_____

57. Angelo, a 22-year-old man, comes to the office for a checkup. While interviewing him, he tells you that he drinks a lot on the weekends, but it's "no big deal." What three things could you say to Angelo that may help him understand that excessive alcohol is a big deal?

_____

_____

_____

_____

58. Dr. Mercer has given Joe, an overweight patient, clearance to start exercising. He told him to include workouts that will target each of the components of physical fitness. Joe feels overwhelmed. When talking to Joe, describe how you would explain the three components of physical fitness and how each one will help his body and health.

_____

_____

_____

_____

59. Your patient Carolyn is working with a nutritionist to improve her health. The nutritionist told her it is okay to take vitamins C and B every day; however, she indicated that Carolyn should not take vitamin E every day. During her office visit, Carolyn asks you why she should not take vitamin E every day because she thought it was necessary to take all vitamins every day. What would you say to Carolyn?

_____

_____

_____

_____

60. A patient is upset because he has been placed on a special therapeutic diet because of his high blood pressure. He doesn't understand why he needs to stop eating some of his favorite foods, and he is worried he will not be successful in changing his diet. How can you encourage him to follow the physician's order to improve his health?

_____

_____

_____

_____

61. Your 17-year-old patient comes into the physician's office because he has a bad cough. This is the second time this winter that he has seen the physician for respiratory problems. When you review the patient's chart, you see that he had asthma when he was younger. You ask the patient if he smokes and he says that he does occasionally with his friends but also indicates that he is "not a smoker" because he's not addicted to nicotine. He also notes that he would prefer that his parents not know that he smokes, even occasionally. What should you say to this patient about his breathing issues? Would it be appropriate to tell his parents? Why or why not?

_____

_____

_____

_____

PSY PROCEDURE 16-1 | **Teach a Patient How to Read Food Labels**

Name: _____ Date: _____ Time: _____ Grade: _____

EQUIPMENT/SUPPLIES: Two boxes of the same item, one low calorie or "lite," the other regular; measuring cup; two bowls

STANDARDS: Given the needed equipment and a place to work, the student will perform this skill with _____ % accuracy in a total of _____ minutes. *(Your instructor will tell you what the percentage and time limits will be before you begin.)*

KEY: 4 = Satisfactory 0 = Unsatisfactory NA = This step is not counted

PROCEDURE STEPS	SELF	PARTNER	INSTRUCTOR
1. Identify the patient	❏	❏	❏
2. Introduce yourself and explain the procedure, including the rationale	❏	❏	❏
3. Have the patient look at the labels comparing the two food items	❏	❏	❏
4. Ask the patient to pour out a normal serving	❏	❏	❏
5. Measure the exact serving size printed on the label	❏	❏	❏
6. Compare the two. Discuss the difference, if any	❏	❏	❏
7. Explain to the patient the sections of the label: serving size and servings per package	❏	❏	❏
8. Explain the column for the amount in serving	❏	❏	❏
9. Explain the column for percent daily value (formerly RDA)	❏	❏	❏
10. Explain calories and calories from fat	❏	❏	❏
11. Have the patient calculate the percentage of fat calories and compare it with the label	❏	❏	❏
12. Read down the label and discuss each nutrient, pointing out the amounts and percentages	❏	❏	❏
13. Have the patient compare the two labels and tell you how many total carbohydrates are in each label, sugars, protein, etc.	❏	❏	❏
14. **AFF** Explain how to respond to a patient who has religious or personal beliefs against eating specific food groups, such as meats	❏	❏	❏

_____

_____

_____

_____

PSY PROCEDURE 16-1	Teach a Patient How to Read Food Labels (continued)			
15. Ask the patient if she has any questions		❑	❑	❑
16. Log into the Electronic Medical Record (EMR) using your username and secure password OR obtain the paper medical record from a secure location and assure it is kept away from public access				
17. Chart the verbal and written instructions given to the patient. When finished, log out of the EMR and/or replace the paper medical record in an appropriate and secure location		❑	❑	❑

CALCULATION

Total Possible Points: _____

Total Points Earned: _____ Multiplied by 100 = _____ Divided by Total Possible Points = _____ %

PASS   FAIL   COMMENTS:
❑   ❑

Student's signature _____ Date _____

Partner's signature _____ Date _____

Instructor's signature _____ Date _____

PSY PROCEDURE 16-2 **Develop a Meal Plan Utilizing Basic Principles of Nutrition; Instruct a Patient according to Patient's Special Dietary Needs**

Name: _____ **Date:** _____ **Time:** _____ **Grade:** _____

EQUIPMENT/SUPPLIES: Reference materials related to dietary choices that include nutritional components (i.e., calories and nutrient amounts such as protein, fat, and carbohydrates), a physician order, and the patient medical record.

STANDARDS: Given the needed equipment and a place to work, the student will perform this skill with _____ % accuracy in a total of _____ minutes. *(Your instructor will tell you what the percentage and time limits will be before you begin.)*

KEY: 4 = Satisfactory   0 = Unsatisfactory   NA = This step is not counted

PROCEDURE STEPS	SELF	PARTNER	INSTRUCTOR
1. Review the physician order to determine the specific nutritional information necessary for patient instruction	❏	❏	❏
2. Identify the patient	❏	❏	❏
3. Introduce yourself and explain the procedure, including the rationale	❏	❏	❏
4. Develop a meal plan based on a regular (i.e., no special dietary needs) 2,000-calorie diet and include information on basic nutrition (nutrients, serving sizes, and calories). Printable materials may be used during instruction from the choosemyplate.gov website if approved by the physician	❏	❏	❏
5. Observe the patient during instruction for nonverbal signs such as confusion, interest or disinterest, emotions, etc.	❏	❏	❏
6. Explain how to respond to a patient who verbalizes concern about the ability to purchase fresh fruits and vegetables due to lack of monetary resources and reliance on public transportation to shop for groceries	❏	❏	❏
7. Instruct a patient according to one of the following special dietary needs as ordered by the physician: **a.** low sodium **b.** low fat **c.** low carbohydrate **d.** high protein **e.** restricted calorie (i.e., 500, 1,800, etc.) **f.** lactose free **g.** gluten free **h.** high fiber	❏	❏	❏
8. Ask the patient questions during instruction and allow the opportunity for them to ask questions during instruction and at the end	❏	❏	❏
9. Explain how to respond to a patient who has a religious or personal belief against specific food groups, such as being a vegetarian	❏	❏	❏

	PROCEDURE 16-2	Develop a Meal Plan Utilizing Basic Principles of Nutrition; Instruct a Patient according to Patient's Special Dietary Needs (continued)

10. Log into the Electronic Medical Record (EMR) using your username and secure password OR obtain the paper medical record from a secure location and assure it is kept away from public access	❑	❑	❑
11. Chart the verbal and written instructions given to the patient. When finished, log out of the EMR and/or replace the paper medical record in an appropriate and secure location	❑	❑	❑

_____

_____

_____

_____

CALCULATION

Total Possible Points: _____

Total Points Earned: _____ Multiplied by 100 = _____ Divided by Total Possible Points = _____ %

PASS   FAIL   COMMENTS:
❑   ❑

Student's signature _____ Date _____

Partner's signature _____ Date _____

Instructor's signature _____ Date _____

CHAPTER 17

Medical Asepsis and Infection Control

LEARNING OUTCOMES

COG Cognitive Domain*

1. Spell and define key terms
2. *Identify the infection cycle, including the infectious agent, reservoir, susceptible host, means of transmission, portals of entry, and portals of exit*
3. *Identify major types of infectious agents*
4. *Identify different methods of controlling the growth of microorganisms*
5. *Identify the following as practiced within an ambulatory care setting: a. medical asepsis b. surgical asepsis*
6. List the various ways microbes are transmitted
7. *Identify the principles of standard precautions*
8. Compare the effectiveness in reducing or destroying microorganisms using the various levels of infection control
9. Identify personal safety precautions as established by the Occupational Safety and Health Administration (OSHA)
10. *Identify personal protective equipment (PPE)*
11. *Identify the implications for failure to comply with the Centers for Disease Control (CDC) regulations in healthcare settings*
12. List the required components of an exposure control plan
13. Explain the facts pertaining to the transmission and prevention of the hepatitis B virus and the human immunodeficiency virus in the medical office

PSY Psychomotor Domain*

1. *Perform a medical aseptic handwashing procedure (Procedure 17-1)*
2. *Select appropriate PPE and remove contaminated gloves (Procedure 17-2)*
3. Clean and decontaminate biohazardous spills (Procedure 17-3)
4. *Participate in bloodborne pathogen training (Procedure 17-4)*

AFF Affective Domain*

1. *Demonstrate critical thinking skills*
2. *Demonstrate self-awareness*

MAERB Standards are italicized.

ABHES Competencies

1. Define and use medical abbreviations when appropriate and acceptable
2. Practice standard precautions and perform disinfection/sterilization techniques

Name: _____   Date: _____   Grade: _____

COG MULTIPLE CHOICE

Circle the letter preceding the correct answer.

Scenario for Questions 1 through 3: Susan enters the examination room, where a patient is being seen for flu-like symptoms. While Susan takes the patient's blood pressure, the patient suddenly coughs near her face. Three days later, Susan has the same signs and symptoms as the patient.

1. Which of the following terms best describes the patient in the infection cycle?
   a. Reservoir host
   b. Disease portal
   c. Pathogen portal
   d. Susceptible host
   e. Disease transmitter

2. Which of the following procedures could Susan have performed that might have helped to minimize her chances of contracting the patient's disease?
   a. Ask the patient to look the other way while coughing
   b. Put on a facemask before entering the exam room
   c. Run out of the room right after the patient coughed
   d. Wash her face right after the coughing episode
   e. Sterilize the examination room

3. What type of transmission process occurred during Susan's contact with the patient?
   a. Direct
   b. Vector
   c. Viable
   d. Manual
   e. Indirect

4. *Clostridium tetani* causes tetanus. Because it does not require oxygen to survive, this microbe is an example of an:
   a. anoxic bacteria.
   b. aerobic bacteria.
   c. anaerobic bacteria.
   d. anaerolytic bacteria.
   e. aerosolized bacteria.

5. Which of the following groups of conditions best favors microbial growth?
   a. Cold, light, and dry
   b. Dry, dark, and warm
   c. Dark, moist, and cool
   d. Warm, moist, and light
   e. Moist, warm, and dark

6. *Escherichia coli* is normally found in the intestinal tract. *Escherichia coli* can be transmitted to the urinary tract, causing an infection. When in the urinary tract, *E. coli* is an example of:
   a. viral flora.
   b. normal flora.
   c. resident flora.
   d. resistant flora.
   e. transient flora.

7. Which of the following practices is most important for maintaining medical asepsis?
   a. Airing out examination rooms after each patient
   b. Receiving all available vaccinations on an annual basis
   c. Wearing gloves before and after handling medical tools
   d. Wearing a gown if you are concerned about bodily fluids
   e. Washing your hands before and after each patient contact

8. To minimize infection, an endoscope should be:
   a. rinsed.
   b. sanitized.
   c. sterilized.
   d. disinfected.
   e. germicided.

9. At which temperature do most pathogenic microorganisms thrive?
   a. Below 32°F
   b. Above 212°F
   c. Around body temperature
   d. Around room temperature
   e. At any temperature

10. What level of disinfection would be appropriate to use when cleaning a speculum?
    a. None
    b. Low
    c. Intermediate
    d. High
    e. Sterilization

11. Which of the following job responsibilities has the highest risk exposure in the group?
    a. Measuring a patient's body temperature
    b. Covering a urine-filled specimen jar
    c. Drawing blood for lab analysis
    d. Auscultating a patient's blood pressure
    e. Irrigating a patient's ear for excess earwax

12. OSHA is responsible for:
   a. certifying all medical doctors.
   b. vaccinating school-age children.
   c. ensuring the safety of all workers.
   d. analyzing medical laboratory samples.
   e. caring for people with contagious diseases.

13. Jeremy approaches you and says that he just accidentally stuck himself with a needle while drawing a blood sample from a patient. He points to his thumb, where you can see a puncture. There is no bleeding. Which of the following actions should you take *first*?
   a. Direct Jeremy to wash his hands with soap and water
   b. Lance the puncture with a scalpel to induce bleeding
   c. Help him complete an exposure report right away
   d. Call the physician in the office to ask for advice
   e. Drive him to an occupational health clinic

14. One example of PPE includes:
   a. name tag.
   b. stethoscope.
   c. face shield.
   d. scrub pants.
   e. syringe.

15. A patient arrives at the urgent care center complaining of nausea. As you begin to assess her, she begins to vomit bright red blood. Which of the following sets of PPE would be *most* appropriate to wear under these circumstances?
   a. Gown, gloves, and booties
   b. Eyewear, gown, and uniform
   c. Face shield and safety glasses
   d. Gloves, face shield, and gown
   e. Face shield, gown, and booties

16. Which of the following statements is *true* regarding hepatitis B virus (HBV)?
   a. HBV dies quickly outside the host body
   b. There are no effective treatments for HBV
   c. There is no vaccine protection against HBV
   d. HBV is transmitted through blood contact, such as a needle puncture
   e. It is easier to contract human immunodeficiency virus (HIV) than HBV

17. Which of the following is *not* part of the body's natural defenses against disease?
   a. Plasma in blood
   b. Mucus in the nose
   c. Lysozyme in tears
   d. Saliva in the mouth
   e. Acid in the stomach

18. A vial of blood fell on the floor, the glass broke, and the contents spilled on the floor. Proper cleaning of this spill includes:
   a. depositing the blood-soaked towels into a biohazard container.
   b. pouring hot water carefully onto the spill to avoid any splash.
   c. notifying the physician.
   d. allowing the blood to dry before cleaning.
   e. trying to piece the vial back together.

19. If a biohazard container becomes contaminated on the outside, you should:
   a. fill out a biohazard report form.
   b. immediately wash the surface in a sink.
   c. dispose of the container in a trash facility outside.
   d. place the container inside another approved container.
   e. call the biohazard removal company as soon as possible.

20. You should change your gloves *after*:
   a. touching a patient's saliva.
   b. measuring a patient's weight.
   c. auscultating a blood pressure.
   d. palpating a patient's abdomen.
   e. taking a patient's temperature.

COG **MATCHING**

Grade: _____

Match each key term with its description.

Key Terms

21. _____ aerobe
22. _____ asymptomatic
23. _____ disinfection
24. _____ germicide
25. _____ immunization
26. _____ microorganisms
27. _____ pathogens
28. _____ resistance
29. _____ spore
30. _____ sanitation
31. _____ standard precautions
32. _____ virulen

Definitions

a. the killing or rendering inert of most, but not all, pathogenic microorganisms

b. disease-causing microorganisms

c. bacterial life form that resists destruction by heat, drying, or chemicals

d. highly pathogenic and disease producing; describes a microorganism

e. chemical that kills most pathogenic microorganisms; disinfectant

f. maintenance of a healthful, disease-free environment

g. microscopic living organisms

h. usual steps to prevent injury or disease

i. without any symptoms

j. body's immune response to prevent infections by invading pathogenic microorganisms

k. microorganism that requires oxygen to live and reproduce

l. act or process of rendering an individual immune to specific disease

COG **IDENTIFICATION**

Grade: _____

33. Indicate whether the following microorganisms are resident or transient flora by writing RF (resident flora) or TF (transient flora) on the line preceding the name of the microbe and its location on or in the body.

a. _____ *Escherichia coli* (large intestine)

b. _____ *Staphylococcus aureus* (subcutaneous tissue)

c. _____ *Escherichia coli* (peritoneum)

d. _____ *Staphylococcus aureus* (epidermis; skin)

e. _____ *Helicobacter pylori* (digestive tract)

34. Indicate whether the following situations could be a direct or indirect mode of disease transmission by writing D (direct) or I (indirect) on the line preceding the situation.

a. _____ Shaking hands with someone

b. _____ Getting a mosquito bite

c. _____ Cleaning up a broken blood tube on the floor without gloves

d. _____ Sneezing

e. _____ Removing a tick from your leg

f. _____ Sharing a soda with a friend using the same straw

35. What type of PPE might be appropriate for a medical assistant to wear when facing specific types of bodily fluids? Place a checkmark on the line under each of the types of PPE, if any, that you would use based on the patient's presentation in the exam room.

Patient Presentation	Gloves	Protective Eyewear	Mask	Gown
a. Abdominal pain, vomiting				
b. Abdominal pain				
c. Headache, coughing				
d. Confusion, nausea, diarrhea				
e. Fever, nonproductive cough				
f. Generalized weakness				

OOG SHORT ANSWER

Grade: _____

36. Your body is in a constant state of war—battling pathogens that are intent on getting into your body to grow and reproduce. Fortunately, your body has a variety of mechanisms to fight off pathogens. For each of the body structures below, explain how it fights the pathogens to protect the body.

a. Nose cilia: _____

b. Mucus: _____

c. Skin: _____

d. Urination: _____

e. Tears: _____

f. Saliva: _____

g. Stomach: _____

37. A nondisposable vaginal speculum has just been used by the physician on a patient. After the exam is over and the patient leaves, how do you prepare this equipment for the next patient?

_____

_____

_____

_____

38. Name four factors that affect the disinfection process.

_____

_____

_____

_____

39. You accidentally stick yourself with a bloody needle. After washing the site, describe what you should do next.

_____

_____

_____

_____

COG TRUE OR FALSE? Grade: _____

40. Indicate whether the statements are true or false by placing the letter T (true) or F (false) on the line preceding the statement.

a. _____ Adhering to "clean technique," or medical asepsis, ensures that an object or area is free from all microorganisms.

b. _____ Sterilization is the highest level of infection control.

c. _____ Low-level disinfection destroys bacteria but not viruses.

d. _____ There are three levels of disinfection: minor, moderate, and severe.

e. _____ Handwashing is a form of surgical or sterile asepsis.

COG AFF CASE STUDIES FOR CRITICAL THINKING Grade: _____

41. Mei Lin is a clinical medical assistant who works in an outpatient clinic. Today she arrives at work with a minor cold. Over the course of an hour, she sees four patients. She draws a blood sample from one patient and retrieves a urine sample from another patient. During the hour, she sneezes three times. She is preparing to leave for her lunch break. How many times should she have washed her hands during this time period?

_____

_____

_____

_____

42. Your patient is a 24-year-old female who has been diagnosed with bacterial pneumonia. The physician has ordered antibiotic therapy and bed rest. When leaving the office, she tells you that she is concerned about the fact that she has a 7-month-old baby at home. What information could you give her to clearly explain what steps she can take to avoid transmitting her illness to her child?

_____

_____

_____

_____

43. An established patient in your office is a 38-year-old female with AIDS. One of your coworkers, Steve, is afraid of interacting with this patient and has made disparaging remarks about her in the back office. You worry that Steve's attitude will affect patient care and you decide to talk to him privately. What points will you make? Should you also talk with your supervisor about Steve? Why or why not?

_____

_____

_____

_____

44. The test results for 15-year-old Ashley Lewis come in and show that she is positive for hepatitis C. Her mother phones and asks you for the results. Is it appropriate for you to give her mother the test results? Why or why not? How would you handle this call?

_____

_____

_____

_____

45. A middle-aged male comes into the medical office with a low-grade fever and productive cough that has lasted several weeks. The physician orders a chest x-ray to aid in diagnosis. After the patient leaves to get his chest x-ray, you begin to clean the room for the next patient. What level of disinfection will you use? What product(s) will you use? Provide detailed information about your actions, including dilution instructions, if appropriate.

_____

_____

_____

_____

46. You work in a pediatrician's office and have been working extra hours to save for a new, more reliable vehicle. Between work and school, you are tired and rundown. This morning, you woke up with a sore throat and headache. The last thing you want to do is call in sick because you need the money and you want your supervisor to think you are reliable. What should you do? Explain your answer.

_____

_____

_____

_____

PSY PROCEDURE 17-1	**Perform Medical Aseptic Handwashing Procedure**

Name: _____ **Date:** _____ **Time:** _____ **Grade:** _____

EQUIPMENT/SUPPLIES: Liquid soap, disposable paper towels, a waste can

STANDARDS: Given the needed equipment and a place to work, the student will perform this skill with _____ % accuracy in a total of _____ minutes. *(Your instructor will tell you what the percentage and time limits will be before you begin.)*

KEY: 4 = Satisfactory 0 = Unsatisfactory NA = This step is not counted

PROCEDURE STEPS	SELF	PARTNER	INSTRUCTOR
1. Remove all rings and wristwatch	❏	❏	❏
2. Stand close to the sink without touching it	❏	❏	❏
3. Turn on the faucet and adjust the temperature of the water to warm	❏	❏	❏
4. Wet hands and wrists, apply soap, and work into a lather	❏	❏	❏
5. Rub palms together and rub soap between your fingers at least 10 times	❏	❏	❏
6. Scrub one palm with fingertips, work soap under nails, and then reverse hands	❏	❏	❏
7. Rinse hands and wrists under warm running water	❏	❏	❏
8. Hold hands lower than elbows and avoid touching the inside of the sink	❏	❏	❏
9. Clean under the nails by scraping the fingernails of one hand against the soapy palm of the other hand for 10 seconds. Repeat with other hand	❏	❏	❏
10. Reapply liquid soap and rewash hands and wrists	❏	❏	❏
11. Rinse hands again while holding hands lower than the wrists and elbows	❏	❏	❏
12. Use a dry paper towel to dry your hands and wrists gently	❏	❏	❏
13. Use a dry paper towel to turn off the faucets and discard the paper towel	❏	❏	❏

_____

_____

_____

_____

PSY PROCEDURE 17-1 | **Perform Medical Aseptic Handwashing Procedure** (continued)

CALCULATION

Total Possible Points: _____

Total Points Earned: _____ Multiplied by 100 = _____ Divided by Total Possible Points = _____ %

PASS **FAIL** **COMMENTS:**
❑ ❑

Student's signature _____ Date _____

Partner's signature _____ Date _____

Instructor's signature _____ Date _____

PSY PROCEDURE 17-2 **Select Appropriate Personal Protective Equipment and Remove Contaminated Gloves**

Name: _____ **Date:** _____ **Time:** _____ **Grade:** _____

EQUIPMENT/SUPPLIES: PPE (Clean examination gloves; goggles or disposable masks with eye/splash guard; disposable masks; disposable gown); biohazard waste container

STANDARDS: Given the needed equipment and a place to work, the student will perform this skill with _____ % accuracy in a total of _____ minutes. *(Your instructor will tell you what the percentage and time limits will be before you begin.)*

KEY: 4 = Satisfactory 0 = Unsatisfactory NA = This step is not counted

PROCEDURE STEPS	SELF	PARTNER	INSTRUCTOR
1. Given a potentially biohazardous situation, choose the correct PPE: **a.** Cleaning up spilled urine **b.** Irrigating a wound **c.** Giving an injection **d.** Disinfecting examination tables	❏	❏	❏
2. Apply appropriately chosen PPE. If a gown, mask, and goggles are necessary, apply the gown and mask/goggles first. Choose the appropriate size gloves for your hands and put them on last	❏	❏	❏
3. Make sure clothing is protected if a gown is worn and no skin is showing	❏	❏	❏
4. After the procedure is finished, appropriately remove PPE by removing the gloves first, next the gown, and last the goggles and mask or face shield	❏	❏	❏
5. To remove gloves, grasp the glove of your nondominant hand at the palm and pull the glove away	❏	❏	❏
6. Slide your hand out of the glove, rolling the glove into the palm of the gloved dominant hand	❏	❏	❏
7. Holding the soiled glove in the palm of your gloved hand, slip your ungloved fingers under the cuff of the glove you are still wearing, being careful not to touch the outside of the glove	❏	❏	❏
8. Stretch the glove of the dominant hand up and away from your hand while turning it inside out, with the already removed glove balled up inside	❏	❏	❏
9. Both gloves should now be removed, with the first glove inside the second glove and the second glove inside out	❏	❏	❏
10. Discard both gloves as one unit into a biohazard waste receptacle	❏	❏	❏

PSY PROCEDURE 17-2 | **Select Appropriate Personal Protective Equipment and Remove Contaminated Gloves** (continued)

Step			
11. If only gloves were worn as PPE, wash your hands	❏	❏	❏
12. If other PPE were worn (i.e., gown, mask, goggles), remove gloves following the procedure above and untie the gown carefully at the neck. Pull the neck strings of the gown toward the front of the body with the arms straight. Pull each arm out of the sleeve, making the sleeves inside out. Continue removing the gown, rolling it into a ball, touching only the uncontaminated inside of the gown with the hands. Drop the rolled gown in a biohazard waste container	❏	❏	❏
13. Remove the goggles, face shield, and/or mask. Dispose of any disposable items appropriately. If goggles are nondisposable, place in a designated area for disinfecting	❏	❏	❏
14. Wash your hands	❏	❏	❏

_____

_____

_____

_____

CALCULATION

Total Possible Points: _____

Total Points Earned: _____ Multiplied by 100 = _____ Divided by Total Possible Points = _____ %

PASS   FAIL   COMMENTS:
  ❏   ❏

Student's signature _____ Date _____

Partner's signature _____ Date _____

Instructor's signature _____ Date _____

PSY PROCEDURE 17-3   Cleaning Biohazardous Spills

Name: _____ Date: _____ Time: _____ Grade: _____

EQUIPMENT/SUPPLIES: Commercially prepared germicide *or* 1:10 bleach solution, gloves, disposable towels, chemical absorbent, biohazardous waste bag, protective eye wear (goggles or mask and face shield), disposable shoe coverings, disposable gown or apron made of plastic or other material that is impervious to soaking up contaminated fluids

STANDARDS: Given the needed equipment and a place to work, the student will perform this skill with _____ % accuracy in a total of _____ minutes. *(Your instructor will tell you what the percentage and time limits will be before you begin.)*

KEY: 4 = Satisfactory   0 = Unsatisfactory   NA = This step is not counted

PROCEDURE STEPS	SELF	PARTNER	INSTRUCTOR
1. Put on gloves. Wear protective eyewear, gown or apron, and shoe coverings if you anticipate any splashing	❏	❏	❏
2. Apply chemical absorbent material to the spill as indicated by office policy. Clean up the spill with disposable paper towels, being careful not to splash	❏	❏	❏
3. Dispose of paper towels and absorbent material in a biohazard waste bag	❏	❏	❏
4. Spray the area with commercial germicide or bleach solution and wipe with disposable paper towels. Discard towels in a biohazard bag	❏	❏	❏
5. With your gloves on, remove the protective eyewear and discard or disinfect per office policy. Remove the gown or apron and shoe coverings and put in the biohazard bag if disposable or the biohazard laundry bag for reusable linens	❏	❏	❏
6. Place the biohazard bag in an appropriate waste receptacle for removal according to your facility's policy	❏	❏	❏
7. Remove your gloves and wash your hands thoroughly	❏	❏	❏

_____

_____

_____

_____

PSY PROCEDURE 17-3 **Cleaning Biohazardous Spills** (continued)

CALCULATION

Total Possible Points: _____

Total Points Earned: _____ Multiplied by 100 = _____ Divided by Total Possible Points = _____ %

PASS **FAIL** **COMMENTS:**
❏ ❏

Student's signature _____ Date _____

Partner's signature _____ Date _____

Instructor's signature _____ Date _____

PSY PROCEDURE 17-4 **Bloodborne Pathogen Training**

Name: _____ Date: _____ Time: _____ Grade: _____

EQUIPMENT/SUPPLIES: A commercial kit that includes presentation materials with current OSHA guidelines regarding bloodborne pathogen training; participation log documenting training, including date.

STANDARDS: Given the needed equipment and a place to work, the student will perform this skill with _____ % accuracy in a total of _____ minutes. *(Your instructor will tell you what the percentage and time limits will be before you begin.)*

KEY: 4 = Satisfactory 0 = Unsatisfactory NA = This step is not counted

PROCEDURE STEPS	SELF	PARTNER	INSTRUCTOR
1. Plan ahead to attend the training as scheduled by your facility	❏	❏	❏
2. Come to the training on time and prepared to take notes and ask questions	❏	❏	❏

3. The training includes information about the following:
  a. Bloodborne pathogens and diseases
  b. Exposure control plan
  c. Postexposure evaluation and follow-up procedures
	❏	❏	❏

4. After participating in the training, you should be able to define bloodborne pathogens and the diseases that may affect humans from these pathogens, procedures to follow in case of an accidental exposure, and engineering and workplace controls to reduce the likelihood of contamination	❏	❏	❏
5. Sign and date the Bloodborne Pathogen Training log to document your attendance	❏	❏	❏

_____

_____

_____

_____

_____

CALCULATION

Total Possible Points: _____

Total Points Earned: _____ Multiplied by 100 = _____ Divided by Total Possible Points = _____ %

PASS **FAIL** **COMMENTS:**
❏ ❏

Student's signature _____ Date _____

Partner's signature _____ Date _____

Instructor's signature _____ Date _____

CHAPTER 18

Medical History and Patient Assessment

LEARNING OUTCOMES

COG Cognitive Domain*

1. Spell and define key terms
2. *Identify communication barriers*
3. *Identify techniques for overcoming communication barriers*
4. Give examples of the type of information included in each section of the patient history
5. Identify guidelines for conducting a patient interview using principles of verbal and nonverbal communication
6. *Identify subjective and objective information*
7. Discuss open-ended and closed-ended questions and explain when to use each type during the patient interview
8. *Identify the medical assistant's role in telehealth*

PSY Psychomotor Domain*

1. Use feedback techniques to obtain patient information, including: (a) reflection, (b) restatement, and (c) clarification

2. *Correctly use and pronounce medical terminology in healthcare interactions*
3. *Respond to nonverbal communication*
4. Obtain and record a patient history (Procedure 18-1)
5. Accurately document a chief complaint and present illness (Procedure 18-2)
6. *Participate in a telehealth interaction with a patient (Procedure 18-3)*

AFF Affective Domain*

1. *Demonstrate critical thinking skills*
2. *Demonstrate empathy for patient concerns*
3. *Recognize personal boundaries*
4. *Respect diversity*
5. *Demonstrate tactfulness*
6. *Respect self-awareness*

MAERB Standards are italicized.

ABHES Competencies

1. Demonstrate an understanding of the core competencies for interprofessional collaborative practice, i.e., values/ethics; roles/responsibilities; inter-professional communication; teamwork
2. Partner with healthcare teams to attain optimal patient health outcomes
3. Display effective interpersonal skills with patients and healthcare team members
4. Demonstrate cultural awareness

285

Name: _____   Date: _____   Grade: _____

COG MULTIPLE CHOICE

Circle the letter preceding the correct answer.

1. The best place to interview a patient is:
   a. over the phone.
   b. at the patient's home.
   c. in the reception area.
   d. in an examination room.
   e. in the physician's office.

2. Which of the following would appear in the past history (PH) section of a patient's medical history?
   a. Hospitalizations
   b. Chief complaint
   c. Insurance carrier
   d. Review of systems
   e. Deaths in the immediate family

3. You are collecting the medical history of a patient. The patient discloses that her brother, sister, paternal grandfather, and paternal aunt are overweight. For this patient, obesity is considered to be:
   a. familial.
   b. historic.
   c. hereditary.
   d. homeopathic.
   e. demographic.

4. Under HIPAA, who may access a patient's medical records?
   a. Any healthcare provider
   b. The patient's family and friends
   c. Anyone who fills out the proper forms
   d. Only the patient's primary care physician
   e. Only healthcare providers directly involved in the patient's care

5. During an interview, your patient tells you that she drinks alcohol four to five times a week. This information should be included in the:
   a. chief complaint.
   b. past history.
   c. present illness.
   d. social history.
   e. family history.

6. Which of the following is included in the patient's present illness (PI)?
   a. Self-care activities
   b. Hereditary diseases
   c. Signs and symptoms
   d. Preventative medicine
   e. Name, address, and phone number

7. Who completes the patient's medical history form?
   a. The patient only
   b. The patient's insurance provider
   c. The patient's immediate family
   d. The patient, the medical assistant, and the physician
   e. The patient's former physician or primary care provider

8. A homeopathic remedy for a headache could be a(n):
   a. prescription painkiller.
   b. extended period of rest.
   c. 1,000 mg dose of acetaminophen.
   d. icepack on the forehead for 10 minutes.
   e. small dose of an agent that causes headache.

9. An open-ended question is one that:
   a. determines the patient's level of pain.
   b. determines where something happened.
   c. is rhetorical and does not require an answer.
   d. can be answered with a "yes" or a "no" response.
   e. requires the responder to answer using more than one word.

10. One sign of illness might be:
   a. coughing.
   b. headache.
   c. dizziness.
   d. nausea.
   e. muscle pain.

11. Which of the following is a close-ended question?
   a. "What is the reason for your appointment today?"
   b. "Tell me what makes the pain worse?"
   c. "Does the pain leave and return throughout the day?"
   d. "How would you describe the pain you are feeling?"
   e. "What have you done to help eliminate the pain?"

12. At the beginning of an interview, you can establish a trusting, professional relationship with the patient by:
   a. thoroughly introducing yourself.
   b. listing the physician's credentials.
   c. observing the patient's signs of illness.
   d. conducting the review of systems (ROS).
   e. disclosing the patient's weight in private.

13. If you suspect that the patient you are assessing is the victim of abuse, you should:
   a. report your suspicions to the local police station.
   b. record your suspicion of abuse in the patient's chief complaint (CC).
   c. ask the patient if they are being abused with a close-ended question.
   d. document the objective signs and notify the physician of your suspicions.
   e. review the patient's medical history for signs of an abusive spouse or parent.

14. Which of the following is included in the identifying database of a patient's medical history?
   a. The patient's emergency contact
   b. The patient's Social Security number
   c. The patient's reason for visiting the office
   d. The patient's signs and symptoms of illness
   e. The patient's family's addresses

15. One example of a symptom of an illness is:
   a. rash.
   b. cough.
   c. nausea.
   d. vomiting.
   e. wheezing.

16. The patient's PI includes which of the following?
   a. Social history
   b. Family history
   c. Chronology of the illness
   d. Demographic information
   e. History of hospitalizations

17. Before you proceed with a patient interview, you should obtain:
   a. signs and symptoms.
   b. social and family history.
   c. the duration of pain and self-treatment information.
   d. the chief complaint and patient's present illness.
   e. the location of pain and self-treatment information.

18. Which of the following is a poor interview technique?
   a. Asking open-ended questions
   b. Noting observable information
   c. Suggesting expected symptoms
   d. Introducing yourself to the patient
   e. Reading through the patient's medical history beforehand

19. You think that a patient has a disease that was passed down from her parents. Where could you look to find information on the patient's parents?
   a. Medical history forms
   b. History of self-treatment
   c. Demographic information
   d. Notes during the patient interview
   e. Chief complaints from previous visits

20. While obtaining a patient's present illness, you need to find out:
   a. where she lives.
   b. the chief complaint.
   c. if she smokes tobacco.
   d. the severity of the pain.
   e. any hereditary disease(s) she has.

COG MATCHING

Grade: _____

Match each key term with its definition.

Key Terms
21. _____ assessment
22. _____ chief complaint
23. _____ demographic
24. _____ familial
25. _____ hereditary
26. _____ homeopathic
27. _____ medical history
28. _____ over the counter
29. _____ signs
30. _____ symptoms

Definitions
a. relating to the statistical characteristics of populations
b. subjective indications of disease or bodily dysfunction as sensed by the patient
c. process of gathering information about a patient and the presenting condition
d. a record containing information about a patient's past and present health status
e. traits or disorders that are passed from parent to offspring
f. objective indications of disease or bodily dysfunction as observed or measured by the healthcare professional
g. the main reason for a patient's visit to the medical office
h. medications and natural drugs that are available without a prescription
i. traits that tend to occur often within a particular family
j. describing a type of alternative medicine in which patients are treated with small doses of substances that produce similar symptoms and use the body's own healing abilities

COG IDENTIFICATION

Grade: _____

31. Indicate whether the following patient interview questions during a patient assessment are helpful or not helpful by writing H (helpful) or NH (not helpful) on the line preceding the question.

   a. _____ "Do you feel pain?"

   b. _____ "How often does the pain occur?"

   c. _____ "What were you doing when the pain started?"

   d. _____ "Have you taken ibuprofen for the pain?"

   e. _____ "Does lying down lessen the pain you feel?"

32. Two types of home remedies are over-the-counter medications and homeopathic medications. Determine whether the items below are over-the-counter or homeopathic medications by writing OTC (over-the-counter) or H (homeopathic) on the line next to the item.

   a. _____ 1,000 mg of acetaminophen to relieve the pain of a sprained ankle

   b. _____ A small dose of mercury to treat symptoms similar to mercury poisoning

   c. _____ Ingesting ipecacuanha, a root that causes vomiting, in order to treat vomiting

   d. _____ A cooling topical ointment applied to skin afflicted by sunburn

33. As a medical assistant, you will have many responsibilities. Place a check mark on the line next to the actions that you may perform as a medical assistant.

   a. _____ Documenting the patient's chief complaint (CC)

   b. _____ Assessing the patient's present illness (PI) during a patient interview

   c. _____ Going over the medical file to the patient's family and friends

   d. _____ Reviewing the patient's medical history before interviewing the patient

   e. _____ Recording judgments based on the patient's appearance in the patient's record

   f. _____ Advising the patient about which over-the-counter or homeopathic treatments to use

COG COMPLETION

Grade: _____

34. Using any available resources, find information about influenza. On the lines below, list three signs and three symptoms that a patient may have influenza (or the flu).

Signs	Symptoms
a.	a.
b.	b.
c.	c.

35. The section of the patient history that reviews each body system and invites the patient to share any information that they may have forgotten to mention earlier is called

_____

36. The _____ section covers the health status of the patient's immediate family members.

37. Information needed for administrative purposes, such as the patient's name, address, and telephone number, is included in the _____ section.

38. Important information about the patient's lifestyle is documented in the _____ section.

39. The section of the patient history that focuses on the patient's prior health status is called _____.

⬤OG **SHORT ANSWER**   Grade: _____

40. What is the purpose of gathering a patient's social history?

_____

_____

_____

_____

41. When are close-ended questions appropriate during a patient interview? Give one example of an appropriate close-ended question.

_____

_____

_____

_____

42. During a patient interview, you learn that the patient is an extreme sports enthusiast and works in a coal mine. Where should you record this information in the patient's medical history forms?

_____

_____

_____

_____

43. Why is the reception area a poor place to interview a patient? What would be a better location for interviewing a patient?

_____

_____

_____

_____

44. What are two ways in which a patient's medical history is gathered in the medical office?

_____

_____

_____

_____

45. What should you say to the patient when introducing yourself? Why is a thorough introduction important?

_____

_____

_____

_____

COG TRUE OR FALSE?

Grade: _____

Indicate whether the statements are true or false by placing the letter T (true) or F (false) on the line preceding the statement.

46. _____ Unlike OTC medications, homeopathic medications are only available by prescription.

47. _____ Nausea is a sign of food poisoning.

48. _____ It is always the patient's responsibility to fill out his medical history completely and accurately.

49. _____ The chief complaint is always a description of a patient's signs and symptoms.

50. _____ Obtaining a urine specimen from the patient may be part of the chief complaint.

51. _____ It is appropriate to assist an older adult who cannot hold a pen due to arthritis with filling out the medical history form.

52. _____ Entries made in the patient record should be signed and dated.

53. _____ It is the responsibility of the receptionist to make sure the demographic information is complete.

COG AFF CASE STUDIES FOR CRITICAL THINKING

Grade: _____

54. You are interviewing a patient, Mr. Gibson. You learn that Mr. Gibson is a 55-year-old male. He is starting a new job as a childcare provider and needs to submit a physical examination to his new place of employment. Mr. Gibson's father died of colon cancer when he was 60 years old, and Mr. Gibson's wife is a smoker. Mr. Gibson says he feels healthy and has not had any health-related problems in the last few years. What should you record as the chief complaint in Mr. Gibson's medical record?

_____

_____

_____

_____

55. Mrs. Frank is a returning patient at Dr. Mohammad's office. She is 89 years old and needs the assistance of a wheelchair. What are some important considerations that you should make when showing Mrs. Frank to an exam room, gathering her medical history, and performing a patient assessment? How would those considerations change if the patient was a 2-year-old child?

_____

_____

_____

_____

56. Your patient is a 49-year-old female who speaks very little English. She is a returning patient, so her medical history is already on file at the office. You have called a coworker who can act as a translator, but he will not arrive at the office for an hour. Meanwhile, the patient is clearly uncomfortable. She appears sweaty and lethargic. She leans on you as you escort her to an examination room. Describe how you can determine the patient's chief complaint and present illness so that you and the physician can begin to help her.

_____

_____

_____

_____

57. Alicia, a medical assistant in Dr. Howard's office, has recorded the following in a patient assessment:
"CC: Pt. c/o fatigue, depressed mood, and inability to stay asleep at night. He has taken Tylenol PM for two nights with "no effect" on sleep and has not eaten for 2 days because of lack of appetite, which is likely caused by his depression. His face is pale and his skin clammy." Was there anything in this documentation that should not have been recorded? Explain your answer.

_____

_____

_____

_____

58. Giles is a medical assistant in Dr. Yardley's office. Giles enters the examination room to interview a patient. Giles notices that the patient is lying on the examination table, holding his abdomen. He is holding a black trash bin that contains a small amount of his vomit. The patient is flushed and sweating. Before even speaking to the patient, Giles has realized some of the patient's signs and symptoms of illness. Explain the significance of signs and symptoms and then fill in this patient's signs and symptoms in the chart below.

Signs	Symptoms
a.	a.
b.	b.
c.	c.

59. There are two patients waiting in examination rooms to see the physician. Patient A is a new patient, and Patient B is coming into the office for a complete physical examination. When sorting these patients to determine who should be taken back to the exam room first, what factors should be considered?

_____

_____

_____

_____

60. What are your ethical and legal responsibilities as a medical assistant concerning a patient's medical history records?

_____

_____

_____

_____

61. Your patient is a 17-year-old male. His symptoms are shortness of breath and fatigue. During the interview, you learn that his father and older brother are obese. You also learn that both of his grandfathers died of complications resulting from heart disease. Although this patient is not overweight, he tells you that he does not have time to exercise but would like to avoid gaining weight, especially when he enters college this fall. What changes does the patient need to make in his lifestyle in order to improve his health and avoid obesity and heart disease? Should you make suggestions for the members of his family who are obese? Why or why not?

_____

_____

_____

_____

62. Ms. Butler, 20 years old, received a pregnancy test during a visit to the physician's office. A week later, Mr. Gordon, a 25-year-old male, comes into the office demanding to see the results of Ms. Butler's test. He tells you that he is her boyfriend and that if Ms. Butler is pregnant, he deserves to know. What would you say to Mr. Gordon?

_____

_____

_____

_____

63. On your way to the exam room, you notice a coworker weighing another patient on the scales located in the hallway. As the patient steps onto the scale, your coworker moves the weights on the scale and then reads the patient's weight out loud. The patient appears embarrassed. What would you say, if anything, to your coworker? Why or why not?

_____

_____

_____

_____

PSY PROCEDURE 18-1 **Obtain and Record a Patient History**

Name: _____ Date: _____ Time: _____ Grade: _____

EQUIPMENT/SUPPLIES: Paper medical history form or questionnaire, black or blue pen

STANDARDS: Given the needed equipment and a place to work, the student will perform this skill with _____ % accuracy in a total of _____ minutes. *(Your instructor will tell you what the percentage and time limits will be before you begin.)*

KEY: 4 = Satisfactory   0 = Unsatisfactory   NA = This step is not counted

PROCEDURE STEPS	SELF	PARTNER	INSTRUCTOR
1. Gather the supplies	❏	❏	❏
2. Review the medical history form for completeness	❏	❏	❏
3. Take the patient to a private area or the examination room and assist them with completing the form	❏	❏	❏
4. Sit across from the patient at eye level and maintain eye contact	❏	❏	❏
5. Introduce yourself and explain the purpose of the interview	❏	❏	❏
6. Using language the patient can understand, ask the appropriate questions, and document the patient's responses. Be sure to determine the patient's CC and PI	❏	❏	❏
7. Use feedback techniques, including: 　**a.** Reflection. 　**b.** Restatement. 　**c.** Clarification.	❏	❏	❏
8. Regardless of the confidences shared by the patient, avoid projecting a judgmental attitude with words or actions	❏	❏	❏
9. **AFF** Explain how to respond to a patient who does not speak English	❏	❏	❏
10. **AFF** Explain to the patient what to expect during examinations or procedures at that visit	❏	❏	❏
11. Review the history form for completion and accuracy	❏	❏	❏
12. Thank the patient for cooperating during the interview, and offer to answer any questions	❏	❏	❏
13. Describe examples of applying local, state, and federal healthcare legislation and regulation in the medical office	❏	❏	❏

(continues)

PSY PROCEDURE 18-1   **Obtain and Record a Patient History** (continued)

_____

_____

_____

_____

_____

CALCULATION

Total Possible Points: _____

Total Points Earned: _____ Multiplied by 100 = _____ Divided by Total Possible Points = _____ %

PASS   FAIL   COMMENTS:
  ❏   ❏

Student's signature _____ Date _____

Partner's signature _____ Date _____

Instructor's signature _____ Date _____

PSY PROCEDURE 18-2 | **Document a Chief Complaint and Present Illness**

Name: _____ Date: _____ Time: _____ Grade: _____

EQUIPMENT/SUPPLIES: A paper or electronic medical record, including a cumulative problem list or progress notes form, black or blue ink pen

STANDARDS: Given the needed equipment and a place to work, the student will perform this skill with _____ % accuracy in a total of _____ minutes. *(Your instructor will tell you what the percentage and time limits will be before you begin.)*

KEY: 4 = Satisfactory   0 = Unsatisfactory   NA = This step is not counted

PROCEDURE STEPS	SELF	PARTNER	INSTRUCTOR
1. Gather the supplies, including the medical record containing the cumulative problem list or progress note form	❏	❏	❏
2. Review the new or established patient's medical history form	❏	❏	❏
3. Greet and identify the patient while escorting them to the examination room. Close the door	❏	❏	❏
4. Use open-ended questions to find out why the patient is seeking medical care; maintain eye contact	❏	❏	❏
5. When reviewing medical history, including medications with the patient, pronounce all terms and medications accurately	❏	❏	❏
6. **AFF** Explain how to respond to a patient who has dementia and whose facial expression shows confusion	❏	❏	❏
7. Determine the PI using open-ended and close-ended questions	❏	❏	❏
8. Document the CC and PI correctly on the cumulative problem list or progress report form	❏	❏	❏
9. How would you respond to a patient who is moving to another town and asks about having their medical records transferred to a physician in another town?	❏	❏	❏
10. Thank the patient for cooperating, and explain that the physician will soon be in to examine the patient	❏	❏	❏

_____

_____

_____

_____

(continues)

PSY PROCEDURE 18-2 | **Document a Chief Complaint and Present Illness** (continued)

CALCULATION

Total Possible Points: _____

Total Points Earned: _____ Multiplied by 100 = _____ Divided by Total Possible Points = _____ %

PASS **FAIL** **COMMENTS:**

❏ ❏

Student's signature _____ Date _____

Partner's signature _____ Date _____

Instructor's signature _____ Date _____

PSY PROCEDURE 18-3 **Document a Telehealth Encounter**

Name: _____ Date: _____ Time: _____ Grade: _____

EQUIPMENT/SUPPLIES: Computer and electronic medical record such as Caretracker

STANDARDS: Given the needed equipment and a place to work, the student will perform this skill with _____ % accuracy in a total of _____ minutes. *(Your instructor will tell you what the percentage and time limits will be before you begin.)*

KEY: 4 = Satisfactory   0 = Unsatisfactory   NA = This step is not counted

PROCEDURE STEPS	SELF	PARTNER	INSTRUCTOR
1. Go to a private room with limited background noise, adequate lighting, Internet accessibility, and a computer with audio and video capabilities	❏	❏	❏
2. Determine if patient consent is needed for the visit based on state informed consent laws	❏	❏	❏
3. Enter the telecommunication platform to be used for the visit and greet the patient	❏	❏	❏
4. Verify the patient's name and another piece of identifying information in order to access the correct medical record. The patient should provide any proof of identification and/or insurance information by holding the identification or cards in front of the camera while the medical assistant verifies and/or takes a screenshot	❏	❏	❏
5. Verify the patient is in a private, well-lit location for the visit and not a public space or driving a vehicle	❏	❏	❏
6. Obtain the patient's chief complaint and document in the medical record	❏	❏	❏
7. **AFF** Explain how you would respond if a patient had a family member present during the telehealth visit	❏	❏	❏

_____

_____

_____

_____

CALCULATION

Total Possible Points: _____

Total Points Earned: _____ Multiplied by 100 = _____ Divided by Total Possible Points = _____ %

PASS   FAIL   COMMENTS:
  ❏   ❏

Student's signature _____ Date _____

Partner's signature _____ Date _____

Instructor's signature _____ Date _____

CHAPTER 19

Anthropometric Measurements and Vital Signs

LEARNING OUTCOMES

COG Cognitive Domain*

1. Spell and define key terms
2. Explain the procedures for measuring a patient's height and weight
3. Identify and describe the types of thermometers
4. Compare the procedures for measuring a patient's temperature using the oral, rectal, axillary, and tympanic methods
5. List the fever process, including the stages of fever
6. Describe the procedure for measuring a patient's pulse and respiratory rates
7. Identify the various sites on the body used for palpating a pulse
8. Define Korotkoff sounds and the five phases of blood pressure
9. Identify factors that may influence the blood pressure
10. Explain the factors to consider when choosing the correct blood pressure cuff size

PSY Psychomotor Domain*

1. *Accurately measure and record a patient's weight (adult)* (Procedure 19-1)

2. *Accurately measure and record a patient's height* (Procedure 19-2)
3. Accurately measure and record a patient's rectal temperature (Procedure 19-3)
4. Accurately measure and record a patient's axillary temperature (Procedure 19-4)
5. Accurately measure and record a patient's temperature using an electronic thermometer (Procedure 19-5)
6. Accurately measure and record a patient's temperature using a tympanic thermometer (Procedure 19-6)
7. *Accurately measure and record a patient's temperature using a temporal artery thermometer* (Procedure 19-7)
8. *Accurately measure and record a patient's radial pulse* (Procedure 19-8)
9. *Accurately measure and record a patient's respirations* (Procedure 19-9)
10. *Accurately measure and record a patient's blood pressure* (Procedure 19-10)
11. *Instruct and prepare a patient for a procedure or a treatment*

12. *Document patient care accurately in the medical record*
13. *Coach patients regarding medical encounters*

AFF Affective Domain*

1. *Demonstrate critical thinking skills*
2. *Reassure patients*
3. *Demonstrate empathy for patients' concerns*
4. *Demonstrate active listening*
5. *Respect diversity*
6. *Recognize personal boundaries*
7. *Demonstrate tactfulness*
8. *Demonstrate self-awareness*

*MAERB standards are italicized.

ABHES Competencies

1. Obtain vital signs, obtain patient history, and formulate a chief complaint
2. Follow documentation guidelines
3. Display effective interpersonal skills with patients and healthcare team members
4. Demonstrate cultural awareness

Name: _____   Date: _____   Grade: _____

⬛ MULTIPLE CHOICE

Circle the letter preceding the correct answer.

1. Anthropometric measurements:
   a. include vital signs.
   b. include height and weight.
   c. don't include height in adults.
   d. are taken only at the first visit.
   e. are used only as baseline information.

2. What are the cardinal signs?
   a. Height and weight
   b. Baseline measurements
   c. Pulse, respiration, and blood pressure
   d. Pulse, respiration, blood pressure, and temperature
   e. Temperature, pulse, blood pressure, respiration, and cardiac output

3. When you greet a patient, what should you always do before taking any measurements?
   a. Put on gloves
   b. Identify the patient
   c. Get a family history
   d. Get a medical history
   e. Determine whether the patient speaks English

4. After getting an accurate weight measurement, what is the next thing you should do?
   a. Remove the paper towel
   b. Write down the measurement
   c. Assist the patient off the scale
   d. Tell the patient their weight
   e. Convert the measurement to kilograms

5. If the balance bar of a balance beam scale points to the midpoint when the large counterweight is at 100, and the small counterweight is 2 lines to the right of the mark for 30, what is the patient's weight?
   a. 32 pounds
   b. 73 pounds
   c. 128 pounds
   d. 132 pounds
   e. 264 pounds

6. To get an accurate height measurement, you should:
   a. wash your hands and put down a paper towel.
   b. have the patient stand barefoot with heels together.
   c. have the patient face the ruler and look straight ahead.
   d. put the measuring bar on the patient's hair and deduct an inch.
   e. record the measurement before helping the patient off the scale.

7. An axillary temperature would be a good measurement to take when:
   a. the patient is very talkative.
   b. there are no more disposable plastic sheaths.
   c. the office is so full that there is little privacy.
   d. the patient is wearing many layers of clothing.
   e. you need to know the temperature as quickly as possible.

8. One difference between using electronic thermometers and using glass thermometers is the:
   a. use of gloves for rectal measurements.
   b. use of a disposable cover for the thermometer.
   c. color code for oral and rectal measurements.
   d. wait time before the thermometer is removed.
   e. receptacle for disposable covers after measurements.

9. The three stages of fever are:
   a. abrupt onset, course, and lysis.
   b. onset, various course, and lysis.
   c. onset, sustained fever, and crisis.
   d. abrupt or gradual onset, course, and resolution.
   e. onset, fluctuating course, and abrupt resolution.

10. Which method would you use to take a brachial pulse?
    a. Palpation alone
    b. Auscultation alone
    c. Palpation and/or auscultation
    d. Palpation and/or use of a Doppler unit
    e. Auscultation and/or use of a Doppler unit

11. Which method would you use to take an apical pulse?
    a. Palpation alone
    b. Auscultation alone
    c. Palpation and/or auscultation
    d. Palpation and/or use of a Doppler unit
    e. Auscultation and/or use of a Doppler unit

12. Which statement is true of a respiratory rate?
    a. It increases when a patient is lying down
    b. It is the number of expirations in 60 seconds
    c. It is the number of complete inspirations per minute
    d. It should be taken while the patient is not aware of it
    e. It is the number of inspirations and expirations in 30 seconds

13. Abnormal breathing may be characterized by:
   a. inhalations that are medium and rhythmic.
   b. inhalations and exhalations that are regular and consistent.
   c. air moving in and out, heard with a stethoscope.
   d. breathing that is shallow or wheezing.
   e. a rate of 16 to 20.

14. Hyperpnea is:
   a. no respiration.
   b. shallow respirations.
   c. abnormally deep, gasping breaths.
   d. inability to breathe while lying down.
   e. a respiratory rate that is too high for oxygen demand.

15. The Korotkoff sound that signals systolic blood pressure is:
   a. faint tapping.
   b. soft swishing.
   c. soft tapping that becomes faint.
   d. rhythmic, sharp, distinct tapping.
   e. sharp tapping that becomes soft swishing.

16. Which group of factors is likely to affect blood pressure?
   a. Age, exercise, occupation
   b. Activity, stress, tobacco use
   c. Alcohol, education, prescriptions
   d. Body position, height, history of heart conditions
   e. Dietary habits, wealth, family history of heart disease

17. Which blood pressure cuff is the correct size?
   a. One that has the Velcro in places that match up
   b. One with a length that wraps three times around the arm
   c. One with a width that goes halfway around the upper arm
   d. One with a width that wraps all the way around the lower arm
   e. One with a length that wraps one and a half times around the arm

18. Which measurement is a normal axillary temperature?
   a. 36.4°C
   b. 37.0°C
   c. 37.6°C
   d. 98.6°F
   e. 99.6°F

19. A tympanic thermometer measures temperature:
   a. in the ear.
   b. in the mouth.
   c. under the armpit.
   d. on the temple.
   e. in the rectum.

20. Diaphoresis is:
   a. sweating.
   b. constant fever.
   c. elevated blood pressure.
   d. needing to sit upright to breathe.
   e. blood pressure that drops upon standing.

OOG MATCHING

Grade: _____

Match each key term with its definition.

Key Terms

21. _____ afebrile
22. _____ anthropometric
23. _____ apnea
24. _____ baseline
25. _____ calibrated
26. _____ cardiac cycle
27. _____ cardinal signs
28. _____ diastole
29. _____ diaphoresis
30. _____ dyspnea
31. _____ febrile
32. _____ hyperpnea
33. _____ hyperpyrexia
34. _____ hypertension
35. _____ hyperventilation
36. _____ hypopnea
37. _____ intermittent
38. _____ orthopnea
39. _____ palpation
40. _____ postural hypotension
41. _____ pyrexia
42. _____ relapsing fever
43. _____ remittent fever
44. _____ sphygmomanometer
45. _____ sustained fever
46. _____ systole

Definitions

a. profuse sweating
b. fever that is fluctuating
c. no respiration
d. fever that is constant
e. shallow respirations
f. occurring at intervals
g. elevated blood pressure
h. pertaining to measurements of the human body
i. difficult or labored breathing
j. device used to measure blood pressure
k. abnormally deep, gasping breaths
l. phase in which the heart contracts
m. having a temperature above normal
n. original or initial measure with which other measurements will be compared
o. having a temperature within normal limits
p. extremely high temperature, from 105° to 106°F
q. marked in units of measurement
r. phase in which the heart pauses briefly to rest and refill
s. fever of 102°F or higher rectally or 101°F or higher orally
t. act of pressing an artery against an underlying firm surface
u. a sudden drop in blood pressure upon standing
v. fever returning after an extended period of normal readings
w. respiratory rate that greatly exceeds the body's oxygen demand
x. the period from the beginning of one heartbeat to the beginning of the next
y. inability to breathe lying down
z. measurements of vital signs

OOG IDENTIFICATION

Grade: _____

47. Place a check mark on the line next to each factor that can affect blood pressure.

a. _____ Activity

b. _____ Age

c. _____ Alcohol use

d. _____ Arteriosclerosis

e. _____ Atherosclerosis

f. _____ Body position

g. _____ Dietary habits

h. _____ Economic status

i. _____ Education

j. _____ Exercise

k. _____ Family history of heart conditions

l. _____ General health of the patient

m. _____ Height

n. _____ History of heart conditions

o. _____ Medications

p. _____ Occupation

q. _____ Stress

r. _____ Tobacco use

COG COMPLETION

Grade: _____

48. Indicate whether the following measurements are anthropometric, cardinal signs, performed at the first office visit (baseline), or performed at every office visit. Place a checkmark in the appropriate column. Measurements may have more than one check mark.

	Anthropometric	Baseline (First Time)	Every Time	Cardinal Sign
a. Blood pressure				
b. Cardiac output				
c. Height				
d. Pulse rate				
e. Respiratory rate				
f. Temperature				
g. Weight				

49. The steps for weighing a patient with a balance beam scale are listed below, but they are not in the correct order. Starting with the number one (1), number the steps in the correct order.

_____ Record the weight

_____ Memorize the weight

_____ Help the patient off the scale

_____ Help the patient onto the scale

_____ Be sure the counterweights are both at zero

_____ Be sure the counterweights are both at zero

_____ Slide the larger counterweight toward zero until it rests securely in a notch

_____ Slide the smaller counterweight toward zero until the balance bar is exactly at the midpoint

_____ Slide the larger counterweight away from zero until the balance bar moves below the midpoint

_____ Slide the smaller counterweight away from zero until the balance bar moves below the midpoint

_____ Add the readings from the two counterweight bars, counting each line after the smaller counterweight as ¼ pound

50. For each step listed in measuring a patient's height, circle the correct word or phrase from the two options given in parentheses.

    a. Wash your hands if the height is measured at (a different time from/the same time as) the weight

    b. The patient should (remove/wear) shoes

    c. The patient should stand straight with heels (a hand's width apart/together)

    d. The patient's eyes should be looking (at the floor/straight ahead)

    e. A better measurement is usually taken with the patient's (back/front) to the ruler

    f. Position the measuring bar perpendicular to the (ruler/top of the head)

    g. Slowly lower the measuring bar until it touches the patient's (hair/head)

    h. Measure at the (point of movement/top of the ruler)

    i. A measurement of 66 inches should be recorded as (5 feet, 6 inches/66 inches)

COG **SHORT ANSWER**

Grade: _____

51. What does the hypothalamus do when it senses that the body is too warm?

_____

_____

_____

_____

52. What happens when the body temperature is too cool?

_____

_____

_____

_____

53. What factors aside from illness affect body temperature?

_____

_____

_____

_____

54. List and describe the three stages of fever. Include the variations in the time and their related terms.

_____

_____

_____

_____

55. If the patient has 19 full inspirations and 18 full expirations in 1 minute, what is the patient's respiratory rate?

_____

_____

_____

_____

56. At which sound is the systolic blood pressure recorded?

_____

_____

_____

_____

57. At which sound is the diastolic blood pressure recorded?

_____

_____

_____

_____

COG TRUE OR FALSE?

Grade: _____

58. Indicate whether the statements are true or false by placing the letter T (true) or F (false) on the line preceding the statement.

a. _____ The weight scale should be kept in the waiting room for ease of access

b. _____ An axillary temperature can be taken with either an oral or a rectal thermometer

c. _____ In pediatric offices, temperatures are almost always taken rectally

d. _____ If a glass mercury thermometer breaks, you should soak up the mercury immediately with tissues and put them in the trash before the mercury sinks into any surfaces

AFF CASE STUDIES FOR CRITICAL THINKING

Grade: _____

59. Ms. Green arrived at the office late for her appointment, frantic and explaining that her alarm clock had not gone off. She discovered that her car was almost out of gas, and she had to stop to refuel. Once she got to the clinic, she could not find a parking place in the lot and she had to park two blocks away. How would you expect this to affect her vital signs? Explain why.

_____

_____

_____

_____

60. A patient comes into the office complaining of fever and chills. While taking her vital signs, you notice that her skin feels very warm. When you take her temperature, you find that her oral temperature is 105°F. What should you do?

_____

_____

_____

_____

61. Mr. Juarez, the father of a 6-month-old baby and a 4-year-old child, would like to purchase a thermometer. He is not sure which one to buy and isn't familiar with how to use the different kinds of thermometers. He also isn't aware of the possible variations that may occur in readings. How would you explain the various types of thermometers and temperature readings to him? What would you recommend and why?

_____

_____

_____

_____

62. Mrs. Chin has come into the office complaining of pain in her right foot. You take her vital signs, which are normal, and you help her remove her shoes so that the doctor can examine both feet. You notice a difference in appearance between her two feet, and it occurs to you to check her femoral, popliteal, posterior tibial, and dorsalis pedis pulses. What are you looking for, and what should you look for next?

_____

_____

_____

_____

63. You've noticed that whenever you try to take Mr. Kimble's respiration rate, he always breathes in when you do and breathes out when you do. You're concerned that you're not assessing Mr. Kimble's breathing accurately, and you know that he has had asthma on occasion. What can you do to get an accurate reading?

_____

_____

_____

_____

PSY PROCEDURE 19-1 Measure and Record a Patient's Weight

Name: _____ Date: _____ Time: _____ Grade: _____

EQUIPMENT/SUPPLIES: Calibrated balance beam scale, digital scale or dial scale; paper towel

STANDARDS: Given the needed equipment and a place to work, the student will perform this skill with _____ % accuracy in a total of _____ minutes. *(Your instructor will tell you what the percentage and time limits will be before you begin.)*

KEY: 4 = Satisfactory   0 = Unsatisfactory   NA = This step is not counted

PROCEDURE STEPS	SELF	PARTNER	INSTRUCTOR
1. Wash your hands	❏	❏	❏
2. Ensure that the scale is properly balanced at zero	❏	❏	❏
3. Greet and identify the patient. Explain the procedure	❏	❏	❏
4. Escort the patient to the scale and place a paper towel on the scale	❏	❏	❏
5. Have the patient remove shoes and heavy outerwear and put down their purse	❏	❏	❏
6. Assist patient onto the scale facing forward and standing on paper towel without touching or holding on to anything if possible, while watching for difficulties with balance	❏	❏	❏
7. Weigh the patient: **a.** Balance beam scale: Slide counterweights on bottom and top bars (start with heavier bars) from zero to approximate weight. Each counterweight should rest securely in the notch with indicator mark at proper calibration. To obtain measurement, balance bar must hang freely at exact midpoint. To calculate weight, add top reading to bottom one. (Example: If bottom counterweight reads 100 and lighter one reads 16 plus three small lines, record weight as 116¾ pounds) **b.** Digital scale: Read and record weight displayed on digital screen **c.** Dial scale: Indicator arrow rests at patient's weight. Read this number directly above the dial	❏	❏	❏
8. Return the bars on the top and bottom to zero	❏	❏	❏
9. Assist the patient from the scale if necessary and discard the paper towel	❏	❏	❏
10. Record the patient's weight	❏	❏	❏
11. **AFF** Explain how to respond to a patient who is visually impaired	❏	❏	❏

_____

_____

_____

_____

PSY PROCEDURE 19-1 **Measure and Record a Patient's Weight** (continued)

CALCULATION

Total Possible Points: _____

Total Points Earned: _____ Multiplied by 100 = _____ Divided by Total Possible Points = _____ %

PASS **FAIL** **COMMENTS:**
❏ ❏

Student's signature _____ Date _____

Partner's signature _____ Date _____

Instructor's signature _____ Date _____

PSY PROCEDURE 19-2 **Measure and Record a Patient's Height**

Name: _____ Date: _____ Time: _____ Grade: _____

EQUIPMENT/SUPPLIES: A scale with a ruler

STANDARDS: Given the needed equipment and a place to work, the student will perform this skill with _____ % accuracy in a total of _____ minutes. *(Your instructor will tell you what the percentage and time limits will be before you begin.)*

KEY: 4 = Satisfactory 0 = Unsatisfactory NA = This step is not counted

PROCEDURE STEPS	SELF	PARTNER	INSTRUCTOR
1. Wash your hands if this procedure is not done at the same time as the weight	❏	❏	❏
2. Have the patient remove shoes and stand straight and erect on the scale, with heels together and eyes straight ahead. (Patient may face the ruler, but a better measurement is made with the patient's back to the ruler)	❏	❏	❏
3. With the measuring bar perpendicular to the ruler, slowly lower it until it firmly touches the patient's head. Press lightly if the hair is full or high	❏	❏	❏
4. Read the measurement at the point of movement on the ruler. If measurements are in inches, convert to feet and inches (e.g., if the bar reads 65 plus two smaller lines, read it at 65½. Remember that 12 inches equals 1 foot; therefore, the patient is 5 feet, 5½ inches tall)	❏	❏	❏
5. Assist the patient from the scale if necessary; watch for signs of difficulty with balance	❏	❏	❏
6. Record the weight and height measurements in the medical record	❏	❏	❏
7. **AFF** Explain how to respond to a patient who has dementia	❏	❏	❏

_____

_____

_____

_____

_____

CALCULATION

Total Possible Points: _____

Total Points Earned: _____ Multiplied by 100 = _____ Divided by Total Possible Points = _____ %

PASS   FAIL   COMMENTS:
❏   ❏

Student's signature _____ Date _____

Partner's signature _____ Date _____

Instructor's signature _____ Date _____

PSY PROCEDURE 19-3 | **Measure and Record a Rectal Temperature**

Name: _____ Date: _____ Time: _____ Grade: _____

EQUIPMENT/SUPPLIES: Electronic thermometer with rectal probe; tissues or cotton balls; disposable plastic sheaths; surgical lubricant; biohazard waste container; gloves.

STANDARDS: Given the needed equipment and a place to work, the student will perform this skill with ____ % accuracy in a total of ____ minutes. *(Your instructor will tell you what the percentage and time limits will be before you begin.)*

KEY: 4 = Satisfactory 0 = Unsatisfactory NA = This step is not counted

PROCEDURE STEPS	SELF	PARTNER	INSTRUCTOR
1. Wash your hands and assemble the necessary supplies	❏	❏	❏
2. Insert the thermometer into a plastic sheath	❏	❏	❏
3. Spread lubricant onto a tissue and then from the tissue onto the sheath of the thermometer	❏	❏	❏
4. Greet and identify the patient and explain the procedure	❏	❏	❏
5. Ensure the patient's privacy by placing the patient in a side-lying position facing the examination room door and draping appropriately	❏	❏	❏
6. Apply gloves and visualize the anus by lifting the top buttock with your nondominant hand	❏	❏	❏
7. Gently insert the thermometer past the sphincter muscle about 1½ inches for an adult, 1 inch for a child, and ½ inch for an infant	❏	❏	❏
8. Release the upper buttock and hold the thermometer in place with your dominant hand for 3 minutes. Replace the drape without moving the dominant hand	❏	❏	❏
9. The electronic thermometer will signal when the reading is obtained. Discard the sheath into an appropriate waste container and note the reading	❏	❏	❏
10. Replace the electronic thermometer into the charger as necessary	❏	❏	❏
11. Remove your gloves and wash your hands	❏	❏	❏
12. Record the procedure and mark the letter R next to the reading, indicating that the temperature was taken rectally	❏	❏	❏
13. **AFF** Explain how to respond to a patient who is developmentally challenged	❏	❏	❏

_____

_____

_____

_____

PSY PROCEDURE 19-3 **Measure and Record a Rectal Temperature** (continued)

CALCULATION

Total Possible Points: _____

Total Points Earned: _____ Multiplied by 100 = _____ Divided by Total Possible Points = _____ %

PASS   **FAIL**   **COMMENTS:**
❑   ❑

Student's signature _____   Date _____

Partner's signature _____   Date _____

Instructor's signature _____   Date _____

PSY PROCEDURE 19-4 Measure and Record an Axillary Temperature

Name: _____ **Date:** _____ **Time:** _____ **Grade:** _____

EQUIPMENT/SUPPLIES: Electronic thermometer (oral or rectal); tissues or cotton balls; disposable plastic sheaths; biohazard waste container.

STANDARDS: Given the needed equipment and a place to work, the student will perform this skill with _____ % accuracy in a total of _____ minutes. *(Your instructor will tell you what the percentage and time limits will be before you begin.)*

KEY: 4 = Satisfactory 0 = Unsatisfactory NA = This step is not counted

PROCEDURE STEPS	SELF	PARTNER	INSTRUCTOR
1. Wash your hands and assemble the necessary supplies	❏	❏	❏
2. Insert the electronic thermometer probe into a plastic sheath	❏	❏	❏
3. Expose the patient's axilla without exposing more of the chest or upper body than is necessary	❏	❏	❏
4. Place the tip of the thermometer deep in the axilla and bring the patient's arm down, crossing the forearm over the chest. Drape the patient as appropriate for privacy	❏	❏	❏
5. The electronic thermometer will signal when the reading is obtained. Discard the sheath into an appropriate waste container and note the reading	❏	❏	❏
6. Replace the electronic thermometer into the charger as necessary	❏	❏	❏
7. Wash your hands	❏	❏	❏
8. Record the procedure and mark a letter A next to the reading, indicating that the reading is axillary	❏	❏	❏
9. AFF Explain how to respond to a patient who is from a different generation	❏	❏	❏

_____

_____

_____

_____

PSY PROCEDURE 19-4 **Measure and Record an Axillary Temperature** (continued)

CALCULATION

Total Possible Points: _____

Total Points Earned: _____ Multiplied by 100 = _____ Divided by Total Possible Points = _____ %

PASS   FAIL   COMMENTS:
 ❏   ❏

Student's signature _____   Date _____

Partner's signature _____   Date _____

Instructor's signature _____   Date _____

PSY	PROCEDURE 19-5	Measure and Record a Patient's Oral Temperature Using an Electronic Thermometer

Name: _____ **Date:** _____ **Time:** _____ **Grade:** _____

EQUIPMENT/SUPPLIES: Electronic thermometer with oral or rectal probe, disposable probe covers, biohazard waste container, gloves for taking an oral temperature

STANDARDS: Given the needed equipment and a place to work, the student will perform this skill with _____ % accuracy in a total of _____ minutes. *(Your instructor will tell you what the percentage and time limits will be before you begin.)*

KEY: 4 = Satisfactory 0 = Unsatisfactory NA = This step is not counted

PROCEDURE STEPS	SELF	PARTNER	INSTRUCTOR
1. Wash your hands and assemble the necessary supplies	❏	❏	❏
2. Greet and identify the patient and explain the procedure	❏	❏	❏
3. Attach the appropriate probe to the battery-powered unit	❏	❏	❏
4. Insert the probe into a probe cover	❏	❏	❏
5. Position the thermometer appropriately for the method. To take an oral temperature, place the end of the thermometer under the patient's tongue to either side of the frenulum	❏	❏	❏
6. Wait for the electronic thermometer unit to "beep" when it senses no signs of the temperature rising further. This usually occurs within 20 to 30 seconds	❏	❏	❏
7. After the beep, remove the probe and note the reading on the digital display screen on the unit before replacing the probe into the unit	❏	❏	❏
8. Discard the probe cover by pressing a button, usually on the end of the probe, while holding the probe over a biohazard container. After noting the temperature, replace the probe into the unit	❏	❏	❏
9. Remove your gloves, if used, wash your hands, and record the procedure	❏	❏	❏
10. Return the unit and probe to the charging base	❏	❏	❏
11. **AFF** Explain how to respond to a patient who is hearing impaired	❏	❏	❏

_____

_____

_____

_____

PSY PROCEDURE 19-5 | **Measure and Record a Patient's Oral Temperature Using an Electronic Thermometer** (continued)

CALCULATION

Total Possible Points: _____

Total Points Earned: _____ Multiplied by 100 = _____ Divided by Total Possible Points = _____ %

PASS   FAIL   COMMENTS:
❏   ❏

Student's signature _____   Date _____

Partner's signature _____   Date _____

Instructor's signature _____   Date _____

PSY PROCEDURE 19-6 Measure and Record a Patient's Temperature Using a Tympanic Thermometer

Name: _____ **Date:** _____ **Time:** _____ **Grade:** _____

EQUIPMENT/SUPPLIES: Tympanic thermometer, disposable probe covers, biohazard waste container

STANDARDS: Given the needed equipment and a place to work, the student will perform this skill with _____ % accuracy in a total of _____ minutes. *(Your instructor will tell you what the percentage and time limits will be before you begin.)*

KEY: 4 = Satisfactory 0 = Unsatisfactory NA = This step is not counted

PROCEDURE STEPS	SELF	PARTNER	INSTRUCTOR
1. Wash your hands and assemble the necessary supplies	❏	❏	❏
2. Greet and identify the patient and explain the procedure	❏	❏	❏
3. Insert the ear probe into a probe cover	❏	❏	❏
4. Place the end of the ear probe into the patient's ear canal with your dominant hand while straightening out the ear canal with your nondominant hand	❏	❏	❏
5. With the ear probe properly placed in the ear canal, press the button on the thermometer. The reading is displayed on the digital display screen in about 2 seconds	❏	❏	❏
6. Remove the probe and note the reading. Discard the probe cover into an appropriate waste container	❏	❏	❏
7. Wash your hands and record the procedure	❏	❏	❏
8. Return the unit to the charging base	❏	❏	❏
9. **AFF** Explain how to respond to a patient who is deaf	❏	❏	❏

_____

_____

_____

_____

_____

CALCULATION

Total Possible Points: _____

Total Points Earned: _____ Multiplied by 100 = _____ Divided by Total Possible Points = _____ %

PASS **FAIL** **COMMENTS:**
❏ ❏

Student's signature _____ Date _____

Partner's signature _____ Date _____

Instructor's signature _____ Date _____

PSY PROCEDURE 19-7 Measure and Record a Patient's Temperature Using a Temporal Artery Thermometer

Name: _____ **Date:** _____ **Time:** _____ **Grade:** _____

EQUIPMENT/SUPPLIES: Temporal artery thermometer, antiseptic wipes

STANDARDS: Given the needed equipment and a place to work, the student will perform this skill with _____ % accuracy in a total of _____ minutes. *(Your instructor will tell you what the percentage and time limits will be before you begin.)*

KEY: 4 = Satisfactory 0 = Unsatisfactory NA = This step is not counted

PROCEDURE STEPS	SELF	PARTNER	INSTRUCTOR
1. Wash your hands and assemble the necessary supplies	❑	❑	❑
2. Greet and identify the patient and explain the procedure	❑	❑	❑
3. Place the probe end of the hand-held unit on the forehead of the patient. Make sure the patient's skin is dry	❑	❑	❑
4. With the thermometer against the forehead, depress the on/off button, move the thermometer across and down the forehead, and release the on/off button with the unit over the temporal artery	❑	❑	❑
5. The reading is displayed on the digital display screen in 1 to 2 seconds	❑	❑	❑
6. Properly disinfect the end of the thermometer according to manufacturer instructions	❑	❑	❑
7. Wash your hands and record the procedure	❑	❑	❑
8. Return the unit to the charging base	❑	❑	❑
9. **AFF** Explain how to respond to a patient who is visually impaired	❑	❑	❑

_____

_____

_____

_____

CALCULATION

Total Possible Points: _____

Total Points Earned: _____ Multiplied by 100 = _____ Divided by Total Possible Points = _____ %

PASS FAIL COMMENTS:
❑   ❑

Student's signature _____ Date _____

Partner's signature _____ Date _____

Instructor's signature _____ Date _____

PSY PROCEDURE 19-8 Measure and Record a Patient's Radial Pulse

Name: _____ **Date:** _____ **Time:** _____ **Grade:** _____

EQUIPMENT/SUPPLIES: A watch with a sweeping second hand

STANDARDS: Given the needed equipment and a place to work, the student will perform this skill with _____ % accuracy in a total of _____ minutes. *(Your instructor will tell you what the percentage and time limits will be before you begin.)*

KEY: 4 = Satisfactory   0 = Unsatisfactory   NA = This step is not counted

PROCEDURE STEPS	SELF	PARTNER	INSTRUCTOR
1. Wash your hands	❑	❑	❑
2. Greet and identify the patient and explain the procedure	❑	❑	❑
3. Position the patient with the arm relaxed and supported either on the lap of the patient or on a table	❑	❑	❑
4. With the index, middle, and ring fingers of your dominant hand, press with your fingertips firmly enough to feel the pulse but gently enough not to obliterate it	❑	❑	❑
5. If the pulse is regular, count it for 30 seconds, watching the second hand of your watch. Multiply the number of pulsations by 2 since the pulse is always recorded as beats per minute. If the pulse is irregular, count it for a full 60 seconds	❑	❑	❑
6. Record the rate in the medical record with the other vital signs. Also note the rhythm if irregular and the volume if thready or bounding	❑	❑	❑
7. **AFF** Explain how to respond to a patient who is developmentally challenged	❑	❑	❑

_____

_____

_____

_____

CALCULATION

Total Possible Points: _____

Total Points Earned: _____ Multiplied by 100 = _____ Divided by Total Possible Points = _____ %

PASS   FAIL   COMMENTS:
❑   ❑

Student's signature _____ Date _____

Partner's signature _____ Date _____

Instructor's signature _____ Date _____

PSY PROCEDURE 19-9   **Measure and Record a Patient's Respirations**

Name: _____   Date: _____   Time: _____   Grade: _____

EQUIPMENT/SUPPLIES: A watch with a sweeping second hand

STANDARDS: Given the needed equipment and a place to work, the student will perform this skill with _____ % accuracy in a total of _____ minutes. *(Your instructor will tell you what the percentage and time limits will be before you begin.)*

KEY: 4 = Satisfactory   0 = Unsatisfactory   NA = This step is not counted

PROCEDURE STEPS	SELF	PARTNER	INSTRUCTOR
1. Wash your hands	❏	❏	❏
2. Greet and identify the patient and explain the procedure	❏	❏	❏
3. After counting the radial pulse and still watching your second hand, count a complete rise and fall of the chest as one respiration. Note: Some patients have abdominal movement rather than chest movement during respirations. Observe carefully for the easiest area to assess for the most accurate reading	❏	❏	❏
4. If the breathing pattern is regular, count the respiratory rate for 30 seconds and multiply by 2. If the pattern is irregular, count for a full 60 seconds	❏	❏	❏
5. Record the respiratory rate in the medical record with the other vital signs. Also, note whether the rhythm is irregular, along with any unusual or abnormal sounds such as wheezing	❏	❏	❏
6. **AFF** Explain how to respond to a patient who has dementia	❏	❏	❏

_____

_____

_____

_____

CALCULATION

Total Possible Points: _____

Total Points Earned: _____ Multiplied by 100 = _____ Divided by Total Possible Points = _____ %

PASS   FAIL   COMMENTS:
❏   ❏

Student's signature _____   Date _____

Partner's signature _____   Date _____

Instructor's signature _____   Date _____

PSY PROCEDURE 19-10 | **Measure and Record a Patient's Blood Pressure**

Name: _____ Date: _____ Time: _____ Grade: _____

EQUIPMENT/SUPPLIES: Sphygmomanometer, stethoscope

STANDARDS: Given the needed equipment and a place to work, the student will perform this skill with _____ % accuracy in a total of _____ minutes. *(Your instructor will tell you what the percentage and time limits will be before you begin.)*

KEY: 4 = Satisfactory   0 = Unsatisfactory   NA = This step is not counted

PROCEDURE STEPS	SELF	PARTNER	INSTRUCTOR
1. Wash your hands	❏	❏	❏
2. Greet and identify the patient and explain the procedure	❏	❏	❏
3. Position the patient with the arm to be used supported with the forearm on the lap or a table and slightly flexed, with the palm upward. The upper arm should be level with the patient's heart	❏	❏	❏
4. Expose the patient's upper arm	❏	❏	❏
5. Palpate the brachial pulse in the antecubital area and center the deflated cuff directly over the brachial artery. The lower edge of the cuff should be 1 to 2 inches above the antecubital area	❏	❏	❏
6. Wrap the cuff smoothly and snugly around the arm and secure it with the Velcro edges	❏	❏	❏
7. With the air pump in your dominant hand and the valve between your thumb and forefinger, turn the screw clockwise to tighten. Do not tighten it to the point that it will be difficult to release	❏	❏	❏
8. While palpating the brachial pulse with your nondominant hand, inflate the cuff and note the point or number on the dial or mercury column at which you no longer feel the brachial pulse	❏	❏	❏
9. Deflate the cuff by turning the valve counterclockwise. Wait at least 30 seconds before reinflating the cuff	❏	❏	❏
10. Place the stethoscope earpieces in your ears with the openings pointed slightly forward. Stand about 3 feet from the manometer with the gauge at eye level. Your stethoscope tubing should hang freely without touching or rubbing against any part of the cuff	❏	❏	❏
11. Place the diaphragm of the stethoscope against the brachial artery and hold it in place with the nondominant hand without pressing too hard	❏	❏	❏
12. With your dominant hand, turn the screw on the valve just enough to close the valve; inflate the cuff. Pump the valve bulb to about 30 mm Hg above the number felt during Step 8	❏	❏	❏

PSY PROCEDURE 19-10 | **Measure and Record a Patient's Blood Pressure** (continued)

13. Once the cuff is appropriately inflated, turn the valve counterclockwise to release air at about 2 to 4 mm Hg per second	❏	❏	❏
14. Listening carefully, note the point on the gauge at which you hear the first clear tapping sound. This is the systolic sound, or Korotkoff I	❏	❏	❏
15. Maintaining control of the valve screw, continue to listen and deflate the cuff. When you hear the last sound, note the reading and quickly deflate the cuff. Note: Never immediately reinflate the cuff if you are unsure of the reading. Totally deflate the cuff and wait 1 to 2 minutes before repeating the procedure	❏	❏	❏
16. Remove the cuff and press the air from the bladder of the cuff	❏	❏	❏
17. If this is the first recording or a new patient, the physician may also want a reading in the other arm or in another position	❏	❏	❏
18. Put the equipment away and wash your hands	❏	❏	❏
19. Record the reading with the systolic over the diastolic pressure, noting which arm was used (120/80 LA). Also, record the patient's position if other than sitting	❏	❏	❏
20. **AFF** Explain how to respond to a patient who is from a different culture	❏	❏	❏

_____

_____

_____

_____

_____

CALCULATION

Total Possible Points: _____

Total Points Earned: _____ Multiplied by 100 = _____ Divided by Total Possible Points = _____ %

PASS   FAIL   COMMENTS:
❏   ❏

Student's signature _____ Date _____

Partner's signature _____ Date _____

Instructor's signature _____ Date _____

CHAPTER 20

Assisting with the Physical Examination

LEARNING OUTCOMES

COG Cognitive Domain*

1. Spell and define the key terms
2. Identify and state the use of the basic and specialized instruments and supplies used in the physical examination
3. Describe the four methods used to examine the patient
4. State your responsibilities before, during, and after the physical examination
5. List the basic sequence of the physical examination
6. *Identify the normal function of each body system*

PSY Psychomotor Domain*

1. Assist with the adult physical examination (Procedure 20-1)
2. *Assist provider with a patient exam*
3. *Coach patients regarding medical encounters*
4. *Document patient care accurately in the medical record*

AFF Affective Domain*

1. *Demonstrate critical thinking skills*
2. *Reassure patients*
3. *Demonstrate empathy—for patient's concerns*
4. *Demonstrate active listening*

5. *Respect diversity*
6. *Recognize personal boundaries*
7. *Demonstrate tactfulness*
8. *Demonstrate self-awareness*
9. Protect the integrity of the medical record

*MAERB standards are italicized.

ABHES Competencies

1. Prepare and maintain examination and treatment area
2. Prepare patient for examinations and treatments
3. Assist physician with routine and specialty examinations and treatments

Name: _____ Date: _____ Grade: _____

▣ MULTIPLE CHOICE

Circle the letter preceding the correct answer.

1. Which of these instruments would a physician use to examine a patient's throat?
  a. Stethoscope
  b. Laryngeal mirror
  c. Percussion hammer
  d. Ayre spatula
  e. Tuning fork

2. The purpose of a regular physical examination is to:
  a. identify a disease or condition based on patient symptoms.
  b. compare symptoms of several diseases that the patient may exhibit.
  c. look for late warning signs of disease.
  d. maintain the patient's health and prevent disease.
  e. ensure the patient is maintaining a healthy diet and exercise regime.

3. Which of the following tasks would be performed by a medical assistant?
  a. Collecting specimens for diagnostic testing
  b. Diagnosing a patient
  c. Prescribing treatment for a patient
  d. Performing a physical examination
  e. Testing a patient's reflexes

4. Which of the following statements is true about physical examinations?
  a. Patients aged 20 to 40 years should have a physical examination every year
  b. It is not necessary to have a physical examination until you are over age 40 years
  c. Women should have physical examinations more frequently than men
  d. Patients aged 20 to 40 years should have a physical examination every 1 to 3 years
  e. Patients over the age of 60 years should have a physical examination every 6 months

5. In which information-gathering technique might a physician use their sense of smell?
  a. Palpation
  b. Percussion
  c. Inspection
  d. Auscultation
  e. Visualization

6. If a physician notices asymmetry in a patient's features, it means that the patient:
  a. is normal and has nothing wrong.
  b. has features that are of unequal size or shape.
  c. has features that are abnormally large.
  d. will need immediate surgery.
  e. has perfectly even features.

7. Which part of the body can be auscultated?
  a. Lungs
  b. Legs
  c. Spine
  d. Feet
  e. Ears

8. The best position in which to place a female patient for a genital and rectal examination is the:
  a. Sims position.
  b. Fowler position.
  c. lithotomy position.
  d. Trendelenburg position.
  e. prone position.

9. A patient may be asked to walk around during a physical examination in order to:
  a. raise the pulse rate.
  b. observe gait and coordination.
  c. loosen the muscles in the legs.
  d. assess posture.
  e. demonstrate balance.

10. Women over age 40 years should receive mammograms every:
  a. 6 months.
  b. 2 years.
  c. 5 years.
  d. 1 year.
  e. 3 months.

11. How would a physician use a tuning fork to test a patient's hearing?
  a. By striking the prongs against the patient's leg and holding the handle in front of the patient's ear
  b. By holding the prongs behind the patient's ear and tapping the handle against their head
  c. By striking the prongs against the hand and holding the handle against the skull near the patient's ear
  d. By repeatedly tapping the prongs against the skull near the patient's ear
  e. By tapping the prongs on the table and inserting the handle into the patient's ear

12. Which of these may be an early warning sign of cancer?
   a. Obvious change in a wart or mole
   b. Dizziness or fainting spells
   c. Loss of appetite
   d. Inability to focus attention
   e. Sudden weight gain

13. How would a physician most likely be able to diagnose a hernia?
   a. Inspection
   b. Percussion
   c. Auscultation
   d. Palpation
   e. Visualization

Scenario for questions 14–16: A patient arrives for her physical checkup. While you are obtaining the patient's history, she mentions to you that she is taking several over-the-counter medications.

14. What is the correct procedure?
   a. Tell the physician immediately.
   b. Tell the patient that it will not affect her physical examination.
   c. Make a note of the medications the patient is taking in her medical record.
   d. Ask the patient to reschedule the physical examination when she has stopped taking the medications for at least a week.
   e. Prepare the necessary materials for a blood test.

15. During the patient's physical examination, the physician asks you to hand her the instruments needed to examine the patient's eyes. You should give her a(n):
   a. otoscope and penlight.
   b. stethoscope and speculum.
   c. ophthalmoscope and penlight.
   d. laryngoscope and gloves.
   e. anoscope and speculum.

16. Once the examination is over, you escort the patient to the front desk. After she has left the office, what do you do with her medical record?
   a. Check that the data have been accurately documented and release it to the billing department
   b. Check that the data have been accurately documented and file the medical report under the patient's name
   c. Pass the medical report on to the physician to check for any errors
   d. Give the medical report directly to the billing department to maintain confidentiality
   e. File the medical report under the patient's name for easy retrieval

17. What is the difference between an otoscope and an audioscope?
   a. An otoscope is used to screen patients for hearing loss, whereas an audioscope is used to assess the internal structures of the ear.
   b. An audioscope is used to screen patients for hearing loss, whereas an otoscope is used to assess the internal structures of the ear.
   c. An otoscope is made of stainless steel, whereas an audioscope is made of plastic.
   d. An audioscope is made of plastic, whereas an otoscope is made of stainless steel.
   e. An otoscope is an older version of an audioscope and is not used much anymore.

18. A baseline examination is a(n):
   a. examination to determine the cause of an illness.
   b. full medical examination for people over age 50 years.
   c. initial examination to give physicians information about the patient.
   d. examination based on the patient's symptoms.
   e. examination of the abdominal regions of the patient.

19. Which of the following materials should be stored in a room away from the examination room?
   a. Gloves
   b. Tongue depressors
   c. Tape measure
   d. Cotton tipped applicators
   e. Syringes

20. What does the "P" stand for in PERRLA?
   a. Position
   b. Protrusion
   c. Posture
   d. Pupil
   e. Perception

COG **MATCHING**

Match each key term with its definition.

Key Terms

21. _____ auscultation
22. _____ Babinski reflex
23. _____ bimanual
24. _____ bruit
25. _____ cerumen
26. _____ extraocular
27. _____ hernia
28. _____ occult
29. _____ Papanicolaou (Pap) test
30. _____ PERRLA
31. _____ range of motion (ROM)
32. _____ sclera
33. _____ speculum
34. _____ transillumination
35. _____ tympanic membrane
36. _____ clinical diagnosis
37. _____ differential diagnosis
38. _____ gait
39. _____ lubricant
40. _____ manipulation
41. _____ nasal septum
42. _____ rectovaginal
43. _____ peripheral
44. _____ applicator
45. _____ symmetry
46. _____ asymmetry

Definitions

a. an instrument used for examining body cavities
b. thin, semitransparent membrane in the middle ear that transmits vibrations
c. a reflex noted by the extension of the great toe and abduction of the other toes
d. a test in which cells from the cervix are examined microscopically for abnormalities
e. an examination performed with both hands
f. the extent of movement in the joints
g. abnormal sound or murmur in the blood vessels
h. white fibrous tissue covering the eye
i. passage of light through body tissues for the purpose of examination
j. blood present in stool that is not visibly apparent
k. a diagnosis based only on a patient's symptoms
l. act of listening to the sounds within the body to evaluate the heart, lungs, intestines, or fetal heart tones
m. an acronym that means pupils are equal, round, and reactive to light and accommodation
n. earwax
o. a protrusion of an organ through a weakened muscle wall
p. outside of the eye
q. a diagnosis made by comparing symptoms of several diseases
r. the passive movement of the joints to determine the extent of movement
s. pertaining to the rectum and vagina
t. equality in size and shape or position of parts on opposite sides of the body
u. a water-soluble agent that reduces friction
v. device for applying local treatments and tests
w. inequality in size and shape on opposite sides of the body
x. pertaining to or situated away from the center
y. partition dividing the nostrils
z. a manner of walking

COG **MATCHING**

Match each physical examination technique with its description by placing the letter preceding the definition on the line next to the correct basic examination technique.

Techniques

47. _____ inspection
48. _____ palpation
49. _____ percussion
50. _____ auscultation

Descriptions

a. touching or moving body areas with fingers or hands
b. looking at areas of the body to observe physical features
c. listening to the sounds of the body
d. tapping the body with the hand or an instrument to produce sounds

COG MATCHING

Grade: _____

Match each medical instrument with its description by placing the letter preceding the definition on the line next to the correct instrument.

Instruments
51. _____ tuning fork
52. _____ ophthalmoscope
53. _____ anoscope
54. _____ stethoscope
55. _____ laryngeal mirror
56. _____ headlight

Descriptions
a. an instrument used for listening to body sounds and taking blood pressure
b. an instrument used to examine the interior structures of the eyes
c. an instrument with two prongs used to test hearing
d. a light attached to a headband that provides direct light on the area being examined
e. an instrument used to examine areas of the patient's throat and larynx
f. a short, stainless steel or plastic speculum used to inspect the anal canal

COG IDENTIFICATION

Grade: _____

Anticipating what the physician will need during a patient examination is a skill that the competent medical assistant must develop. Indicate which of the following instruments would the physician most likely ask for to examine the patient in each situation. Place a check mark on the line next to the possible instrument (more than one instrument may apply).

57. A patient comes into the physician's office complaining of ringing in her ears.

a. _____ percussion hammer

b. _____ tuning fork

c. _____ laryngeal mirror

d. _____ otoscope

e. _____ ophthalmoscope

58. A male patient complains of weakness in his legs.

a. _____ percussion hammer

b. _____ tuning fork

c. _____ laryngeal mirror

d. _____ otoscope

e. _____ ophthalmoscope

59. A young female patient complains of a headache and fever.

a. _____ percussion hammer

b. _____ tuning fork

c. _____ laryngeal mirror

d. _____ otoscope

e. _____ ophthalmoscope

60. Listed below are the body areas inspected by the physician during a physical examination, but they are not in the correct order. Starting with the number one (1), number the body areas in the correct order in which they are examined.

_____ Eyes and ears

_____ Legs

_____ Head and neck

_____ Chest, breasts, and abdomen

_____ Nose and sinuses

_____ Reflexes

_____ Posture, gait, balance, and strength

_____ Mouth and throat

_____ Genitalia and rectum

61. Place a check mark on the line next to each factor that may be a warning sign for cancer. Check all that apply.

_____ an itchy rash on the arms and legs

_____ a nagging cough or hoarse voice

_____ unusual bleeding or discharge

_____ stiffness in joints

_____ a sore that will not heal

_____ frequent upper respiratory infections

_____ pain in any body area

62. As a medical assistant, you will be required to assist the physician before, during, and after physical examinations. Read the list of tasks below and place a letter on the line preceding the task indicating whether you would perform the task before (B), during (D), or after (A) the examination.

a. _____ Escort the patient to the front desk.

b. _____ Obtain a urine specimen from the patient, if required.

c. _____ Adjust the drape on the patient to expose the necessary body part.

d. _____ Ask the patient about medication used on a regular basis.

e. _____ Check the patient's medical record to ensure all the information has been accurately documented.

f. _____ Place the patient's chart outside the examining room door.

g. _____ Offer reassurance to the patient and check for signs of anxiety.

COG **SHORT ANSWER**   Grade: _____

63. A patient calls the physician's office and explains that her daughter cries continuously, has been vomiting regularly, and stumbles a lot. Which of these do you recommend and why?

    a. Tell her that it is probably a bug and to keep her child home from school for a couple of days.

    _____

    _____

    _____

    _____

    b. Advise that she keep an eye on the child and inform the physician if there is any change.

    _____

    _____

    _____

    _____

    c. Tell her to have the child examined immediately.

    _____

    _____

    _____

    _____

64. A patient comes into the physician's office with an open wound. When obtaining the patient's medical records, you discover that he last had a tetanus booster 4 years ago. What is the correct procedure and why?

    a. Recommend the patient has another tetanus booster.

    _____

    _____

    _____

    _____

    b. Tell the patient he does not need immunizing for another 6 years.

    _____

    _____

    _____

    _____

    c. Tell the patient he should have a booster if he is traveling abroad.

    _____

    _____

    _____

    _____

65. Dr. O'Brien tells you that a patient's eardrum is infected. What are the symptoms that could have led Dr. O'Brien to this diagnosis?

_____

_____

_____

_____

66. As a medical assistant, you are responsible for checking each examination room at the beginning of the day to make sure that it is ready for patients. List three things that need to be done to ensure that a room is ready.

_____

_____

_____

_____

COG TRUE OR FALSE?

Grade: _____

Indicate whether the statements are true or false by placing the letter T (true) or F (false) on the line preceding the statement.

67. _____ A normal tympanic membrane will be light pink and curve slightly outward.

68. _____ Patients should have a baseline electrocardiogram (ECG) when they turn age 60 years.

69. _____ The instruments used to examine the rectum and colon are all one standard size.

70. _____ The medical assistant is responsible for preparing the examination room, preparing the patient, assisting the physician, and cleaning the equipment and examination room.

COG AFF CASE STUDIES FOR CRITICAL THINKING

Grade: _____

71. A 19-year-old patient has never had a Pap smear before and does not understand what the test is for, or what is going to happen during the procedure. The physician asks you to explain the process to her in simple terms. List some key aspects of a Pap smear and explain the purpose of the procedure to this patient in a way that she will understand.

_____

_____

_____

_____

72. Alicia is assisting a male physician with performing a gynecologic examination. Midway through the examination, she is paged to assist another medical procedure. Explain what she should do and why.

_____

_____

_____

73. Your patient is a 35-year-old male who has a long family history of cancer. The patient is terrified of developing cancer and has been to see the physician several times for minor false alarms. Prepare an information sheet for the patient, explaining the early warning signs of cancer. What else can you do to alleviate the fear in this patient?

_____

_____

_____

_____

74. You are assisting with the physical examination of a 55-year-old male. When the physician begins to prepare for the rectal examination, the patient refuses and says that it is unnecessary and that he is fine. What would be the most appropriate thing to do at this point?

_____

_____

_____

_____

75. At the beginning of the day, you are preparing the examination rooms with a fellow medical assistant. You are both in a hurry because the first patients are arriving and the physicians are waiting for you to finish. Your fellow medical assistant suggests that you don't need to check the batteries in the equipment because everything worked well yesterday. What would you do or say?

_____

_____

_____

_____

76. While you are escorting a patient to the front desk, the patient asks you whether an over-the-counter medication will affect her prescribed treatment. You are familiar with both drugs. What is the correct response?

_____

_____

_____

_____

77. You are assisting a physician during a genital and pelvic examination on a female disabled patient who cannot be placed into the lithotomy position. What is the correct course of action?

_____

_____

_____

_____

PSY PROCEDURE 20-1 | **Assisting with the Adult Physical Examination**

Name: _____ Date: _____ Time: _____ Grade: _____

Equipment/SUPPLIES: A variety of instruments and supplies, including the stethoscope, ophthalmoscope, otoscope, penlight, tuning fork, nasal speculum, tongue blade, percussion hammer, gloves, water-soluble lubricant, an examinations light, and patient gown and draping supplies

STANDARDS: Given the needed equipment and a place to work, the student will perform this skill with _____ % accuracy in a total of _____ minutes. *(Your instructor will tell you what the percentage and time limits will be before you begin.)*

KEY: 4 = Satisfactory 0 = Unsatisfactory NA = This step is not counted

PROCEDURE STEPS	SELF	PARTNER	INSTRUCTOR
1. Wash your hands	❑	❑	❑
2. Prepare the examination room and assemble the equipment	❑	❑	❑
3. Greet the patient by name and escort him or her to the examining room	❑	❑	❑
4. Explain the procedure	❑	❑	❑
5. Obtain and record the medical history and chief complaint	❑	❑	❑
6. Take and record the vital signs, height, weight, and visual acuity	❑	❑	❑
7. If anticipated, instruct the patient to obtain a urine specimen and escort them to the bathroom	❑	❑	❑
8. Once inside the examination room, instruct the patient in disrobing, including directions on how to put the gown on (open in the front or back). Leave the room unless the patient needs assistance	❑	❑	❑
9. **AFF** Explain how to respond to a patient who has cultural or religious beliefs and is uncomfortable about disrobing	❑	❑	❑
10. Assist patient into a sitting position on the edge of the examination table. Cover the lap and legs with a drape	❑	❑	❑
11. **AFF** Place the medical record outside the examination room and notify the physician that the patient is ready. If your office uses an electronic medical record, assure you have entered and updated all information necessary and log off the computer before leaving the room	❑	❑	❑
12. Assist the physician by handing them the instruments as needed and positioning the patient appropriately	❑	❑	❑
13. Help the patient return to a sitting position	❑	❑	❑
14. Perform any follow-up procedures or treatments	❑	❑	❑
15. Leave the room while the patient dresses unless assistance is needed	❑	❑	❑

PSY PROCEDURE 20-1	**Assisting with the Adult Physical Examination** (continued)		

16. Return to the examination room after the patient has dressed to:
   a. answer questions.
   b. reinforce instructions.
   c. provide patient education.
	❑	❑	❑

17. Escort the patient to the front desk	❑	❑	❑
18. Properly clean or dispose of all used equipment and supplies	❑	❑	❑
19. Clean the room with a disinfectant and prepare for the next patient	❑	❑	❑

20. Wash your hands
   a. Record any instructions that were ordered for the patient
   b. Note if any specimens were obtained
   c. Indicate the results of the test or note the laboratory where the specimens are being sent for testing
	❑	❑	❑

_____

_____

_____

_____

CALCULATION

Total Possible Points: _____

Total Points Earned: _____ Multiplied by 100 = _____ Divided by Total Possible Points = _____ %

PASS   **FAIL**   **COMMENTS:**
  ❑   ❑

Student's signature _____ Date _____

Partner's signature _____ Date _____

Instructor's signature _____ Date _____

CHAPTER 21

Sterilization and Surgical Instruments

LEARNING OUTCOMES

COG Cognitive Domain*

1. Spell and define the key terms
2. *Identify the following as practiced within an ambulatory care setting: surgical asepsis*
3. *Identify quality assurance practices in health care*
4. Describe several methods of sterilization
5. Categorize surgical instruments based on use and identify each by its characteristics
6. Identify surgical instruments specific to designated specialties
7. State the difference between reusable and disposable instruments

8. Explain how to handle and store instruments, equipment, and supplies
9. Describe the necessity and steps for maintaining documents and records of maintenance for instruments and equipment

PSY Psychomotor Domain*

1. Sanitize equipment and instruments (Procedure 21-1)
2. *Prepare items for autoclaving*
3. Properly wrap instruments for autoclaving (Procedure 21-2)
4. *Perform sterilization procedures*

5. Perform sterilization technique and operate an autoclave (Procedure 21-3)
6. *Perform a quality-control measure*

MAERB Standards are Italicized.

ABHES Competencies

1. Practice standard precautions and perform disinfection/ sterilization techniques.
2. Practice quality control

Name: _____   Date: _____   Grade: _____

COG MULTIPLE CHOICE

Circle the letter preceding the correct answer:

1. A sterile field is defined as an area:
   a. where the autoclave is kept.
   b. that is free of all microorganisms.
   c. where sterilized instruments are stored.
   d. that has been cleaned with a chemical disinfectant.
   e. in which only sanitized equipment can be used.

2. Instruments that are sterilized in the autoclave maintain their sterility for:
   a. 15 days.
   b. 20 days.
   c. 25 days.
   d. 30 days.
   e. 35 days.

3. Autoclave tape indicates that an object:
   a. has not been sterilized.
   b. contains a specific type of microorganism.
   c. has been exposed to steam in the autoclave.
   d. needs to be placed on its side in the autoclave.
   e. did not reach the proper pressure and temperature in the autoclave.

4. Material used to wrap items that are being sterilized in the autoclave must be:
   a. permeable to steam but not contaminants.
   b. permeable to distilled water but not tap water.
   c. permeable to heat but not formaldehyde.
   d. permeable to ethylene oxide but not pathogens.
   e. permeable to contaminants but not microorganisms.

5. Which of the following should be included in an equipment record?
   a. Expiration date
   b. Date of purchase
   c. Physician's name
   d. The office's address
   e. Date of last sterilization

6. Which of the following should be included in a sterilization record?
   a. Location of the item
   b. Number of items in the load
   c. Method of sterilization used
   d. Reason for the service request
   e. Results of the sterilization indicator

7. One instrument commonly used in urology is a(n):
   a. curet.
   b. tonometer.
   c. urethral sound.
   d. sigmoidoscope.
   e. uterine dilator.

8. Forceps are used to:
   a. cut sutures.
   b. dissect tissue.
   c. make incisions.
   d. guide instruments.
   e. compress or join tissue.

9. All packs containing bowls or containers should be placed in the autoclave:
   a. upright.
   b. under a cloth.
   c. on their sides.
   d. stacked on top of each other.
   e. with their sterilization indicators facing up.

10. Consult the material safety data sheet (MSDS) before:
    a. handling a chemical spill.
    b. reading a sterilization indicator.
    c. sterilizing an instrument in the autoclave.
    d. requesting service for a piece of equipment.
    e. disposing of a used scalpel handle and blade.

11. Why does the autoclave use pressure in the sterilization process?
    a. Pathogens and microorganisms thrive in low-pressure environments.
    b. High pressure makes the wrapping permeable to steam and not contaminants.
    c. Pressure must be applied to distilled water in order to release sterilizing agents.
    d. High pressure prevents microorganisms from penetrating the objects being sterilized.
    e. High pressure allows the steam to reach the high temperatures needed for sterilization.

12. Which of the following instruments are used to hold sterile drapes in place during surgical procedures?
    a. Directors
    b. Serrations
    c. Towel clamps
    d. Curved scissors
    e. Alligator biopsies

13. Notched mechanisms that hold the tips of the forceps together tightly are called:
    a. springs.
    b. sutures.
    c. ratchets.
    d. serrations.
    e. clamps.

14. After use, scalpel blades should be:
    a. sterilized in the autoclave.
    b. discarded in a sharps container.
    c. reattached to a scalpel handle.
    d. processed in a laboratory.
    e. wrapped in cotton muslin.

15. The instrument used to hold open layers of tissue to expose the areas underneath during a surgical procedure is a:
    a. retractor.
    b. scalpel.
    c. director.
    d. clamp.
    e. forceps.

16. Ratcheted instruments should be stored:
    a. open.
    b. closed.
    c. hanging.
    d. standing.
    e. upside down.

17. Medical asepsis is intended to prevent the spread of microbes from:
    a. one patient to another.
    b. the autoclave to the patient.
    c. the instruments to the physician.
    d. the inside to the outside of the body.
    e. the physician to the medical assistant.

18. A punch biopsy is used to:
    a. diagnose glaucoma.
    b. dissect delicate tissues.
    c. explore bladder depths.
    d. remove tissue for microscopic study.
    e. guide an instrument during a procedure.

19. The best way to test the effectiveness of an autoclave is to use:
    a. thermometers.
    b. wax pellets.
    c. autoclave tape.
    d. color indicators.
    e. strips with heat-resistant spores.

20. Which is a step in operating the autoclave?
    a. Stacking items on top of each other
    b. Filling the reservoir tank with tap water
    c. Filling the reservoir a little past the fill line
    d. Removing items from the autoclave the moment they are done
    e. Setting the timer after the correct temperature has been reached

OOG MATCHING

Grade: _____

Match each key term with its definition.

Key Terms

21. _____ autoclave
22. _____ disinfection
23. _____ ethylene oxide
24. _____ forceps
25. _____ hemostat
26. _____ needle holder
27. _____ obturator
28. _____ ratchet
29. _____ sanitation
30. _____ sanitize
31. _____ scalpel
32. _____ scissors
33. _____ serration
34. _____ sound
35. _____ sterilization

Definitions

a. surgical instrument used to grasp, hold, compress, pull, or join tissue, equipment, or supplies

b. a long instrument used to explore or dilate body cavities

c. a gas used to sterilize surgical instruments and other supplies

d. appliance used to sterilize medical instruments with steam under pressure

e. a surgical instrument with slender jaws that is used to grasp blood vessels

f. groove, either straight or crisscross, etched or cut into the blade or tip of an instrument to improve its bite or grasp

g. a notched mechanism that clicks into position to maintain tension on the opposing blades or tips of the instrument

h. killing or rendering inert most but not all pathogenic microorganisms

i. to reduce the number of microorganisms on a surface by use of low-level disinfectant practices

j. a sharp instrument composed of two opposing cutting blades, held together by a central pin on which the blades pivot

k. a type of forceps that is used to hold and pass suture through tissue

l. a small pointed knife with a convex edge for surgical procedures

m. a process, act, or technique for destroying microorganisms using heat, water, chemicals, or gases

n. the maintenance of a healthful, disease-free environment

o. a smooth, rounded, removable inner portion of a hollow tube that allows for easier insertion

OOG MATCHING

Grade: _____

Match each instrument with its description.

Instruments

36. _____ forceps
37. _____ scissors
38. _____ scalpels
39. _____ clamps
40. _____ retractors

Descriptions

a. dissect delicate tissue

b. hold sterile drapes in place

c. grasp tissue for dissection

d. make an incision

e. transfer sterile supplies

f. cut off a bandage

g. excise tissue

h. hold open layers of tissue

OOG IDENTIFICATION

Grade: _____

41. Complete this table, which identifies four types of scissors and their use.

Type	Use
bandage scissors	a.
b.	dissect superficial and delicate tissues
straight scissors	c.
d.	remove sutures

42. Complete the chart below by identifying one instrument used in each specialty.

Specialty	Instrument
Obstetrics, gynecology	a.
Orthopedics	b.
Urology	c.
Proctology	d.
Otology, rhinology	e.
Ophthalmology	f.
Dermatology	g.

43. Complete this table, which describes the most effective method of sterilizing various instruments and materials.

Method of Sterilization	Most Effective for
a.	minor surgical instruments surgical storage trays and containers bowls for holding sterile equipment
b.	instruments or equipment subject to water damage
c.	instruments or equipment subject to heat damage

COG SHORT ANSWER

Grade: _____

44. Describe the process by which an autoclave sterilizes instruments.

_____

_____

_____

_____

45. What is the purpose of sterilization indicators? What factors may alter the results of a sterilization indicator?

_____

_____

_____

_____

46. What components must be properly set in order for the autoclave to work effectively?

_____

_____

_____

_____

47. List the guidelines that you should follow when handling and storing sharp instruments.

_____

_____

_____

_____

48. What is the purpose of autoclave tape?

_____

_____

_____

_____

49. Which method of sterilization is more effective: boiling water or the autoclave? Why?

_____

_____

_____

_____

50. Compare the qualities of medical asepsis and surgical asepsis.

_____

_____

_____

_____

COG TRUE OR FALSE?   Grade: _____

Indicate whether the statements are true or false by placing the letter T (true) or F (false) on the line preceding the statement.

51. _____ Equipment must be sanitized before it is sterilized.

52. _____ Autoclave indicator tape is 100% effective in indicating whether a package is sterile.

53. _____ It is the medical assistant's responsibility to maintain complete and accurate records of sterilized equipment.

54. _____ The handle and blade of a reusable steel scalpel may be reused after being properly sterilized.

COG AFF **CASE STUDIES FOR CRITICAL THINKING** _____ Grade: _____

55. You are one of two medical assistants working in a small office that specializes in ophthalmology. There is one examination room. The office sees about 50 patients a week, with an average of three patients a week needing minor ophthalmologic procedures. The physician has asked you to order new instruments for the office for the next month. What are two of the instruments that you will order? What factors will you need to consider when placing the order?

_____

_____

_____

_____

56. Your medical office has one autoclave along with two pairs of sterilized suture scissors and adequate numbers of other instruments. In the morning, the physician uses one pair of suture scissors to perform a minor procedure. He tosses the scissors into a sink when he is finished, damaging the instrument. At noon, the autoclave suddenly malfunctions, and you put in a service request to repair it. In the afternoon, a patient comes into the office complaining that her sutures are painful. The physician decides that he must remove them right away. Right before the procedure begins, the physician drops the only sterile pair of suture scissors in the office before he can use them. Describe two possible plans of action you can take to help the patient who is still in pain.

_____

_____

_____

_____

57. The physician has just completed a procedure in which he used a disposable scalpel. How should you dispose of this instrument and why? Would it be appropriate to autoclave this scalpel to save money? Why or why not?

_____

_____

_____

_____

58. Your patient is about to undergo a minor office surgery and is concerned because she once received a facial piercing that led to a massive infection due to improperly sterilized instruments. Now, she is worried about the cleanliness of your office. How would you explain the precautions your office takes to ensure that all instruments and equipment are safe and sterile in language that the patient can understand?

_____

_____

_____

_____

59. A package arrives at your office and you and your coworker are unable to open it. After looking around the immediate area, your coworker leaves the room and comes back with a pair of sterile operating scissors to open the package. Should you allow your coworker to use the scissors to open the package? What reason would you give your coworker for allowing or not allowing them to use the scissors?

_____

_____

_____

_____

60. Your office uses formaldehyde to sterilize some instruments. While transporting the instruments soaking in formaldehyde, you accidentally spill the formaldehyde. You are in a hurry and consider leaving the small amount of chemical on the floor until later. Would this be an appropriate action to take? Why or why not? How would you clean up this spill?

_____

_____

_____

_____

PSY PROCEDURE 21-1 | Sanitize Equipment and Instruments

Name: _____ Date: _____ Time: _____ Grade: _____

EQUIPMENT/SUPPLIES: Instruments or equipment to be sanitized, gloves, eye protection, impervious gown, soap and water, small hand-held scrub brush

STANDARDS: Given the needed equipment and a place to work, the student will perform this skill with _____ % accuracy in a total of _____ minutes. *(Your instructor will tell you what the percentage and time limits will be before you begin.)*

KEY: 4 = Satisfactory   0 = Unsatisfactory   NA = This step is not counted

PROCEDURE STEPS	SELF	PARTNER	INSTRUCTOR
1. Put on gloves, gown, and eye protection	❏	❏	❏
2. For equipment that requires assembly, take removable sections apart	❏	❏	❏
3. Check the operation and integrity of the equipment	❏	❏	❏
4. Rinse the instrument with cool water	❏	❏	❏
5. Force streams of soapy water through any tubular or grooved instruments	❏	❏	❏
6. Use a hot, soapy solution to dissolve fats or lubricants left on the surface	❏	❏	❏

7. Soak for 5 to 10 minutes
  a. Use friction (brush or gauze) to wipe down the instruments
  b. Check jaws or scissors/forceps to ensure that all debris has been removed
	❏	❏	❏

8. Rinse well	❏	❏	❏
9. Dry well before autoclaving if sterilizing or soaking in disinfecting solution	❏	❏	❏
10. Items (brushes, gauze, solution) used in sanitation process must be disinfected or discarded	❏	❏	❏

CALCULATION

Total Possible Points: _____

Total Points Earned: _____ Multiplied by 100 = _____ Divided by Total Possible Points = _____ %

PASS   FAIL   COMMENTS:
  ❏   ❏

Student's signature _____ Date _____

Partner's signature _____ Date _____

Instructor's signature _____ Date _____

PSY PROCEDURE 21-2   Wrap Instruments Properly for Autoclaving

Name: _____   **Date:** _____   **Time:** _____   **Grade:** _____

EQUIPMENT/SUPPLIES: Sanitized and wrapped instruments or equipment, distilled water, autoclave operating manual

STANDARDS: Given the needed equipment and a place to work, the student will perform this skill with _____ % accuracy in a total of _____ minutes. *(Your instructor will tell you what the percentage and time limits will be before you begin.)*

KEY: 4 = Satisfactory   0 = Unsatisfactory   NA = This step is not counted

PROCEDURE STEPS	SELF	PARTNER	INSTRUCTOR
1. Assemble the equipment and supplies	❏	❏	❏
2. Check the instruments being wrapped for working order. Explain what to do if an instrument is found not to be in good working order	❏	❏	❏
3. Obtain correct material for wrapping instruments to be autoclaved	❏	❏	❏
4. Tear off one to two pieces of autoclave tape. On one piece, label the contents of the pack, the date, and your initials	❏	❏	❏
5. Lay the wrap diagonally on a flat, clean, dry surface 　**a.** Place the instrument in the center, with ratchets or handles in the open position 　**b.** Include a sterilization indicator	❏	❏	❏
6. Fold the first flap up at the bottom of the diagonal wrap. Fold back the corner to make a tab	❏	❏	❏
7. Fold left corner of the wrap toward the center. Fold back the corner to make a tab	❏	❏	❏
8. Fold the right corner of the wrap toward the center. Fold back the corner to make a tab	❏	❏	❏
9. Fold the top corner down, making the tab tuck under the material	❏	❏	❏
10. Secure the package with labeled autoclave tape	❏	❏	❏

CALCULATION

Total Possible Points: _____

Total Points Earned: _____ Multiplied by 100 = _____ Divided by Total Possible Points = _____ %

PASS   FAIL   COMMENTS:
❏   ❏

Student's signature _____   Date _____

Partner's signature _____   Date _____

Instructor's signature _____   Date _____

PSY PROCEDURE 21-3 | **Perform Sterilization Technique and Operate an Autoclave**

Name: _____ Date: _____ Time: _____ Grade: _____

EQUIPMENT/SUPPLIES: Sanitized and wrapped instruments or equipment, distilled water, autoclave, autoclave operating manual

STANDARDS: Given the needed equipment and a place to work, the student will perform this skill with _____ % accuracy in a total of _____ minutes. *(Your instructor will tell you what the percentage and time limits will be before you begin.)*

KEY: 4 = Satisfactory 0 = Unsatisfactory NA = This step is not counted

PROCEDURE STEPS	SELF	PARTNER	INSTRUCTOR
1. Assemble the equipment, including the wrapped articles with a sterilization indicator in each package according to office policy	❏	❏	❏
2. Check the water level of the autoclave reservoir and add more, if needed	❏	❏	❏
3. Add water to the internal chamber of the autoclave to the fill line	❏	❏	❏
4. Properly load the autoclave	❏	❏	❏
5. Read the instructions, close the door, and secure or lock it. Turn the machine on	❏	❏	❏
6. Set the timer at the appropriate time and for the proper length of time	❏	❏	❏
7. When the timer indicates that the cycle is over, vent the chamber	❏	❏	❏
8. When the load has cooled, remove the items. Check the separately wrapped sterilization indicator, if used, for proper sterilization	❏	❏	❏
9. Store the items in a clean, dry, dust-free area	❏	❏	❏
10. Explain how to clean the autoclave	❏	❏	❏

CALCULATION

Total Possible Points: _____

Total Points Earned: _____ Multiplied by 100 = _____ Divided by Total Possible Points = _____ %

PASS   FAIL   COMMENTS:
  ❏   ❏

Student's signature _____ Date _____

Partner's signature _____ Date _____

Instructor's signature _____ Date _____

CHAPTER 22

Assisting with Minor Office Surgery

LEARNING OUTCOMES

COG Cognitive Domain*

1. Spell and define key terms
2. List your responsibilities before, during, and after minor office surgery
3. Identify the guidelines for preparing and maintaining sterility of the field and surgical equipment during a minor office procedure
4. State your responsibility in relation to informed consent and patient preparation
5. Explain the purpose of local anesthetics and list three commonly used in the medical office
6. Describe the types of needles and sutures and the uses of each
7. Describe the various methods of skin closure used in the medical office
8. Explain your responsibility during surgical specimen collection
9. List the types of laser surgery and electrosurgery used in the medical office and explain the precautions for each
10. Describe the guidelines for applying a sterile dressing

PSY Psychomotor Domain*

1. Open sterile surgical packs (Procedure 22-1)
   a. *Prepare a sterile field*

2. Use sterile transfer forceps (Procedure 22-2)
3. Add sterile solution to a sterile field (Procedure 22-3)
   a. *Prepare a sterile field*
   b. *Perform within a sterile field*
4. Perform skin preparation and hair removal (Procedure 22-4)
   a. *Instruct and prepare a patient for a procedure or a treatment*
5. Apply sterile gloves (Procedure 22-5)
6. Apply a sterile dressing (Procedure 22-6)
   a. *Instruct and prepare a patient for a procedure or a treatment*
   b. *Prepare a sterile field*
   c. *Perform within a sterile field*
   d. *Perform wound care*
   e. *Demonstrate proper disposal of biohazardous material: sharps and regulated waste*
   f. Coach patients appropriately considering cultural diversity, developmental life stage, and communication barriers
   g. *Document patient care accurately in the medical record*
7. Change an existing sterile dressing (Procedure 22-7)
   a. *Instruct and prepare a patient for a procedure or treatment*
   b. *Prepare a sterile field*
   c. *Perform within a sterile field*
   d. *Perform a dressing change*
   e. *Perform wound care*

f. *Demonstrate proper disposal of biohazardous material: sharps and regulated waste*
g. *Coach patients appropriately considering cultural diversity, developmental life stage, and communication barriers*
h. *Document patient care accurately in the medical record*
8. Assist with excisional surgery (Procedure 22-8)
   a. *Instruct and prepare a patient for a procedure or a treatment*
   b. *Prepare a sterile field*
   c. *Perform within a sterile field*
   d. *Perform wound care*
   e. *Demonstrate proper disposal of biohazardous material: sharps and regulated waste*
   f. Coach patients appropriately considering cultural diversity, developmental life stage, and communication barriers
   g. *Document patient care accurately in the medical record*
9. Assist with incision and drainage (Procedure 22-9)
   a. *Instruct and prepare a patient for a procedure or a treatment*
   b. *Prepare a sterile field*
   c. *Perform within a sterile field*
   d. *Perform wound care*
   e. *Demonstrate proper disposal of biohazardous material: sharps and regulated waste*

    f. Coach patients appropriately considering cultural diversity, developmental life stage, and communication barriers

    g. *Document patient care accurately in the medical record*

10. Remove sutures (Procedure 22-10)

    a. *Instruct and prepare a patient for a procedure or a treatment*

    b. *Demonstrate proper disposal of biohazardous material: sharps and regulated waste*

    c. Coach patients appropriately considering cultural diversity, developmental life stage, and communication barriers

    d. *Document patient care accurately in the medical record*

11. Remove staples (Procedure 22-11)

    a. *Instruct and prepare a patient for a procedure or a treatment*

    b. *Demonstrate proper disposal of biohazardous material: sharps and regulated waste*

    c. Coach patients appropriately considering cultural diversity, developmental life stage, and communication barriers

    d. *Document patient care accurately in the medical record*

AFF Affective Domain*

1. *Demonstrate critical thinking skills*
2. *Reassure patients*
3. *Demonstrate empathy for patients' concerns*
4. *Demonstrate active listening*
5. *Respect diversity*
6. *Recognize personal boundaries*
7. *Demonstrate tactfulness*
8. *Demonstrate self-awareness*
9. Protect the integrity of the medical record

***MAERB Standards are Italicized.**

ABHES Competencies

1. Perform specialty procedures, including but not limited to, minor surgery, cardiac, respiratory, OB-GYN, neurologic, and gastroenterology
2. Display effective interpersonal skills with patients and healthcare team members
3. Demonstrate cultural awareness
4. Dispose of biohazardous materials
5. Practice standard precautions and perform disinfection/sterilization techniques
6. Follow documentation guidelines

Name: _____   Date: _____   Grade: _____

COG MULTIPLE CHOICE

Circle the letter preceding the correct answer.

1. Which of the following statements is true about working in a sterile field?
   a. Sterile packages should be kept damp
   b. Your back must be kept to the sterile field at all times
   c. A 3-inch border around the field is considered contaminated
   d. All sterile items should be held above waist level
   e. Cover your mouth when coughing near the sterile field

2. Why is a fenestrated drape helpful during surgery?
   a. It is made of lightweight fabric
   b. It has an opening to expose the operative site
   c. It can be used as a blanket to keep the patient warm
   d. It does not need to be sterilized before surgery
   e. It allows for easy cleanup after the surgery

3. Epinephrine is added to local anesthetics during surgery to:
   a. ensure sterilization.
   b. protect the tips of the fingers.
   c. lengthen the anesthetic's effectiveness.
   d. prevent vasoconstriction.
   e. create rapid absorption.

4. Which needles are used most frequently in the medical office?
   a. Curved swaged needles
   b. Traumatic needles
   c. Straight needles
   d. Domestic needles
   e. Keith needles

5. A preservative is added to specimen containers to be sent to a pathologist to:
   a. help the pathologist see the specimen.
   b. delay decomposition.
   c. identify the patient.
   d. make the specimen grow.
   e. prevent contamination.

6. Which type of electrosurgery destroys tissue with controlled electric sparks?
   a. Electrocautery
   b. Electrodesiccation
   c. Electrosection
   d. Fulguration
   e. Electrophysiology

7. Why is it important to know if a patient has a pacemaker before performing electrosurgery?
   a. Metal implants can become very hot and malfunction during the procedure
   b. The electrical charge can cause the electrosurgical device to malfunction
   c. The patient needs to sign a separate consent form if he has any heart problems
   d. The patient can receive an electric shock from the equipment
   e. The implants may counteract the electrosurgery results

Scenario for Questions 8 and 9: A female patient returns to the office to have sutures removed from her forearm. When you remove the dressing, you notice that there is a small amount of clear drainage.

8. The patient's drainage is:
   a. purulent.
   b. sanguineous.
   c. serous.
   d. copious.
   e. serosanguineous.

9. Before you remove the patient's sutures, you should:
   a. apply a local anesthetic to numb the area.
   b. offer the patient pain medication to reduce discomfort.
   c. place an ice pack on the patient's forearm.
   d. advise the patient that she should feel a pulling sensation but not pain.
   e. gently tug on the ends of the suture to make sure they are secure.

10. Which of the following is characteristic of healing by primary intention?
    a. Clean incision
    b. Gaping, irregular wound
    c. Increased granulation
    d. Wide scar
    e. Indirect edge joining

11. What happens during phase II of wound healing?
    a. Fibroblasts build scar tissue to guard the area
    b. The scab dries and pulls the edges of the wound together
    c. Circulation increases and brings white blood cells to the area
    d. Serum and red blood cells form a fibrin to plug the wound
    e. An antiseptic sterilizes the area from possible contamination

12. How must the physician care for an abscess in order for it to heal properly?
    a. Drain the infected material from the site
    b. Suture the site closed
    c. Cover the site with a sterile dressing
    d. Perform cryosurgery to remove the site
    e. Perform a skin graft to cover the site

13. Which of the following items should be added to the label on a specimen container?
    a. The contents of the container
    b. The office number
    c. The patient's age
    d. The patient's gender
    e. The date

14. Which of the following is true about laser surgery?
    a. The Argon laser is the only laser used for coagulation
    b. Colored filters allow the physician to see the path of the laser
    c. Most lasers are used simply as markers for surgery
    d. Laser incisions generally bleed more than regular incisions
    e. Everyone in the room must wear goggles to protect their eyes

15. What is the best way to prepare a patient for surgery?
    a. Remind the patient of procedures by calling a few days before the surgery
    b. Tell the patient all of the instructions during the visit before the surgery
    c. Send the patient home with written instructions on what to do
    d. Instruct the patient to call the day of the procedure for instructions
    e. Have the patient tell a second person about what she needs to do

16. Which of the following supplies must be added at the time of setup for a surgery?
    a. Liquids in open containers
    b. Sterile transfer forceps
    c. Peel-back envelopes
    d. Sterile gloves
    e. Fenestrated drape

17. Absorbable sutures are most frequently used:
    a. in medical offices for wound sutures.
    b. in hospitals for deep-tissue surgery.
    c. in hospitals for surface-tissue surgery.
    d. when patients are young and heal easily.
    e. whenever a wound needs to be sutured.

18. Which of the following might contaminate a sterile dressing?
    a. A patient accidentally bumps into another person
    b. The wound still has sutures underneath
    c. The weather outside has been rainy and damp
    d. The patient adjusted the dressing at home
    e. The patient has had a cold for the past week

19. A child came in with a slight cut on his leg, but there is little tension on the skin, and the cut is clean. The physician believes the wound will heal on its own, with time, and wants to approximate the edges of the wound so that it will heal with minimum scarring. Which of the following would be best to use to close the child's wound?
    a. Adhesive skin closures
    b. Fine absorptive sutures
    c. Traumatic sutures
    d. Staples
    e. Nothing

20. The last step in any surgical procedure is to:
    a. assist the patient to leave.
    b. instruct the patient on postoperative procedures.
    c. remove all biohazardous materials.
    d. wash your hands.
    e. record the procedure.

OOG **MATCHING**

Grade: _____

Place the letter preceding the definition on the line next to the term.

Key Terms
21. _____ approximate
22. _____ atraumatic
23. _____ bandage
24. _____ cautery
25. _____ coagulate
26. _____ cryosurgery
27. _____ dehiscence
28. _____ dressing
29. _____ electrode
30. _____ fulgurate
31. _____ keratosis
32. _____ lentigines
33. _____ preservative
34. _____ purulent
35. _____ swaged needle
36. _____ traumatic

Definitions
a. separation or opening of the edges of a wound
b. a medium for conducting or detecting electrical current
c. tissue surfaces that are as close together as possible
d. a covering applied directly to a wound to apply pressure, support, absorb secretions, protect from trauma, slow or stop bleeding, or hide disfigurement
e. a means or device that destroys tissue using an electric current, freezing, or burning
f. causing or relating to tissue damage
g. a swaged type of needle that does not require threading
h. to destroy tissue by electrodesiccation
i. a soft material applied to a body part to immobilize the body part or control bleeding
j. to change from a liquid to a solid or semisolid mass
k. brown skin macules occurring after exposure to the sun; freckles
l. drainage from a wound that is white, green, or yellow, signaling an infection
m. a metal needle fused to suture material
n. a skin condition characterized by overgrowth and thickening
o. a substance that delays decomposition
p. surgery in which abnormal tissue is removed by freezing

OOG **MATCHING**

Grade: _____

Place the letter preceding the description on the line next to the procedure.

Procedures
37. _____ electrocautery
38. _____ electrodesiccation
39. _____ electrosection
40. _____ fulguration

Descriptions
a. destroys tissue with controlled electric sparks
b. causes quick coagulation of small blood vessels with the heat created by the electric current
c. is used for incision or excision of tissue
d. dries and separates tissue with an electric current

COG IDENTIFICATION

Grade: _____

41. As a medical assistant, you may be called on to assist a physician with minor office surgery. Review the list of tasks below and determine which tasks you are responsible for as a medical assistant. Place a check in the "Yes" column for those duties you will assist with as a medical assistant, and place a check in the "No" column for those tasks that you would not be able to perform.

Task	Yes	No
a. Remind the patient of the physician's presurgery instructions, such as fasting		
b. Prepare the treatment room, including the supplies and equipment		
c. Obtain the informed consent document from the patient		
d. Inject the patient with local anesthesia, if necessary		
e. Choose the size of the suture to be used to close the wound		
f. Apply a dressing or bandage to the wound		
g. Instruct the patient about postoperative wound care		
h. Prescribe pain medication for the patient to take at home		
i. Prepare lab paperwork for any specimens that must be sent out to the lab		
j. Patient materials		
k. Clean and sterilize the room for the next patient		

42. A patient comes into the physician's office with a large wound on his leg. The physician asks you to assist with minor surgery to care for the wound. Because you must help maintain a sterile field before and during the procedure, review the list of actions below and indicate whether sterility (S) was maintained or if there has been any possible contamination (C).

a. _____ The sterile package was moist before the surgery started

b. _____ The physician spills a few drops of sterile water onto the sterile field

c. _____ You hold the sterile items for the physician above waist level

d. _____ The physician rests the sterile items in the middle of the sterile field

e. _____ You ask the physician a question over the sterile field

f. _____ The physician leaves the room and places a drape over the field

g. _____ The physician passes soiled gauze over the sterile field and asks you to dispose of it properly

43. As a medical assistant, you may be responsible for preparing and maintaining sterile packs. Determine if the packs listed below are appropriately sterilized (S) or if they need to be repackaged (R) and sterilized again.

a. _____ No moisture is present on the pack

b. _____ The package was sterilized onsite 15 days ago

c. _____ The wrapper is ripped down one side

d. _____ The sterilization indicator has changed color

e. _____ An item from the package fell out onto the floor when you picked it up

44. Which of the following information must be stated on the informed consent document? Circle the letter preceding all items that apply.

    a. The name of the procedure

    b. The tools used in the procedure

    c. The purpose of the procedure

    d. The expected results

    e. The patient's Social Security number

    f. Possible side effects

    g. The length of the procedure

    h. Potential risks and complications

    i. The date of the follow-up appointment

45. Listed below are the steps that a medical assistant should take to clean the examination room and prepare it for the next patient after a minor office surgical procedure. However, the steps below are not listed in the correct order. Review the steps and then place a number on the line next to each step to show the correct order in which they should occur with number 1 being the first step taken.

    a. _____ Put on gloves

    b. _____ Remove papers and sheets from the table and discard properly

    c. _____ Replace the table sheet paper for the next patient

    d. _____ Wipe down the examination table, surgical stand, sink, counter, and other surfaces used during the procedure with a disinfectant and allow them to dry

COG SHORT ANSWER

Grade: _____

46. List the three ways in which you may add the contents of peel-back packages to a sterile field.

    a. _____

    b. _____

    c. _____

47. Name four anesthetics that are commonly used in a medical office.

    a. _____

    b. _____

    c. _____

    d. _____

48. Name three ways in which needles can be classified.

a. _____

b. _____

c. _____

COG TRUE OR FALSE?

Grade: _____

Indicate whether the statements are true or false by placing the letter T (true) or F (false) on the line preceding the statement.

49. _____ Anesthesia with epinephrine is approved for use on the tips of the fingers, toes, nose, and penis.

50. _____ Atraumatic needles need to be threaded by the physician before they can be used.

51. _____ Nonabsorbable sutures must be removed after healing.

52. _____ All metal must be removed from a patient before electrosurgery.

COG AFF CASE STUDIES FOR CRITICAL THINKING

Grade: _____

53. The physician asks you to position a patient for surgery in the lithotomy position. You know that the physician has to meet with another patient before he will come into the room to perform the surgery. What can you do to keep the patient comfortable before the physician is ready to begin? List three things you can do, and explain why they are important.

_____

_____

_____

_____

54. There is a delay in the office, and all of the appointments are running 30 minutes late. The patients are becoming upset, and the office manager said that you should work quickly to try to get back on schedule. You assist the physician with the removal of a small wart from a patient's neck. After the surgery is completed, you need to meet with a new patient to go over the new patient interview and paperwork. But it's also your job to label the specimen and complete the paperwork to send it to the lab. It's almost lunchtime, and you know the lab won't get to it right away. Which task should you complete first—meeting with the patient or preparing the specimen for the lab? Explain your answer.

_____

_____

_____

_____

55. Dante is a clinical medical assistant who is assisting a physician with minor office surgery. Dr. Yan asks him to prepare the local anesthesia. Dante chooses the anesthetic and draws the medication into a syringe. Next, he places the filled syringe on the sterile tray. Were these actions appropriate? Why or why not? Should Dr. Yan put on sterile gloves before or after she administers the anesthesia? Explain your answer.

_____

_____

_____

_____

56. A homeless patient comes into the urgent care office with a cut on his chin. Which size suture would the physician likely want for this procedure in order to reduce the size of the scar—a size 3 suture or a size 23-0 suture? The patient seems confused and smells of alcohol. How would you handle this situation before, during, and after the procedure?

_____

_____

_____

_____

57. Ghani is a clinical medical assistant. On Monday, he assisted the physician while she sutured a deep wound on a 7-year-old boy's leg. A few hours after the surgery, the mother brings the boy back to the office because she is concerned the site is infected. When Ghani inspects the sterile dressing, he notes that there is a moderate amount of pink drainage. What does this drainage indicate about the healing process? Is the mother's concern legitimate? How would you respond to her?

_____

_____

_____

_____

58. Your patient is a 79-year-old female who has had a large mole excised from her forearm. The cyst is being sent out for pathology to rule out skin cancer. You give her extra bandages so she can change the dressing herself and explain that the physician wants to see her back in the office in 1 week. She is very hard of hearing and lives alone. What instructions would you need to explain to the patient about caring for the wound? How would you handle this situation?

_____

_____

_____

_____

59. Your patient is a 13-year-old boy who received staples for a wound he got in a biking accident. While you are removing the staples, he asks why staples are being used, and not stitches. Explain the difference between sutures and staples, and when it is more appropriate to use each.

_____

_____

_____

60. A 15-year-old patient has a mole on her face that needs to be removed. She feels anxious about having to wear a large dressing to cover the wound on her face while it heals. In addition, she is nervous about the possibilities of scarring, and she is worried that the mole is cancerous. How would you handle this situation? What would you say to her to ease her mind before and after the procedure?

_____

_____

_____

_____

61. You are working with another medical assistant to prepare a sterile field for surgery. You are almost finished setting up the sterile field when your coworker sneezes over the sterile field. She says that it's only allergies and that she's not contagious, so the field isn't contaminated. She assures you that you don't need to start your work over again. How would you handle this situation? What would you say to your coworker? What should you do next?

_____

_____

_____

_____

PSY PROCEDURE 22-1 **Opening Sterile Surgical Packs**

Name: _____ Date: _____ Time: _____ Grade: _____

EQUIPMENT/SUPPLIES: Surgical pack, surgical or Mayo stand

STANDARDS: Given the needed equipment and a place to work, the student will perform this skill with _____ % accuracy in a total of _____ minutes. *(Your instructor will tell you what the percentage and time limits will be before you begin.)*

KEY: 4 = Satisfactory 0 = Unsatisfactory NA = This step is not counted

PROCEDURE STEPS	SELF	PARTNER	INSTRUCTOR
1. Wash your hands	❏	❏	❏
2. Verify the procedure to be performed and remove the appropriate tray or item from the storage area. Check the label for contents and expiration date. Check the package for tears and moisture	❏	❏	❏
3. Place the package, with the label facing up, on a clean, dry, flat surface such as a Mayo or surgical stand	❏	❏	❏
4. Without tearing the wrapper, carefully remove the sealing tape. With commercial packages, carefully remove the outer protective wrapper	❏	❏	❏
5. Loosen the first flap of the folded wrapper by pulling it up, out, and away; let it fall over the far side of the table or stand	❏	❏	❏
6. Open the side flaps in a similar manner, using your left hand for the left flap and your right hand for the right flap. Touch only the unsterile outer surface; do not touch the sterile inner surface	❏	❏	❏
7. Pull the remaining flap down and toward you by grasping the outside surface only. The outer surface of the wrapper is now against the surgical stand; the sterile inside of the wrapper forms the sterile field	❏	❏	❏
8. Open the side flaps in a similar manner. Do not touch the sterile inner surface	❏	❏	❏
9. Pull the remaining flap down and toward you	❏	❏	❏
10. Repeat Steps 4 through 6 for packages with a second or inside wrapper	❏	❏	❏
11. If you must leave the area after opening the field, cover the tray with a sterile drape			

(continues)

PSY PROCEDURE 22-1 **Opening Sterile Surgical Packs** (continued)

CALCULATION

Total Possible Points: _____

Total Points Earned: _____ Multiplied by 100 = _____ Divided by Total Possible Points = _____ %

PASS   **FAIL**   **COMMENTS:**
❏   ❏

Student's signature _____   Date _____

Partner's signature _____   Date _____

Instructor's signature _____   Date _____

PSY PROCEDURE 22-2 **Using Sterile Transfer Forceps**

Name: _____ Date: _____ Time: _____ Grade: _____

EQUIPMENT/SUPPLIES: Sterile transfer forceps in a container with sterilization solution, sterile field, sterile items to be transferred

STANDARDS: Given the needed equipment and a place to work, the student will perform this skill with _____ % accuracy in a total of _____ minutes. *(Your instructor will tell you what the percentage and time limits will be before you begin.)*

KEY: 4 = Satisfactory 0 = Unsatisfactory NA = This step is not counted

PROCEDURE STEPS	SELF	PARTNER	INSTRUCTOR
1. Slowly lift the forceps straight up and out of the container without touching the inside above the level of the solution or outside of the container	❏	❏	❏
2. Hold the forceps with the tips down at all times	❏	❏	❏
3. Keep the forceps above waist level	❏	❏	❏
4. With the forceps, pick up the articles to be transferred and drop them onto the sterile field, but do not let the forceps come into contact with the sterile field	❏	❏	❏
5. Carefully place the forceps back into the sterilization solution	❏	❏	❏

CALCULATION

Total Possible Points: _____

Total Points Earned: _____ Multiplied by 100 = _____ Divided by Total Possible Points = _____ %

PASS FAIL COMMENTS:
❏ ❏

Student's signature _____ Date _____

Partner's signature _____ Date _____

Instructor's signature _____ Date _____

PSY PROCEDURE 22-3 | **Adding Sterile Solution to a Sterile Field**

Name: _____ Date: _____ Time: _____ Grade: _____

EQUIPMENT/SUPPLIES: Sterile setup, container of sterile solution, sterile bowl or cup

STANDARDS: Given the needed equipment and a place to work, the student will perform this skill with _____ % accuracy in a total of _____ minutes. *(Your instructor will tell you what the percentage and time limits will be before you begin.)*

KEY: 4 = Satisfactory 0 = Unsatisfactory NA = This step is not counted

PROCEDURE STEPS	SELF	PARTNER	INSTRUCTOR
1. Identify the correct solution by carefully reading the label	❏	❏	❏
2. Check the expiration date on the label	❏	❏	❏
3. If adding medications into the solution, show medication label to the physician	❏	❏	❏
4. Remove the cap or stopper; avoid contamination of the inside of the cap	❏	❏	❏
5. If it is necessary to put the cap down, place on side table with opened end facing up	❏	❏	❏
6. Retain bottle to track amount added to field	❏	❏	❏
7. Grasp container with label against the palm of your hand	❏	❏	❏
8. Pour a small amount of the solution into a separate container or waste receptacle	❏	❏	❏
9. Slowly pour the desired amount of solution into the sterile container	❏	❏	❏
10. Recheck the label for the contents and expiration date and replace the cap	❏	❏	❏
11. Return the solution to its proper storage area or discard the container after rechecking the label	❏	❏	❏

CALCULATION

Total Possible Points: _____

Total Points Earned: _____ Multiplied by 100 = _____ Divided by Total Possible Points = _____ %

PASS **FAIL** **COMMENTS:**
❏ ❏

Student's signature _____ Date _____

Partner's signature _____ Date _____

Instructor's signature _____ Date _____

PSY PROCEDURE 22-4 Performing Skin Preparation and Hair Removal

Name: _____ Date: _____ Time: _____ Grade: _____

EQUIPMENT/SUPPLIES: Nonsterile gloves; shaving cream, lotion, or soap; new disposable razor; gauze or cotton balls; warm water; antiseptic; sponge forceps

STANDARDS: Given the needed equipment and a place to work, the student will perform this skill with _____ % accuracy in a total of _____ minutes. *(Your instructor will tell you what the percentage and time limits will be before you begin.)*

KEY: 4 = Satisfactory   0 = Unsatisfactory   NA = This step is not counted

PROCEDURE STEPS	SELF	PARTNER	INSTRUCTOR
1. Wash your hands	❑	❑	❑
2. Assemble the equipment	❑	❑	❑
3. Greet and identify the patient; explain the procedure and answer any questions	❑	❑	❑
4. Put on gloves	❑	❑	❑
5. Prepare the patient's skin	❑	❑	❑
6. If the patient's skin is to be shaved, apply shaving cream or soapy lather **a.** Pull the skin taut and shave in the direction of hair growth **b.** Rinse and pat the shaved area dry thoroughly using a gauze square	❑	❑	❑
7. If the patient's skin is not to be shaved, wash with soap and water; rinse well and pat the area dry thoroughly using a gauze square	❑	❑	❑
8. Apply antiseptic solution to the operative area using sterile gauze sponges **a.** Wipe skin in circular motions starting at the operative site and working outward **b.** Discard each sponge after a complete sweep has been made **c.** If circles are not appropriate, the sponge may be wiped straight outward from the operative site and discarded **d.** Repeat the procedure until the entire area has been thoroughly cleaned	❑	❑	❑
9. Instruct the patient not to touch or cover the prepared area	❑	❑	❑
10. Explain how to respond to a patient who is developmentally challenged	❑	❑	❑

_____

_____

_____

_____

(continues)

PSY PROCEDURE 22-4	Performing Skin Preparation and Hair Removal (continued)		
11. Remove your gloves and wash your hands	❑	❑	❑
12. Inform the physician that the patient is ready for the surgical procedure	❑	❑	❑
13. Drape the prepared area with a sterile drape if the physician will be delayed by more than 10 or 15 minutes	❑	❑	❑

CALCULATION

Total Possible Points: _____

Total Points Earned: _____ Multiplied by 100 = _____ Divided by Total Possible Points = _____ %

PASS   FAIL   COMMENTS:
 ❑   ❑

Student's signature _____ Date _____

Partner's signature _____ Date _____

Instructor's signature _____ Date _____

PSY PROCEDURE 22-5 **Applying Sterile Gloves**

Name: _____ **Date:** _____ **Time:** _____ **Grade:** _____

EQUIPMENT/SUPPLIES: One package of sterile gloves in the appropriate size

STANDARDS: Given the needed equipment and a place to work, the student will perform this skill with _____ % accuracy in a total of _____ minutes. *(Your instructor will tell you what the percentage and time limits will be before you begin.)*

KEY: 4 = Satisfactory   0 = Unsatisfactory   NA = This step is not counted

PROCEDURE STEPS	SELF	PARTNER	INSTRUCTOR
1. Remove rings and other jewelry	❑	❑	❑
2. Wash your hands	❑	❑	❑
3. Place prepackaged gloves on a clean, dry, flat surface with the cuffed end toward you **a.** Pull the outer wrapping apart to expose the sterile inner wrap **b.** With the cuffs toward you, fold back the inner wrap to expose the gloves	❑	❑	❑
4. Grasping the edges of the outer paper, open the package out to its fullest	❑	❑	❑
5. Use your nondominant hand to pick up the dominant hand glove **a.** Grasp the folded edge of the cuff and lift it up and away from the paper **b.** Curl your fingers and thumb together and insert them into the glove **c.** Straighten your fingers and pull the glove on with your nondominant hand still grasping the cuff	❑	❑	❑
6. Unfold the cuff by pinching the inside surface and pull it toward your wrist	❑	❑	❑
7. Place the fingers of your gloved hand under the cuff of the remaining glove **a.** Lift the glove up and away from the wrapper **b.** Slide your ungloved hand carefully into the glove with your fingers and thumb curled together **c.** Straighten your fingers and pull the glove up and over your wrist by carefully unfolding the cuff	❑	❑	❑
8. Settle the gloves comfortably onto your fingers by lacing your fingers together	❑	❑	❑
9. Remove contaminated sterile gloves and discard them appropriately. Wash your hands	❑	❑	❑

(continues)

PSY PROCEDURE 22-5 **Applying Sterile Gloves** (continued)

CALCULATION

Total Possible Points: _____

Total Points Earned: _____ Multiplied by 100 = _____ Divided by Total Possible Points = _____ %

PASS **FAIL** **COMMENTS:**
❏ ❏

Student's signature _____ Date _____

Partner's signature _____ Date _____

Instructor's signature _____ Date _____

PROCEDURE 22-6   Applying a Sterile Dressing

PSY

Name: _____   Date: _____   Time: _____   Grade: _____

EQUIPMENT/SUPPLIES: Sterile gloves, sterile gauze dressings, scissors, bandage tape, any medication to be applied to the dressing if ordered by the physician

STANDARDS: Given the needed equipment and a place to work, the student will perform this skill with _____ % accuracy in a total of _____ minutes. *(Your instructor will tell you what the percentage and time limits will be before you begin.)*

KEY: 4 = Satisfactory   0 = Unsatisfactory   NA = This step is not counted

PROCEDURE STEPS	SELF	PARTNER	INSTRUCTOR
1. Wash your hands	❑	❑	❑
2. Assemble the equipment and supplies	❑	❑	❑
3. Greet and identify the patient	❑	❑	❑
4. Ask about any tape allergies before deciding on what type of tape to use	❑	❑	❑
5. Cut or tear lengths of tape to secure the dressing	❑	❑	❑
6. Explain the procedure and instruct the patient to remain still; avoid coughing, sneezing, or talking until the procedure is complete	❑	❑	❑
7. Open the dressing pack to create a sterile field, maintaining sterile asepsis **a.** If sterile gloves are to be used, open and place near the dressing pack **b.** If using a sterile transfer forceps, place it near the other supplies	❑	❑	❑
8. Apply topical medication to the sterile dressing that will cover the wound	❑	❑	❑
9. Apply the number of dressings necessary to properly cover and protect the wound	❑	❑	❑
10. Apply sufficient cut lengths of tape over the dressing to secure	❑	❑	❑
11. Remove contaminated gloves and discard in the proper receptacle. Wash your hands	❑	❑	❑
12. Provide patient education and supplies as appropriate	❑	❑	❑
13. **AFF** Explain how to respond to a patient who is visually impaired	❑	❑	❑

_____

_____

_____

_____

(continues)

PSY PROCEDURE 22-6 **Applying a Sterile Dressing** (continued)			
14. Clean and sanitize the room and equipment	❑	❑	❑
15. Record the procedure	❑	❑	❑

CALCULATION

Total Possible Points: _____

Total Points Earned: _____ Multiplied by 100 = _____ Divided by Total Possible Points = _____ %

PASS **FAIL** **COMMENTS:**
❑ ❑

Student's signature _____ Date _____

Partner's signature _____ Date _____

Instructor's signature _____ Date _____

PSY PROCEDURE 22-7 | **Changing an Existing Sterile Dressing**

Name: _____ Date: _____ Time: _____ Grade: _____

EQUIPMENT/SUPPLIES: Sterile gloves, nonsterile gloves, sterile dressing, prepackaged skin antiseptic swabs (or sterile antiseptic solution poured into a sterile basin and sterile cotton balls or gauze), tape, approved biohazard containers

STANDARDS: Given the needed equipment and a place to work, the student will perform this skill with _____ % accuracy in a total of _____ minutes. *(Your instructor will tell you what the percentage and time limits will be before you begin.)*

KEY: 4 = Satisfactory 0 = Unsatisfactory NA = This step is not counted

PROCEDURE STEPS	SELF	PARTNER	INSTRUCTOR
1. Wash your hands	❏	❏	❏
2. Assemble the equipment and supplies	❏	❏	❏
3. Greet and identify the patient; explain the procedure and answer any questions	❏	❏	❏
4. Prepare a sterile field including opening sterile dressings	❏	❏	❏
5. Open a sterile basin and use the inside of the wrapper as the sterile field **a.** Flip the sterile gauze or cotton balls into the basin **b.** Pour antiseptic solution appropriately into the basin **c.** If using prepackaged antiseptic swabs, carefully open an adequate number **d.** Set swabs aside without contaminating them	❏	❏	❏
6. Instruct the patient not to talk, cough, sneeze, laugh, or move during the procedure	❏	❏	❏
7. **AFF** Explain how to respond to a patient who has dementia	❏	❏	❏
_____ _____ _____ _____			
8. Wear clean gloves and carefully remove tape from the wound dressing by pulling it toward the wound **a.** Remove the old dressing **b.** Discard the soiled dressing into a biohazard container	❏	❏	❏
9. Inspect wound for the degree of healing, amount and type of drainage, and appearance of wound edges	❏	❏	❏

(continues)

PSY PROCEDURE 22-7 **Changing an Existing Sterile Dressing** (continued)

10. Observing medical asepsis, remove and discard your gloves	❑	❑	❑
11. Using proper technique, apply sterile gloves	❑	❑	❑
12. Clean the wound with the antiseptic solution ordered by the physician	❑	❑	❑
13. Clean in a straight motion with the cotton or gauze or the prepackaged antiseptic swab. Discard the wipe (cotton ball, swab) after each use	❑	❑	❑
14. Remove your gloves and wash your hands	❑	❑	❑
15. Change the dressing using the procedure for sterile dressing application (Procedure 22-6) and using sterile gloves (Procedure 22-5) or sterile transfer forceps (Procedure 22-2)	❑	❑	❑
16. Record the procedure	❑	❑	❑

CALCULATION

Total Possible Points: _____

Total Points Earned: _____ Multiplied by 100 = _____ Divided by Total Possible Points = _____ %

PASS **FAIL** **COMMENTS:**
  ❑   ❑

Student's signature _____ Date _____

Partner's signature _____ Date _____

Instructor's signature _____ Date _____

PSY PROCEDURE 22-8 **Assisting with Excisional Surgery**

Name: _____ Date: _____ Time: _____ Grade: _____

EQUIPMENT/SUPPLIES: Sterile gloves, local anesthetic, antiseptic wipes, adhesive tape, specimen container with completed laboratory request; *On the field*: basin for solutions, gauze sponges and cotton balls, antiseptic solution, sterile drape, dissecting scissors, disposable scalpel, blade of physician's choice, mosquito forceps, tissue forceps, needle holder, suture, and needle of physician's choice

STANDARDS: Given the needed equipment and a place to work, the student will perform this skill with _____ % accuracy in a total of _____ minutes. *(Your instructor will tell you what the percentage and time limits will be before you begin.)*

KEY:　　　4 = Satisfactory　　　0 = Unsatisfactory　　　NA = This step is not counted

PROCEDURE STEPS	SELF	PARTNER	INSTRUCTOR
1. Wash your hands	❏	❏	❏
2. Assemble the equipment appropriate for the procedure and according to physician preference	❏	❏	❏
3. Greet and identify the patient; explain the procedure and answer any questions	❏	❏	❏
4. Set up a sterile field on a surgical stand with additional equipment close at hand	❏	❏	❏
5. Cover the field with a sterile drape until the physician arrives	❏	❏	❏
6. Position the patient appropriately	❏	❏	❏
7. Put on sterile gloves (Procedure 22-5) or use sterile transfer forceps (Procedure 22-2) and cleanse the patient's skin (Procedure 22-4)	❏	❏	❏
8. Be ready to assist during the procedure: adding supplies as needed, assisting the physician, and comforting the patient	❏	❏	❏
9. Assist with collecting tissue specimen in an appropriate container	❏	❏	❏
10. At the end of the procedure, wash your hands and dress the wound using sterile technique (Procedure 22-6)	❏	❏	❏
11. Thank the patient and give appropriate instructions	❏	❏	❏
12. **AFF** Explain how to respond to a patient who is hearing impaired	❏	❏	❏

_____

_____

_____

_____

(continues)

PSY PROCEDURE 22-8	Assisting with Excisional Surgery (continued)		
13. Sanitize the examining room in preparation for the next patient	❏	❏	❏
14. Discard all disposables in the appropriate biohazard containers	❏	❏	❏
15. Record the procedure	❏	❏	❏

CALCULATION

Total Possible Points: _____

Total Points Earned: _____ Multiplied by 100 = _____ Divided by Total Possible Points = _____ %

PASS   **FAIL**   **COMMENTS:**
❏   ❏

Student's signature _____ Date _____

Partner's signature _____ Date _____

Instructor's signature _____ Date _____

PSY PROCEDURE 22-9 **Assisting with Incision and Drainage**

Name: _____ Date: _____ Time: _____ Grade: _____

EQUIPMENT/SUPPLIES: Sterile gloves, local anesthetic, antiseptic wipes, adhesive tape, sterile dressings, packing gauze, a culture tube if the wound may be cultured; *On the field*: basin for solutions, gauze sponges and cotton balls, antiseptic solution, sterile drape, syringes and needles for local anesthetic, commercial I&D sterile setup *or* scalpel, dissecting scissors, hemostats, tissue forceps, 4 × 4 gauze sponges, and probe (optional)

STANDARDS: Given the needed equipment and a place to work, the student will perform this skill with _____ % accuracy in a total of _____ minutes. *(Your instructor will tell you what the percentage and time limits will be before you begin.)*

KEY: 4 = Satisfactory 0 = Unsatisfactory NA = This step is not counted

PROCEDURE STEPS	SELF	PARTNER	INSTRUCTOR
1. Wash your hands	❏	❏	❏
2. Assemble the equipment appropriate for the procedure and according to physician preference	❏	❏	❏
3. Greet and identify the patient. Explain the procedure and answer any questions	❏	❏	❏
4. Set up a sterile field on a surgical stand with additional equipment close at hand	❏	❏	❏
5. Cover the field with a sterile drape until the physician arrives	❏	❏	❏
6. Position the patient appropriately	❏	❏	❏
7. Put on sterile gloves (Procedure 22-5) or use sterile transfer forceps (Procedure 22-2) and cleanse the patient's skin (Procedure 22-4)	❏	❏	❏
8. Be ready to assist during the procedure: adding supplies as needed, assisting the physician, comforting the patient	❏	❏	❏
9. Assist with collecting culturette specimen for culture and sensitivity	❏	❏	❏
10. At the end of procedure, remove gloves, wash your hands, and dress the wound using a sterile technique (Procedure 22-6)	❏	❏	❏
11. Thank the patient and give appropriate instructions	❏	❏	❏
12. Sanitize the examining room in preparation for the next patient	❏	❏	❏
13. Discard all disposables in appropriate biohazard containers	❏	❏	❏
14. Record the procedure	❏	❏	❏

(continues)

PSY   PROCEDURE 22-9   **Assisting with Incision and Drainage** (continued)

CALCULATION

Total Possible Points: _____

Total Points Earned: _____ Multiplied by 100 = _____ Divided by Total Possible Points = _____ %

PASS   FAIL   COMMENTS:
❏   ❏

Student's signature _____   Date _____

Partner's signature _____   Date _____

Instructor's signature _____   Date _____

PSY PROCEDURE 22-10 **Removing Sutures**

Name: _____ Date: _____ Time: _____ Grade: _____

EQUIPMENT/SUPPLIES: Skin antiseptic, sterile gloves, prepackaged suture removal kit or thumb forceps, suture scissors, gauze

STANDARDS: Given the needed equipment and a place to work, the student will perform this skill with _____ % accuracy in a total of _____ minutes. *(Your instructor will tell you what the percentage and time limits will be before you begin.)*

KEY: 4 = Satisfactory 0 = Unsatisfactory NA = This step is not counted

PROCEDURE STEPS	SELF	PARTNER	INSTRUCTOR
1. Wash your hands and apply clean examination gloves	❑	❑	❑
2. Assemble the equipment	❑	❑	❑
3. Greet and identify the patient; explain the procedure and answer any questions	❑	❑	❑
4. If dressings have not been removed previously, remove them from the wound area **a.** Properly dispose of the soiled dressings in the biohazard trash container **b.** Remove your gloves and wash your hands	❑	❑	❑
5. Cover the field with a sterile drape until the physician arrives	❑	❑	❑
6. Open suture removal packet using sterile asepsis	❑	❑	❑
7. Put on sterile gloves **a.** With the thumb forceps, grasp the end of the knot closest to the skin surface and lift it slightly and gently up from the skin **b.** Cut the suture below the knot as close to the skin as possible **c.** Use the thumb forceps to pull the suture out of the skin with a smooth motion	❑	❑	❑
8. Place the suture on the gauze sponge; repeat the procedure for each suture to be removed	❑	❑	❑
9. Clean the site with an antiseptic solution and cover it with a sterile dressing	❑	❑	❑
10. Thank the patient	❑	❑	❑
11. **AFF** Explain how to respond to a patient who is developmentally challenged	❑	❑	❑

_____

_____

_____

_____

(continues)

PSY   PROCEDURE 22-10   **Removing Sutures** (continued)

12. Properly dispose of the equipment and supplies	❏	❏	❏
13. Clean the work area, remove your gloves, and wash your hands	❏	❏	❏
14. Record the procedure, including the time, location of sutures, the number removed, and the condition of the wound	❏	❏	❏

CALCULATION

Total Possible Points: _____

Total Points Earned: _____ Multiplied by 100 = _____ Divided by Total Possible Points = _____ %

PASS   FAIL   COMMENTS:
   ❏   ❏

Student's signature _____ Date _____

Partner's signature _____ Date _____

Instructor's signature _____ Date _____

PSY PROCEDURE 22-11 **Removing Staples**

Name: _____ Date: _____ Time: _____ Grade: _____

EQUIPMENT/SUPPLIES: Antiseptic solution or wipes, gauze squares, sponge forceps, prepackaged sterile staple removal instrument, examination gloves, sterile gloves

STANDARDS: Given the needed equipment and a place to work, the student will perform this skill with _____ % accuracy in a total of _____ minutes. *(Your instructor will tell you what the percentage and time limits will be before you begin.)*

KEY: 4 = Satisfactory 0 = Unsatisfactory NA = This step is not counted

PROCEDURE STEPS	SELF	PARTNER	INSTRUCTOR
1. Wash your hands	❏	❏	❏
2. Assemble the equipment	❏	❏	❏
3. Greet and identify the patient; explain the procedure and answer any questions	❏	❏	❏
4. If the dressing has not been removed, put on clean examination gloves and do so	❏	❏	❏
5. Dispose of the dressing properly in a biohazard container	❏	❏	❏
6. Clean the incision with antiseptic solution	❏	❏	❏
7. Pat dry using dry sterile gauze sponges	❏	❏	❏
8. Put on sterile gloves	❏	❏	❏
9. Gently slide the end of the staple remover under each staple to be removed; press the handles together to lift the ends of the staple out of the skin and remove the staple	❏	❏	❏
10. Place each staple on a gauze square as it is removed	❏	❏	❏
11. When all staples are removed, clean the incision as instructed for all procedures	❏	❏	❏
12. Pat dry and dress the site if ordered to do so by the physician	❏	❏	❏
13. Thank the patient and properly care for, or dispose of, all equipment and supplies	❏	❏	❏
14. **AFF** Explain how to respond to a patient who is visually impaired	❏	❏	❏

_____

_____

_____

_____

(continues)

PSY PROCEDURE 22-11	**Removing Staples** (continued)			
15. Clean the work area, remove your gloves, and wash your hands		❑	❑	❑
16. Record the procedure		❑	❑	❑

CALCULATION

Total Possible Points: _____

Total Points Earned: _____ Multiplied by 100 = _____ Divided by Total Possible Points = _____ %

PASS   FAIL   COMMENTS:
❑   ❑

Student's signature _____   Date _____

Partner's signature _____   Date _____

Instructor's signature _____   Date _____

CHAPTER 23

Pharmacology

LEARNING OUTCOMES

Cognitive Domain*

1. Spell and define key terms
2. Describe the relationship between anatomy and physiology of all body systems and medications used for treatment in each
3. Identify chemical, trade, and generic drug names
4. Discuss all levels of government legislation and regulation as they apply to medical assisting practice, including FDA and DEA regulations
5. Explain the various drug actions and interactions, including pharmacodynamics and pharmacokinetics
6. *Identify the classifications of medications, including indications for use, desired effects, side effects, and adverse reactions*
7. Name the sources for locating information on pharmacology

MAERB Standards are Italicized

ABHES Competencies

1. Identify drug classifications, usual dose, side effects, and contraindications of the top most commonly used medications
2. Prescriptions: Identify parts of prescriptions; identify appropriate abbreviations that are accepted in prescription writing; comply with legal aspects of creating prescriptions, including federal and state laws
3. Properly utilize *Physicians' Desk Reference*, drug handbook, and other drug references to identify a drug's classification, usual dosage, usual side effects, and contradictions
4. Define and use medical abbreviations when appropriate and acceptable

Name: _____   Date: _____   Grade: _____

⬤⬤ MULTIPLE CHOICE

Circle the letter preceding the correct answer.

1. A physician needs to register with the U.S. Attorney General:
  a. every 3 years.
  b. every 2 years.
  c. every 4 years.
  d. only once; registration is for life.
  e. every year.

2. When a drug is contraindicated, it:
  a. is not properly eliminated.
  b. is distributed throughout the bloodstream.
  c. should not be used.
  d. is detected in urine excretion.
  e. should be retested for accuracy.

3. Emetics are used to:
  a. dilate bronchi.
  b. prevent symptoms of menopause.
  c. control diabetes.
  d. dissolve blood clots.
  e. promote vomiting.

4. Which substance is an example of a Schedule I controlled substance?
  a. Morphine
  b. Ritalin
  c. Amphetamines
  d. Opium
  e. Tylenol with codeine

5. Which drug below is an example of an antipyretic?
  a. Aspirin
  b. Dramamine
  c. Lanoxin
  d. Zantac
  e. Benylin

6. A symptom of an allergic reaction is:
  a. nausea.
  b. drowsiness.
  c. dryness of mouth.
  d. hives.
  e. fever.

7. Two drugs when taken together that can create synergism are:
  a. sedatives and barbiturates.
  b. antacids and antibiotics.
  c. diuretics and decongestants.
  d. antibiotics and antifungals.
  e. antihypertensives and expectorants.

8. The DEA is a branch of the:
  a. BNDD.
  b. DOJ.
  c. FDA.
  d. AMA.
  e. AHFS.

9. All drugs cause:
  a. cellular and physiologic change.
  b. cellular and psychological change.
  c. physiologic and psychological change.
  d. physiologic changes.
  e. cellular, physiologic, and psychological change.

10. Green leafy vegetables can sometimes interact with:
  a. coumadin.
  b. verapamil.
  c. ibuprofen.
  d. amoxicillin.
  e. phenobarbital.

11. Drugs with a potential for abuse and currently accepted for medicinal use are:
  a. Schedule I drugs.
  b. Schedule II drugs.
  c. Schedule III drugs.
  d. Schedule IV drugs.
  e. Schedules I and IV drugs.

12. A drug is given a brand name when it:
  a. is first developed in laboratories.
  b. is used in field testing and studies.
  c. is assigned a sponsor for the research.
  d. is approved by the FDA.
  e. is available for commercial use.

Scenario for questions 13 and 14: A teenage patient has called in saying that the pharmacy will not refill her painkiller prescription. It has been just over a month since she last refilled her prescription.

13. What is the first step you should take?
  a. Check her records to see how many more refills she has left.
  b. Inform the physician about the situation for directions.
  c. Call the pharmacy to find out how many refills she has gotten.
  d. Write out another prescription and fax it to the pharmacy.
  e. Inform the patient that she has no more refills remaining.

14. The patient still has three remaining refills on her prescription. After you call the pharmacy; however, you are informed that the patient has been purchasing over-the-counter painkillers along with her prescription. There is suspicion that the patient might be selling her medication and taking over-the-counter drugs. What do you do?
    a. Call the patient and confront her about the purchases.
    b. Discuss the possibility of drug abuse with the physician.
    c. Call the police immediately and report the patient.
    d. Tell the pharmacy to give her the prescriptions anyway.
    e. Gather information and report your findings.

15. The study of how drugs act on the body, including cells, tissues, and organs, is:
    a. pharmacokinetics.
    b. pharmacodynamics.
    c. synergism.
    d. antagonism.
    e. potentiation.

16. What kind of drug is used to increase the size of arterial blood vessels?
    a. Anticonvulsants
    b. Emetics
    c. Cholinergics
    d. Antihypertensives
    e. Immunologic agents

17. Which of the following is a trait of a Schedule I drug?
    a. No accepted safety standards
    b. Cannot be prescribed by a physician
    c. Lowest potential for abuse
    d. May be filled up to five times in 6 months
    e. Requires a handwritten prescription

18. When you are administering a controlled substance in a medical office, you must include:
    a. a drug schedule.
    b. the time of administration.
    c. patient allergies.
    d. your name.
    e. location.

19. If a patient is receiving a medication that has a high incidence of allergic reactions, how long should the patient wait before leaving the office?
    a. No wait time necessary
    b. 5 to 10 minutes
    c. 20 to 30 minutes
    d. 30 minutes to an hour
    e. Overnight observation

20. The chemical name of a drug is the:
    a. last name a drug is given before it is put on the market.
    b. description of the chemical compounds found in the drug.
    c. name given to the drug during research and development.
    d. name given to the drug by the FDA and AMA.
    e. name of the chemical the drug supplements in the body.

COG MATCHING

Grade: _____

Match each key term with its definition.

Key Terms

21. _____ allergy
22. _____ anaphylaxis
23. _____ antagonism
24. _____ chemical name
25. _____ contraindication
26. _____ drug
27. _____ generic name
28. _____ interaction
29. _____ pharmacodynamics
30. _____ pharmacokinetics
31. _____ pharmacology
32. _____ potentiation
33. _____ synergism
34. _____ trade name

Definitions

a. effects, positive and negative, of two or more drugs taken by a patient
b. situation or condition that prohibits the prescribing or administering of a drug or medication
c. any substance that may modify one or more of the functions of an organism
d. study of drugs and their origin, nature, properties, and effects upon living organisms
e. exact chemical descriptor of a drug
f. official name given to a drug whose patent has expired
g. name given to a medication by the company that owns the patent
h. study of the effects and reactions of drugs within the body
i. study of the action of drugs within the body from administration to excretion
j. harmonious action of two agents, such as drugs or organs, producing an effect that neither could produce alone or that is greater than the total effects of each agent operating by itself
k. mutual opposition or contrary action with something else; opposite of synergism
l. describes the action of two drugs taken together in which the combined effects are greater than the sum of the independent effects
m. acquired abnormal response to a substance (allergen) that does not ordinarily cause a reaction
n. severe allergic reaction that may result in death

COG MATCHING

Grade: _____

Match each drug term with its description.

Drug Terms

35. _____ therapeutic classification
36. _____ idiosyncratic reaction
37. _____ indications
38. _____ teratogenic category
39. _____ hypersensitivity
40. _____ contraindications
41. _____ adverse reactions

Descriptions

a. relates the level of risk to fetal or maternal health (These rank from Category A through D, with increasing danger at each level. Category X indicates that the particular drug should never be given during pregnancy)
b. refers to an excessive reaction to a particular drug; also known as a *drug allergy* (The body must build this response; the first exposures may or may not indicate that a problem is developing)
c. indicates conditions or instances for which the particular drug should not be used
d. states the purpose for the drug's use (e.g., cardiotonic, anti-infective, antiarrhythmic)
e. refers to an abnormal or unexpected reaction to a drug peculiar to the individual patient; not technically an allergy
f. gives diseases for which the particular drug would be prescribed
g. refers to undesirable side effects of a particular drug

⬛ IDENTIFICATION

Grade: _____

42. Identify whether the following descriptions describe the chemical, generic, or trade name of a drug by writing C (chemical), G (generic), or T (trade) on the line preceding the description.

a. _____ The name of a drug that begins with a lowercase letter

b. _____ The name assigned to a drug during research and development

c. _____ The name given to a drug when it is available for commercial use

d. _____ The first name given to any medication

e. _____ The name that is registered by the U.S. patent office

f. _____ The name that identifies the chemical components of the drug

43. Determine if the information below can be found in the *Physicians' Desk Reference (PDR)* or the *United States Pharmacopeia Dispensing Information (USPDI)*. Place a check mark in the appropriate box below.

	Physicians' Desk Reference	United States Pharmacopeia Dispensing Information
a. Drug sources		
b. Indications		
c. Dosages		
d. Pictures		
e. Chemistry		
f. Physical properties		
g. Side effects		
h. Tests for identity		
i. Storage		
j. Contraindications		

44. Indicate where the following elements of a prescription go in sequential order.

Patient's name and address	Line 1: _____
Date	Line 2. _____
Inscription	Line 3. _____
Superscription	Line 4. _____
Subscription	Line 5. _____
Physician's signature	Line 6. _____
Signature	Line 7. _____
Generic	Line 8. _____
Refills	Line 9. _____

45. Indicate each drug's controlled substance category by writing I, II, III, IV, or V on the line preceding the drug name.

a. _____ morphine

b. _____ Tylenol with codeine

c. _____ cocaine

d. _____ codeine in cough medications

e. _____ marijuana

f. _____ Valium

g. _____ LSD

h. _____ Ritalin

i. _____ Librium

COG COMPLETION

Grade: _____

46. Each of the following statements about inventory of controlled substances is incorrect or incomplete. Rewrite each statement to make it correct or complete.

a. List only category III controlled substances on the appropriate inventory form.

_____

b. When you receive controlled substances, make sure that only the physician signs the receipt.

_____

c. Keep all controlled substance inventory forms for 10 years.

_____

d. When a controlled substance leaves the medical office inventory, record the following information: drug name and patient.

_____

e. Notify the office manager immediately if these drugs are lost or stolen.

_____

f. Store controlled substances in the same cabinet as other medications and supplies.

_____

COG SHORT ANSWER

Grade: _____

47. What are pharmacodynamics and pharmacokinetics? Explain the relationship between these two processes.

_____

_____

_____

_____

48. What four processes are connected to pharmacokinetics?

_____

_____

_____

_____

49. Why is it important for patients to know about food–drug interactions?

_____

_____

_____

_____

50. Explain the difference between drug side effects and allergic reactions.

_____

_____

_____

_____

51. List three common and predictable drug side effects.

_____

_____

_____

_____

52. Compare and contrast the different types of drug interactions, including synergism, antagonism, and potentiation.

_____

_____

_____

_____

53. Compare the effect or action of the following therapeutic classifications: stimulants, diuretics, emetics, and immunologic agents.

_____

_____

_____

_____

COG TRUE OR FALSE?

Grade: _____

Indicate whether the statements are true or false by placing the letter T (true) or F (false) in the blank preceding the statement.

54. _____ The DEA is concerned with controlled substances only.

55. _____ Drugs are derived from natural and synthetic sources.

56. _____ Children have a slower response to drug intakes.

57. _____ Allergic reactions are always immediate.

58. _____ Side effects from drugs are often life threatening.

59. _____ A drug is a chemical substance that affects body function or functions.

60. _____ A drug administered for a systemic effect is applied topically.

61. _____ Women may react differently to certain drugs than men.

62. _____ Medications should always be taken on a full stomach.

COG AFF CASE STUDIES FOR CRITICAL THINKING

Grade: _____

63. You are doing an inventory of the controlled substances in your office and notice that the office's supply of morphine is off count. You double-check all written records of medications given for administration and still cannot account for the missing morphine. After realizing this, you immediately tell the physician. The physician tells you not to worry about it. Three weeks later you notice that more morphine is missing. What do you do?

_____

_____

_____

_____

64. A patient just received a shot of penicillin. Before the shot was administered, you advised the patient that she needs to remain in the physician's office for 30 minutes before leaving. However, the patient just remembered that she must pick her mother up for an appointment that her mother needs to attend. The patient is adamant that she must leave right away so as not to be late. How would you respond to this patient?

_____

_____

_____

_____

65. You have an elderly patient who is taking Lasix for his high blood pressure. This patient has recently called in to the office complaining of muscle weakness. What classification is the drug Lasix? What is possibly causing the patient's muscle weakness? How would you respond to this patient?

_____

_____

_____

_____

66. You have a patient with hepatic disease. After she consults with the physician, she asks you some general questions to clarify how her body processes medication. Think about the pharmacokinetic effects of drugs on her body. What processes would you discuss with her about her condition and medications?

_____

_____

_____

_____

67. Your patient tells you that she feels like she is coming down with a cold and has had a sore throat since yesterday. She also tells you that her friend gave her some leftover antibiotics that she did not finish when she had strep throat last month. How would you respond to this patient? Is this important information for the physician to know? Why or why not?

_____

_____

_____

_____

68. Louise asks Mr. Fujiwara about his medical history and if he has any allergies to any medications. Mr. Fujiwara says that he has an allergy to aspirin. Louise marks Mr. Fujiwara's drug allergy prominently on the front of his medication record before giving the record to the physician. What else should the medical assistant do?

_____

_____

_____

_____

CHAPTER 24

Preparing and Administering Medications

LEARNING OUTCOMES

COG Cognitive Domain*

1. Spell and define the key terms
2. Demonstrate knowledge of basic math computations
3. *Define basic units of measurement in:*
   a. *the metric system*
   b. *the household system*
4. Convert among measurement systems
5. *Identify abbreviations and use in calculating medication dosages*
6. List the safety guidelines for medication administration
7. Explain the differences among various parenteral and nonparenteral routes of medication administration
8. Describe the parts of a syringe and needle and name those parts that must be kept sterile
9. List the various needle lengths, gauges, and preferred site for each type of injection
10. Compare the types of injections and locate the sites where each may be administered safely
11. Describe principles of intravenous therapy

PSY Psychomotor Domain*

1. Administer oral medications (Procedure 24-1)

    a. *Perform patient screening following established protocols*
    b. *Verify the rules of medication administration (right patient, right medication, right dose, right route, right time, right documentation)*
    c. *Administer oral medications*
    d. *Document patient care accurately in the medical record*

2. Prepare injections (Procedure 24-2)

3. Administer an intradermal injection (Procedure 24-3)

    a. *Verify the rules of medication administration (right patient, right medication, right dose, right route, right time, right documentation)*
    b. *Select proper sites for administration of parenteral medications*
    c. *Instruct and prepare patient for a procedure or treatment*
    d. *Calculate proper dosage of medication for administration*
    e. *Administer parenteral (excluding IV) medications*
    f. *Demonstrate proper disposal of biohazard material: a. sharps b. regulated waste*
    g. *Document patient care accurately in the medical record*

4. Administer a subcutaneous injection (Procedure 24-4)

    a. *Verify the rules of medication administration (right patient, right medication, right dose, right route, right time, right documentation)*
    b. *Select proper sites for administration of parenteral medications*
    c. *Instruct and prepare the patient for a procedure or treatment*
    d. *Calculate proper dosage of medication for administration*
    e. *Administer parenteral (excluding IV) medications*
    f. *Demonstrate proper disposal of biohazard material: a. sharps b. regulated waste*
    g. *Document patient care accurately in the medical record*

5. Administer an intramuscular injection (Procedure 24-5)

    a. *Verify the rules of medication administration (right patient, right medication, right dose, right route, right time, right documentation)*
    b. *Select proper sites for administration of parenteral medications*
    c. *Instruct and prepare patient for a procedure or treatment*

    d. *Calculate proper dosage of medication for administration*

    e. *Administer parenteral (excluding IV) medications*

    f. *Demonstrate proper disposal of biohazard material: a. sharps b. regulated waste*

    g. *Document patient care accurately in the medical record*

6. Administer an intramuscular injection using the Z-track method (Procedure 24-6)

    a. *Verify the rules of medication administration (right patient, right medication, right dose, right route, right time, right documentation)*

    b. *Select proper sites for administration of parenteral medications*

    c. *Instruct and prepare patient for a procedure or treatment*

    d. *Calculate proper dosage of medication for administration*

    e. *Administer parenteral (excluding IV) medications*

    f. *Demonstrate proper disposal of biohazard material: a. sharps b. regulated waste*

    g. *Document patient care accurately in the medical record*

7. Apply transdermal medications (Procedure 24-7)

8. *Complete an incident report related to an error in patient care* (Procedure 24-8)

AFF Affective Domain*

1. *Demonstrate critical thinking skills*
2. *Reassure patients*
3. *Demonstrate empathy for patients' concerns*
4. *Demonstrate active listening*
5. *Respect diversity*
6. *Recognize personal boundaries*
7. *Demonstrate tactfulness*
8. *Demonstrate self-awareness*
9. Protect the integrity of the medical record

MAERB Standards are Italicized

ABHES Competencies

1. Demonstrate accurate occupational math and metric conversions for proper medication administration
2. Practice standard precautions and perform disinfection/sterilization techniques
3. Prepare and administer oral and parenteral medications and monitor intravenous infusions
4. Follow documentation guidelines
5. Dispose of biohazardous materials
6. Demonstrate cultural awareness

Name: _____   Date: _____   Grade: _____

COG MULTIPLE CHOICE

Circle the letter preceding the correct answer.

1. When administering an unfamiliar drug, you should look up information on:
   a. alternate formulations.
   b. the chemical name.
   c. generic alternatives.
   d. how the medication is stored.
   e. the route of administration.

2. When preparing medications you should:
   a. use previous medications and dosages listed on the patient's chart as a safety check.
   b. use a resource like the Internet to cross reference generic and brand names for medications.
   c. work in a quiet, well-lit area.
   d. crush tablets so patients can swallow them easily.
   e. recap used needles to protect against accidental jabs.

3. Patient safety is protected by ensuring:
   a. a nurse prepares the medication for you to administer.
   b. you are administering the right drug to the right patient.
   c. medications are delivered to the right room for administration by the nurse.
   d. you are using the right type of syringe.
   e. you write down and document medications before you give them.

4. When dispensing drugs, make sure you convert the dosage ordered to the:
   a. apothecary system.
   b. household system.
   c. imperial units.
   d. system and units noted on the medication label.
   e. metric units.

5. The basic unit of weight in the metric system is the:
   a. grain.
   b. gram.
   c. liter.
   d. newton.
   e. pound.

6. What number do you multiply the base metric unit by if the prefix is "milli"?
   a. 1,000
   b. 1,000,000
   c. 0.000001
   d. 0.001
   e. 0.01

7. Which of these measurements equals 2 cc?
   a. 2 mg
   b. 20 mg
   c. 2 mL
   d. 30 g
   e. 120 mg

8. Which of these measurements equals 45 mL?
   a. 0.75 fl oz
   b. 1.5 fl oz
   c. 3.0 fl oz
   d. 4.5 fl oz
   e. 20.5 fl oz

9. The physician orders chloroquine syrup 100 mg oral for a 20-kg child. The concentration of the syrup is 50 mg/mL. How much medication do you give the child?
   a. 0.5 mL
   b. 2 mL
   c. 10 mL
   d. 40 mL
   e. 250 mL

10. Which method is the most accurate means of calculating pediatric dosages?
    a. Body weight method
    b. The Clarke rule
    c. The Fried rule
    d. BSA method
    e. The Young rule

11. Medicine administered under the tongue follows the:
    a. buccal route.
    b. dental route.
    c. dermal route.
    d. oral route.
    e. sublingual route.

12. Which item below could be a multiple-dose dispenser?
    a. Ampule
    b. Cartridge
    c. Carpuject
    d. Tubex
    e. Vial

13. How large is a tuberculin syringe?
    a. 10 U
    b. 5 mL
    c. 3 mL
    d. 1 mL
    e. 0.1 mL

14. A possible site for an intradermal injection is the:
   a. antecubital fossa.
   b. anterior forearm.
   c. upper arm.
   d. deltoid.
   e. vastus lateralis.

Scenario for questions 15 and 16: You are directed to set up an IV line delivering RL 30 mL/hour TKO with a 10-gtt/mL system.

15. How many drips per minute should the IV deliver?
   a. 1 gtt/minute
   b. 3 gtt/minute
   c. 5 gtt/minute
   d. 10 gtt/minute
   e. 20 gtt/minute

16. A good site for the angiocatheter would be the:
   a. antecubital fossa.
   b. anterior forearm.
   c. upper arm.
   d. deltoid.
   e. vastus lateralis.

17. A good place to administer a 0.25-mL IM injection on a child is the:
   a. antecubital fossa.
   b. anterior forearm.
   c. upper arm.
   d. deltoid.
   e. vastus lateralis.

18. The physician orders Demerol 150 mg IM for a patient. The vial label indicates a total of 20 mL of medication with 100 mg/mL. Find the dosage.
   a. 0.67 mL
   b. 1.5 mL
   c. 2.5 mL
   d. 7.5 mL
   e. 30 mL

19. A good site to inject a medication ordered SC would be the:
   a. antecubital fossa.
   b. anterior forearm.
   c. upper arm.
   d. deltoid.
   e. vastus lateralis.

20. You are told to administer a medicine by the otic route. This medicine should be administered into:
   a. the ears.
   b. inhaler.
   c. the eyes
   d. the mouth.
   e. the nose.

OG MATCHING

Match each key term with its definition.

Key Terms

21. _____ ampule
22. _____ apothecary system of measurement
23. _____ buccal
24. _____ diluent
25. _____ gauge
26. _____ induration
27. _____ infiltration
28. _____ Mantoux
29. _____ metric system
30. _____ nebulizer
31. _____ ophthalmic
32. _____ otic
33. _____ parenteral
34. _____ sublingual
35. _____ topical
36. _____ vial

Definitions

a. leakage of intravenous fluids into surrounding tissues
b. administration of medication between the cheek and gum of the mouth
c. all systemic administration routes excluding the gastrointestinal tract
d. a system of measurement that uses grams, liters, and meters
e. diameter of a needle lumen
f. device for administering respiratory medications as a fine inhaled spray
g. a tuberculosis screening test
h. small glass container that must be broken at the neck so that the solution can be aspirated into the syringe
i. administration route to a local spot on the outside of the body
j. administration route to the eyes
k. a system of measures based on drops, minims, grains, drams, and ounces
l. administration route to or by way of the ears
m. hardened area at the injection site after an intradermal screening test for tuberculosis
n. administration beneath the tongue
o. glass or plastic container sealed at the top by a rubber stopper
p. specified liquid used to reconstitute powder medications for injection

OG MATCHING

Match the injection route to the proper location for administration. There may be more than one location for each injection.

Injection Routes

37. _____ intradermal (ID)
38. _____ adult intramuscular (IM)
39. _____ juvenile (<2 years old) intramuscular (IM)
40. _____ Z-track intramuscular (IM)
41. _____ subcutaneous (SC)

Locations

a. abdomen
b. anterior forearm
c. back
d. deltoid
e. dorsogluteal
f. rectus femoris
g. thigh
h. upper arm
i. vastus lateralis
j. ventrogluteal

Grade: _____

42. When preparing medications, the patient's safety relies on good communication between the physician and yourself. Identify the safety rules you should use to prevent communication errors by placing a check mark on the line under "Yes" if the statement is a safety rule and check "No" if the rule does not apply.

Rule	Yes	No
a. Confirm all medications verbally. Do not try to interpret the physician's handwriting.		
b. Use previous medications and dosages listed on the patient's chart as a safety check.		
c. Check with the physician if you have any doubt about a medication or an order.		

43. Once you have correctly interpreted the medication order from the physician, you must locate and identify the correct drugs to dispense or administer. Choose the rules that prevent errors with identifying the correct medications by placing a check mark on the line under "Yes" if the statement is a safety rule and check "No" if the rule does not apply.

Rule	Yes	No
a. Check the label when taking the medication from the shelf, when preparing it, and again when replacing it on the shelf or disposing of the empty container.		
b. Peel off the label from the medication and place it in the patient's record.		
c. Place the order and the medication side by side to compare for accuracy.		
d. Only fill prescriptions written using brand names.		
e. Read labels carefully. Do not scan labels or medication orders.		
f. Use a resource like the Internet to cross-reference generic and brand names for medications.		
g. It is always safer to give a medication poured or drawn up by someone more experienced.		

44. Once you have correctly interpreted the medication order from the physician and identified the correct medication, you must safely dispense and/or administer the medication. Identify which rules prevent mistakes in dispensing and administering medications by placing a check mark on the line under "Yes" if the statement is a safety rule and check "No" if the rule does not apply.

Rule	Yes	No
a. Know the policies of your office regarding the administration of medications.		
b. Never question the physician's written orders.		
c. Prepare medications in the presence of the patient so you can discuss what you are doing and answer the patient's questions.		
d. Check the strength of the medication (e.g., 250 vs. 500 mg) and the route of administration.		
e. If you are interrupted, return the medicine to its original container so you can correctly identify it when you come back and finish.		
f. Work in a quiet, well-lit area.		
g. Check the patient's medical record for allergies to the actual medication or its components before administering.		

45. Indicate whether the following are parenteral or enteral by writing P (parenteral) or E (enteral) on the line preceding the route.

a. _____ buccal

b. _____ inhalation

c. _____ intramuscular

d. _____ intravenous

e. _____ oral

f. _____ rectal

g. _____ subcutaneous

h. _____ sublingual

i. _____ transdermal

46. Identify the medical term for the route for administration by placing the term on the line next to the administration method.

a. ear drops _____

b. eye drops _____

c. nitroglycerine patch _____

d. lotion _____

e. TB test _____

f. nebulizer _____

g. suppositories _____

h. cough syrup _____

COG COMPLETION

Grade: _____

For each of the dosage calculations, show your work and circle your answer.

47. The physician orders enoxaparin 40 mg SC. The label on the package reads 150 mg/mL. Find the correct dosage for this patient.

_____

_____

_____

_____

48. You are directed to give a heroin addict 30 mg of methadone PO. The medication comes in tablets labeled 20 mg/tablet. How many tablets would you give the patient?

_____

_____

_____

_____

49. As ordered by the physician, your patient needs 300,000 units of penicillin G IM. The label on the medication vial reads "Penicillin G 1 million units/2 mL." How many mL would you need to give?

_____

_____

_____

_____

50. The physician has written an order for you to give 40 mg of prednisone PO now before the patient leaves the office. You have on hand two strengths of prednisone: 10 mg/tablet and 5 mg/tablet. Choose the appropriate strength and calculate the number of tablets you would give to the patient.

_____

_____

_____

_____

51. Your patient has been ordered by the physician to receive 40 mg of furosemide IM. The ampule states "Furosemide 20 mg/mL." How much medication should you draw up to administer?

_____

_____

_____

_____

52. The patient seen in your office today is ordered by the physician to receive 750 mg of Rocephin™ deep IM. The label on the vial states "Rocephin 1 g/2 cc." How much would you give?

_____

_____

_____

_____

53. The physician has ordered your patient to take doxycycline 100 mg BID for 7 days. She would like the patient to have a dose before leaving the office. The medication label on the doxycycline in your office reads "Doxycycline 50 mg/capsule." How many would you give to the patient?

_____

_____

_____

_____

54. Your patient arrives at the office with nausea and vomiting. The physician orders you to give 12.5 mg of Phenergan™ IM. The vial states "Phenergan 25 mg/mL." How much would you give to the patient?

_____

_____

_____

_____

55. An order has been written by the physician for you to administer 7 mg of warfarin PO to your patient. You have three bottles of warfarin available: 2 mg/tablet; 2.5 mg/tablet; and 5 mg/tablet. Which tablet strength would you choose and how many tablets would you give the patient to ensure 7 mg were taken?

_____

_____

_____

_____

COG SHORT ANSWER

Grade: _____

56. What are the primary differences between enteral, parenteral, and topical medications?

_____

_____

_____

_____

57. List the four parts of a syringe that must be kept sterile.

_____

_____

_____

_____

58. What size needle (gauge and length) would you use for the following administration routes?

Route	Gauge	Length
a. IM		
b. SC		
c. ID		

COG TRUE OR FALSE?

Grade: _____

Indicate whether the statements are true or false by placing the letter T (true) or F (false) on the line preceding the statement.

59. _____ It is normal for frightened patients to have trouble breathing after taking a medication.

60. _____ A sip of water will help a patient take nitroglycerine sublingually.

61. _____ During SC and IM injections, a small amount of blood appears in the syringe when there is good penetration.

62. _____ Redness, swelling, pain, and discomfort are normal complications of IV therapy.

63. _____ Check the medication's expiration date, and use outdated medications first.

64. _____ Be alert for color changes, precipitation, odor, or any indication that the medication's properties have changed and discard appropriately.

65. _____ Keep narcotics on your person so others do not have access to them.

66. _____ Do not leave the medication cabinet unlocked when it is not in use.

67. _____ Never give keys for the medication cabinet to an unauthorized person.

COG AFF CASE STUDIES FOR CRITICAL THINKING

Grade: _____

68. The parent of an 18-month old insists that you give the IM immunization in the child's "hip." How would you respond to the parent's request?

_____

_____

_____

_____

69. The patient you are monitoring is receiving intravenous fluids for rehydration. Unfortunately, the insertion site in the left anterior forearm has developed complications and must be removed. How would you respond to the patient who does not understand why the IV must be removed?

_____

_____

_____

_____

70. One of the physicians in your medical office would like to change office policy so that no abbreviations are used in the patients' medical charts for fear of potentially harmful errors. The office is divided on the issue. What is your opinion and why?

_____

_____

_____

_____

71. You are directed to give a Z-track IM injection to a patient. The patient's spouse observes you deliberately draw a bubble into the syringe and panics because you are about to inject air into the patient. How do you address the spouse's concerns?

_____

_____

_____

_____

PSY PROCEDURE 24-1 — Administer Oral Medications

Name: _____ Date: _____ Time: _____ Grade: _____

EQUIPMENT/SUPPLIES: Physician's order, oral medication, disposable calibrated cup, glass of water, patient's medical record

STANDARDS: Given the needed equipment and a place to work, the student will perform this skill with _____ % accuracy in a total of _____ minutes. *(Your instructor will tell you what the percentage and time limits will be before you begin.)*

KEY: 4 = Satisfactory   0 = Unsatisfactory   NA = This step is not counted

PROCEDURE STEPS	SELF	PARTNER	INSTRUCTOR
1. Wash your hands	❑	❑	❑

2. Review the physician's medication order and select the correct oral medication
  a. Compare the label with the physician's instructions
  b. Note the expiration date
  c. Check the label three times: when taking it from the shelf, while pouring, and when returning to the shelf
	❑	❑	❑

3. Calculate the correct dosage to be given if necessary	❑	❑	❑
4. If using a multidose container, remove cap from container. For single-dose medications, obtain the correct amount of medication.	❑	❑	❑

5. Remove the correct dose of medication
  a. For solid medications:
    (1) Pour the capsule/tablet into the bottle cap
    (2) Transfer the medication to a disposable cup
  b. For liquid medications:
    (1) Open the bottle lid: place it on a flat surface with the open end up
    (2) Palm the label to prevent liquids from dripping onto the label
    (3) With the opposite hand, place the thumbnail at the correct calibration
    (4) Pour the medication until the proper amount is in the cup
	❑	❑	❑

6. Greet and identify the patient. Explain the procedure	❑	❑	❑
7. Ask the patient about medication allergies that might not be noted on the chart	❑	❑	❑
8. Give the patient a glass of water, unless contraindicated. Hand the patient the disposable cup containing the medication or pour the tablets or capsules into the patient's hand	❑	❑	❑
9. Remain with the patient to be sure that all of the medication is swallowed **a.** Observe any unusual reactions and report them to the physician	❑	❑	❑
10. Thank the patient and give any appropriate instructions	❑	❑	❑

PSY PROCEDURE 24-1   **Administer Oral Medications** (continued)

11. **AFF** Explain how to respond to a patient who is hearing impaired	❑	❑	❑
12. Wash your hands	❑	❑	❑
13. **AFF** Log into the Electronic Medical Record (EMR) using your username and secure password OR obtain the paper medical record from a secure location and assure it is kept away from public access. Record the procedure noting the date, time, name of medication, dose administered, route of administration, and your name	❑	❑	❑
14. When finished, log out of the EMR and/or replace the paper medical record in an appropriate and secure location	❑	❑	❑

CALCULATION

Total Possible Points: _____

Total Points Earned: _____ Multiplied by 100 = _____ Divided by Total Possible Points = _____ %

PASS   **FAIL**   **COMMENTS:**
❑   ❑

Student's signature _____ Date _____

Partner's signature _____ Date _____

Instructor's signature _____ Date _____

PSY PROCEDURE 24-2   **Prepare Injections**

Name: _____ Date: _____ Time: _____ Grade: _____

EQUIPMENT/SUPPLIES: Physician's order, medication for injection in ampule or vial, antiseptic wipes, gloves, appropriate-size needle and syringe, small gauze pad, biohazard sharps container, patient's medical record

STANDARDS: Given the needed equipment and a place to work, the student will perform this skill with _____ % accuracy in a total of _____ minutes. *(Your instructor will tell you what the percentage and time limits will be before you begin.)*

KEY: 4 = Satisfactory   0 = Unsatisfactory   NA = This step is not counted

PROCEDURE STEPS	SELF	PARTNER	INSTRUCTOR
1. Wash your hands	❏	❏	❏

2. Review the physician's medication order and select the correct medication
  a. Compare the label with the physician's instructions. Note the expiration date
  b. Check the label three times: when taking it from the shelf, while drawing it up into the syringe, and when returning to the shelf
	❏	❏	❏

3. Calculate the correct dosage to be given, if necessary	❏	❏	❏
4. Choose the needle and syringe according to the route of administration, type of medication, and size of the patient	❏	❏	❏
5. Open the needle and syringe package. Assemble if necessary. Secure the needle to the syringe	❏	❏	❏

6. Withdraw the correct amount of medication:
  a. From an ampule:
    (1) Tap the stem of the ampule lightly
    (2) Place a piece of gauze around the ampule neck
    (3) Grasp the gauze and ampule firmly. Snap the stem off the ampule
    (4) Dispose of the ampule top in a biohazard sharps container
    (5) Insert the needle lumen below the level of the medication
    (6) Withdraw the medication
    (7) Dispose of the ampule in a biohazard sharps container
    (8) Remove any air bubbles in the syringe
    (9) Draw back on the plunger to add a small amount of air; then gently push the plunger forward to eject the air out of the syringe
	❏	❏	❏

PSY PROCEDURE 24-2   **Prepare Injections** (continued)

b. From a vial:	❏	❏	❏
(1) Using the antiseptic wipe, cleanse the rubber stopper of the vial			
(2) Pull air into the syringe with the amount equivalent to the amount of medication to be removed from the vial			
(3) Insert the needle into the vial top. Inject the air from the syringe			
(4) With the needle inside the vial, invert the vial			
(5) Hold the syringe at eye level			
(6) Aspirate the desired amount of medication into the syringe			
(7) Displace any air bubbles in the syringe by gently tapping the barrel			
(8) Remove the air by pushing the plunger slowly and forcing the air into the vial			
7. Carefully recap the needle using one-hand technique	❏	❏	❏

_____

_____

_____

_____

CALCULATION

Total Possible Points: _____

Total Points Earned: _____ Multiplied by 100 = _____ Divided by Total Possible Points = _____ %

PASS   **FAIL**   **COMMENTS:**
 ❏   ❏

Student's signature _____ Date _____

Partner's signature _____ Date _____

Instructor's signature _____ Date _____

PSY PROCEDURE 24-3 **Administer an Intradermal Injection**

Name: _____ Date: _____ Time: _____ Grade: _____

EQUIPMENT/SUPPLIES: Physician's order, medication for injection in ampule or vial, antiseptic wipes, gloves, appropriate-size needle and syringe, small gauze pad, biohazard sharps container, patient's medical record

STANDARDS: Given the needed equipment and a place to work, the student will perform this skill with _____ % accuracy in a total of _____ minutes. *(Your instructor will tell you what the percentage and time limits will be before you begin.)*

KEY: 4 = Satisfactory 0 = Unsatisfactory NA = This step is not counted

PROCEDURE STEPS	SELF	PARTNER	INSTRUCTOR
1. Wash your hands **a.** Review the physician's medication order and select the correct medication **b.** Compare the label with the physician's instructions. Note the expiration date **c.** Check the label three times: when taking it from the shelf, while drawing it up into the syringe, and when returning it to the shelf	❑	❑	❑
2. Prepare the injection according to the steps in Procedure 24-2	❑	❑	❑
3. Greet and identify the patient. Explain the procedure	❑	❑	❑
4. Ask patient about medication allergies	❑	❑	❑
5. Select the appropriate site for the injection	❑	❑	❑
6. Prepare the site by cleansing with an antiseptic wipe	❑	❑	❑
7. Put on gloves. Remove the needle guard	❑	❑	❑
8. Using your nondominant hand, pull the patient's skin taut	❑	❑	❑
9. With the bevel of the needle facing upward, insert the needle at a 10- to 15-degree angle into the upper layer of the skin **a.** When the bevel of the needle is under the skin, stop inserting the needle **b.** The needle will be slightly visible below the surface of the skin **c.** It is not necessary to aspirate when performing an intradermal injection	❑	❑	❑
10. Inject the medication slowly by depressing the plunger **a.** A wheal will form as the medication enters the dermal layer of the skin **b.** Hold the syringe steady for proper administration	❑	❑	❑
11. Remove the needle from the skin at the same angle at which it was inserted **a.** Do not use an antiseptic wipe or gauze pad over the site. **b.** Do not press or massage the site. Do not apply an adhesive bandage	❑	❑	❑

PSY PROCEDURE 24-3   **Administer an Intradermal Injection** (continued)

12. Do not recap the needle	❏	❏	❏
13. Dispose of the needle and syringe in an approved biohazard sharps container	❏	❏	❏
14. **AFF** Explain how to respond to a patient with dementia	❏	❏	❏

_____

_____

_____

_____

15. Remove your gloves and wash your hands	❏	❏	❏
16. Depending on the type of skin test administered, the length of time required for the body tissues to react, and the policies of the medical office, perform one of the following: **a.** Read the test results. Inspect and palpate the site for the presence and amount of induration **b.** Tell the patient when to return (date and time) to the office to have the results read **c.** Instruct the patient to read the results at home **d.** Make sure the patient understands the instructions	❏	❏	❏
17. **AFF** Log into the Electronic Medical Record (EMR) using your username and secure password OR obtain the paper medical record from a secure location and assure it is kept away from public access. Record the procedure noting the date, time, name of medication, dose administered, route of administration, patient instructions, and your name	❏	❏	❏
18. When finished, log out of the EMR and/or replace the paper medical record in an appropriate and secure location	❏	❏	❏

CALCULATION

Total Possible Points: _____

Total Points Earned: _____ Multiplied by 100 = _____ Divided by Total Possible Points = _____ %

PASS   FAIL   COMMENTS:
❏   ❏

Student's signature _____ Date _____

Partner's signature _____ Date _____

Instructor's signature _____ Date _____

PSY PROCEDURE 24-4 — Administer a Subcutaneous Injection

Name: _____ Date: _____ Time: _____ Grade: _____

EQUIPMENT/SUPPLIES: Physician's order, medication for injection in ampule or vial, antiseptic wipes, gloves, appropriate-size needle and syringe, small gauze pad, biohazard sharps container, patient's medical record

STANDARDS: Given the needed equipment and a place to work, the student will perform this skill with _____ % accuracy in a total of _____ minutes. *(Your instructor will tell you what the percentage and time limits will be before you begin.)*

KEY: 4 = Satisfactory   0 = Unsatisfactory   NA = This step is not counted

PROCEDURE STEPS	SELF	PARTNER	INSTRUCTOR

1. Wash your hands
  a. Review the physician's medication order and select the correct medication
  b. Compare the label with the physician's instructions. Note the expiration date
  c. Check the label three times: when taking it from the shelf, while drawing it up into the syringe, and when returning it to the shelf
	❏	❏	❏

2. Prepare the injection according to the steps in Procedure 24-2	❏	❏	❏
3. Greet and identify the patient. Explain the procedure	❏	❏	❏
4. Ask the patient about medication allergies	❏	❏	❏
5. Select the appropriate site for the injection	❏	❏	❏
6. Prepare the site by cleansing with an antiseptic	❏	❏	❏
7. Put on gloves	❏	❏	❏
8. Using your nondominant hand, hold the skin surrounding the injection site	❏	❏	❏
9. With a firm motion, insert the needle into the tissue at a 45-degree angle to the skin surface	❏	❏	❏
10. Hold the barrel between the thumb and the index finger of your dominant hand	❏	❏	❏
11. Insert the needle completely to the hub	❏	❏	❏
12. Remove your nondominant hand from the skin	❏	❏	❏
13. Holding the syringe steady, pull back on the syringe gently. If blood appears in the hub or the syringe, do not inject the medication; remove the needle and prepare a new injection	❏	❏	❏
14. Inject the medication slowly by depressing the plunger	❏	❏	❏

PSY PROCEDURE 24-4 **Administer a Subcutaneous Injection** (continued)

15. Place a gauze pad over the injection site and remove the needle
   a. Gently massage the injection site with the gauze pad
   b. Do not recap the used needle; place it in the biohazard sharps container
   c. Apply an adhesive bandage if needed
	❏	❏	❏

16. Remove your gloves and wash your hands	❏	❏	❏
17. **AFF** Explain how to respond to a patient who is deaf	❏	❏	❏

18. An injection given for allergy desensitization requires:
   a. Keeping the patient in the office for at least 30 minutes for observation
   b. Notifying the doctor of any reaction. (Be alert, anaphylaxis is possible)
	❏	❏	❏

19. **AFF** Log into the Electronic Medical Record (EMR) using your username and secure password OR obtain the paper medical record from a secure location and assure it is kept away from public access. Record the procedure noting the date, time, name of medication, dose administered, route of administration, and your name	❏	❏	❏
20. When finished, log out of the EMR and/or replace the paper medical record in an appropriate and secure location	❏	❏	❏

CALCULATION

Total Possible Points: _____

Total Points Earned: _____ Multiplied by 100 = _____ Divided by Total Possible Points = _____ %

PASS   **FAIL**   **COMMENTS:**
   ❏   ❏

Student's signature _____ Date _____

Partner's signature _____ Date _____

Instructor's signature _____ Date _____

PSY PROCEDURE 24-5 | Administer an Intramuscular Injection

Name: _____ Date: _____ Time: _____ Grade: _____

EQUIPMENT/SUPPLIES: Physician's order, medication for injection in ampule or vial, antiseptic wipes, gloves, appropriate-size needle and syringe, small gauze pad, biohazard sharps container, patient's medical record

STANDARDS: Given the needed equipment and a place to work, the student will perform this skill with _____ % accuracy in a total of _____ minutes. *(Your instructor will tell you what the percentage and time limits will be before you begin.)*

KEY: 4 = Satisfactory 0 = Unsatisfactory NA = This step is not counted

PROCEDURE STEPS	SELF	PARTNER	INSTRUCTOR
1. Wash your hands **a.** Review the physician's order and select the correct medication **b.** Compare the label with the physician's instructions. Note the expiration date **c.** Check the label three times: when taking it from the shelf, while drawing it up into the syringe, and when returning to the shelf	❑	❑	❑
2. Prepare the injection according to the steps in Procedure 24-2	❑	❑	❑
3. Greet and identify the patient. Explain the procedure	❑	❑	❑
4. Ask the patient about medication allergies	❑	❑	❑
5. Select the appropriate site for the injection	❑	❑	❑
6. Prepare the site by cleansing with an antiseptic wipe	❑	❑	❑
7. Put on gloves	❑	❑	❑
8. Using your nondominant hand, hold the skin surrounding the injection site	❑	❑	❑
9. While holding the syringe like a dart, use a quick, firm motion to insert the needle at a 90-degree angle to the skin surface. Hold the barrel between the thumb and the index finger of the dominant hand and insert the needle completely to the hub	❑	❑	❑
10. Holding the syringe steady, pull back on the syringe gently. If blood appears in the hub or the syringe, do not inject the medication; remove the needle and prepare a new injection	❑	❑	❑
11. Inject the medication slowly by depressing the plunger	❑	❑	❑
12. Place a gauze pad over the injection site and remove the needle **a.** Gently massage the injection site with the gauze pad **b.** Do not recap the used needle. Place in biohazard sharps container **c.** Apply an adhesive bandage if needed	❑	❑	❑
13. **AFF** Explain how to respond to a patient who is visually impaired	❑	❑	❑

PSY PROCEDURE 24-5 **Administer an Intramuscular Injection** (continued)

_____

_____

_____

_____

_____

14. Remove your gloves and wash your hands	❏	❏	❏
15. Notify the doctor of any reaction. (Be alert, anaphylaxis is possible)	❏	❏	❏
16. **ARF** Log into the Electronic Medical Record (EMR) using your username and secure password OR obtain the paper medical record from a secure location and assure it is kept away from public access. Record the procedure noting the date, time, name of medication, dose administered, route of administration, and your name	❏	❏	❏
17. When finished, log out of the EMR and/or replace the paper medical record in an appropriate and secure location	❏	❏	❏

CALCULATION

Total Possible Points: _____

Total Points Earned: _____ Multiplied by 100 = _____ Divided by Total Possible Points = _____ %

PASS **FAIL** **COMMENTS:**
❏   ❏

Student's signature _____ Date _____

Partner's signature _____ Date _____

Instructor's signature _____ Date _____

PSY PROCEDURE 24-6 **Administer an Intramuscular Injection Using the Z-Track Method**

Name: _____ Date: _____ Time: _____ Grade: _____

EQUIPMENT/SUPPLIES: Physician's order, medication for injection in ampule or vial, antiseptic wipes, gloves, appropriate-size needle and syringe, small gauze pad, biohazard sharps container, patient's medical record

STANDARDS: Given the needed equipment and a place to work, the student will perform this skill with _____ % accuracy in a total of _____ minutes. *(Your instructor will tell you what the percentage and time limits will be before you begin.)*

KEY: 4 = Satisfactory 0 = Unsatisfactory NA = This step is not counted

PROCEDURE STEPS	SELF	PARTNER	INSTRUCTOR
1. Follow steps 1 through 7 as described in Procedure 24-5	❏	❏	❏
2. Pull the top layer of skin to the side and hold it with your nondominant hand throughout the injection	❏	❏	❏
3. While holding the syringe like a dart, use a quick, firm motion to insert the needle at a 90-degree angle to the skin surface **a.** Hold the barrel between the thumb and index finger of the dominant hand **b.** Insert the needle completely to the hub	❏	❏	❏
4. Aspirate by withdrawing the plunger slightly **a.** If no blood appears, push the plunger in slowly and steadily **b.** Count to 10 before withdrawing the needle	❏	❏	❏
5. Place a gauze pad over the injection site and remove the needle **a.** Gently massage the injection site with the gauze pad **b.** Do not recap the used needle. Place in the biohazard sharps container **c.** Apply an adhesive bandage, if needed	❏	❏	❏
6. Remove your gloves and wash your hands	❏	❏	❏
7. Notify the doctor of any reaction. (Be alert, anaphylaxis is possible)	❏	❏	❏
8. **AFF** Log into the Electronic Medical Record (EMR) using your username and secure password OR obtain the paper medical record from a secure location and assure it is kept away from public access. Record the procedure noting the date, time, name of medication, dose administered, route of administration, and your name. If instructions were given to the patient, document these also	❏	❏	❏
9. When finished, log out of the EMR and/or replace the paper medical record in an appropriate and secure location.	❏	❏	❏

PSY PROCEDURE 24-6 | **Administer an Intramuscular Injection Using the Z-Track Method** (continued)

CALCULATION

Total Possible Points: _____

Total Points Earned: _____ Multiplied by 100 = _____ Divided by Total Possible Points = _____ %

PASS   FAIL   COMMENTS:
  ❑   ❑

Student's signature _____   Date _____

Partner's signature _____   Date _____

Instructor's signature _____   Date _____

PSY PROCEDURE 24-7 **Apply Transdermal Medications**

Name: _____ Date: _____ Time: _____ Grade: _____

EQUIPMENT/SUPPLIES: Physician's order, medication, gloves, patient's medical record

STANDARDS: Given the needed equipment and a place to work, the student will perform this skill with _____ % accuracy in a total of _____ minutes. *(Your instructor will tell you what the percentage and time limits will be before you begin.)*

KEY: 4 = Satisfactory   0 = Unsatisfactory   NA = This step is not counted

PROCEDURE STEPS	SELF	PARTNER	INSTRUCTOR
1. Wash your hands	❑	❑	❑
2. Review the physician's medication order and select the correct medication **a.** Compare the label with the physician's instructions. Note the expiration date **b.** Check the label three times: when taking it from the shelf, before taking it into the patient exam room, and before applying it to the patient's skin	❑	❑	❑
3. Greet and identify the patient. Explain the procedure	❑	❑	❑
4. Ask the patient about medication allergies that might not be noted on the medical record	❑	❑	❑
5. Select the appropriate site and perform any necessary skin preparation. The sites are usually the upper arm, the chest or back surface, or behind the ear **a.** Ensure that the skin is clean, dry, and free from any irritation **b.** Do not shave areas with excessive hair; trim the hair closely with scissors	❑	❑	❑
6. If there is a transdermal patch already in place, remove it carefully while wearing gloves. Discard the patch in the trash container. Inspect the site for irritation	❑	❑	❑
7. Open the medication package by pulling the two sides apart. Do not touch the area of medication	❑	❑	❑
8. Apply the medicated patch to the patient's skin, following the manufacturer's directions **a.** Press the adhesive edges down firmly all around, starting at the center and pressing outward **b.** If the edges do not stick, fasten with tape	❑	❑	❑
9. **AFF** Explain how to respond to a patient who is uncomfortable, exposing skin on areas such as the chest or arms due to cultural or religious beliefs	❑	❑	❑

PSY PROCEDURE 24-7 **Apply Transdermal Medications** (continued)

_____

_____

_____

_____

10. Wash your hands	❏	❏	❏
11. **AFF** Log into the Electronic Medical Record (EMR) using your username and secure password OR obtain the paper medical record from a secure location and assure it is kept away from public access. Record the procedure noting the date, time, name of medication, dose administered, route of administration, site of the new patch, and your name	❏	❏	❏
12. When finished, log out of the EMR and/or replace the paper medical record in an appropriate and secure location	❏	❏	❏

_____

_____

_____

_____

CALCULATION

Total Possible Points: _____

Total Points Earned: _____ Multiplied by 100 = _____ Divided by Total Possible Points = _____ %

PASS   FAIL   COMMENTS:
❏   ❏

Student's signature _____ Date _____

Partner's signature _____ Date _____

Instructor's signature _____ Date _____

PSY PROCEDURE 24-8 | **Complete an Incident Report Related to an Error in Patient Care**

Name: _____ **Date:** _____ **Time:** _____ **Grade:** _____

EQUIPMENT/SUPPLIES: An incident form

STANDARDS: Given the needed equipment and a place to work, the student will perform this skill with _____ % accuracy in a total of _____ minutes. *(Your instructor will tell you what the percentage and time limits will be before you begin.)*

KEY: 4 = Satisfactory 0 = Unsatisfactory NA = This step is not counted

PROCEDURE STEPS	SELF	PARTNER	INSTRUCTOR
1. Recognize the error in patient care (i.e., medication administration) and notify the physician immediately after assessing the patient and providing emergency procedures if appropriate	❑	❑	❑
2. Once the patient is assessed and necessary interventions taken per physician instructions, complete an incident report form.	❑	❑	❑
3. Sign and date the incident report form and file with the office or practice manager	❑	❑	❑
4. **AFF** Advise the patient on any follow-up procedures as instructed by the physician	❑	❑	❑

CALCULATION

Total Possible Points: _____

Total Points Earned: _____ Multiplied by 100 = _____ Divided by Total Possible Points = _____ %

PASS **FAIL** **COMMENTS:**
❑   ❑

Student's signature _____ Date _____

Partner's signature _____ Date _____

Instructor's signature _____ Date _____

Great Falls Medical Center Physician Offices

Employee Incident/Injury Report Form

Employee Name:	Title:
Location:	Date and Time of Injury/Illness:
Person or Employee the Injury/Illness Reported to:	Title of Person or Employee Injury or Illness Reported to:

Describe the details of your accident, injury, or illness. Be as specific as possible:

Explain what you were doing at the time of your accident, injury, or illness:

For injuries, list the part or parts of your body that were injured. Be specific (i.e., right index finger, left ankle, etc...):

If there was a delay in reporting the injury or illness, explain the reason for this delay:

Names and Titles of Any Witnesses to your Injury or Illness:

Employee Signature:	Date:

CHAPTER 25

Diagnostic Imaging

© VASNABADA/Shutterstock

LEARNING OUTCOMES

COG Cognitive Domain*

1. Spell and define the key terms
2. Explain the theory and function of x-rays and x-ray machines
3. State the principles of radiology
4. Describe routine and contrast media, fluoroscopy, computed tomography, sonography, magnetic resonance imaging, nuclear medicine, and mammographic examinations
5. Explain the role of the medical assistant in radiologic procedures
6. *Identify a. body planes b. directional terms c. quadrants d. body cavities*
7. Identify critical information required for scheduling patient procedures

PSY Psychomotor Domain*

1. Assist with x-ray procedures (Procedure 25-1)
   a. *Instruct and prepare a patient for a procedure or treatment*
   b. *Document patient care accurately in the medical record*

AFF Affective Domain*

1. *Demonstrate critical thinking skills*
2. *Reassure patients*
3. *Demonstrate empathy for patients' concerns*
4. *Demonstrate active listening*
5. *Respect diversity*
6. *Recognize personal boundaries*
7. *Demonstrate tactfulness*

8. *Demonstrate self-awareness*
9. Protect the integrity of the medical record

MAERB Standards are Italicized.

ABHES Competencies

1. Partner with health care teams to attain optimal patient health outcomes
2. Display effective interpersonal skills with patients and healthcare team members.
3. Demonstrate cultural awareness
4. Make adaptations for patients with special needs (psychological or physical limitations)

Name: _____   Date: _____   Grade: _____

OG MULTIPLE CHOICE

Circle the letter preceding the correct answer.

1. Which term below means lying face downward?
   a. Supine
   b. Prone
   c. Decubitus
   d. Recumbent
   e. Relaxed

2. Which of the following is a form of nuclear medicine?
   a. Radiopaque
   b. Barium
   c. Iodine
   d. Radionuclides
   e. Radiolucent

3. Noises heard during an x-ray exposure may come from:
   a. the x-ray tube.
   b. x-rays.
   c. the positioning aid.
   d. high voltage.
   e. the sheet of film.

4. Which of the following is an example of radiopaque tissue?
   a. Lungs
   b. Bone
   c. Muscle
   d. Fat
   e. Veins

5. A minimum of two x-rays should be taken at:
   a. 180 degrees of each other.
   b. 30 degrees of each other.
   c. 70 degrees of each other.
   d. 90 degrees of each other.
   e. 50 degrees of each other.

6. A type of radiography that creates cross-sectional images of the body is:
   a. fluoroscopy.
   b. echogram.
   c. computerized tomography.
   d. ultrasound.
   e. mammography.

7. Which of the following forms of radiography do not use x-rays?
   a. MRI
   b. Nuclear medicine
   c. Fluoroscopy
   d. Teleradiology
   e. Tomography

8. Which procedure creates an image that depends on the chemical makeup of the body?
   a. Tomography
   b. Fluoroscopy
   c. MRI
   d. Mammography
   e. Nuclear medicine

9. Sonograms create images using:
   a. radioactive material.
   b. contrast media.
   c. magnetic resonance.
   d. chemotherapy.
   e. sound waves.

10. X-rays can be harmful to infants and young children because:
    a. their immune systems are not fully developed.
    b. their cells divide at a rapid pace.
    c. they have less muscle mass than adults.
    d. they have a smaller body mass.
    e. they have less body fat than adults.

11. Which of the following procedures may be done in a confined space?
    a. MRI
    b. Nuclear medicine
    c. Fluoroscopy
    d. Teleradiology
    e. Tomography

12. A physician who specializes in interpreting the images on the processed film is a(n):
   a. pulmonologist.
   b. internist.
   c. immunologist.
   d. ophthalmologist.
   e. radiologist.

Scenario for questions 13 and 14: A patient has come in for an x-ray. The physician wants you to get a clear image of the patient's liver.

13. What is another possible way to view the patient's liver without injections?
   a. Mammography
   b. Sonography
   c. Fluoroscopy
   d. Teleradiology
   e. Tomography

14. Which position would allow the best images of the liver?
   a. Supine
   b. Decubitus
   c. Posterior
   d. Left anterior oblique
   e. Right anterior oblique

15. Who owns the x-ray film after it has been developed?
   a. The patient
   b. The physician who ordered the x-rays
   c. The physician who will use the x-rays
   d. The lab that developed the film
   e. The site where the film was taken and developed.

16. You should wear a dosimeter to:
   a. lower the level of radiation.
   b. protect against radiation effects.
   c. monitor personal radiation exposure.
   d. enhance radiography images.
   e. collect data on different procedures.

17. Why do some tests require patients to be NPO before an administration of barium PO?
   a. Gastric juices may interfere with the readings
   b. A full stomach may distort or alter an image
   c. Patients are not allowed to relieve themselves
   d. Undigested food might counteract contrast media
   e. Instruments might become soiled during the procedure

18. Images that partially block x-rays are called:
   a. radiographs.
   b. radiolucent.
   c. radiopaque.
   d. radionuclides.
   e. radiograms.

19. Why is radiology used as a form of cancer treatment?
   a. X-rays show the exact location of cancer
   b. Radioactive cells produce more white blood cells
   c. Radiation can destroy or weaken cancer cells
   d. Radiation makes cancerous tumors benign
   e. Chemotherapy is not as effective as radiation

20. When explaining procedures to patients:
   a. let the physician go into detail.
   b. answer all of the questions they ask.
   c. do not worry them with potential risk.
   d. soothe their fears without telling them anything.
   e. allow only the nurse to explain the procedure.

COG MATCHING

Grade: _____

Match each key term with its definition.

Key Terms

21. _____ cassette
22. _____ contrast medium
23. _____ film
24. _____ fluoroscopy
25. _____ magnetic resonance imaging
26. _____ nuclear medicine
27. _____ radiograph
28. _____ radiography
29. _____ radiologist
30. _____ radiology
31. _____ radiolucent
32. _____ radionuclide
33. _____ radiopaque
34. _____ teleradiology
35. _____ tomography
36. _____ ultrasound
37. _____ x-rays

Definitions

a. invisible electromagnetic radiation waves used in diagnosis and treatment of various disorders

b. a lightproof holder in which film is exposed

c. imaging technique that uses a strong magnetic field

d. a radioactive material with a short life that is used in small amounts in nuclear medicine studies

e. physician who interprets images to provide diagnostic information

f. imaging technique that uses sound waves to diagnose or monitor various body structures

g. not permeable to passage of x-rays

h. processed film that contains a visible image

i. a substance ingested or injected into the body to facilitate imaging of internal structures

j. the use of computed imaging and information systems to transmit diagnostic images to distant locations

k. a procedure in which the x-ray tube and film move in relation to each other during exposure, blurring out all structures except those in the focal plane

l. a raw material on which x-rays are projected through the body; prior to processing, this does not contain a visible image

m. permitting the passage of x-rays

n. a special x-ray technique for examining a body part by immediate projection onto a fluorescent screen

o. the branch of medicine involving diagnostic and therapeutic applications of x-rays

p. a branch of medicine that uses radioactive isotopes to diagnose and treat disease

q. the art and science of producing diagnostic images with x-rays

COG MATCHING

Grade: _____

Match the different types of radiography techniques with their individual characteristics.

Techniques

38. _____ Fluoroscopy
39. _____ Tomography
40. _____ Mammography
41. _____ Ultrasound
42. _____ Magnetic resonance imaging
43. _____ Radiation therapy

Characteristics

a. the image depends on the chemical makeup of the body, commonly used in prenatal testing

b. can create three-dimensional images, so that organs can be viewed from all angles

c. the area of the body exposed must be defined exactly so that each treatment is identical

d. used as an aid to other types of treatment, such as reducing fractures and implanting devices such as pacemakers

e. a vital adjunct to biopsy

f. designed to concentrate on specific areas of the body

COG SHORT ANSWER

Grade: _____

44. List the four processes by which radiographic film is produced.

_____

_____

_____

_____

45. List five radiation safety procedures for patients.

_____

_____

_____

_____

46. Fill in the full names for the abbreviations below.

a. PET _____

b. SPECT _____

c. ALARA _____

47. Name two contrast mediums.

_____

_____

_____

_____

48. What are the three ways contrast media may be introduced into the body?

_____

_____

_____

_____

49. Name four types of interventional radiological procedures.

_____

_____

_____

_____

50. List five side effects of radiation therapy.

_____

_____

_____

_____

51. What is the difference between radiolucent and radiopaque tissues? How do these tissues appear differently on a radiograph? Give an example of each.

_____

_____

_____

_____

52. Why do x-ray examinations require a minimum of two exposures?

_____

_____

_____

_____

53. Why is it imperative to have an esophagogastroduodenoscopy done before other barium studies?

_____

_____

_____

_____

54. Compare and contrast fluoroscopy with tomography. How do these procedures use movement?

_____

_____

_____

_____

55. You have a patient who will have a radiographic exam using contrast media next week. You find out this patient has an allergy to shellfish. What should you do?

_____

_____

_____

_____

COG TRUE OR FALSE?

Grade: _____

Indicate whether the statements are true or false by placing the letter T (true) or F (false) on the line preceding the statement.

56. _____ A patient may hear noises during an x-ray procedure.

57. _____ A mammogram is a minimally invasive procedure.

58. _____ You need to be proficient in the operation of your facility's equipment.

59. _____ The best way to explain procedures to a patient is with lots of detail.

COG **AFF** **CASE STUDIES FOR CRITICAL THINKING** _____ Grade: _____

60. Mrs. Kay has had several radiographic and contrast media studies over the past 5 years. She is now moving to another state and wants to know how to get copies of the films and reports to her new physician. What will you tell her about transferring these records?

_____

_____

_____

_____

61. You have a patient with a fear of enclosed spaces who is not able to have an open MRI at your outpatient radiographic center. How would you console this patient and explain x-ray procedures?

_____

_____

_____

_____

62. You have a patient coming in for radiation therapy who has been experiencing side effects such as weight loss, loss of appetite, and hair loss. She has concerns about the radiation therapy that she has been receiving and feels that it may be too much for her body. What would you say to her to help her better understand the situation?

_____

_____

_____

_____

63. You have a patient who has had radiographs taken with a referring physician. This patient has already spoken to his referral physician about the finding in his x-rays and would now like to consult with his primary care physician. However, the referring physician has not yet sent a summary of findings. Your patient is very anxious. What should you say?

_____

_____

_____

_____

PSY PROCEDURE 25-1 | **Assist with X-Ray Procedures**

Name: _____ Date: _____ Time: _____ Grade: _____

EQUIPMENT/SUPPLIES: Patient gown and drape

STANDARDS: Given the needed equipment and a place to work, the student will perform this skill with _____ % accuracy in a total of _____ minutes. *(Your instructor will tell you what the percentage and time limits will be before you begin.)*

KEY: 4 = Satisfactory 0 = Unsatisfactory NA = This step is not counted

PROCEDURE STEPS	SELF	PARTNER	INSTRUCTOR
1. Wash your hands	❏	❏	❏
2. Greet the patient by name, introduce yourself, and escort them to the room where the x-ray equipment is maintained	❏	❏	❏
3. Ask female patients about the possibility of pregnancy. If the patient is unsure or indicates pregnancy in any trimester, consult with the physician before proceeding with the x-ray procedure	❏	❏	❏
4. **AFF** Explain how to respond to a patient who speaks English as a second language	❏	❏	❏
_____ _____ _____ _____			
5. After explaining what clothing should be removed, if any, give the patient a gown and privacy	❏	❏	❏
6. Notify the x-ray technician or physician that the patient is ready for the x-ray procedure. Stay behind the lead-lined wall during the x-ray procedure to avoid exposure to x-rays during the procedure	❏	❏	❏
7. After the x-ray, ask the patient to remain in the room until the film has been developed and checked for accuracy and readability	❏	❏	❏
8. Once you have determined that the exposed film is adequate for the physician to view for diagnosis, have the patient get dressed and escort them to the front desk	❏	❏	❏
9. **AFF** Log into the Electronic Medical Record (EMR) using your username and secure password OR obtain the paper medical record from a secure location and assure it is kept away from public access	❏	❏	❏
10. When finished, log out of the EMR and/or replace the paper medical record in an appropriate and secure location	❏	❏	❏

PSY PROCEDURE 25-1 **Assist with X-Ray Procedures** (continued)

CALCULATION

Total Possible Points: _____

Total Points Earned: _____ Multiplied by 100 = _____ Divided by Total Possible Points = _____ %

PASS **FAIL** **COMMENTS:**
❑ ❑

Student's signature _____ Date _____

Partner's signature _____ Date _____

Instructor's signature _____ Date _____

CHAPTER 26

Medical Office Emergencies

LEARNING OUTCOMES

COG Cognitive Domain*

1. Spell and define key terms
2. List principles and steps of professional/provider CPR
3. *Identify basic principles of first aid*
4. Identify the five types of shock and the management of each
5. Describe how burns are classified and managed
6. Explain the management of allergic reactions
7. Describe the management of poisoning and the role of the poison control center
8. List the three types of hyperthermic emergencies and the treatment for each type
9. Discuss the treatment of hypothermia
10. Describe the role of the medical assistant in managing psychiatric emergencies

PSY Psychomotor Domain*

1. Administer oxygen (Procedure 26-1)

2. Perform cardiopulmonary resuscitation (Procedure 26-2)
   a. *Provide up-to-date documentation of provider/professional level CPR*
3. Use an automatic external defibrillator (Procedure 26-3)
4. Manage a foreign body airway obstruction (Procedure 26-4)
5. Control bleeding (Procedure 26-5)
   a. *Perform first aid procedures for bleeding*
6. Respond to medical emergencies other than bleeding, cardiac/respiratory arrest, or foreign body airway obstruction (Procedure 26-6)
   a. *Perform first aid procedures for seizures, shock, and syncope*
   b. Perform first aid procedure for fractures
7. *Document patient care accurately in the medical record*

AFF Affective Domain*

1. *Demonstrate critical thinking skills*

2. *Reassure patients*
3. *Demonstrate empathy for patients' concerns*
4. *Demonstrate active listening*
5. *Respect diversity*
6. *Recognize personal boundaries*
7. *Demonstrate tactfulness*
8. *Demonstrate self-awareness*
9. Protect the integrity of the medical record

MAERB Standards are Italicized.

ABHES Competencies

1. Follow documentation guidelines
2. Recognize and respond to medical office emergencies
3. Make adaptations for patients with special needs (psychological or physical limitations)
4. Practice standard precautions and perform disinfection/sterilization techniques
5. Display effective interpersonal skills with patients and healthcare team members
6. Demonstrate cultural awareness

Name: _____   Date: _____   Grade: _____

COG MULTIPLE CHOICE

Circle the letter preceding the correct answer.

1. During a primary assessment, you should check:
   a. AVPU.
   b. pupils.
   c. responsiveness.
   d. vital signs.
   e. patient identification.

2. What signs and symptoms are consistent with heat stroke?
   a. Cyanotic skin
   b. Pale wet skin
   c. Ecchymosis
   d. Dry, flushed skin
   e. Waxy, gray skin

3. Superficial burns are categorized as:
   a. first degree.
   b. second degree.
   c. third degree.
   d. partial thickness.
   e. full thickness.

4. Which is an example of a closed wound?
   a. Abrasion
   b. Avulsion
   c. Contusion
   d. Laceration
   e. Ecchymosis

5. What is the BSA of the anterior portion of an adult's trunk?
   a. 1%
   b. 9%
   c. 13.5%
   d. 18%
   e. 36%

6. A patient with pneumonia is at risk for:
   a. hypothermia.
   b. hypovolemic shock.
   c. septic shock.
   d. seizures.
   e. hyperthermia.

7. The first step to take when discovering an unresponsive patient is to:
   a. begin CPR.
   b. check circulation.
   c. establish an airway.
   d. go find help.
   e. identify the patient.

8. During a physical examination of an emergency patient's abdomen, check for:
   a. cerebral fluid.
   b. distal pulses.
   c. paradoxical movement.
   d. tenderness, rigidity, and distension.
   e. lethargy and slow movements.

9. A potential complication from a splint could be:
   a. compartment syndrome.
   b. dislocation.
   c. hematoma.
   d. injury from sharp bone fragments.
   e. tissue ischemia and infarction.

10. Circulation after splinting can be tested using:
    a. blood pressure.
    b. brachial pulse.
    c. carotid pulse.
    d. distal pulse.
    e. femoral pulse.

Scenario for questions 11 and 12: A patient complains about tightness in the chest, a feeling of warmth, and itching. After a minute, the patient's breathing is labored.

11. You are most likely watching the early warning signs of:
    a. an allergic reaction.
    b. cardiogenic shock.
    c. a myocardial infarction.
    d. poisoning.
    e. ecchymosis.

12. What action is contraindicated if this patient goes into shock?
    a. Cardiac monitoring
    b. Epinephrine (1:1,000)
    c. Establishing an IV line
    d. Intubation
    e. Providing high-flow oxygen

13. If a patient is having a seizure, you should:
    a. force something into the patient's mouth to protect the tongue.
    b. maintain spine immobilization.
    c. protect the patient from injury.
    d. restrain the patient.
    e. assist patient to supine position.

14. What is the difference between an emotional crisis and a psychiatric emergency?
    a. A psychiatric emergency results from substance abuse
    b. A patient in a psychiatric emergency poses a physical threat to himself or others
    c. An emotional crisis is a case of bipolar disorder
    d. A psychiatric emergency involves a patient diagnosed with a psychiatric disorder
    e. An emotional crisis does not include delusions

15. A patient suffering hypothermia should be given:
    a. alcohol to promote circulation.
    b. hot chocolate to provide sugar.
    c. IV fluids for rehydration.
    d. warm coffee to raise their level of consciousness.
    e. dry heat to warm the surface.

16. What agency should be contacted first when a patient is exposed to a toxic substance?
    a. AMAA
    b. EMS
    c. MSDS
    d. Centers for Disease Control
    e. Poison Control Center

17. Which form of shock is an acute allergic reaction?
    a. Neurogenic shock
    b. Anaphylactic shock
    c. Cardiogenic shock
    d. Septic shock
    e. Hypovolemic shock

18. What does the "V" in AVPU stand for?
    a. Vocalization
    b. Vital signs
    c. Viscosity
    d. Voice recognition
    e. Verbal response

19. To manage open soft tissue injuries, you should:
    a. leave them open to the air.
    b. wrap loosely in bandages.
    c. immediately stitch closed.
    d. elevate the wound.
    e. apply direct pressure.

20. Which of the following items should be included in an emergency kit?
    a. Alcohol wipes
    b. Syringe
    c. Penicillin
    d. Oscilloscope
    e. Sample containers

COG MATCHING

Grade: _____

Match each key term with its definition.

Key Terms

21. _____ allergen
22. _____ anaphylactic shock
23. _____ cardiogenic shock
24. _____ contusion
25. _____ ecchymosis
26. _____ full-thickness burn
27. _____ heat cramps
28. _____ heat stroke
29. _____ hematoma
30. _____ hyperthermia
31. _____ hypothermia
32. _____ hypovolemic shock
33. _____ infarction
34. _____ ischemia
35. _____ melena
36. _____ neurogenic shock
37. _____ partial-thickness burn
38. _____ seizure
39. _____ septic shock
40. _____ shock
41. _____ splint
42. _____ superficial burn

Definitions

a. an abnormal discharge of electrical activity in the brain, resulting in erratic muscle movements, strange sensations, or a complete loss of consciousness

b. black, tarry stools caused by digested blood from the gastrointestinal tract

c. severe allergic reaction within minutes to hours after exposure to a foreign substance

d. an emergency where the body cannot compensate for elevated temperatures

e. a bruise or collection of blood under the skin or in damaged tissue

f. a burn limited to the epidermis

g. any device used to immobilize a sprain, strain, fracture, or dislocated limb

h. shock that results from dysfunction of the nervous system following a spinal cord injury

i. muscle cramping that follows a period of physical exertion and profuse sweating in a hot environment

j. a penetrating burn that has destroyed all skin layers

k. a characteristic black and blue mark from blood accumulation

l. below-normal body temperature

m. the general condition of excessive body heat

n. a blood clot that forms at an injury site

o. a burn that involves epidermis and varying levels of the dermis

p. a decrease in oxygen to tissue

q. a substance that causes manifestations of an allergy

r. shock that results from general infection in the bloodstream

s. shock caused by loss of blood or other body fluids

t. death of tissue due to lack of oxygen

u. condition resulting from the lack of oxygen to individual cells of the body

v. type of shock in which the left ventricle fails to pump enough blood for the body to function

COG IDENTIFICATION

Grade: _____

43. As a medical assistant, you may be called on to assist during an emergency. Review the list of tasks below and determine which tasks you may be responsible for as a medical assistant. Place a check mark in the "Yes" column for those duties you might assist with as a medical assistant and place a check mark in the "No" column for those tasks that are not the responsibility of the medical assistant.

Task	Yes	No
a. Obtain important patient information		
b. Perform CPR		
c. Set and splint bone fractures		
d. Remove foreign body airway obstructions		
e. Remain calm and react competently and professionally during a psychiatric crisis		

f. Coordinate multiple ongoing events while rendering patient care in a cardiac emergency		
g. Negotiate with or attempt to calm a violent patient during a psychiatric crisis		
h. Know what emergency system is used in the community		
i. Provide immediate care to the patient while the physician is notified		
j. Perform rapid sequence intubation (RSI) on a patient who is suffering respiratory failure		
k. Administer first aid		
l. Document all actions taken		
m. Complete routine scheduled tasks		
n. Assist EMS personnel as necessary		
o. Examine the patient for EMS personnel		
p. Direct care of the patient for EMS personnel		
q. Remove any obstacles that prevent speedy evacuation of the patient by stretcher		
r. Direct family members to the reception area or a private room		

44. Identify the type of shock described in the following scenarios.

    a. A very ill patient has been complaining of increasing pain in the pelvis and legs. Blood is present in the urine. The patient's temperature was elevated but is dropping.

    _____

    b. An elderly patient falls on her back while attempting to get out of bed. Her heart rate becomes rapid and thready, and her blood pressure drops quickly.

    _____

    c. A patient presents with fluid in the lungs, difficulty breathing, and chest pain.

    _____

    d. A patient presents with labored breathing, grunting, wheezing, and swelling followed by fainting.

    _____

    e. A child is brought in for diarrhea. She has poor skin turgor and capillary refill. Her mental status appears to be deteriorating.

    _____

45. Put a check mark on the line next to the correct signs and symptoms of shock.

a. _____ low blood pressure

b. _____ high blood pressure

c. _____ calm or lethargic

d. _____ restlessness or signs of fear

e. _____ thirst

f. _____ polyuria

g. _____ hunger

h. _____ nausea

i. _____ hot, sweaty skin

j. _____ cool, clammy skin

k. _____ pale skin with cyanosis (bluish color) at the lips and earlobes

l. _____ flushed skin

m. _____ rapid and weak pulse

n. _____ bounding pulse

46. Classify the type, severity, and coverage of the burns in each of these scenarios.

a. A contractor installing medical equipment accidentally touches exposed wires. He has burns on his right arm, but no sensation of pain.

- Type:

  _____

- Severity:

  _____

- Coverage:

  _____

b. A child spills bleach on one leg. The leg is blistering and causing severe pain.

- Type:

  _____

- Severity:

  _____

- Coverage:

  _____

c. A man watches a welder install handrails on your office's handicapped ramp. Now his face is red and painful, and his eyes have a painful itching sensation.

- Type:

_____

- Severity:

_____

- Coverage:

_____

d. A patient spills hot coffee while driving to your office, painfully blistering his genital area.

- Type:

_____

- Severity:

_____

- Coverage:

_____

47. Identify the hyperthermic and hypothermic emergencies from the list below and match them with the proper treatment. Place the number preceding the correct treatment on the line next to the heat or cold emergency.

a. _____ heat cramps

1. Remove wet clothing.
Cover the patient.
Give warm fluids by mouth if the patient is alert and oriented.

b. _____ frostbite

2. Move the patient to a cool area.
Remove clothing that may be keeping in the heat.
Place cool, wet clothes or a wet sheet on the scalp, neck, axilla, and groin.
Administer oxygen as directed by the physician and apply a cardiac monitor.
Notify the EMS for transportation to the hospital as directed by the physician.

c. _____ heat stroke

3. Immerse the affected tissue in lukewarm water (41°C, 105°F) until the area becomes pliable and the color and sensation return.
Do not apply dry heat.
Do not massage the area; massage may cause further tissue damage.
Avoid breaking any blisters that may form.
Notify the EMS for transportation to a hospital.

d. _____ hypothermia

4. Move the patient to a cool area.
Give fluids (commercial electrolyte solution) by mouth if uncomplicated.
Give IV fluids if patient presents with nausea.

48. What are your responsibilities for managing an allergic reaction? Circle the letter preceding all tasks that apply.

   a. Leave the patient to bring the emergency kit or cart, oxygen, and to get a physician to evaluate the patient

   b. Assist the patient to a supine position

   c. Scrub the patient's skin to remove allergens and urticaria

   d. Assess the patient's respiratory and circulatory status by obtaining the blood pressure, pulse, and respiratory rates

   e. Observe skin color and warmth

   f. If the patient complains of being cold or is shivering, cover them with a blanket

   g. Intubate the patient

   h. Upon the direction of the physician, start an intravenous line and administer oxygen

   i. Administer medications as ordered by the physician

   j. Document vital signs and any medications and treatments given, noting the time each set of vital signs is taken or medications are administered

   k. Communicate relevant information to the EMS personnel, including copies of the progress notes or medication record as needed

COG SHORT ANSWER

Grade: _____

49. List nine interventions or steps to manage burns.

_____

_____

_____

_____

50. A sullen and moody patient suddenly becomes threatening. Name three things the medical assistant should do.

_____

_____

_____

_____

51. What six pieces of information should be included in your office's emergency plan?

_____

_____

_____

_____

52. What are the elements of the AVPU scale for assessing a patient's level of consciousness?

A	
V	
P	
U	

53. List the first three steps you should use to control bleeding from an open wound.

_____

_____

_____

_____

54. You enter an exam room and unexpectedly find someone sprawled on the floor. What four things do you check on your primary assessment?

_____

_____

_____

_____

55. At what point do you assess the general appearance of the patient?

_____

_____

_____

_____

56. A patient is found unconscious. You do not suspect trauma. In what order would you perform the physical examination?

_____

_____

_____

_____

57. An examination of the eyes can be done according to the acronym "PEARL," meaning *Pupils Equal And Reactive to Light.* What does this examination reveal?

_____

_____

_____

_____

58. A 55-year-old male begins complaining about nausea. He is clearly anxious or agitated. What could this be an early symptom of?

_____

_____

_____

_____

COG TRUE OR FALSE?

Grade: _____

Indicate whether the statements are true or false by placing the letter T (true) or F (false) on the line preceding the statement.

59. _____ During a primary assessment, you find a patient has inadequate respirations. You should proceed to the secondary assessment and physical examination to find out why

60. _____ An impaled object should not be removed but requires careful immobilization of the patient and the injured area of the body

61. _____ An allergic reaction will be evident immediately after exposure to an allergen

62. _____ Closed wounds are not life threatening

COG AFF CASE STUDIES FOR CRITICAL THINKING

Grade: _____

63. A male older adult falls in an exam room. He is conscious, but agitated and anxious. You are the first to discover him struggling on the floor. What is the only duty you will perform until others arrive, and why?

_____

_____

_____

_____

64. A patient in your office is in respiratory arrest. The physician is attending this patient. You have collected notes on the patient's vitals and SAMPLE history (signs and symptoms, allergies, medications, past pertinent history, last oral intake, and the events that led to the problem). A family member of the patient is present and is growing upset and intrusive. The EMTs arrive on the scene. What is your immediate responsibility? Explain.

_____

_____

_____

_____

65. A teenage patient is given an instant cold pack for an injury to the mouth. A few minutes later, you discover the teenager misunderstood and drank the contents of the cold pack. What information do you need to collect to prepare for a call to the poison control center?

---

66. Dante commutes to your office by public transportation. On a particularly cold day, Dante arrives late with cool, pale skin. He is lethargic and confused, with slow and shallow respirations and a slow and faint pulse. Describe what actions are appropriate.

---

67. You have just had a patient suffer anaphylactic shock and respiratory arrest due to an unsuspected penicillin allergy. EMS has transported the patient to a local hospital. The following week, the patient calls to ask what she can do to prevent this from happening in the future. What would you tell this patient? Are there any future precautions this patient should take? If so, what?

---

68. You have a 35-year-old patient who has religious reservations about some medical procedures. Normally, you and the physician carefully explain procedures to this patient so she has the opportunity to make informed consent decisions. Now she is lying unconscious in front of you with a medical emergency. How do you handle informed consent with an unconscious patient?

---

69. You have an elderly patient with a "do not resuscitate" order, because he does not want to receive CPR in the event of a heart attack. During treatment for another condition, he collapses in apparent anaphylactic shock. Do you provide emergency medical assistance?

PSY PROCEDURE 26-1 Administer Oxygen

Name: _____ Date: _____ Time: _____ Grade: _____

EQUIPMENT/SUPPLIES: Oxygen tank with a regulator and flow meter, an oxygen delivery system (nasal cannula or mask)

STANDARDS: Given the needed equipment and a place to work, the student will perform this skill with _____ % accuracy in a total of _____ minutes. *(Your instructor will tell you what the percentage and time limits will be before you begin.)*

KEY: 4 = Satisfactory   0 = Unsatisfactory   NA = This step is not counted

PROCEDURE STEPS	SELF	PARTNER	INSTRUCTOR
1. Wash your hands	❏	❏	❏
2. Check the physician order for the amount of oxygen and the delivery method (nasal cannula, mask)	❏	❏	❏
3. Obtain the oxygen tank and nasal cannula or mask	❏	❏	❏
4. Greet and identify the patient	❏	❏	❏
5. **AFF** Explain how to respond to a patient who has dementia	❏	❏	❏
6. Connect the distal end of the nasal cannula or mask tubing to the adapter on the oxygen tank regulator, which is attached to the oxygen tank	❏	❏	❏
7. Place the oxygen delivery device in the patient's nares (nasal cannula) or over the patient's nose and mouth (mask)	❏	❏	❏
8. Turn the regulator dial to the liters per minute ordered by the physician	❏	❏	❏
9. **AFF** Log into the Electronic Medical Record (EMR) using your username and secure password OR obtain the paper medical record from a secure location and assure it is kept away from public access	❏	❏	❏
10. Record the procedure in the patient's medical record	❏	❏	❏
11. When finished, log out of the EMR and/or replace the medical record in an appropriate and secure location to protect patient privacy	❏	❏	❏

CALCULATION

Total Possible Points: _____

Total Points Earned: _____ Multiplied by 100 = _____ Divided by Total Possible Points = _____ %

PASS   FAIL   COMMENTS:
  ❏   ❏

Student's signature _____ Date _____

Partner's signature _____ Date _____

Instructor's signature _____ Date _____

PSY PROCEDURE 26-2 | Perform Cardiopulmonary Resuscitation (Adult)

Name: _____ Date: _____ Time: _____ Grade: _____

EQUIPMENT/SUPPLIES: CPR mannequin, mouth-to-mouth barrier device, gloves

STANDARDS: Given the needed equipment and a place to work, the student will perform this skill with _____ % accuracy in a total of _____ minutes. *(Your instructor will tell you what the percentage and time limits will be before you begin.)*

NOTE: All healthcare professionals should receive training for proficiency in CPR in an approved program. This skill sheet is not intended to substitute for proficiency training with a mannequin and structured protocol.

KEY: 4 = Satisfactory   0 = Unsatisfactory   NA = This step is not counted

PROCEDURE STEPS	SELF	PARTNER	INSTRUCTOR
1. Determine unresponsiveness by shaking the patient and shouting, "Are you okay?"	❏	❏	❏
2. Instruct another staff member to get the physician, emergency cart/supplies, and AED	❏	❏	❏
3. Put on clean exam gloves	❏	❏	❏
4. If the patient does not respond, assess for cardiac function by feeling for a pulse using the carotid artery at the side of the patient's neck	❏	❏	❏
5. If no pulse is present, follow the protocol for chest compressions according to the standards for training provided by an approved basic life support provider	❏	❏	❏
6. After 30 compressions, check for airway patency and respiratory effort using the head-tilt, chin-lift maneuver with the patient in the supine position	❏	❏	❏
7. After opening the airway, begin rescue breathing by placing a mask over the patient's mouth and nose and giving two slow breaths, causing the chest to rise without overfilling the lungs	❏	❏	❏
8. Continue chest compressions and rescue breathing at a ratio of 30:1 until relieved by another healthcare provider or EMS arrives	❏	❏	❏
9. Utilize the recovery position if the patient regains consciousness or a pulse and adequate breathing	❏	❏	❏
10. Document the procedure and copy any records necessary for transport with EMS	❏	❏	❏

(continues)

CALCULATION

Total Possible Points: _____

Total Points Earned: _____ Multiplied by 100 = _____ Divided by Total Possible Points = _____ %

PASS   **FAIL**   **COMMENTS:**
❏   ❏

Student's signature _____   Date _____

Partner's signature _____   Date _____

Instructor's signature _____   Date _____

PSY PROCEDURE 26-3 **Use an Automatic External Defibrillator (Adult)**

Name: _____ Date: _____ Time: _____ Grade: _____

EQUIPMENT/SUPPLIES: Practice mannequin, training automatic external defibrillator with chest pads and connection cables, scissors, gauze, gloves

STANDARDS: Given the needed equipment and a place to work, the student will perform this skill with _____ % accuracy in a total of _____ minutes. *(Your instructor will tell you what the percentage and time limits will be before you begin.)*

NOTE: All healthcare professionals should receive training for proficiency in CPR and using an AED in an approved program. This skill sheet is not intended to substitute for proficiency training with a mannequin and structured protocol.

KEY: 4 = Satisfactory   0 = Unsatisfactory   NA = This step is not counted

PROCEDURE STEPS	SELF	PARTNER	INSTRUCTOR
1. Determine unresponsiveness by shaking the patient and shouting, "Are you okay?"	❏	❏	❏
2. Instruct another staff member to get the physician, emergency cart/supplies, and AED	❏	❏	❏
3. While the other staff member continues CPR, remove the patient's shirt and prepare the chest for the AED electrodes: **a.** If there are medication patches on the chest where the electrodes will be placed, remove them and wipe away any excess medication with a towel **b.** If there is excess hair on the chest that will prevent the AED electrodes from sticking, apply one set of electrodes and quickly remove, pulling any hair from the chest **c.** If the chest is wet, dry with a towel or other cloth before applying the electrodes	❏	❏	❏
4. After removing the paper on the back of the AED electrodes, apply the electrodes to the chest area: one to the upper right chest area and the other on the lower left chest area	❏	❏	❏
5. Explain what should be done in the event that the patient has an implantable device in the area where the chest electrodes should be applied	❏	❏	❏
6. With the electrodes securely on the chest, connect the wire from the electrodes to the AED unit and turn the AED on	❏	❏	❏
7. Advise everyone to not touch the patient while the AED is analyzing the heart rhythm	❏	❏	❏
8. If no shock is advised by the AED, resume CPR	❏	❏	❏
9. If a shock is advised by the AED, make sure no one is touching the patient before pressing the appropriate button on the AED	❏	❏	❏
10. After a shock is delivered by the AED, resume CPR until the AED advises you that the heart rhythm is being analyzed again	❏	❏	❏

(continues)

PSY PROCEDURE 26-3	**Use an Automatic External Defibrillator (Adult)** (continued)		
11. Do not touch the patient while the heart rhythm is being reanalyzed at any point during the procedure	❑	❑	❑
12. Continue to follow the instructions given by the AED and the physician until EMS has been notified and has arrived	❑	❑	❑
13. Document the procedure and copy any records necessary for transport with EMS	❑	❑	❑

CALCULATION

Total Possible Points: _____

Total Points Earned: _____ Multiplied by 100 = _____ Divided by Total Possible Points = _____ %

PASS   FAIL   COMMENTS:
  ❑   ❑

Student's signature _____ Date _____

Partner's signature _____ Date _____

Instructor's signature _____ Date _____

PROCEDURE 26-4 Manage a Foreign Body Airway Obstruction (Adult)

PSY

Name: _____ Date: _____ Time: _____ Grade: _____

EQUIPMENT/SUPPLIES: Practice mannequin, mouth-to-mouth barrier device, gloves

STANDARDS: Given the needed equipment and a place to work, the student will perform this skill with _____ % accuracy in a total of _____ minutes. *(Your instructor will tell you what the percentage and time limits will be before you begin.)*

NOTE: All healthcare professionals should receive training for proficiency in managing a foreign body airway obstruction in an approved program. This skill sheet is not intended to substitute for proficiency training with a mannequin and structured protocol.

KEY: 4 = Satisfactory 0 = Unsatisfactory NA = This step is not counted

PROCEDURE STEPS	SELF	PARTNER	INSTRUCTOR
1. If the patient is conscious and appears to be choking, ask the patient, "Are you choking?"	❏	❏	❏
2. Do not perform abdominal thrusts if the patient can speak or cough because these are signs that the obstruction is not complete	❏	❏	❏
3. If the patient cannot speak or cough but has indicated that they are choking, move behind the patient, wrapping your arms around their abdomen	❏	❏	❏
4. Place the fist of your dominant hand with the thumb against the patient's abdomen, between the navel and xiphoid process	❏	❏	❏
5. Put your other hand against your dominant hand and give quick, upward thrusts, forceful enough to dislodge the obstruction in the airway	❏	❏	❏
6. If the patient is obese or pregnant, place your hands against the middle of the sternum, above the xiphoid process, and proceed with quick thrusts inward	❏	❏	❏
7. Continue with the abdominal thrusts until the object is expelled and the patient can breathe or the patient becomes unconscious	❏	❏	❏
8. If the patient becomes unconscious or is found unconscious, open the airway and give two rescue breaths	❏	❏	❏
9. If rescue breaths are obstructed, reposition the head, and try again	❏	❏	❏
10. If rescue breaths continue to be obstructed after repositioning, begin abdominal thrusts by placing your palm against the patient's abdomen with your fingers facing their head (you may need to straddle the patient's hips). The palm of the hand should be located between the navel and the xiphoid process	❏	❏	❏
11. Lace the fingers of the other hand into the fingers of the hand on the abdomen and give five abdominal thrusts	❏	❏	❏

(continues)

PSY PROCEDURE 26-4	Manage a Foreign Body Airway Obstruction (Adult) (continued)		
12. After five abdominal thrusts, open the patient's mouth using a tongue-jaw lift maneuver and do a finger- sweep of the mouth, removing any objects that may have been dislodged	❑	❑	❑
13. If an item has been dislodged and can be removed easily, remove the object and attempt rescue breaths. Continue rescue breaths and chest compressions as necessary and appropriate	❑	❑	❑
14. If the item has not been dislodged, attempt rescue breaths. If rescue breaths are successful, continue rescue breathing and chest compressions as necessary and appropriate	❑	❑	❑
15. If the item has not been dislodged and rescue breaths are not successful, continue with abdominal thrusts	❑	❑	❑
16. Repeat the pattern of abdominal thrusts, finger -sweep, and rescue breaths and follow the physician's orders until EMS is notified and arrives	❑	❑	❑
17. Document the procedure and copy any records necessary for transport with EMS	❑	❑	❑

CALCULATION

Total Possible Points: _____

Total Points Earned: _____ Multiplied by 100 = _____ Divided by Total Possible Points = _____ %

PASS **FAIL** **COMMENTS:**
❑ ❑

Student's signature _____ Date _____

Partner's signature _____ Date _____

Instructor's signature _____ Date _____

PSY P R O C E D U R E 2 6 - 5 **Control Bleeding**

Name: _____ Date: _____ Time: _____ Grade: _____

EQUIPMENT/SUPPLIES: Gloves, sterile gauze pads

STANDARDS: Given the needed equipment and a place to work, the student will perform this skill with _____ % accuracy in a total of _____ minutes. *(Your instructor will tell you what the percentage and time limits will be before you begin.)*

KEY: 4 = Satisfactory 0 = Unsatisfactory NA = This step is not counted

PROCEDURE STEPS	SELF	PARTNER	INSTRUCTOR
1. Identify the patient and assess the extent of the bleeding and type of accident	❏	❏	❏
2. Take the patient to an examination room and notify the physician, if appropriate	❏	❏	❏
3. Give the patient some gauze pads and have them apply pressure to the area while you put on a pair of clean examination gloves and open additional sterile gauze pads	❏	❏	❏
4. Observe the patient for signs of dizziness or lightheadedness. Have the patient lie down	❏	❏	❏
5. Using several sterile gauze pads, apply direct pressure to the wound	❏	❏	❏
6. Maintain pressure until the bleeding stops	❏	❏	❏
7. If the bleeding continues or seeps through the gauze, apply additional gauze on top of the saturated gauze while continuing to apply direct pressure	❏	❏	❏
8. If directed by the physician to do so, apply pressure to the artery delivering blood to this area while continuing to apply direct pressure to the wound to control bleeding	❏	❏	❏
9. Once the bleeding is controlled, prepare to assist the physician with a minor office surgical procedure to close the wound	❏	❏	❏
10. Continue to monitor the patient for signs of shock and be prepared to treat the patient appropriately	❏	❏	❏
11. Document the treatment in the patient's medical record	❏	❏	❏

CALCULATION

Total Possible Points: _____

Total Points Earned: _____ Multiplied by 100 = _____ Divided by Total Possible Points = _____ %

PASS   FAIL   COMMENTS:
❏   ❏

Student's signature _____ Date _____

Partner's signature _____ Date _____

Instructor's signature _____ Date _____

PSY PROCEDURE 26-6 | **Respond to Medical Emergencies Other than Bleeding, Cardiac/Respiratory Arrest, or Foreign Body Airway Obstruction**

Name: _____ Date: _____ Time: _____ Grade: _____

EQUIPMENT/SUPPLIES: A medical emergency kit that contains a minimum of personal protective equipment including gloves, low-dose aspirin tablets, 2 × 2 and 4 × 4 sterile gauze pads, vinegar or acetic acid solution, blood pressure cuff and stethoscope, sterile water or saline for irrigation, ice bags, and towel or rolled gauze bandage material

STANDARDS: Given the needed equipment and a place to work, the student will perform this skill with _____ % accuracy in a total of _____ minutes. *(Your instructor will tell you what the percentage and time limits will be before you begin.)*

KEY: 4 = Satisfactory 0 = Unsatisfactory NA = This step is not counted

PROCEDURE STEPS	SELF	PARTNER	INSTRUCTOR
1. Identify the patient and assess the type of emergency involved	❑	❑	❑
2. Escort the patient to an examination room	❑	❑	❑
3. Have another staff member get the physician, medical emergency cart/supplies, and AED	❑	❑	❑
4. Apply clean examination gloves and other PPE as appropriate	❑	❑	❑
5. Assist the patient to the exam table and have them lie down	❑	❑	❑

6. Treat the patient according to the physician's instructions and the most current guidelines for first aid procedures for the following:
 a. Chest pain
 b. Snakebite
 c. Jellyfish sting
 d. Dental injuries
   (1) Chipped tooth
   (2) Cracked or broken tooth
   (3) Tooth removed
   (4) Broken jaw
 e. Fracture Injuries
 f. Seizure
 g. Shock
 h. Syncope
	❑	❑	❑

7. If the patient develops cardiac or respiratory arrest, follow the procedure for CPR according to the most recent standards and guidelines	❑	❑	❑
8. Document the treatment in the patient's medical record	❑	❑	❑

PSY PROCEDURE 26-6 | **Respond to Medical Emergencies Other than Bleeding, Cardiac/Respiratory Arrest, or Foreign Body Airway Obstruction** (continued)

CALCULATION

Total Possible Points: _____

Total Points Earned: _____ Multiplied by 100 = _____ Divided by Total Possible Points = _____ %

PASS   FAIL   COMMENTS:
❏   ❏

Student's signature _____ Date _____

Partner's signature _____ Date _____

Instructor's signature _____ Date _____

CHAPTER 27

Disaster Preparedness and the Medical Assistant

LEARNING OUTCOMES

COG Cognitive Domain*

1. Spell and define the key terms
2. Describe what is meant by a disaster and disaster preparedness
3. List several types of disasters
4. *Identify critical elements of an emergency plan for response to a natural disaster or other emergency*
5. *Identify emergency practices for evacuation of a healthcare setting*
6. Identify emergency preparedness plans in your community
7. Discuss potential role(s) of the medical assistant in emergency preparedness

PSY Psychomotor Domain*

1. Respond to a simulated disaster (Procedure 27-1)
   a. Participate in a mock exposure event with documentation of specific steps

b. *Evaluate an environment to identify unsafe conditions*
   c. Report relevant information concisely and accurately
2. Maintain a list of community resources for emergency preparedness (Procedure 27-2)
3. Develop a personal safety plan (Procedure 27-3)

AFF Affective Domain*

1. *Demonstrate critical thinking skills*
2. *Reassure patients*
3. *Demonstrate empathy for patients' concerns*
4. *Demonstrate active listening*
5. *Respect diversity*
6. *Recognize personal boundaries*
7. *Demonstrate tactfulness*
8. *Demonstrate self-awareness*

MAERB Standards are Italicized.

ABHES Competencies

1. Follow documentation guidelines
2. Follow established policies when initiating or terminating medical treatment
3. Adapt care to address developmental stages of life
4. Partner with healthcare teams to attain optimal patient health outcomes
5. Display effective interpersonal skills with patients and healthcare team members
6. Demonstrate cultural awareness

Name: _____   Date: _____   Grade: _____

COG MULTIPLE CHOICE

Circle the letter preceding the correct answer.

1. The 2001 discovery of anthrax in an envelope to be delivered to a U.S. Congressman is an example of a(n):
   a. bioterrorist attack.
   b. epidemic.
   c. pandemic.
   d. ergonomics.
   e. ADF.

2. An effective disaster plan for the medical office should include the input of which individuals?
   a. The physician or physicians
   b. The practice manager
   c. The medical assistants
   d. The receptionist
   e. All of the above

3. Which of these is not an example of a natural disaster?
   a. Flood
   b. Tornado
   c. Air quality advisory
   d. Hurricane
   e. Earthquake

4. An emergency action plan should include all of the following except:
   a. contact information for poison control.
   b. emergency procedures.
   c. the location of the emergency supplies.
   d. patient information sheets.
   e. contact information for local hospitals.

5. A well-written emergency plan is essential to being prepared for a disaster. What qualities are inherent in a well-written emergency plan?
   a. It is easy to read and include pictures
   b. It is flexible and easily implemented
   c. It is based on research and has references
   d. It should include enough information to fill a 3-inch binder
   e. It is written based on the reading level of the office personnel

6. A location in or near the medical office should be identified to coordinate activities in a disaster, commonly known as a/n:
   a. central activities center.
   b. common planning center.
   c. central operation center.
   d. command center.
   e. operation command center.

7. An example of a manmade disaster includes all of the following except:
   a. drought.
   b. bioterrorism.
   c. a nuclear accident.
   d. chemical contamination of a water source.
   e. none of the above.

8. A bioterrorism agent that is easily available, can be transferred to people easily, and has the potential to cause injury and death to large amounts of people and other animals is included in which category?
   a. Category A
   b. Category B
   c. Category C
   d. Category D
   e. Category E

9. A disease that infects many people in a small geographic area is known as a/n:
   a. pandemic.
   b. Category C agent.
   c. infectious pathogen.
   d. bioterrorist.
   e. epidemic.

10. The role of the medical assistant in planning for emergencies and disasters includes assisting the physician with all of the following except:
    a. performing CPR, if needed.
    b. transferring patients or victims.
    c. preparing and administering medications.
    d. diagnosing and treating illness and injuries caused by the emergency.
    e. collecting information and communicating clearly with everyone involved.

Scenario for Questions 11 through 15: A tornado just came through the neighborhood where you are working in a family practice office. Although your office was not hit, several businesses around your office were damaged or destroyed. People are running into your office yelling for help for other victims who cannot get to the office or they are injured and bleeding themselves.

11. Your priority in assisting patients and victims in the office includes:
    a. asking nonpatients coming into the office to wait outside until the EMS arrives.
    b. remaining calm and implementing the emergency plan quickly and efficiently.
    c. asking the practice manager if you can leave to check on your family.
    d. standing outside to direct traffic and flag down emergency medical services.
    e. gathering equipment and supplies that may be needed for any injuries.

12. This is an example of which type of disaster?
    a. A pandemic
    b. A water emergency
    c. A bioterrorism disaster
    d. A manmade disaster
    e. A natural disaster

13. Your role in assisting in this disaster includes which of the following:
    a. Gathering medical information from patients and victims
    b. Assisting the physician with procedures and treatments
    c. Administering tetanus to everyone who is injured before they are seen by the physician.
    d. A and B.
    e. All of the above.

14. Because you are actively involved in assisting during this disaster, you are considered a
    a. first-level victim.
    b. secondary-level victim.
    c. third-level victim.
    d. fourth-level victim.
    e. fifth-level victim.

15. One month after the disaster, you notice your coworker is unusually irritable and is unable to concentrate on simple tasks, making mistakes throughout the day. These behaviors are not typical of her personality and may be signs of:
    a. depression.
    b. posttraumatic stress disorder.
    c. a sleeping disorder.
    d. an anxiety disorder.
    e. a possible infectious disease contracted during the emergency.

⬛COG **MATCHING**

Grade: _____

Match each key term with its definition.

Key Terms

16. _____ bioterrorism
17. _____ disaster
18. _____ epidemic
19. _____ pandemic
20. _____ PTSD

Definitions

a. a disease that affects numerous people within a specific geographical area
b. a sudden and unplanned event that has the potential to cause damage to property or life; may be caused by an accident or by nature, including weather events such as a hurricane.
c. a condition in some individuals who are affected by acute traumatic stress.
d. intentional release of a biologic agent with the intent to harm individuals.
e. a disease that affects numerous people in many areas of the world at the same time.

⬛COG **IDENTIFICATION**

Grade: _____

21. You may be called upon to assist before, during, and after a disaster. Place a check mark in the "Yes" column for those duties you might assist with as a medical assistant and place a check mark in the "No" column for those tasks that are not the responsibility of the medical assistant with regard to disaster preparedness.

Task	Yes	No
a. Obtain important patient information		
b. Perform first aid and CPR procedures		
c. Suture small lacerations		
d. Obtain vital signs		
e. Remain calm and react competently and professionally		
f. Coordinate multiple ongoing events		
g. Prescribe antibiotics to patients who may be infected		
h. Know what emergency system is used in the community		
i. Provide immediate care to the patient while the physician is notified		
j. Advise victims with minor injuries to go home and take over-the-counter (OTC) medications for discomfort		
k. Work as a law enforcement officer to manage victims exhibiting dangerous behaviors		
l. Create medical records and document all actions taken		
m. Manage the temporary medical clinic		
n. Assist EMS personnel as necessary		

COG SHORT ANSWER

Grade: _____

22. What six pieces of information should be included in your office's emergency plan?

_____

_____

_____

_____

23. During a disaster, medical assistants must be able to coordinate multiple ongoing events while rendering patient care. What are the key components to managing a chaotic situation during a disaster?

_____

_____

_____

_____

24. Explain the purpose of a Central Operation Center.

_____

_____

_____

_____

25. How does the CDC determine that a biologic agent is a weapon?

_____

_____

_____

_____

COG TRUE OR FALSE?

Grade: _____

Indicate whether the statements are true or false by placing the letter T (true) or F (false) on the line preceding the statement.

26. _____ A pandemic is a disease that affects many people within a very specific, localized geographic area.

27. _____ Having an alternative source of electricity is essential during a disaster.

28. _____ When evacuating an office during an emergency, you must first recognize the emergency as one that requires the removal from the area.

29. _____ Psychological first aid requires that you discuss all aspects of the disaster with coworkers and patients, even if they do not wish to discuss the details.

30. _____ The primary defense mechanism used by individuals after a disaster is anxiety.

COG IDENTIFICATION

Grade: _____

31. Place a checkmark in the appropriate box to indicate whether the statement should be considered to develop an evacuation plan for the medical office.

Consideration for Evacuation Plan?	Yes	No
a. Assign staff members to perform surgical procedures on victims who need immediate first aid		
b. Identify evacuation routes		
c. Make sure everyone understands they are not to discuss patient/staff illness or injury during the evacuation		
d. Identify who is responsible for ordering the evacuation		
e. Do not allow anyone to reenter the facility after the disaster when the safety of everyone reentering the office has been established		
f. Determine a location to move to and a backup site		
g. Define responsibilities of each staff member		
h. Do not waste time making sure patients and staff are accounted for during and after the evacuation		
i. Decide what supplies or equipment you will need to transport		

AFF CASE STUDIES FOR CRITICAL THINKING

Grade: _____

32. You have been assigned to put together an emergency kit for the family practice office where you work. Which items should you include in this kit?

_____

_____

_____

_____

33. There has just been an earthquake where you live and the medical office has stopped shaking, leaving patients and staff wondering what happened. There are items on the floor throughout the office that were shaken off the shelves and walls. What is your immediate responsibility? Explain.

_____

_____

_____

_____

34. An environmental safety plan was written for the office where you work and it includes emergency procedures for all chemicals used in your office. When reviewing this plan, you notice that it does not include a plan to train employees on environmental safety guidelines. Is this important to include in the plan? Why or why not?

_____

_____

_____

_____

35. The practice manager at your office has scheduled a meeting to "test" the office emergency plan. He has asked the local fire department to assist in this training. How can you "test" an emergency plan and why would the local fire department be involved?

_____

_____

_____

_____

36. A tornado hit the community where you work 1 month ago, and there was significant property damage, injuries, and fatalities. A patient comes into the office today and complains that she is unable to sleep for more than 3 hours at a time as she "wakes up" frequently hearing tornado sirens and reliving the storm. What would you tell this patient?

_____

_____

_____

_____

PSY PROCEDURE 27-1 **Respond to a Simulated Disaster**

Name: _____ Date: _____ Time: _____ Grade: _____

EQUIPMENT/SUPPLIES: Phone, disaster drill manual for a medical office, paper medical record forms and folders, pen, portable emergency kit.

STANDARDS: Given the needed equipment and a place to work, the student will perform this skill with _____ % accuracy in a total of _____ minutes. *(Your instructor will tell you what the percentage and time limits will be before you begin.)*

KEY: 4 = Satisfactory 0 = Unsatisfactory NA = This step is not counted

PROCEDURE STEPS	SELF	PARTNER	INSTRUCTOR
1. Develop and/or review an emergency/disaster procedure manual	❏	❏	❏
2. Assume the role of an employee, patient, or visitor in a medical office	❏	❏	❏
3. During a "normal" workday, a disaster occurs without warning	❏	❏	❏
4. Follow the protocol and procedures for the disaster according to the emergency/disaster plan	❏	❏	❏
5. After the mock disaster drill, discuss the event, including the strengths and weaknesses of the emergency plan	❏	❏	❏
6. AFF Complete a reflection paper about the mock disaster, including your feelings, perceptions, and thoughts before, during, and after the mock disaster	❏	❏	❏

CALCULATION

Total Possible Points: _____

Total Points Earned: _____ Multiplied by 100 = _____ Divided by Total Possible Points = _____ %

PASS **FAIL** **COMMENTS:**
❏ ❏

Student's signature _____ Date _____

Partner's signature _____ Date _____

Instructor's signature _____ Date _____

PSY PROCEDURE 27-2 **Maintain a List of Community Resources for Emergency Preparedness**

Name: _____ Date: _____ Time: _____ Grade: _____

EQUIPMENT/SUPPLIES: Phone, computer with Internet access, paper and pen, binder.

STANDARDS: Given the needed equipment and a place to work, the student will perform this skill with _____ % accuracy in a total of _____ minutes. *(Your instructor will tell you what the percentage and time limits will be before you begin.)*

KEY: 4 = Satisfactory 0 = Unsatisfactory NA = This step is not counted

PROCEDURE STEPS	SELF	PARTNER	INSTRUCTOR
1. Determine the geographic area of your community, including the city or town, county, and surrounding counties or towns as appropriate	❑	❑	❑
2. Complete an Internet search of the possible resources available in your community, beginning with the local resources	❑	❑	❑
3. Create a list of resources, including the name of the agency, resources available, phone numbers, addresses, and web address, if available	❑	❑	❑
4. Organize the resources you find in a binder or other notebook for easy reference	❑	❑	❑

CALCULATION

Total Possible Points: _____

Total Points Earned: _____ Multiplied by 100 = _____ Divided by Total Possible Points = _____ %

PASS **FAIL** **COMMENTS:**
❑ ❑

Student's signature _____ Date _____

Partner's signature _____ Date _____

Instructor's signature _____ Date _____

| | PROCEDURE 27-3 | **Develop a Personal Safety Plan** |

PSY

Name: _____ **Date:** _____ **Time:** _____ **Grade:** _____

EQUIPMENT/SUPPLIES: Phone, computer with Internet access, paper and pen, binder.

STANDARDS: Given the needed equipment and a place to work, the student will perform this skill with _____ % accuracy in a total of _____ minutes. *(Your instructor will tell you what the percentage and time limits will be before you begin.)*

KEY: 4 = Satisfactory   0 = Unsatisfactory   NA = This step is not counted

PROCEDURE STEPS	SELF	PARTNER	INSTRUCTOR
1. Download an electronic version of a family or personal safety plan template from a reputable website	❏	❏	❏
2. Gather information needed for inclusion in the safety plan	❏	❏	❏
3. Speak with family members and decide how you will contact each other in the event of a disaster. Include the location where you will go and/or meet	❏	❏	❏
4. Once the personal or family plan is developed, keep a copy in the emergency supply kit or another safe place	❏	❏	❏

CALCULATION

Total Possible Points: _____

Total Points Earned: _____ Multiplied by 100 = _____ Divided by Total Possible Points = _____ %

PASS   FAIL   COMMENTS:
❏   ❏

Student's signature _____ Date _____

Partner's signature _____ Date _____

Instructor's signature _____ Date _____

UNIT FIVE

Clinical Duties Related to Medical Specialties

CHAPTER 28

Dermatology

LEARNING OUTCOMES

COG Cognitive Domain*

1. Spell key terms
2. *Identify the following as related to body systems:*
   a. *Medical terms*
   b. *Abbreviations*
3. *Identify structural organization of the human body*
4. *Identify body systems*
5. Identify the anatomical location of major organs in each body system
6. *Identify the normal function of each body system*
7. *Identify common pathology related to each body system including*
   a. *Signs*
   b. *Symptoms*
   c. *Etiology*
   d. *Diagnostic measures*
   e. *Treatment modalities*
8. Describe common skin disorders
9. Explain the difference between bandages and dressings and give the purpose of each
10. Identify the guidelines for applying bandages

PSY Psychomotor Domain*

1. Apply a warm or cold compress (Procedure 28-1)
   a. *Instruct and prepare a patient for a procedure or a treatment*
   b. *Assist provider with a patient exam*
   c. *Document patient care accurately in the medical record*

2. Assist with therapeutic soaks (Procedure 28-2)
   a. *Instruct and prepare a patient for a procedure or treatment*
   b. *Assist provider with a patient exam*
   c. *Document patient care accurately in the medical record*
3. Apply a tubular gauze bandage (Procedure 28-3)
   a. *Instruct and prepare a patient for a procedure or treatment*
   b. *Assist provider with a patient exam*
   c. *Document patient care accurately in the medical record*

AFF Affective Domain*

1. *Demonstrate critical thinking skills*
2. *Reassure patients*
3. *Demonstrate empathy for patients' concerns*
4. *Demonstrate active listening*
5. *Respect diversity*
6. *Recognize personal boundaries*
7. *Demonstrate tactfulness*
8. *Demonstrate self-awareness*
9. Protect the integrity of the medical record

MAERB Standards are Italicized.

ABHES Competencies

1. Apply medical terminology for each specialty.
2. Assist provider with specialty examinations, including cardiac, respiratory, OB-GYN, neurologic, and gastroenterology procedures

3. Perform specialty procedures including but not limited to minor surgery, cardiac, respiratory, OB-GYN, neurologic, and gastroenterology
4. Follow established policies when initiating or terminating medical treatment
5. Adapt care to address the developmental stages of life
6. Partner with healthcare teams to attain optimal patient health outcomes
7. Display effective interpersonal skills with patients and healthcare team members
8. Demonstrate cultural awareness

Name: _____   Date: _____   Grade: _____

COG MULTIPLE CHOICE

Circle the letter preceding the correct answer.

1. Which of the following groups of people are most likely to develop impetigo?
   a. Older adults
   b. Women
   c. Young children
   d. Men
   e. Teenagers

2. What type of infection is herpes simplex?
   a. Bacterial
   b. Fungal
   c. Parasitic
   d. Viral
   e. Genetic

3. Public showers and swimming pools are common places to pick up fungal infections because:
   a. fungi thrive in moist conditions.
   b. areas that are highly populated increase the risk factor.
   c. sharing towels passes fungal infections from one person to another.
   d. fungi grow quickly on tile surfaces.
   e. antifungal medications do not work once they come into contact with water.

4. Which of these skin disorders may be caused by food allergies?
   a. Keloids
   b. Intertrigo
   c. Alopecia
   d. Eczema
   e. Seborrheic dermatitis

5. Which of the following statements is true about albinism?
   a. Respiratory problems are common among sufferers of albinism
   b. Albinism is treated with benzoyl peroxide
   c. Albinism usually occurs in exposed areas of the skin
   d. People who suffer from albinism should have regular checkups
   e. People who suffer from albinism should take particular care of their eyes in the sun

6. Which statements are true about decubitus ulcers?
   a. They are frequently diagnosed in school-aged children
   b. They are most common in aged, debilitated, and immobilized patients
   c. They are highly contagious
   d. They generally occur on the chin and forehead
   e. They are effectively treated with antifungal creams

7. When bandaging a patient, you should:
   a. fasten bandages only with safety pins.
   b. complete surgical asepsis before you begin.
   c. keep the area to be bandaged warm.
   d. leave fingers and toes exposed when possible.
   e. wrap the bandage as tightly as possible to prevent it from coming loose.

8. A person suffering from high stress levels is most likely to develop:
   a. urticaria.
   b. acne vulgaris.
   c. impetigo.
   d. leukoderma.
   e. herpes zoster.

9. How many people in the United States will typically develop malignant melanoma?
   a. 1 in 5
   b. 1 in 500
   c. 1 in 105
   d. 1 in 1,005
   e. 1 in 5,000

10. Which of the following conditions would be treated with topical antifungal cream?
    a. Folliculitis
    b. Vitiligo
    c. Tinea versicolor
    d. Urticaria
    e. Decubitus ulcers

11. What should patients do if they have an absence of melanin in their skin?
    a. Avoid coming into contact with other people
    b. Protect their skin from the sun
    c. Seek immediate medical assistance
    d. Take supplementary vitamin pills
    e. Stop sharing towels and bedding

Scenario for Questions 12 and 13: A male patient comes into the physician's office to have a wart removed from his finger. While you are preparing him for the procedure, he tells you that he regularly gets verrucae on his feet.

12. How would you advise the patient to avoid further viral infections?
    a. Wash all bedding and clothing at high temperatures
    b. Avoid sharing combs and toiletries with anyone
    c. Avoid coming into direct contact with skin lesions
    d. Wear comfortable footwear and avoid walking long distances
    e. Frequently wash hands with antibacterial soap

13. The patient should look for over-the-counter wart medication that contains:
    a. podophyllum resin.
    b. acyclovir.
    c. selenium sulfide.
    d. permethrin.
    e. prednisone.

14. Before you apply a bandage to an open wound, you should:
    a. moisten the bandage.
    b. keep the bandage at room temperature.
    c. apply pressure to the wound.
    d. apply a sterile dressing to the wound.
    e. check to see how the patient would like the bandage fastened.

15. How can you tell that a patient is suffering from stage I decubitus ulcers?
    a. The skin is blistered, peeling, or cracked
    b. Red skin does not return to normal when massaged
    c. The skin is scaly, dry, and flaky
    d. The skin is extremely itchy
    e. The patient is unable to feel pressure on the area

16. When a physician performs a shave biopsy, he:
    a. cuts the lesion off just above the skin line.
    b. removes a small section from the center of the lesion.
    c. removes the entire lesion for evaluation.
    d. cuts the lesion off just below the skin line.
    e. removes a small section from the edge of the lesion.

17. Which of these is thought to be a cause of skin cancer in areas not exposed to the sun?
    a. Chemicals in toiletries
    b. Pet allergies
    c. Frequent irritation
    d. Second-hand smoke
    e. Excessive scratching

18. Treatment of impetigo involves:
    a. washing the area two to three times a day followed by application of topical antibiotics.
    b. cleaning with alcohol sponges twice a day.
    c. washing towels, washcloths, and bed linens daily.
    d. oral antibiotics for severe cases.
    e. the physician removing the infected area.

19. Which of the following statements is true about nevi?
    a. Nevi are usually malignant
    b. Nevi are usually found on the back or legs
    c. It is common for nevi to bleed occasionally
    d. Nevi are congenital pigmented skin blemishes
    e. Nevi are extremely rare in young patients

20. Which part of the body is affected by tinea capitis?
    a. Hands
    b. Feet
    c. Hair follicles
    d. Groin
    e. Scalp

⬤OG MATCHING

Place the letter preceding the definition on the line next to the term.

Key Terms

21. _____ alopecia
22. _____ bulla
23. _____ carbuncle
24. _____ cellulitis
25. _____ dermatophytosis
26. _____ eczema
27. _____ erythema
28. _____ folliculitis
29. _____ furuncle
30. _____ herpes simplex
31. _____ herpes zoster
32. _____ impetigo
33. _____ macule
34. _____ neoplasm
35. _____ pediculosis
36. _____ pruritus
37. _____ psoriasis
38. _____ seborrhea
39. _____ urticaria
40. _____ verruca
41. _____ vesicle
42. _____ pustule

Definitions

a. a highly infectious skin infection causing erythema and progressing to honey-colored crusts
b. redness of the skin
c. an inflammation of hair follicles
d. a small, flat discoloration of the skin
e. an abnormal growth of new tissue; tumor
f. an infection of an interconnected group of hair follicles or several furuncles forming a mass
g. an inflammation or infection of the skin and deeper tissues that may result in tissue destruction if not treated properly
h. an infection caused by the herpes simplex virus
i. hives
j. an infection caused by reactivation of varicella zoster virus, which causes chicken pox
k. a wart
l. a large blister or vesicle
m. an infestation with parasitic lice
n. baldness
o. superficial dermatitis
p. itching
q. an overproduction of sebum by the sebaceous glands
r. an infection in a hair follicle or gland; characterized by pain, redness, and swelling with necrosis of tissue in the center
s. a skin lesion that appears as a small sac containing fluid; a blister
t. a fungal infection of the skin
u. a vesicle filled with pus
v. a chronic skin disorder that appears as red patches covered with thick, dry, silvery scales

⬤OG MATCHING

Place the letter of the description on the line preceding the skin disorder.

Disorders

43. _____ vitiligo
44. _____ decubitus ulcer
45. _____ corn
46. _____ acne vulgaris
47. _____ carbuncle
48. _____ squamous cell carcinoma
49. _____ seborrheic dermatitis

Descriptions

a. a skin disease characterized by pimples, comedones, and cysts
b. a pigmentation disorder thought to be an autoimmune disorder in patients with an inherited predisposition
c. an infection in an interconnected group of hair follicles
d. a skin inflammation caused by an overproduction of sebum that affects the scalp, eyelids, face, back, umbilicus, and body folds
e. a hard, raised thickening of the stratum corneum on the toes
f. an ulcerative lesion caused by impaired blood supply and insufficient oxygen to an area
g. a type of skin cancer that is a slow-growing, malignant tumor

OOG MATCHING

Grade: _____

Place the letter of the description on the line preceding the type of bandage.

Bandages

50. _____ roller bandages
51. _____ elastic bandages
52. _____ tubular gauze bandages

Descriptions

a. These bandages can be given to the patient to take home to wash and reuse. You should be careful when applying them so as not to compromise circulation.
b. These bandages are made of soft, woven materials and are available in various lengths and widths. They can be either sterile or clean.
c. These bandages are very stretchy and are used to enclose fingers, toes, arms, legs, head, and trunk.

OOG MATCHING

Grade: _____

Although medical assistants do not prescribe treatments, match each of the following skin disorders with the most likely physician-prescribed treatment. Place the letter of the possible treatment on the line next to the skin disorder.

Disorders

53. _____ decubitus ulcers
54. _____ basal cell carcinoma
55. _____ cellulitis
56. _____ folliculitis
57. _____ verruca
58. _____ urticaria

Treatments

a. saline soaks or compresses
b. antihistamines
c. antibiotic powder
d. surgical removal
e. keratolytic agents
f. antibiotics

PSY IDENTIFICATION

Grade: _____

59. Which of the following skin disorders cannot be treated? Circle the correct answer.
    a. Impetigo
    b. Folliculitis
    c. Albinism
    d. Malignant melanoma
    e. Decubitus ulcers

60. How would a physician be able to confirm a suspected case of malignant melanoma? Circle the correct answer.
    a. Wood light analysis
    b. Inspection
    c. Urine test

61. As a medical assistant, you will be responsible for helping the physician perform physical examinations of the skin. Review the list of tasks below and determine which tasks you may be responsible for as a medical assistant. Place a check mark in the "Yes" column for duties that you might assist with and a check mark in the "No" column for tasks that someone else would complete.

Task	Yes	No
a. Assemble the equipment required by the physician		
b. Perform a skin biopsy		
c. Inject local anesthetic when needed		
d. Direct specimens to the appropriate laboratories		
e. Clean and disinfect the examination room		
f. Diagnose and treat common skin inflammations		
g. Reinforce the physician's instructions about caring for a skin condition at home		

62. You are applying a bandage to a patient. Read the statements below and check the appropriate box to show whether the bandage has been applied correctly or incorrectly.

	Applied Correctly	Applied Incorrectly
a. You have fastened the bandage with adhesive tape		
b. The area that you are about to bandage is clean and damp		
c. You have dressed two burned fingers separately and then bandaged them together		
d. The skin around the bandaged arm is pale and cool		
e. You have bandaged a wounded foot by covering the toes to make it neater		
f. You have bandaged an elbow with extra padding		

63. Place a check mark in the appropriate box to show whether the person described is at a high risk or a low risk of developing impetigo

	High Risk	Low Risk
a. A slightly overweight 34-year-old woman who showers twice a day		
b. A 55-year-old man who works at a hospital laundry room and does not wash his hands		
c. A 22-year-old woman with severe anorexia		
d. An 18-year-old drug addict who lives in an abandoned warehouse		
e. A 40-year-old mother of three who enjoys reading in the tub		

64. Read these descriptions of five of Dr. Marsh's patients and then decide which of his patients is at the highest risk of developing malignant melanoma. Place a check mark on the line preceding the patient descriptions that are at the highest risk

a. _____ Mrs. Pearson, 42-year-old mother of two. Light brown hair, brown eyes, enjoys reading and watching movies

b. _____ Mr. Stevens, 50-year-old widower. Gray hair, brown eyes, enjoys walking and playing golf

c. _____ Jessica Phillips, 24-year-old college student. Red hair, blue eyes, enjoys playing volleyball and surfing

d. _____ Todd Andrews, 18-year-old student. Black hair, green eyes, enjoys running and swimming

e. _____ Mr. Archer, 39-year-old father of three. Blond hair, blue eyes, lives in Minnesota and enjoys skiing

COG SHORT ANSWER

Grade: _____

65. What are the symptoms of psoriasis?

_____

_____

_____

_____

66. A man brings his 85-year-old mother to the physician's office. He tells you that his mother lives in a local care home. When the physician examines the patient, you notice multiple decubitus ulcers on her body. Explain why this would be a particular cause of concern.

_____

_____

_____

_____

67. List the three types of skin biopsy performed by a physician.

_____

_____

_____

_____

68. List the three bacterial skin infections that develop in the hair follicles.

_____

_____

_____

_____

69. A patient has a band of lesions on his back made up of small red papules. What skin disorder does this person most likely have? Explain what causes the condition.

_____

_____

_____

_____

70. A father brings his 8-year-old son to the physician, who diagnoses the child with pediculosis. What advice could you give the father to ensure that no other members of the family become infected? List three things that the father could do to contain the problem.

_____

_____

_____

_____

71. What is the full version of the cancer prevention message, "Slip! Slop! Slap! Wrap!"?

_____

_____

_____

_____

72. The physician suspects that a patient has ringworm. Explain what method the physician would most likely use to confirm the diagnosis?

_____

_____

_____

_____

OOG TRUE OR FALSE?

Grade: _____

73. Indicate whether the statements are true or false by placing the letter T (true) or F (false) on the line preceding the statement.

   a. _____ Before applying a bandage, you should perform surgical asepsis.

   b. _____ Young women are more likely to develop keloids than young men.

   c. _____ A wound culture is obtained by excising the wound.

   d. _____ Erythema is best treated with antihistamines.

OOG AFF CASE STUDIES FOR CRITICAL THINKING

Grade: _____

74. A patient has come into the physician's office for a skin biopsy on his thigh. After the physician has removed the tissue, she asks you to bandage the area. List three things you should do while you are bandaging the patient's thigh to ensure that it is both sterile and secure. Explain why they are important.

   _____

   _____

   _____

   _____

75. There are three patients waiting to be seen by a physician, and all of the appointments are slightly behind schedule. One of the patients is a young man who has clusters of wheals on his left arm. The second patient is a 7-year-old girl who has dry scaly crusts on her face and neck. The third patient is a 5-year-old boy with dried skin flakes and bald patches on his scalp. All three patients are itching, and the receptionist is concerned that they might be contagious. You have only one spare examination room. Which patient would you isolate in the examination room? Explain your answer.

   _____

   _____

   _____

   _____

76. Your patient is a 25-year-old female who has been to see the physician several times for severe sunburn. You know that her lifestyle can lead to long-term skin problems. Explain how you could educate her about staying safe in the sun. Include some of the early warning signs of skin cancer that she should keep an eye out for.

   _____

   _____

   _____

   _____

77. A mother brings her 8-year-old son to the physician's office, and the child is diagnosed with pediculosis. She insists that her child cannot possibly have lice because they live in a very clean home. The mother demands that the physician examines the child again. What do you say to the mother to calm her down? How do you reassure her?

_____

_____

_____

_____

78. A 14-year-old boy comes into the physician's office with severe acne vulgaris on his face and neck. He is embarrassed and depressed about his condition and is worried that it will never get better. He says that he has tried every over-the-counter medication and that this is his last hope. What would you say to this patient?

_____

_____

_____

_____

PSY PROCEDURE 28-1 **Apply a Warm or Cold Compress**

Name: _____ Date: _____ Time: _____ Grade: _____

EQUIPMENT/SUPPLIES: Warm compresses—appropriate solution (water with possible antiseptic, if ordered), warmed to 110°F or recommended temperature; bath thermometer; absorbent material (cloths, gauze); waterproof barriers; hot water bottle (optional); clean or sterile basin; gloves. Cold compresses—appropriate solution; ice bag or cold pack; absorbent material (cloths, gauze); waterproof barriers; gloves

STANDARDS: Given the needed equipment and a place to work, the student will perform this skill with _____ % accuracy in a total of _____ minutes. (*Your instructor will tell you what the percentage and time limits will be before you begin.*)

KEY: 4 = Satisfactory   0 = Unsatisfactory   NA = This step is not counted

PROCEDURE STEPS	SELF	PARTNER	INSTRUCTOR
1. Wash your hands and put on gloves	❑	❑	❑
2. Check the physician's order and assemble the equipment and supplies	❑	❑	❑
3. Pour the appropriate solution into the basin. For hot compresses, check the temperature of the warmed solution	❑	❑	❑
4. Greet and identify the patient. Identify yourself including your title. Explain the procedure	❑	❑	❑
5. Ask the patient to remove appropriate clothing	❑	❑	❑
6. Gown and drape accordingly	❑	❑	❑
7. **AFF** Explain how to respond to a patient who is hearing impaired	❑	❑	❑
_____			
_____			
_____			
_____			
8. Protect the examination table with a waterproof barrier	❑	❑	❑
9. Place absorbent material or gauze into the prepared solution. Wring out excess moisture	❑	❑	❑
10. Place the compress on the patient's skin and ask about comfort of temperature	❑	❑	❑
11. Observe the skin for changes in color	❑	❑	❑
12. Arrange the wet compress over the area	❑	❑	❑
13. Insulate the compress with plastic or another waterproof barrier	❑	❑	❑

(continues)

PSY   PROCEDURE 28-1   **Apply a Warm or Cold Compress** (continued)

14. Check the compress frequently for moisture and temperature
    a. Hot water bottles or ice packs may be used to maintain the temperature
    b. Rewet absorbent material as needed
	❏	❏	❏

15. After the prescribed amount of time, usually 20 to 30 minutes, remove the compress
    a. Discard disposable materials
    b. Disinfect reusable equipment
	❏	❏	❏

16. Remove your gloves and wash your hands	❏	❏	❏

17. Log into the Electronic Medical Record (EMR) using your username and secure password OR obtain the paper medical record from a secure location and assure it is kept away from public access. Document the procedure including:
    a. Length of treatment, type of solution, temperature of solution
    b. Skin color after treatment, assessment of the area, and patient's reactions
	❏	❏	❏

18. When finished, log out of the EMR and/or replace the paper medical record in an appropriate and secure location	❏	❏	❏

CALCULATION

Total Possible Points: _____

Total Points Earned: _____ Multiplied by 100 = _____ Divided by Total Possible Points = _____ %

PASS   FAIL   COMMENTS:
❏   ❏

Student's signature _____ Date _____

Partner's signature _____ Date _____

Instructor's signature _____ Date _____

PSY PROCEDURE 28-2 **Assist with Therapeutic Soaks**

Name: _____ Date: _____ Time: _____ Grade: _____

EQUIPMENT/SUPPLIES: Clean or sterile basin or container to comfortably contain the body part to be soaked; solution, and/or medication; dry towels; bath thermometer; gloves

STANDARDS: Given the needed equipment and a place to work, the student will perform this skill with _____ % accuracy in a total of _____ minutes. *(Your instructor will tell you what the percentage and time limits will be before you begin.)*

KEY: 4 = Satisfactory   0 = Unsatisfactory   NA = This step is not counted

PROCEDURE STEPS	SELF	PARTNER	INSTRUCTOR
1. Wash your hands and apply your gloves	❏	❏	❏
2. Assemble the equipment and supplies, including the appropriately sized basin or container. Pad surfaces of container for comfort	❏	❏	❏
3. Fill the container with solution and check the temperature with a bath thermometer. The temperature should be below 110°F	❏	❏	❏
4. Greet and identify the patient. Identify yourself including your credentials. Explain the procedure	❏	❏	❏
5. **AFF** Explain how to respond to the patient who has dementia	❏	❏	❏
6. Slowly lower the patient's extremity or body part into the container	❏	❏	❏
7. Arrange the part comfortably and in easy alignment	❏	❏	❏
8. Check for pressure areas and pad the edges as needed for comfort	❏	❏	❏
9. Check the solution every 5 to 10 minutes for proper temperature	❏	❏	❏
10. Soak for the prescribed amount of time, usually 15 to 20 minutes	❏	❏	❏
11. Remove the body part from the solution and carefully dry the area with a towel	❏	❏	❏
12. Properly care for the equipment; appropriately dispose of single-use supplies and wash your hands	❏	❏	❏

(continues)

PSY PROCEDURE 28-2 **Assist with Therapeutic Soaks** (continued)			

13. Log into the Electronic Medical Record (EMR) using your username and secure password OR obtain the paper medical record from a secure location and assure it is kept away from public access. Document the procedure including:
   a. Length of treatment, type of solution, temperature of solution
   b. Skin color after treatment, assessment of the area, and patient's reactions
	❏	❏	❏

14. When finished, log out of the EMR and/or replace the paper medical record in an appropriate and secure location	❏	❏	❏

CALCULATION

Total Possible Points: _____

Total Points Earned: _____ Multiplied by 100 = _____ Divided by Total Possible Points = _____ %

PASS   FAIL   COMMENTS:
  ❏   ❏

Student's signature _____ Date _____

Partner's signature _____ Date _____

Instructor's signature _____ Date _____

PSY PROCEDURE 28-3 **Apply a Tubular Gauze Bandage**

Name: _____ Date: _____ Time: _____ Grade: _____

EQUIPMENT/SUPPLIES: Tubular gauze, applicator, tape, scissors

STANDARDS: Given the needed equipment and a place to work, the student will perform this skill with _____ % accuracy in a total of _____ minutes. *(Your instructor will tell you what the percentage and time limits will be before you begin.)*

KEY: 4 = Satisfactory 0 = Unsatisfactory NA = This step is not counted

PROCEDURE STEPS	SELF	PARTNER	INSTRUCTOR
1. Wash your hands and assemble the equipment	❏	❏	❏
2. Greet and identify the patient. Identify yourself, including your credentials. Explain the procedure	❏	❏	❏
3. **AFF** Explain how to respond to a patient who is visually impaired	❏	❏	❏
_____ _____ _____ _____			
4. Choose the appropriate-size tubular gauze applicator and gauze width	❏	❏	❏
5. Select and cut or tear adhesive tape in lengths to secure the gauze ends	❏	❏	❏

6. Place the gauze bandage on the applicator in the following manner:
   a. Be sure that the applicator is upright (open end up) and placed on a flat surface
   b. Pull a sufficient length of gauze from the stock box, ready to cut
   c. Open the end of the length of gauze and slide it over the upper end of the applicator
   d. Push estimated amount of gauze needed for this procedure onto the applicator
   e. Cut the gauze when the required amount of gauze has been transferred to the applicator
	❏	❏	❏

7. Place the applicator over the distal end of the affected part. Hold it in place as you move to Step 7	❏	❏	❏
8. Slide applicator containing the gauze up to the proximal end of the affected part	❏	❏	❏
9. Pull the applicator 1 to 2 inches past the end of the affected part if the part is to be completely covered	❏	❏	❏
10. Turn the applicator one full turn to anchor the bandage	❏	❏	❏

(continues)

PSY   PROCEDURE 28-3   Apply a Tubular Gauze Bandage (continued)

Step			
11. Move the applicator toward the proximal part as before	❏	❏	❏
12. Move the applicator forward about 1 inch beyond the original starting point.	❏	❏	❏
13. Repeat the procedure until the desired coverage is obtained	❏	❏	❏
14. The final layer should end at the proximal part of the affected area. Remove the applicator	❏	❏	❏
15. Secure the bandage in place with adhesive tape or cut the gauze into two tails and tie them at the base of the tear	❏	❏	❏
16. Tie the two tails around the closest proximal joint	❏	❏	❏
17. Use the adhesive tape sparingly to secure the end if not using a tie	❏	❏	❏
18. Properly care for or dispose of equipment and supplies	❏	❏	❏
19. Clean the work area. Wash your hands	❏	❏	❏
20. Log into the Electronic Medical Record (EMR) using your username and secure password OR obtain the paper medical record from a secure location and assure it is kept away from public access	❏	❏	❏
21. When finished, log out of the EMR and/or replace the paper medical record in an appropriate and secure location	❏	❏	❏

CALCULATION

Total Possible Points: ＿＿＿＿＿＿＿

Total Points Earned: ＿＿＿＿＿＿ Multiplied by 100 = ＿＿＿＿＿＿ Divided by Total Possible Points = ＿＿＿＿＿＿ %

PASS   FAIL   COMMENTS:
❏   ❏

Student's signature ＿＿＿＿＿＿＿＿＿＿＿＿ Date ＿＿＿＿＿＿

Partner's signature ＿＿＿＿＿＿＿＿＿＿＿＿ Date ＿＿＿＿＿＿

Instructor's signature ＿＿＿＿＿＿＿＿＿＿＿ Date ＿＿＿＿＿＿

CHAPTER 29

Orthopedics

LEARNING OUTCOMES

COG Cognitive Domain*

1. Spell key terms
2. *Identify the following related to body systems:*
   a. *Medical terms*
   b. *Abbreviations*
3. *Identify the structural organization of the human body*
4. *Identify major organs in each body system*
5. *Identify the anatomical location of major organs in each body system*
6. *Identify the normal function of each body system*
7. *Identify common pathology related to each body system including*
   a. *Signs*
   b. *Symptoms*
   c. *Etiology*
   d. *Diagnostic measures*
   e. *Treatment modalities*
8. Discuss the role of the medical assistant in caring for the patient with a musculoskeletal system disorder
9. Describe the various types of ambulatory aids

PSY Psychomotor Domain*

1. Apply an arm sling (Procedure 29-1)
   a. *Instruct and prepare a patient for a procedure or a treatment*
   b. *Assist provider with a patient exam*
   c. *Document patient care accurately in the medical record*
2. Apply cold packs (Procedure 29-2)
   a. *Instruct and prepare a patient for a procedure or treatment*
   b. *Assist provider with a patient exam*
   c. *Document patient care accurately in the medical record*
3. Use a hot water bottle or commercial hot pack (Procedure 29-3)
   a. *Instruct and prepare a patient for a procedure or treatment*
   b. *Assist provider with a patient exam*
   c. *Document patient care accurately in the medical record*
4. Measure a patient for axillary crutches (Procedure 29-4)
   a. *Instruct and prepare a patient for a procedure or treatment*
   b. *Assist provider with a patient exam*
   c. *Document patient care accurately in the medical record*
5. Instruct a patient in various crutch gaits (Procedure 29-5)
   a. *Instruct and prepare a patient for a procedure or treatment*
   b. *Document patient care accurately in the medical record*

AFF Affective Domain*

1. *Demonstrate critical thinking skills*
2. *Reassure patients*
3. *Demonstrate empathy for patients' concerns*
4. *Demonstrate active listening*
5. *Respect diversity*
6. *Recognize personal boundaries*
7. *Demonstrate tactfulness*
8. *Demonstrate self-awareness*
9. Protect the integrity of the medical record

MAERB Standards are Italicized.

ABHES Competencies

1. List all body systems and their structures and functions
2. Describe common diseases, symptoms, and etiology as they apply to each system
3. Identify diagnostic and treatment modalities as they relate to each body system
4. Apply medical terminology for each specialty
5. Follow documentation guidelines
6. Adapt care to address the developmental stages of life
7. Partner with healthcare teams to attain optimal patient health outcomes
8. Display effective interpersonal skills with patients and healthcare team members
9. Demonstrate cultural awareness
10. Assist provider with specialty examinations including cardiac, respiratory, OB-GYN, neurologic, and gastroenterology
11. Perform specialty procedures including but not limited to minor surgery, cardiac, respiratory, OB-GYN, neurological, and gastroenterology
12. Make adaptations for patients with special needs (psychological or physical limitations)
13. Make adaptations to care for patients across their lifespan

Name: _____   Date: _____   Grade: _____

COG MULTIPLE CHOICE

Circle the letter preceding the correct answer.

1. The rebound phenomenon happens:
    a. when the body secretes callus, which fills in fractures and mends damaged bone.
    b. when the body experiences bulging discs or biomechanical stress as a result of poor posture.
    c. when the body overcompensates for a muscle sprain by increasing use of unaffected muscles.
    d. when the body responds to extremes of temperature for long periods of time by exerting an opposite effect.
    e. when the body releases fat droplets from the yellow marrow of the long bones.

2. In which crutch gait do both legs leave the floor together?
    a. One-arm gait
    b. Two-point gait
    c. Three-point gait
    d. Four-point gait
    e. Swing-through gait

3. A fracture that occurs in flat bones (like those of the skull) and results in a fragment being driven below the surface of the bone is called a(n):
    a. depressed fracture.
    b. impacted fracture.
    c. pathological fracture.
    d. compression fracture.
    e. spiral fracture.

4. A possible cause of gout is:
    a. a liver disorder.
    b. a degenerative strain.
    c. a diet high in purines.
    d. the wear and tear on weight-bearing joints.
    e. the release of fat droplets from the marrow of long bones.

Scenario for Questions 5 and 6: The physician has determined that a male patient will need to wear a short arm cast on his left arm as part of the treatment for his fracture. The physician asks you to help her apply the cast to the patient. You assemble the items needed to apply the cast. As the physician prepares the limb for casting, you soak the casting material and press it until it is no longer dripping. Then, the physician wraps the affected limb with the material. After the cast has dried, the physician asks you to apply an arm sling to the patient's left arm.

5. How should the physician wrap the patient's affected arm with the soaked casting material?
    a. From the axilla to mid palm
    b. From mid palm to the axilla
    c. From the elbow to mid palm
    d. From mid palm to the elbow
    e. From the axilla to the elbow

6. Which of these steps will you follow when applying the arm sling?
    a. Cover the left arm with soft knitted tubular material
    b. Position the hand of the left arm at a 90-degree angle
    c. Instruct the patient in various gaits using auxiliary crutches
    d. Check the patient's circulation by pinching each of his fingers
    e. Insert the elbow of the right arm into the pouch end of the sling

7. Rheumatoid arthritis is a(n):
    a. joint failure.
    b. bone fracture.
    c. skeletal tumor.
    d. autoimmune disease.
    e. spine disorder.

8. Tendonitis that is caused by calcium deposits is called:
    a. fibromyalgia.
    b. iontophoresis.
    c. hardened tendons.
    d. calcific tendonitis.
    e. depository tendonitis.

Scenario for Questions 9 and 10: A 20-year-old female patient is visiting your office because of pain in her knee. During the patient interview, the patient tells you that she experiences pain when walking down stairs and getting out of bed. You learn that she is very active and is a member of her university's track and field team.

9. What musculoskeletal disorder does this patient have?
    a. Plantar fasciitis
    b. Lateral humeral epicondylitis
    c. Dupuytren contracture
    d. Chondromalacia patellae
    e. Ankylosing spondylitis

10. What surgical procedure may need to be performed to repair or remove damaged cartilage if the patient's case is severe?
    a. Arthrogram
    b. Arthroplasty
    c. Arthroscopy
    d. Phonophoresis
    e. Electromyography

11. You should *not* apply cold to:
    a. open wounds.
    b. the pregnant uterus.
    c. acute inflammation.
    d. the very young and older adults.
    e. a contusion.

12. Proper cane length calls for the cane to be level with the user's greater trochanter and for the user's elbow to be bent at a:
    a. 30-degree angle.
    b. 50-degree angle.
    c. 60-degree angle.
    d. 80-degree angle.
    e. 90-degree angle.

13. A subluxation is a(n):
    a. dislocation of a facet joint.
    b. partial dislocation of a joint.
    c. complete dislocation of a joint.
    d. dislocation that damages the tendons.
    e. injury to a joint capsule.

14. How is immobilization during closed reduction achieved?
    a. Casting
    b. Surgery
    c. Exercise
    d. Splinting
    e. Ultrasound

15. You and the physician must wear goggles during a cast removal to protect against:
    a. flying particles.
    b. dangerous waves.
    c. unsanitary material.
    d. bloodborne pathogens.
    e. disease and infection.

16. If a fat embolus becomes lodged in a patient's pulmonary or coronary vessels, the patient may experience:
    a. limited mobility.
    b. pain and swelling.
    c. a warm sensation.
    d. an infarction and death.
    e. swelling and numbness.

17. The most common site of bursitis is the:
    a. foot.
    b. wrist.
    c. elbow.
    d. shoulder.
    e. ankle.

18. Your patient has just received a fiberglass leg cast. Which of the following is a sign that proper circulation is present?
    a. Red, hot toes
    b. Swollen toes
    c. Clammy toes
    d. Cold, blue toes
    e. Warm, pink toes

19. Osteoporosis is a condition in which the bones lack:
    a. bursae.
    b. calcium.
    c. vitamin D.
    d. malignancies.
    e. marrow.

20. Your patient is recovering from a strain in his Achilles tendon. He is unable to use one leg, but he has coordination and upper body strength. Which of the following ambulatory assist devices should this patient use to gain mobility?
    a. Cast
    b. Cane
    c. Sling
    d. Walker
    e. Crutches

COG **MATCHING**

Grade: _____

Place the letter preceding the definition on the line next to the term.

Key Terms

21. _____ ankylosing spondylitis
22. _____ arthrogram
23. _____ arthroscopy
24. _____ arthroplasty
25. _____ bursae
26. _____ callus
27. _____ contracture
28. _____ contusion
29. _____ electromyography
30. _____ embolus
31. _____ goniometer
32. _____ iontophoresis
33. _____ kyphosis
34. _____ lordosis
35. _____ Paget disease
36. _____ phonophoresis
37. _____ prosthesis
38. _____ reduction
39. _____ scoliosis

Definitions

a. introduction of various chemical ions into the skin by means of electrical current

b. a deposit of new bone tissue that forms between the healing ends of broken bones

c. any artificial replacement for a missing body part, such as false teeth or an artificial limb

d. a mass of matter (thrombus, air, fat globule) freely floating in the circulatory system

e. small sacs filled with clear synovial fluid that surround some joints

f. a lateral curve of the spine, usually in the thoracic area, with a corresponding curve in the lumbar region, causing uneven shoulders and hips

g. an abnormal shortening of muscles around a joint caused by atrophy of the muscles and resulting in flexion and fixation

h. an abnormally deep ventral curve at the lumbar flexure of the spine; also known as swayback

i. ultrasound treatment used to force medications into tissues

j. surgical repair of a joint

k. an abnormally deep dorsal curvature of the thoracic spine; also known as humpback or hunchback

l. an examination of the inside of a joint through an arthroscope

m. x-ray of a joint

n. an instrument used to measure the angle of joints for range of motion

o. a collection of blood in tissues after an injury; a bruise

p. correcting a fracture by realigning the bones; may be closed (corrected by manipulation) or open (requires surgery)

q. a stiffening of the spine with inflammation

r. a recording of electrical nerve transmission in skeletal muscles

s. a degenerative bone disease usually in older persons with bone destruction and poor repair

COG **MATCHING**

Grade: _____

Place the letter preceding the condition on the line preceding the ambulatory assist device.

Devices

40. _____ crutches
41. _____ cane
42. _____ walker

Conditions

a. Patient A is a 53-year-old female who has recently undergone hip replacement surgery. She is able to walk and needs only slight assistance until she has fully healed from her surgery.

b. Patient B is a 17-year-old male with a sprained ankle. His condition is temporary, but he needs assistance walking with one affected leg.

c. Patient C is a 79-year-old female with osteoarthritis. She has trouble maintaining her balance when walking.

OOG IDENTIFICATION

Grade: _____

43. Complete this chart to show the different types of fractures.

Type of Fracture	Description
Avulsion	Tearing away of bone fragments caused by sharp twisting force applied to ligaments or tendons attached to bone
Comminuted	**a.**
Compound or open	Broken end of bone punctures and protrudes through skin
b.	Damage to bone caused by strong force on both ends of the bone, such as through a fall
Depressed	Fracture of flat bones (typically the skull), which causes bone fragment to be driven below the surface of the bone
Greenstick	**c.**
Impacted	One bone segment driven into another
d.	Break is slanted across the axis of the bone
Pathological	Related to a disease such as osteoporosis, Paget disease, bone cysts, tumors, or cancers
Simple or closed	**e.**
Spiral	Appears as an S-shaped fracture on radiographs and occurs with torsion or twisting injuries
f.	A fracture at right angles to axis of bone that is usually caused by excessive bending force or direct pressure on bone

44. Complete this chart, which shows the variations of arthritis, the most commonly affected site, and the characteristics of the variation.

Disease	Affected Site	Characteristics
Osteoarthritis	Weight-bearing joints	**a.**
b.	Synovial membrane lining of the joint	Usually begins in non–weight-bearing joints, but can spread to many other joints; results in inflammation, pain, stiffness, and crippling deformities
Ankylosing spondylitis (or Marie-Strümpell disease)	**c.**	Rheumatoid arthritis of the spine; results in extreme forward flexion of the spine and tightness in the hip flexors
d.	Joint, usually the great toe	An overproduction of uric acid leads to a deposit of uric acid crystals in the joint; results in a painful, hot, inflamed joint; can become chronic

45. Review the list of tasks below and determine which tasks you may be responsible for as a medical assistant working in the clinical area. Place a check mark in the "Yes" column for those duties you may be responsible for doing and place a check mark in the "No" column for those tasks that you would not perform.

Task	Yes	No
a. Instruct patients on how to use crutches, a cane, a walker, or a wheelchair.		
b. Inform patients of the potential injury associated with heating pad use.		
c. Perform arthroplasty to repair or remove cartilage damaged by chondromalacia patellae.		
d. Assemble the supplies needed to cast a fractured bone.		
e. Treat tendonitis with a transverse friction massage.		
f. Help older adult patients avoid hip fractures by reviewing fall prevention techniques.		
g. Observe and report signs of a musculoskeletal disorder, such as skin color, temperature, tone, and tenderness.		
h. Give patients specific and detailed instructions for applying heat or cold at home.		
i. Identify the type of fracture and decide on the method of treatment.		

46. Use the word bank to fill in the blanks in this paragraph about bone tumors.
The cause of malignant skeletal tumors is unknown but may be linked to rapid development of _____ during youth. An early sign of bone tumors is bone pain, which is most intense at night. Some bone tumors have the potential to spread to the skin and muscles. Bone tumors are identified by _____ after a bone scan reveals the need for further diagnosis. Treatments include surgery, amputation, and _____.

Word Bank:

biopsy   bone tissue   chemotherapy
CT scan   osteosarcomas

COG SHORT ANSWER

Grade: _____

47. Describe these three abnormal spine curvatures.

   a. Lordosis: _____

   b. Kyphosis: _____

   c. Scoliosis: _____

48. What is the difference between a sprain and a strain? How are they similar?

_____

_____

_____

_____

49. Name four common sites of dislocations.

_____

_____

_____

_____

50. Your patient is complaining of pain in his wrist. You learn that the pain began after he fell from a ladder and used his hand to break his fall. What would be signs that the patient has fractured his arm?

_____

_____

_____

_____

51. What is the difference between a spiral fracture and an avulsion fracture?

_____

_____

_____

_____

52. What test is performed that determines whether back pain results from a herniated intervertebral disc? How is the test done, and what is a positive indicator?

_____

_____

_____

_____

53. Both heat and cold treatments are used to relieve pain, but how do their uses differ?

_____

_____

_____

_____

54. List the five gaits utilized by patients who use crutches to assist them with walking.

_____

_____

_____

_____

55. The physician has just applied a plaster cast to a patient. What instructions and information should you give to the patient regarding her plaster cast?

_____

_____

_____

_____

OG TRUE OR FALSE?

Grade: _____

Indicate whether the statements are true or false by placing the letter T (true) or F (false) on the line preceding the statement.

56. _____ Heat, such as heat from a heating pad or hot water bottle, should not be applied to the uterus of a pregnant woman.

57. _____ A greenstick fracture is a partial or incomplete fracture in which only one side of the bone is broken.

58. _____ The swing-through gait is the gait most commonly used to train patients to use crutches.

59. _____ Fibromyalgia is easy to diagnose because the symptoms are constant and centrally located in one joint socket.

AFF CASE STUDIES FOR CRITICAL THINKING

Grade: _____

60. Deirdre is a 52-year-old patient. She visits the office with a complaint of joint pain. After taking Deirdre's height and weight measurements, you notice that she is 1½ inches shorter than she was just 2 years ago. After speaking with the patient, you learn that she does not exercise. The physician suspects Deirdre may have osteoporosis. What tests might the physician order to confirm his diagnosis? What preventative medicine information might be useful for Deirdre?

_____

_____

_____

_____

61. Maddy, a 9-year-old patient, needs to have her arm put into a cast after it is discovered that she has a greenstick fracture. The physician informs Maddy's mother that he will be using a fiberglass cast to immobilize Maddy's arm. Maddy's mother grows concerned after speaking with the physician. She has heard that fiberglass can be dangerous, and she wonders why the physician does not use a plaster, like the cast she received when she was a child with a fractured arm. Explain to Maddy's mother the benefits of a fiberglass cast over a plaster cast, especially when the patient is a young, active child.

_____

_____

_____

_____

62. Your coworker Ben is moving some boxes from the reception area to a closet in the office. As you walk by, you observe him bending his back and lifting a box with extended arms. You know that this method of lifting could lead to serious back problems, so you decide to speak to Ben about avoiding back strain. What should you say to Ben? How would you respond if he laughs and tells you he is fine?

_____

_____

_____

_____

63. A 46-year-old patient has been advised by the physician to avoid using his strained knee. After you secure an ice pack to the patient's knee, you begin to instruct the patient in how to care for his knee at home. While you are speaking, the patient interrupts you saying that he has had this injury before and will "just throw a heating pad on there" like he has done in the past. How would you respond to the patient?

_____

_____

_____

_____

PSY PROCEDURE 29-1   **Apply an Arm Sling**

Name: _____   **Date:** _____   **Time:** _____   **Grade:** _____

EQUIPMENT/SUPPLIES: A canvas arm sling with adjustable straps.

STANDARDS: Given the needed equipment and a place to work, the student will perform this skill with _____ % accuracy in a total of _____ minutes. *(Your instructor will tell you what the percentage and time limits will be before you begin.)*

KEY: 4 = Satisfactory   0 = Unsatisfactory   NA = This step is not counted

PROCEDURE STEPS	SELF	PARTNER	INSTRUCTOR
1. Wash your hands	❏	❏	❏
2. Assemble the equipment and supplies	❏	❏	❏
3. Greet and identify the patient and explain the procedure. Identify yourself including your credentials	❏	❏	❏
4. **AFF** Explain how to respond to a patient who does not speak English	❏	❏	❏
_____ _____ _____ _____			
5. Position the affected limb with the hand at slightly less than a 90-degree angle	❏	❏	❏
6. Place the affected arm in the sling with the elbow snugly against the back of the sling and the arm extended through the sling with the hand and/or fingers protruding out of the opposite end of the sling	❏	❏	❏
7. Position the strap from the back of the sling around the patient's back, over the opposite shoulder	❏	❏	❏
8. Secure the strap by inserting the end through the two metal rings on the top of the sling and further bringing the end of the strap back, looping it through the top metal ring only	❏	❏	❏
9. Tighten the strap so that the patient's arm in the sling is slightly elevated. Make sure the strap coming around the patient's shoulder and neck is comfortable, padding if necessary to prevent friction and pressure areas	❏	❏	❏
10. Check the patient's level of comfort and distal extremity circulation	❏	❏	❏
11. Wash your hands	❏	❏	❏

PSY PROCEDURE 29-1 **Apply an Arm Sling** (continued)

12. **AFF** Log into the Electronic Medical Record (EMR) using your username and secure password OR obtain the paper medical record from a secure location and assure it is kept away from public access. Document the appliance in the patient's chart	❏	❏	❏
13. When finished, log out of the EMR and/or replace the paper medical record in an appropriate and secure location	❏	❏	❏

CALCULATION

Total Possible Points: _____

Total Points Earned: _____ Multiplied by 100 = _____ Divided by Total Possible Points = _____ %

PASS   FAIL   COMMENTS:
❏   ❏

Student's signature _____ Date _____

Partner's signature _____ Date _____

Instructor's signature _____ Date _____

PSY PROCEDURE 29-2   Apply Cold Packs

Name: _____ Date: _____ Time: _____ Grade: _____

EQUIPMENT/SUPPLIES: Ice bag and ice chips or small cubes, or disposable cold pack; small towel or cover for ice pack; gauze or tape.

STANDARDS: Given the needed equipment and a place to work, the student will perform this skill with _____ % accuracy in a total of _____ minutes. *(Your instructor will tell you what the percentage and time limits will be before you begin.)*

KEY: 4 = Satisfactory   0 = Unsatisfactory   NA = This step is not counted

PROCEDURE STEPS	SELF	PARTNER	INSTRUCTOR
1. Wash your hands	❑	❑	❑
2. Assemble the equipment and supplies, checking the ice bag, if used, for leaks. If using a commercial cold pack, read the manufacturer's directions	❑	❑	❑

3. Fill a nondisposable ice bag about two-thirds full
   a. Press it flat on a surface to express air from the bag
   b. Seal the container
	❑	❑	❑

4. If using a commercial chemical ice pack, activate it now	❑	❑	❑
5. Cover the bag in a towel or other suitable cover	❑	❑	❑
6. Greet and identify the patient. Identify yourself, including your credentials. Explain the procedure	❑	❑	❑
7. **AFF** Explain how to respond to a patient who has cultural or religious beliefs that prohibit disrobing	❑	❑	❑
_____ _____ _____ _____			
8. After assessing skin for color and warmth, place the covered ice pack on the area	❑	❑	❑
9. Secure the ice pack with gauze or tape	❑	❑	❑
10. Apply the treatment for the prescribed amount of time, but no longer than 30 minutes	❑	❑	❑
11. During the treatment, assess the skin under the pack frequently for mottling, pallor, or redness	❑	❑	❑

PSY PROCEDURE 29-2 **Apply Cold Packs** (continued)			
12. Properly care for or dispose of equipment and supplies. Wash your hands	❏	❏	❏
13. AFF Log into the Electronic Medical Record (EMR) using your username and secure password OR obtain the paper medical record from a secure location and assure it is kept away from public access	❏	❏	❏
14. Document the procedure, the site of the application, the results including the condition of the skin after the treatment, and the patient's reactions	❏	❏	❏
15. When finished, log out of the EMR and/or replace the paper medical record in an appropriate and secure location	❏	❏	❏

CALCULATION

Total Possible Points: _____

Total Points Earned: _____ Multiplied by 100 = _____ Divided by Total Possible Points = _____ %

PASS   FAIL   COMMENTS:
❏   ❏

Student's signature _____ Date _____

Partner's signature _____ Date _____

Instructor's signature _____ Date _____

PSY PROCEDURE 29-3   **Use a Hot Water Bottle or Commercial Hot Pack**

Name: _____ Date: _____ Time: _____ Grade: _____

EQUIPMENT/SUPPLIES: A hot water bottle or commercial hot pack, towel or other suitable covering for the hot pack.

STANDARDS: Given the needed equipment and a place to work, the student will perform this skill with _____ % accuracy in a total of _____ minutes. *(Your instructor will tell you what the percentage and time limits will be before you begin.)*

KEY: 4 = Satisfactory   0 = Unsatisfactory   NA = This step is not counted

PROCEDURE STEPS	SELF	PARTNER	INSTRUCTOR
1. Wash your hands	❑	❑	❑
2. Assemble equipment and supplies, checking the hot water bottle for leaks	❑	❑	❑
3. Fill the hot water bottle about two-thirds full with warm (110°F) water **a.** Place the bottle on a flat surface and the opening up; "burp" it by pressing out the air **b.** If using a commercial hot pack, follow the manufacturer's directions for activating it	❑	❑	❑
4. Wrap and secure the pack or bottle before placing it on the patient's skin	❑	❑	❑
5. Greet and identify the patient. Identify yourself, including your credentials. Explain the procedure	❑	❑	❑
6. **AFF** Explain how to respond to a patient who is from a different generation (older) than you are	❑	❑	❑
_____ _____ _____ _____			
7. After assessing the color of the skin where the treatment is to be applied, place the covered hot pack on the area	❑	❑	❑
8. Secure the hot pack with gauze or tape	❑	❑	❑
9. Apply the treatment for the prescribed length of time, but no longer than 30 minutes	❑	❑	❑
10. During treatment, assess the skin every 10 minutes for pallor (an indication of rebound), excessive redness (indicates that temperature may be too high), and swelling (indicates possible tissue damage)	❑	❑	❑

PSY PROCEDURE 29-3 **Use a Hot Water Bottle or Commercial Hot Pack** (continued)

11. Properly care for or dispose of equipment and supplies. Wash your hands	❏	❏	❏
12. **AFF** Log into the Electronic Medical Record (EMR) using your username and secure password OR obtain the paper medical record from a secure location and assure it is kept away from public access	❏	❏	❏
13. Document the procedure, the site of the application, the results including the condition of the skin after the treatment, and the patient's reactions	❏	❏	❏
14. When finished, log out of the EMR and/or replace the paper medical record in an appropriate and secure location	❏	❏	❏

CALCULATION

Total Possible Points: _____

Total Points Earned: _____ Multiplied by 100 = _____ Divided by Total Possible Points = _____ %

PASS   FAIL   COMMENTS:
  ❏   ❏

Student's signature _____   Date _____

Partner's signature _____   Date _____

Instructor's signature _____   Date _____

PSY **PROCEDURE 29-4** **Measure a Patient for Axillary Crutches**

Name: _____ Date: _____ Time: _____ Grade: _____

EQUIPMENT/SUPPLIES: Axillary crutches with tips, pads for the axilla, and hand rests, as needed

STANDARDS: Given the needed equipment and a place to work, the student will perform this skill with _____ % accuracy in a total of _____ minutes. *(Your instructor will tell you what the percentage and time limits will be before you begin.)*

KEY: 4 = Satisfactory 0 = Unsatisfactory NA = This step is not counted

PROCEDURE STEPS	SELF	PARTNER	INSTRUCTOR
1. Wash your hands	❏	❏	❏
2. Assemble the equipment, including the correct-size crutches	❏	❏	❏
3. Greet and identify the patient. Identify yourself, including your credentials. Explain the procedure	❏	❏	❏
4. Ensure that the patient is wearing low-heeled shoes with safety soles	❏	❏	❏
5. Have the patient stand erect. Support the patient as needed	❏	❏	❏
6. **AFF** Explain how to respond to a patient who is hearing impaired	❏	❏	❏
_____ _____ _____ _____			
7. While standing erect, have the patient hold the crutches in the tripod position	❏	❏	❏
8. Adjust the central support in the base **a.** Tighten the bolts for safety when the proper height is reached **b.** Adjust the handgrips. Tighten bolts for safety **c.** If needed, pad axillary bars and handgrips	❏	❏	❏
9. Wash your hands	❏	❏	❏
10. **AFF** Log into the Electronic Medical Record (EMR) using your username and secure password OR obtain the paper medical record from a secure location and assure it is kept away from public access	❏	❏	❏
11. Record the procedure, site of the application, and results, including the condition of the skin after the treatment, the patient's response, the date, time, and your name/credentials	❏	❏	❏

PSY PROCEDURE 29-4	**Measure a Patient for Axillary Crutches** (continued)		

12. When finished, log out of the EMR and/or replace the paper medical record in an appropriate and secure location	❏	❏	❏

CALCULATION

Total Possible Points: _____

Total Points Earned: _____ Multiplied by 100 = _____ Divided by Total Possible Points = _____ %

PASS   FAIL   COMMENTS:
   ❏   ❏

Student's signature _____   Date _____

Partner's signature _____   Date _____

Instructor's signature _____   Date _____

PSY PROCEDURE 29-5 Instruct a Patient in Various Crutch Gaits

Name: _____ Date: _____ Time: _____ Grade: _____

EQUIPMENT/SUPPLIES: Axillary crutches measured appropriately for a patient

STANDARDS: Given the needed equipment and a place to work, the student will perform this skill with _____ % accuracy in a total of _____ minutes. *(Your instructor will tell you what the percentage and time limits will be before you begin.)*

KEY: 4 = Satisfactory   0 = Unsatisfactory   NA = This step is not counted

PROCEDURE STEPS	SELF	PARTNER	INSTRUCTOR
1. Wash your hands	❑	❑	❑
2. Have the patient stand up from a chair: **a.** The patient holds both crutches on the affected side **b.** Then the patient slides to the edge of the chair **c.** The patient pushes down on the chair arm on the unaffected side **d.** Then the patient pushes to stand	❑	❑	❑
3. With one crutch in each hand, rest on the crutches until balance is restored	❑	❑	❑
4. Assist the patient to the tripod position	❑	❑	❑
5. **AFF** Explain how to respond to a patient who is visually impaired	❑	❑	❑
_____ _____ _____ _____			
6. Depending on the patient's weight-bearing ability, coordination, and general state of health, instruct the patient in one or more of the following gaits: **a.** Three-point gait **b.** Two-point gait **c.** Four-point gait **d.** Swing-through gait	❑	❑	❑
7. **AFF** Log into the Electronic Medical Record (EMR) using your username and secure password OR obtain the paper medical record from a secure location and assure it is kept away from public access	❑	❑	❑
8. Record the patient education and instructions	❑	❑	❑
9. When finished, log out of the EMR and/or replace the paper medical record in an appropriate and secure location	❑	❑	❑

FSY PROCEDURE 29-5 | **Instruct a Patient in Various Crutch Gaits** (continued)

CALCULATION

Total Possible Points: _____

Total Points Earned: _____ Multiplied by 100 = _____ Divided by Total Possible Points = _____ %

PASS   FAIL   COMMENTS:
❏   ❏

Student's signature _____   Date _____

Partner's signature _____   Date _____

Instructor's signature _____   Date _____

CHAPTER 30

Ophthalmology and Otolaryngology

LEARNING OUTCOMES

Cognitive Domain*

1. Spell key terms
2. *Identify the following related to body systems:*
   a. *Medical terms*
   b. *Abbreviations*
3. *Identify structural organization of the human body*
4. *Identify major organs in each body system*
5. *Identify the anatomic location of major organs in each body system*
6. *Identify the normal function of each body system*
7. *Identify common pathology related to each body system including*
   a. *Signs*
   b. *Symptoms*
   c. *Etiology*
   d. *Diagnostic measures*
   e. *Treatment modalities*
8. Discuss the role of the medical assistant in caring for the patient with disorders of the eyes or ears

Psychomotor Domain*

1. Measure distance visual acuity with a Snellen chart (Procedure 30-1)
   a. *Instruct and prepare a patient for a procedure or treatment*
   b. *Assist provider with a patient exam*
   c. *Document patient care accurately in the medical record*

2. Measure color perception with an Ishihara color plate book (Procedure 30-2)
   a. *Instruct and prepare a patient for a procedure or treatment*
   b. *Assist provider with a patient exam*
   c. *Document patient care accurately in the medical record*
3. Instill eye medication (Procedure 30-3)
   a. *Instruct and prepare a patient for a procedure or treatment*
   b. *Assist provider with a patient exam*
   c. *Document patient care accurately in the medical record*
4. Irrigate the eye (Procedure 30-4)
   a. *Instruct and prepare a patient for a procedure or treatment*
   b. *Assist provider with a patient exam*
   c. *Document patient care accurately in the medical record*
5. Irrigate the ear (Procedure 30-5)
   a. *Instruct and prepare a patient for a procedure or treatment*
   b. *Assist provider with a patient exam*
   c. *Document patient care accurately in the medical record*
6. Administer an audiometric hearing test (Procedure 30-6)
   a. *Instruct and prepare a patient for a procedure or treatment*
   b. *Assist provider with a patient exam*

   c. *Document patient care accurately in the medical record*
7. Instill ear medication (Procedure 30-7)
   a. *Instruct and prepare a patient for a procedure or treatment*
   b. *Assist provider with a patient exam*
   c. *Document patient care accurately in the medical record*
8. Instill nasal medication (Procedure 30-8)
   a. *Instruct and prepare a patient for a procedure or treatment*
   b. *Assist provider with a patient exam*
   c. *Document patient care accurately in the medical record*

Affective Domain*

1. *Demonstrate critical thinking skills*
2. *Reassure patients*
3. *Demonstrate empathy for patients' concerns*
4. *Demonstrate active listening*
5. *Respect diversity*
6. *Recognize personal boundaries*
7. *Demonstrate tactfulness*
8. *Demonstrate self-awareness*
9. Protect the integrity of the medical record

MAERB Standards are Italicized.

ABHES Competencies

1. List all body systems and their structures and functions
2. Describe common diseases, symptoms, and etiology as they apply to each system
3. Identify diagnostic and treatment modalities as they relate to each body system
4. Apply medical terminology for each specialty
5. Follow documentation guidelines
6. Adapt care to address the developmental stages of life
7. Partner with healthcare teams to attain optimal patient health outcomes
8. Display effective interpersonal skills with patients and healthcare team members
9. Demonstrate cultural awareness
10. Assist provider with specialty examination, including cardiac, respiratory, OB-GYN, neurologic, and gastroenterology
11. Perform specialty procedures, including but not limited to minor surgery, cardiac, respiratory, OB-GYN, neurologic, and gastroenterology
12. Make adaptations for patients with special needs (psychological or physical limitations)
13. Make adaptations to care for patients across their lifespan

Name: _____   Date: _____   Grade: _____

OOG MULTIPLE CHOICE

Circle the letter preceding the correct answer.

1. The Ishihara method is used to test:
   a. hearing.
   b. color vision.
   c. cataract growth.
   d. corneal scarring.
   e. for multiple allergies.

2. A physician who specializes in disorders of the ears, nose, and throat is an:
   a. optician.
   b. ophthalmologist.
   c. optometrist.
   d. otolaryngologist.
   e. otitis externa.

3. A common cause of diminished hearing is:
   a. tinnitus.
   b. nasopharynx.
   c. cerumen.
   d. Ménière disease.
   e. strabismus.

4. Epistaxis is considered severe if bleeding continues how many minutes after treatment has begun?
   a. 5
   b. 10
   c. 15
   d. 20
   e. 30

5. Which of the following statements is true about preventive eye care?
   a. Patients should have regular checkups to maintain healthy eyes
   b. Adults should wear UV-protected sunglasses, but children are not as susceptible
   c. Goggles do not need to be worn if you are wearing your regular glasses
   d. Patients should thoroughly wash hands before rubbing their eyes
   e. Contact lenses cause scarring, so glasses are safer to use

6. It is important to treat sinusitis immediately because:
   a. it can lead to severe cases of upper respiratory infections.
   b. new allergies might develop while the nasal membrane is infected.
   c. mucus may infect areas of throat, nose, and ears, if left unchecked.
   d. vision may be affected from pressure of sinus cavities on the eyes.
   e. complications in the ear and brain may occur, causing damage.

7. One symptom of laryngitis is:
   a. earache.
   b. muscle soreness.
   c. coughing.
   d. inflamed tonsils.
   e. excessive mucus.

8. An infection of any of the lacrimal glands of the eyelids is:
   a. hordeolum.
   b. cataract.
   c. glaucoma.
   d. conjunctivitis.
   e. astigmatism.

9. Which of the following could the physician treat with a warm compress?
   a. Nosebleed
   b. Ear infection
   c. Tonsillitis
   d. Astigmatism
   e. Tinnitus

10. The common term for *otitis externa* is:
   a. pink eye.
   b. nosebleed.
   c. Ménière disease.
   d. swimmer's ear.
   e. presbycusis.

Scenario for Questions 11 and 12: A patient comes in for an annual exam, and the physician diagnoses her with presbycusis and presbyopia. She complains of an intermittent, high whistling in her right ear and cloudy vision in both eyes.

11. Reading the symptoms and diagnosis above, the patient is most likely:
    a. an infant or a toddler.
    b. a young child to early teen.
    c. an older teen to early 30s.
    d. middle aged.
    e. a senior citizen.

12. One possible cause of the cloudy vision is:
    a. presbyopia.
    b. glaucoma.
    c. Ménière disease.
    d. cataracts.
    e. sinusitis.

13. What is a safe way to remove cerumen?
    a. Gently inserting a tissue into the ear canal
    b. Using a cotton swab and digging out as much as possible
    c. Drops of hydrogen peroxide dropped into the ear
    d. Using an otoscope to melt the earwax
    e. Blowing your nose

14. It is important not to use nasal preparations more than four times a day because they:
    a. severely damage your nasal cavity.
    b. may become addictive.
    c. dry out sinuses and cause congestion.
    d. cause irritation to the throat.
    e. can lead to allergies.

15. Color blindness is a result of:
    a. people failing the Ishihara test.
    b. patients being unable to differentiate between colors.
    c. a deficiency in the number of rods in the eye.
    d. a deficiency in the number of cones in the eye.
    e. the size and shape of the eye.

16. What important advice can you give children when dealing with contagious diseases like pink eye?
    a. Keep your hands washed and clean
    b. Do not play with children who are sick
    c. If you sneeze, immediately cover your face with your hand
    d. Do not go to school if you are sick
    e. Try to keep from touching anything others have already touched

17. To test for pharyngitis or tonsillitis, the physician would most likely order:
    a. a blood sample.
    b. a urine sample.
    c. a reflex test.
    d. a throat culture.
    e. radiology.

18. Which form of strabismus is known as *convergent eyes*, in which the eyes are crossed?
    a. Esotropic
    b. Exotropic
    c. Hypotrophic
    d. Hypertrophic
    e. Nonconcomitant

19. The purpose of a hearing aid is to:
    a. fully restore the ability to hear.
    b. assist patients with permanent nerve damage.
    c. amplify sound waves.
    d. differentiate between tones.
    e. permanently correct hearing disabilities.

20. A common treatment for allergic rhinitis is:
    a. sleep.
    b. antihistamine medication.
    c. surgery.
    d. antibiotics.
    e. ear irrigation.

COG MATCHING

_____ Grade: _____

Place the letter preceding the definition on the line next to the term.

Key Terms

21. _____ astigmatism
22. _____ cerumen
23. _____ decibel
24. _____ fluorescein angiography
25. _____ hyperopia
26. _____ intraocular pressure
27. _____ myopia
28. _____ myringotomy
29. _____ ophthalmologist
30. _____ ophthalmoscope
31. _____ optician
32. _____ optometrist
33. _____ otolaryngologist
34. _____ otoscope
35. _____ presbycusis
36. _____ presbyopia
37. _____ refraction
38. _____ retinal degeneration
39. _____ tinnitus
40. _____ tonometry
41. _____ hordeolum
42. _____ strabismus

Definitions

a. physician who specializes in treatment of diseases and disorders of the ears, nose, and throat
b. an extraneous noise heard in one or both ears, described as whirring, ringing, whistling, roaring, etc.; may be continuous or intermittent
c. specialist who can measure for errors of refraction and prescribe lenses but who cannot treat diseases of the eye or perform surgery
d. an instrument used for visual examination of the ear canal and tympanic membrane
e. an incision into the tympanic membrane to relieve pressure
f. unit of intensity of sound
g. an unfocused refraction of light rays on the retina
h. a misalignment of eye movements usually caused by muscle incoordination
i. loss of hearing associated with aging
j. specialist who grinds lenses to correct errors of refraction according to prescriptions
k. yellowish or brownish waxlike secretion in the external ear canal; earwax
l. physician who specializes in treatment of disorders of the eyes
m. farsightedness
n. pathological changes in the cell structure of the retina that impair or destroy its function, resulting in blindness
o. infection of any of the lacrimal glands of the eyelids
p. intravenous injection of fluorescent dye; photographing blood vessels of the eye as dye moves through the vessels
q. measurement of intraocular pressure using a tonometer
r. lighted instrument used to examine the inner surfaces of the eye
s. bending of light rays that enter the pupil to reflect exactly on the fovea centralis, the area of greatest visual acuity
t. pressure within the eyeball
u. vision change (farsightedness) associated with aging
v. nearsightedness

COG IDENTIFICATION

_____ Grade: _____

43. Fill in the chart below with three types of vision testing charts and when you should use each.

Type of Vision Testing Chart	When You Would Use It

44. Identify the seven causes of hearing loss.

a. _____

b. _____

c. _____

d. _____

e. _____

f. _____

g. _____

COG SHORT ANSWER

Grade: _____

45. List five preventive eye care tips that you may be asked to educate patients to follow.

a. _____

b. _____

c. _____

d. _____

e. _____

46. A patient complains of loss of vision and blurring, and cataracts are found in both eyes. How would surgery correct these symptoms?

_____

_____

_____

_____

47. What is the difference between an optometrist and an optician?

_____

_____

_____

_____

48. What is astigmatism?

_____

_____

_____

_____

49. An examination of a patient's eye reveals an irregular corneal surface. What is the method used to diagnose a corneal ulcer?

_____

_____

_____

_____

50. A patient comes in complaining of vertigo, nausea, and slight hearing loss. What might the patient be suffering from?

_____

_____

_____

_____

51. Why is otitis media so common in infants and young children?

_____

_____

_____

_____

52. What is the difference between audiometry and tympanometry?

_____

_____

_____

_____

53. List the initial therapy for common epistaxis.

_____

_____

_____

_____

54. Why is it so important to treat upper respiratory infections?

_____

_____

_____

_____

55. When is the physician likely to suggest that a patient receive a tonsillectomy?

_____

_____

_____

_____

56. What is a way to isolate the protein causing allergic reactions in a patient directly?

_____

_____

_____

_____

57. Where do nasal polyps usually occur?

_____

_____

_____

_____

COG TRUE OR FALSE?

Grade: _____

Indicate whether the statements are true or false by placing the letter T (true) or F (false) on the line preceding the statement.

58. _____ Diagnosis of vision loss of any type is done by testing the hearing using an audiometer.

59. _____ Swimmer's ear goes away on its own and does not need to be treated.

60. _____ Allergic rhinitis is another name for hay fever.

61. _____ A patient with tonsillitis should be told to rest his voice and speak as little as possible.

COG **AFF** CASE STUDIES FOR CRITICAL THINKING

Grade: _____

62. A patient calls in to the physician's office saying that pink eye is going around her son's school. He has not been complaining of pain in either eye, but she has noticed that his eyes are red and that he has been sniffing and coughing lately. She wants to know if she should bring him in for a checkup. What should you tell her?

_____

_____

_____

_____

63. A patient is interested in getting LASIK surgery to correct her nearsightedness. She is 24 years old, and both of her parents have strong prescriptions for nearsightedness as well. She asks you what the surgery will be like, and if there is any chance that her eyes might revert back to their previous state. What is LASIK surgery and what are the advantages and disadvantages of this procedure? Are there any side effects?

_____

_____

_____

_____

64. A middle-aged patient comes in for a routine checkup and mentions a slight loss of hearing since the last exam. What tests would most likely be ordered by the physician to check his hearing? Are there any preventative education tips that you can give him about hearing loss?

_____

_____

_____

_____

65. A swimmer comes into the office complaining of recurrent swimmer's ear. She says she has used cotton swabs in the past to clear her ear canals, and asks if there is any particular medication she can apply to help keep her ear canals clean. How would you respond to this patient?

_____

_____

_____

_____

66. A young man comes in for a routine checkup and mentions that he will soon be learning to drive. However, the physician gives him the Ishihara test, and the teen fails to differentiate between colors. What information can you give him about color blindness, and what encouragement can you give him with regard to his upcoming driving test?

_____

_____

_____

_____

_____

67. A young boy is brought in because he is complaining of headaches in school. The physician determines that the boy needs glasses and that the headaches are from eye strain. However, the boy states that he does not want glasses because he is afraid his classmates will make fun of him. What would you say to him?

_____

_____

_____

_____

_____

PROCEDURE 30-1   Measure Distance Visual Acuity with a Snellen Chart

PSY

Name: _____   Date: _____   Time: _____   Grade: _____

EQUIPMENT/SUPPLIES: Snellen eye chart, paper cup or eye paddle

STANDARDS: Given the needed equipment and a place to work, the student will perform this skill with _____ % accuracy in a total of _____ minutes. *(Your instructor will tell you what the percentage and time limits will be before you begin.)*

KEY: 4 = Satisfactory   0 = Unsatisfactory   NA = This step is not counted

PROCEDURE STEPS	SELF	PARTNER	INSTRUCTOR
1. Wash your hands	❑	❑	❑
2. Prepare the examination area (well lit, distance marker 20 feet from the chart)	❑	❑	❑
3. Make sure the chart is at eye level	❑	❑	❑
4. Greet and identify the patient. Identify yourself and your title. Explain the procedure	❑	❑	❑
5. **AFF** Explain how to respond to a patient who is hearing impaired	❑	❑	❑
_____ _____ _____ _____			
6. Place the patient in a standing or sitting position at the 20-foot marker	❑	❑	❑
7. If they are not wearing glasses, ask the patient about contact lenses. Mark results accordingly	❑	❑	❑
8. Have the patient cover the left eye with the eye paddle	❑	❑	❑
9. Instruct the patient not to close the left eye, but to keep both eyes open during the test	❑	❑	❑
10. Stand beside the chart and point to each row as the patient reads aloud **a.** Point to the lines, starting with the 20/200 line **b.** Record the smallest line that the patient can read with no errors	❑	❑	❑
11. Repeat the procedure with the right eye covered and record	❑	❑	❑

PSY PROCEDURE 30-1	Measure Distance Visual Acuity with a Snellen Chart (continued)			
12. Wash your hands		❏	❏	❏
13. AFF Log into the Electronic Medical Record (EMR) using your username and secure password OR obtain the paper medical record from a secure location and assure it is kept away from public access		❏	❏	❏
14. Record the procedure		❏	❏	❏
15. When finished, log out of the EMR and/or replace the paper medical record in an appropriate and secure location		❏	❏	❏

CALCULATION

Total Possible Points: _____

Total Points Earned: _____ Multiplied by 100 = _____ Divided by Total Possible Points = _____ %

PASS FAIL COMMENTS:
❏ ❏

Student's signature _____ Date _____

Partner's signature _____ Date _____

Instructor's signature _____ Date _____

PSY PROCEDURE 30-2 Measuring Color Perception

Name: _____ Date: _____ Time: _____ Grade: _____

EQUIPMENT/SUPPLIES: Ishihara color plates, gloves

STANDARDS: Given the needed equipment and a place to work, the student will perform this skill with _____ % accuracy in a total of _____ minutes. *(Your instructor will tell you what the percentage and time limits will be before you begin.)*

KEY: 4 = Satisfactory   0 = Unsatisfactory   NA = This step is not counted

PROCEDURE STEPS	SELF	PARTNER	INSTRUCTOR
1. Wash your hands, put on gloves, and obtain the Ishihara color plate book	❏	❏	❏
2. Prepare the examination area (adequate lighting)	❏	❏	❏
3. Greet and identify the patient and yourself, including your title. Explain the procedure	❏	❏	❏
4. **AFF** Explain how to respond to a patient who is developmentally challenged	❏	❏	❏
_____ _____ _____ _____			
5. Hold the first bookplate about 30 inches from the patient	❏	❏	❏

6. Ask if the patient can see the "number" within the series of dots
   a. Record results of test by noting the number or figure the patient reports
   b. If the patient cannot distinguish a pattern, record the plate number–x (e.g., 4–x)
	❏	❏	❏

7. The patient should not take more than 3 seconds when reading the plates
   a. The patient should neither squint nor guess. These indicate that the patient is unsure
   b. Record as plate number–x
	❏	❏	❏

8. Record the results for plates 1 through 10
   a. Plate number 11 requires patient to trace a winding line between Xs
   b. Patients with a color deficit will not be able to trace the line
	❏	❏	❏

9. Store the book in a closed, protected area to preserve the integrity of the colors	❏	❏	❏

PSY PROCEDURE 30-2 **Measuring Color Perception** (continued)			
10. Remove your gloves and wash your hands	❑	❑	❑
11. **AFF** Log into the Electronic Medical Record (EMR) using your username and secure password OR obtain the paper medical record from a secure location and assure it is kept away from public access	❑	❑	❑
12. Record the procedure in the medical record	❑	❑	❑
13. When finished, log out of the EMR and/or replace the paper medical record in an appropriate and secure location	❑	❑	❑

CALCULATION

Total Possible Points: _____

Total Points Earned: _____ Multiplied by 100 = _____ Divided by Total Possible Points = _____ %

PASS   FAIL   COMMENTS:
  ❑   ❑

Student's signature _____   Date _____

Partner's signature _____   Date _____

Instructor's signature _____   Date _____

FSY PROCEDURE 30-3 **Instilling Eye Medication**

Name: _____ **Date:** _____ **Time:** _____ **Grade:** _____

EQUIPMENT/SUPPLIES: Physician's order and patient record, ophthalmic medications, 2 × 2 gauze pad, tissues, gloves

STANDARDS: Given the needed equipment and a place to work, the student will perform this skill with _____ % accuracy in a total of _____ minutes. *(Your instructor will tell you what the percentage and time limits will be before you begin.)*

KEY: 4 = Satisfactory 0 = Unsatisfactory NA = This step is not counted

PROCEDURE STEPS	SELF	PARTNER	INSTRUCTOR
1. Wash your hands	❏	❏	❏
2. Obtain the physician order, the correct medication, sterile gauze, and tissues	❏	❏	❏
3. Greet and identify the patient. Identify yourself, including your title. Explain the procedure	❏	❏	❏
4. Ask the patient about any allergies not recorded in the chart	❏	❏	❏
5. **AFF** Explain how to respond to a patient who does not speak English	❏	❏	❏
_____			
_____			
_____			
_____			
6. Position the patient comfortably	❏	❏	❏
7. Put on gloves. Ask the patient to look upward	❏	❏	❏
8. Use gauze to gently pull lower lid down. Instill the medication: **a.** Ointment **b.** Drops	❏	❏	❏
9. Release the lower lid. Have the patient gently close the eyelid and roll the eyes	❏	❏	❏
10. Wipe off any excess medication with tissue	❏	❏	❏
11. Instruct patient to apply light pressure on the puncta lacrimalia for several minutes	❏	❏	❏
12. Properly care for or dispose of equipment and supplies. Clean the work area	❏	❏	❏

PSY PROCEDURE 30-3 **Instilling Eye Medication** (continued)

13. Wash your hands	❏	❏	❏
14. **AFF** Log into the Electronic Medical Record (EMR) using your username and secure password OR obtain the paper medical record from a secure location and assure it is kept away from public access	❏	❏	❏
15. Record the procedure	❏	❏	❏
16. When finished, log out of the EMR and/or replace the paper medical record in an appropriate and secure location	❏	❏	❏

CALCULATION

Total Possible Points: _____

Total Points Earned: _____ Multiplied by 100 = _____ Divided by Total Possible Points = _____ %

PASS   FAIL   COMMENTS:
 ❏   ❏

Student's signature _____ Date _____

Partner's signature _____ Date _____

Instructor's signature _____ Date _____

PSY PROCEDURE 30-4 Irrigating the Eye

Name: _____ **Date:** _____ **Time:** _____ **Grade:** _____

EQUIPMENT/SUPPLIES: Physician's order and patient record, small basin, irrigating solution and medication, if ordered, protective barrier or towels, emesis basin, sterile bulb syringe or 15- to 20-mL syringe, tissues, gloves

STANDARDS: Given the needed equipment and a place to work, the student will perform this skill with _____ % accuracy in a total of _____ minutes. *(Your instructor will tell you what the percentage and time limits will be before you begin.)*

KEY: 4 = Satisfactory 0 = Unsatisfactory NA = This step is not counted

PROCEDURE STEPS	SELF	PARTNER	INSTRUCTOR
1. Wash your hands and put on your gloves	❏	❏	❏
2. Assemble the equipment, supplies, and medication, if ordered by the physician **a.** Check solution label three times **b.** Make sure that the label indicates for ophthalmic use	❏	❏	❏
3. Greet and identify the patient. Identify yourself and your title. Explain the procedure	❏	❏	❏
4. **AFF** Explain how to respond to a patient who is hard of hearing	❏	❏	❏
_____ _____ _____ _____			
5. Position the patient comfortably **a.** Sitting with head tilted with the affected eye lower **b.** Lying with the affected eye downward	❏	❏	❏
6. Drape patient with the protective barrier or towel to avoid wetting the clothing	❏	❏	❏
7. Place basin against upper cheek near eye with the towel under the basin **a.** Wipe the eye from the inner canthus outward with gauze to remove debris **b.** Separate the eyelids with your thumb and forefinger **c.** Lightly support your hand, holding the syringe, on the bridge of the patient's nose	❏	❏	❏
8. Holding syringe 1 inch above the eye, gently irrigate from inner to outer canthus **a.** Use gentle pressure and do not touch the eye **b.** The physician will order the period of time or amount of solution required	❏	❏	❏

9. Use tissues to wipe any excess solution from the patient's face	❏	❏	❏
10. Properly dispose of equipment or sanitize as recommended	❏	❏	❏
11. Remove your gloves. Wash your hands	❏	❏	❏
12. **AFF** Log into the Electronic Medical Record (EMR) using your username and secure password OR obtain the paper medical record from a secure location and assure it is kept away from public access	❏	❏	❏
13. Record procedure, including amount, type, and strength of solution; which eye was irrigated; and any observations	❏	❏	❏
14. When finished, log out of the EMR and/or replace the paper medical record in an appropriate and secure location	❏	❏	❏

PSY PROCEDURE 30-4 Irrigating the Eye (continued)

CALCULATION

Total Possible Points: _____

Total Points Earned: _____ Multiplied by 100 = _____ Divided by Total Possible Points = _____ %

PASS   FAIL   COMMENTS:
❏   ❏

Student's signature _____ Date _____

Partner's signature _____ Date _____

Instructor's signature _____ Date _____

PSY PROCEDURE 30-5 **Irrigating the Ear**

Name: _____ Date: _____ Time: _____ Grade: _____

EQUIPMENT/SUPPLIES: Physician's order and patient record, emesis basin or ear basin, waterproof barrier or towels, otoscope, irrigation solution, bowl for solution, gauze

STANDARDS: Given the needed equipment and a place to work, the student will perform this skill with _____ % accuracy in a total of _____ minutes. *(Your instructor will tell you what the percentage and time limits will be before you begin.)*

KEY: 4 = Satisfactory   0 = Unsatisfactory   NA = This step is not counted

PROCEDURE STEPS	SELF	PARTNER	INSTRUCTOR
1. Wash your hands	❑	❑	❑
2. Assemble the equipment and supplies	❑	❑	❑
3. Greet and identify the patient. Identify yourself, including your title. Explain the procedure	❑	❑	❑
4. **AFF** Explain how to respond to a patient who has dementia	❑	❑	❑
  _____ _____ _____ _____			
5. Position the patient comfortably in an erect position	❑	❑	❑

6. View the affected ear with an otoscope to locate the foreign matter or cerumen
  a. *Adults:* Gently pull up and back to straighten the auditory canal
  b. *Children:* Gently pull slightly down and back to straighten the auditory canal
	❑	❑	❑

7. Drape the patient with a waterproof barrier or towel	❑	❑	❑
8. Tilt the patient's head toward the affected side	❑	❑	❑
9. Place the drainage basin under the affected ear	❑	❑	❑
10. Fill the irrigating syringe or turn on the irrigating device	❑	❑	❑
11. Gently position the auricle as described above using your non-dominant hand	❑	❑	❑
12. With dominant hand, place the tip of the syringe into the auditory meatus	❑	❑	❑
13. Direct the flow of the solution gently upward toward the roof of the canal	❑	❑	❑

PSY P R O C E D U R E 3 0 - 5   **Irrigating the Ear** (continued)

14. Irrigate for the prescribed period of time or until the desired results are obtained	❏	❏	❏
15. Dry the patient's external ear with gauze	❏	❏	❏
16. Inspect the ear with the otoscope to determine the results	❏	❏	❏
17. Properly care for or dispose of equipment and supplies. Clean the work area	❏	❏	❏
18. Wash your hands	❏	❏	❏
19. **AFF** Log into the Electronic Medical Record (EMR) using your username and secure password OR obtain the paper medical record from a secure location and assure it is kept away from public access	❏	❏	❏
20. Record the procedure in the patient's chart	❏	❏	❏
21. When finished, log out of the EMR and/or replace the paper medical record in an appropriate and secure location	❏	❏	❏

CALCULATION

Total Possible Points: _____

Total Points Earned: _____ Multiplied by 100 = _____ Divided by Total Possible Points = _____ %

PASS   **FAIL**   **COMMENTS:**
  ❏   ❏

Student's signature _____ Date _____

Partner's signature _____ Date _____

Instructor's signature _____ Date _____

PSY PROCEDURE 30-6   Perform an Audiometric Hearing Test

Name: _____ Date: _____ Time: _____ Grade: _____

EQUIPMENT/SUPPLIES: Audiometer, otoscope

STANDARDS: Given the needed equipment and a place to work, the student will perform this skill with _____ % accuracy in a total of _____ minutes. *(Your instructor will tell you what the percentage and time limits will be before you begin.)*

KEY: 4 = Satisfactory   0 = Unsatisfactory   NA = This step is not counted

PROCEDURE STEPS	SELF	PARTNER	INSTRUCTOR
1. Wash your hands	❑	❑	❑
2. Greet and identify the patient. Identify yourself and your title. Explain the procedure	❑	❑	❑
3. **AFF** Explain how to respond to a patient who is visually impaired	❑	❑	❑
_____			
_____			
_____			
_____			
4. Take the patient to a quiet area or room for testing	❑	❑	❑
5. Visually inspect the ear canal and tympanic membrane before the examination	❑	❑	❑
6. Choose the correct size tip for the end of the audiometer	❑	❑	❑
7. Attach a speculum to fit the patient's external auditory meatus	❑	❑	❑
8. With the speculum in the ear canal, retract the pinna: **a.** *Adults:* Gently pull up and back to straighten the auditory canal **b.** *Children:* Gently pull slightly down and back to straighten the auditory canal	❑	❑	❑
9. Follow audiometer instrument directions for use: **a.** Screen right ear **b.** Screen left ear	❑	❑	❑
10. If the patient fails to respond at any frequency, rescreening is required	❑	❑	❑
11. If the patient fails rescreening, notify the physician	❑	❑	❑

PSY PROCEDURE 30-6	**Perform an Audiometric Hearing Test** (continued)			
12. AFF Log into the Electronic Medical Record (EMR) using your username and secure password OR obtain the paper medical record from a secure location and assure it is kept away from public access		❏	❏	❏
13. Record the results in the medical record		❏	❏	❏
14. When finished, log out of the EMR and/or replace the paper medical record in an appropriate and secure location		❏	❏	❏

CALCULATION

Total Possible Points: _____

Total Points Earned: _____ Multiplied by 100 = _____ Divided by Total Possible Points = _____ %

PASS   FAIL   COMMENTS:
  ❏   ❏

Student's signature _____   Date _____

Partner's signature _____   Date _____

Instructor's signature _____   Date _____

PSY PROCEDURE 30-7 Instilling Ear Medication

Name: _____ Date: _____ Time: _____ Grade: _____

EQUIPMENT/SUPPLIES: Physician's order and patient record, otic medication with dropper, cotton balls

STANDARDS: Given the needed equipment and a place to work, the student will perform this skill with _____ % accuracy in a total of _____ minutes. *(Your instructor will tell you what the percentage and time limits will be before you begin.)*

KEY: 4 = Satisfactory   0 = Unsatisfactory   NA = This step is not counted

PROCEDURE STEPS	SELF	PARTNER	INSTRUCTOR
1. Wash your hands	❏	❏	❏
2. Assemble the equipment, supplies, and medication if ordered by the physician **a.** Check solution label three times **b.** Make sure that the label indicates for otic use	❏	❏	❏
3. Greet and identify the patient. Identify yourself, including your title. Explain the procedure	❏	❏	❏
4. Ask the patient about any allergies not documented	❏	❏	❏
5. **AFF** Explain how to respond to a patient who does not speak English	❏	❏	❏
_____ _____ _____ _____			
6. Have the patient seated with the affected ear tilted upward	❏	❏	❏
7. Draw up the ordered amount of medication **a.** Adults: Pull the auricle slightly up and back to straighten the S-shaped canal **b.** Children: Pull the auricle slightly down and back to straighten the S-shaped canal	❏	❏	❏
8. Insert the tip of the dropper without touching the patient's skin **a.** Let the medication flow along the side of the canal **b.** Have the patient sit or lie with affected ear upward for approximately 5 minutes	❏	❏	❏
9. To keep medication in the canal, gently insert a moist cotton ball into the external auditory meatus	❏	❏	❏
10. Properly care for or dispose of equipment and supplies. Clean the work area	❏	❏	❏

PSY PROCEDURE 30-7	**Instilling Ear Medication** (continued)			
11. Wash your hands		❏	❏	❏
12. **AFF** Log into the Electronic Medical Record (EMR) using your username and secure password OR obtain the paper medical record from a secure location and assure it is kept away from public access		❏	❏	❏
13. Record the procedure in the patient record		❏	❏	❏
14. When finished, log out of the EMR and/or replace the paper medical record in an appropriate and secure location		❏	❏	❏

CALCULATION

Total Possible Points: _____

Total Points Earned: _____ Multiplied by 100 = _____ Divided by Total Possible Points = _____ %

PASS   FAIL   COMMENTS:
 ❏   ❏

Student's signature _____ Date _____

Partner's signature _____ Date _____

Instructor's signature _____ Date _____

PSY PROCEDURE 30-8 Instilling Nasal Medication

Name: _____ **Date:** _____ **Time:** _____ **Grade:** _____

EQUIPMENT/SUPPLIES: Physician's order and patient record; nasal medication, drops, or spray; tissues; gloves

STANDARDS: Given the needed equipment and a place to work, the student will perform this skill with _____ % accuracy in a total of _____ minutes. *(Your instructor will tell you what the percentage and time limits will be before you begin.)*

KEY: 4 = Satisfactory 0 = Unsatisfactory NA = This step is not counted

PROCEDURE STEPS	SELF	PARTNER	INSTRUCTOR
1. Wash your hands and put on gloves	❏	❏	❏
2. Assemble the equipment and supplies. Check the medication label three times	❏	❏	❏
3. Greet and identify the patient. Identify yourself, including your title. Explain the procedure	❏	❏	❏
4. Ask patient about any allergies not documented	❏	❏	❏
5. **AFF** Explain how to respond to a patient who has dementia	❏	❏	❏

6. Position the patient in a comfortable recumbent position
  a. Extend the patient's head beyond the edge of the examination table
  b. Or place a pillow under the patient's shoulders
  c. Support the patient's neck to avoid strain as the head is tilted back
	❏	❏	❏

7. Administering nasal medication:
  a. Nasal drops
    (1) Hold the dropper upright just above each nostril
    (2) Drop the medication one drop at a time without touching the nares
    (3) Keep the patient in a recumbent position for 5 minutes
  b. Nasal spray
    (1) Place tip of the bottle at the naris opening without touching the patient
    (2) Spray as the patient takes a deep breath
	❏	❏	❏

8. Wipe any excess medication from the patient's skin with tissues	❏	❏	❏

PSY PROCEDURE 30-8 **Instilling Nasal Medication** (continued)

9. Properly care for or dispose of equipment and supplies. Clean the work area	❏	❏	❏
10. Remove your gloves and wash your hands	❏	❏	❏
11. **AFF** Log into the Electronic Medical Record (EMR) using your username and secure password OR obtain the paper medical record from a secure location and assure it is kept away from public access	❏	❏	❏
12. Record the procedure in the patient's chart	❏	❏	❏
13. When finished, log out of the EMR and/or replace the paper medical record in an appropriate and secure location	❏	❏	❏

CALCULATION

Total Possible Points: _____

Total Points Earned: _____ Multiplied by 100 = _____ Divided by Total Possible Points = _____ %

PASS **FAIL** **COMMENTS:**
❏ ❏

Student's signature _____ Date _____

Partner's signature _____ Date _____

Instructor's signature _____ Date _____

CHAPTER 31

Pulmonary Medicine

LEARNING OUTCOMES

COG Cognitive Domain*

1. Spell key terms
2. *Identify the following related to body systems:*
   a. *Medical terms*
   b. *Abbreviations*
3. *Identify structural organization of the human body*
4. *Identify major organs in each body system*
5. *Identify the anatomical location of major organs in each body system*
6. *Identify the normal function of each body system*
7. *Identify common pathology related to each body system including*
   a. *Signs*
   b. *Symptoms*
   c. *Etiology*
   d. *Diagnostic measures*
   e. *Treatment modalities*
8. Discuss the role of the medical assistant with regard to various diagnostic and therapeutic procedures

PSY Psychomotor Domain*

1. Instruct a patient in the use of the peak flow meter (Procedure 31-1)
   a. *Instruct and prepare a patient for a procedure or treatment*
   b. *Assist provider with a patient exam*
   c. *Document patient care accurately in the medical record*
2. Administer a nebulized breathing treatment (Procedure 31-2)
   a. *Instruct and prepare a patient for a procedure or treatment*

b. *Assist provider with a patient exam*
c. *Document patient care accurately in the medical record*
3. Collecting a Sputum Specimen (Procedure 31-3)
   a. *Instruct and prepare a patient for a procedure or treatment*
   b. *Assist provider with a patient exam*
   c. *Document patient care accurately in the medical record*
4. Perform a pulmonary function test (Procedure 31-4)
   a. *Instruct and prepare a patient for a procedure or treatment*
   b. *Assist provider with a patient exam*
   c. *Document patient care accurately in the medical record*

AFF Affective Domain*

1. *Demonstrate critical thinking skills*
2. *Reassure patients*
3. *Demonstrate empathy for patients' concerns*
4. *Demonstrate active listening*
5. *Respect diversity*
6. *Recognize personal boundaries*
7. *Demonstrate tactfulness*
8. *Demonstrate self-awareness*
9. Protect the integrity of the medical record

MAERB Standards are Italicized.

ABHES Competencies

1. List all body systems and their structures and functions
2. Describe common diseases, symptoms, and etiology as they apply to each system
3. Identify diagnostic and treatment modalities as they relate to each body system
4. Apply medical terminology for each specialty
5. Follow documentation guidelines
6. Adapt care to address the developmental stages of life
7. Partner with healthcare teams to attain optimal patient health outcomes
8. Display effective interpersonal skills with patients and healthcare team members
9. Demonstrate cultural awareness
10. Assist provider with specialty examinations, including cardiac, respiratory, OB-GYN, neurologic, and gastroenterology
11. Perform specialty procedures, including but not limited to minor surgery, cardiac, respiratory, OB-GYN, neurologic, and gastroenterology
12. Make adaptations for patients with special needs (psychological or physical limitations)
13. Make adaptations to care for patients across their lifespan

© YASMARADA/Shutterstock

Name: _____   Date: _____   Grade: _____

⚙️OG MULTIPLE CHOICE

Circle the letter preceding the correct answer.

1. A pulmonary function test measures:
   a. arterial blood gases.
   b. oxygen saturation.
   c. sputum cells.
   d. tidal volume.
   e. fluid in the lungs.

2. A patient in need of an artificial airway will likely undergo:
   a. laryngectomy.
   b. tracheostomy.
   c. chemotherapy.
   d. bronchoscopy.
   e. pneumonectomy.

3. Which procedure necessitates a stethoscope?
   a. Percussion
   b. Palpation
   c. Inspection
   d. Radiation
   e. Auscultation

4. Which of the following would be a normal pulse oximetry reading for someone with no lung disease?
   a. 96%
   b. 94%
   c. 92%
   d. 90%
   e. 88%

5. One lower respiratory disorder is:
   a. laryngitis.
   b. bronchitis.
   c. sinusitis.
   d. pharyngitis.
   e. tonsillitis.

6. Which of the following is anesthetized by cigarette smoke?
   a. Alveoli
   b. Bronchioles
   c. Mucus
   d. Cilia
   e. Trachea

7. The most prominent symptom of bronchitis is:
   a. severe wheezing.
   b. repeated sneezing.
   c. productive cough.
   d. shortness of breath.
   e. coughing blood.

8. Viral pneumonia differs from bacterial pneumonia in that:
   a. it can be treated by antibiotics.
   b. it might result in hospitalization.
   c. it affects gas exchange in the lungs.
   d. it may lead to a fever and cough.
   e. it spreads throughout the lungs.

9. People with asthma have difficulty breathing because their:
   a. airways are narrow.
   b. cilia are inoperative.
   c. alveoli are collapsed.
   d. bronchioles are too wide.
   e. lungs are underdeveloped.

10. A productive cough refers to a cough that produces:
    a. blood.
    b. nasal mucus.
    c. sputum.
    d. oxygen.
    e. antibodies.

11. A type of medication that opens the bronchioles and controls bronchospasms is a(n):
    a. corticosteroid.
    b. bronchodilator.
    c. antibiotic.
    d. antihistamine.
    e. decongestant.

12. The public health department should be alerted about a diagnosis of:
    a. tuberculosis.
    b. pneumonia.
    c. bronchitis.
    d. asthma.
    e. COPD.

13. Which of the following is true of emphysema?
    a. It is not associated with bronchitis
    b. It causes inflammation of the nasal passages
    c. It can be cured with steroids
    d. It is usually reversible
    e. It usually takes many years to develop

14. The purpose of a nebulizer is to:
    a. turn a vaporous medicine into a liquid.
    b. administer an asthma treatment.
    c. turn a liquid medicine into a vapor.
    d. cure COPD.
    e. pump oxygen.

15. Of the following diseases affecting the respiratory system, which, in most cases, is linked to cigarette smoking?
- **a.** Liver cancer
- **b.** Cystic fibrosis
- **c.** Laryngitis
- **d.** Lung cancer
- **e.** Allergic rhinitis

16. In the case of a patient receiving oxygen treatment, a cannula:
- **a.** stores the oxygen.
- **b.** separates oxygen from the air in a room.
- **c.** delivers oxygen to the airways.
- **d.** ensures proper flow of oxygen.
- **e.** prevents accidents caused by oxygen's flammability.

17. COPD patients may take medications that are also prescribed for patients with:
- **a.** influenza.
- **b.** pneumonia.
- **c.** meningitis.
- **d.** lung cancer.
- **e.** asthma.

18. One acute disease of the lower respiratory tract is:
- **a.** asthma.
- **b.** pneumonia.
- **c.** emphysema.
- **d.** sinusitis.
- **e.** COPD.

19. The best way to thin mucus in the airways is:
- **a.** oxygen therapy.
- **b.** steroid medication.
- **c.** to increase oral fluid intake.
- **d.** to consume a balanced diet.
- **e.** frequent exercise.

20. A physician may perform an arterial blood gas test to:
- **a.** determine how much gas is in a patient's lungs.
- **b.** determine whether a patient has a normal respiratory rate.
- **c.** determine when a patient will be ready for respiratory surgery.
- **d.** determine whether a patient will be receptive to oxygen therapy.
- **e.** determine whether the patient's lungs are adequately exchanging gases.

COG MATCHING

Place the letter preceding the definition on the line next to the term.

Key Terms

21. _____ atelectasis
22. _____ chronic obstructive
          pulmonary disease (COPD)
23. _____ dyspnea
24. _____ forced expiratory volume
          (FEV)
25. _____ hemoptysis
26. _____ laryngectomy
27. _____ palliative
28. _____ status asthmaticus
29. _____ thoracentesis
30. _____ tidal volume
31. _____ tracheostomy

Definitions

a. coughing up blood from the respiratory tract
b. easing symptoms without curing
c. a permanent surgical stoma in the neck with an indwelling tube
d. a surgical puncture into the pleural cavity for aspiration of serous fluid or for injection of medication
e. a progressive, irreversible condition with diminished respiratory capacity
f. the volume of air forced out of the lungs
g. difficulty breathing
h. the amount of air inhaled and exhaled during normal respiration
i. an asthma attack that is not responsive to treatment
j. collapsed lung fields; incomplete expansion of the lungs, either partial or complete
k. the surgical removal of the larynx

COG IDENTIFICATION

32. Place a check mark on the line to indicate if each symptom is a possible symptom of laryngeal cancer.

a. _____ hoarseness lasting longer than 3 weeks

b. _____ pain in the throat when drinking hot liquids

c. _____ wheezing

d. _____ a feeling of a lump in the throat

e. _____ chest pain

f. _____ burning in the throat when drinking citrus juice

g. _____ dyspnea

h. _____ night sweats

i. _____ general malaise

33. Which of the following is/are an element/elements of the traditional examination of the chest? Circle the letter preceding all that apply.

a. Palpation

b. Auscultation

c. Sputum culture

d. Chest radiography

e. Inspection

34. Which of the following pulmonary diagnostic methods is considered invasive? Place a check mark on the line next to the appropriate diagnostic methods.

a. _____ Percussion

b. _____ Bronchoscopy

c. _____ Auscultation

d. _____ Sputum culture

e. _____ Posteroanterior x-ray

COG SHORT ANSWER

Grade: _____

35. What is the most common cause of chronic obstructive pulmonary disease?

_____

_____

_____

_____

36. Why is the term _chronic obstructive pulmonary disease_ used to characterize a patient suffering from emphysema and chronic bronchitis?

_____

_____

_____

_____

37. What are two of the most common causes of upper respiratory problems?

_____

_____

_____

_____

38. In the case of a pneumonia patient, what prevents effective gas exchange?

_____

_____

_____

_____

39. What is usually the etiology of chronic bronchitis?

_____

_____

_____

_____

40. What is a symptomatic difference between viral and bacterial pneumonia?

_____

_____

_____

_____

41. What is the role of the medical assistant in the collection and analysis of a sputum specimen?

_____

_____

_____

_____

42. What is the purpose of a peak flow meter?

_____

_____

_____

_____

43. Under what circumstance would a physician perform a laryngectomy?

_____

_____

_____

_____

44. Describe the difference between palliative care and a cure.

_____

_____

_____

_____

45. What measures ought to be taken in the case of an asthmatic patient who does not respond to medication?

_____

_____

_____

_____

46. If a patient is prescribed two bronchodilator inhalers, what is the most likely explanation? Why would two be prescribed?

_____

_____

_____

_____

47. Describe the typical prognosis of a lung cancer patient.

_____

_____

_____

_____

COG TRUE OR FALSE?

Grade: _____

Indicate whether the statements are true or false by placing the letter T (true) or F (false) on the line preceding the statement.

48. _____ An asthma patient will, upon contracting the disease, suffer from it for their entire life.

49. _____ Emphysema entails chronic inflammation of the airways.

50. _____ A patient who tests positive for tuberculosis is contagious.

51. _____ Lung cancer, one of the most common causes of death in men and women, is believed to result usually from cigarette smoking.

COG AFF CASE STUDIES FOR CRITICAL THINKING

Grade: _____

52. Your patient comes to the office with shortness of breath. The physician asks you to perform an arterial blood gas test and send it to the laboratory stat. How would you respond to the physician?

_____

_____

_____

_____

53. A patient with a severe lung disease explains that she has been smoking for decades. You explain that she ought to quit, but she contends that it does not matter. She says she has already damaged her lungs enough that continuing to smoke will do no further harm. How do you respond to this patient?

_____

_____

_____

_____

54. A patient receiving oxygen therapy calls to complain that his machine is not working. He does not know what to do. What suggestions do you have for the patient? What will you do to assist him?

_____

_____

_____

_____

55. Your patient has just been diagnosed with tuberculosis. Explain to him ways in which he should act to protect others while he undergoes treatment.

_____

_____

_____

_____

56. A healthy patient worries that his exposure to the secondhand smoke of his coworkers might cause his health to deteriorate. You are aware of research suggesting that this is so; however, much of the research is controversial. How would you advise the patient?

_____

_____

_____

_____

57. A patient has just been diagnosed with lung cancer that the physician described as "not terribly aggressive and potentially curable." The patient asks you if this means that he will be okay. How do you respond?

_____

_____

_____

_____

PSY PROCEDURE 31-1	**Instruct a Patient on Using the Peak Flow Meter**	

Name: _____ Date: _____ Time: _____ Grade: _____

EQUIPMENT/SUPPLIES: Peak flow meter, recording documentation form

STANDARDS: Given the needed equipment and a place to work, the student will perform this skill with _____ % accuracy in a total of _____ minutes. *(Your instructor will tell you what the percentage and time limits will be before you begin.)*

KEY: 4 = Satisfactory   0 = Unsatisfactory   NA = This step is not counted

PROCEDURE STEPS	SELF	PARTNER	INSTRUCTOR
1. Wash your hands	❏	❏	❏
2. Assemble the peak flow meter, disposable mouthpiece, and patient documentation form	❏	❏	❏
3. Greet and identify the patient. Identify yourself, including your title, and explain the procedure	❏	❏	❏
4. Holding the peak flow meter upright, explain how to read and reset the gauge after each reading	❏	❏	❏
5. **AFF** Explain how to respond to a patient who is visually impaired	❏	❏	❏
_____ _____ _____ _____			
6. Instruct the patient to place the peak flow meter mouthpiece into the mouth, forming a tight seal with the lips. After taking a deep breath, the patient should blow hard into the mouthpiece without blocking the back of the flow meter	❏	❏	❏
7. Note the number on the flow meter denoting the level at which the sliding gauge stopped after the hard blowing into the mouthpiece. Reset the gauge to zero	❏	❏	❏
8. Instruct the patient to perform this procedure a total of three times consecutively, in both the morning and at night, and to record the highest reading on the form	❏	❏	❏
9. Explain to the patient the procedure for cleaning the mouthpiece of the flow meter by washing with soapy water and rinsing without immersing the flow meter in water	❏	❏	❏

(continues)

PSY PROCEDURE 31-1   Instruct a Patient on Using the Peak Flow Meter (continued)

10. AFF Log into the Electronic Medical Record (EMR) using your username and secure password OR obtain the paper medical record from a secure location and assure it is kept away from public access	❏	❏	❏
11. Record the procedure, including the name of the medication and the patient's response	❏	❏	❏
12. When finished, log out of the EMR and/or replace the paper medical record in an appropriate and secure location	❏	❏	❏

CALCULATION

Total Possible Points: _____

Total Points Earned: _____ Multiplied by 100 = _____ Divided by Total Possible Points = _____ %

PASS   FAIL   COMMENTS:
❏   ❏

Student's signature _____ Date _____

Partner's signature _____ Date _____

Instructor's signature _____ Date _____

PSY PROCEDURE 31-2 | **Perform a Nebulized Breathing Treatment**

Name: _____ Date: _____ Time: _____ Grade: _____

EQUIPMENT/SUPPLIES: Physician's order and patient's medical record, inhalation medication, nebulizer disposable setup, nebulizer machine

STANDARDS: Given the needed equipment and a place to work, the student will perform this skill with _____ % accuracy in a total of _____ minutes. *(Your instructor will tell you what the percentage and time limits will be before you begin.)*

KEY: 4 = Satisfactory　　　0 = Unsatisfactory　　　NA = This step is not counted

PROCEDURE STEPS	SELF	PARTNER	INSTRUCTOR
1. Wash your hands	❏	❏	❏
2. Assemble the equipment and medication, checking the medication label three times as indicated when administering any medications	❏	❏	❏
3. Greet and identify the patient. Identify yourself, including your title, and explain the procedure	❏	❏	❏
4. **AFF** Explain how you would respond to a patient who is deaf	❏	❏	❏
_____ _____ _____ _____			
5. Remove the nebulizer treatment cup from the setup and add the medication ordered by the physician	❏	❏	❏
6. Place the top on the cup securely, attach the "T" piece to the top of the cup, and position the mouthpiece firmly on one end of the "T" piece	❏	❏	❏
7. Attach one end of the tubing securely to the connector on the cup and the other end to the connector on the nebulizer machine	❏	❏	❏
8. Ask the patient to place the mouthpiece into the mouth and make a seal with the lips, without biting the mouthpiece. Instruct the patient to breathe normally during the treatment, occasionally taking a deep breath	❏	❏	❏
9. Turn the machine on using the on/off switch. The medication in the reservoir cup will become a fine mist that is inhaled by the patient breathing through the mouthpiece	❏	❏	❏

(continues)

PSY PROCEDURE 31-2   **Perform a Nebulized Breathing Treatment** (continued)

10. Before, during, and after the breathing treatment, take and record the patient's pulse	❏	❏	❏
11. When the treatment is over and the medication is gone from the cup, turn the machine off and have the patient remove the mouthpiece	❏	❏	❏
12. Disconnect the disposable treatment setup and dispose of all parts into a biohazard container. Put away the machine properly	❏	❏	❏
13. Wash your hands	❏	❏	❏
14. **AFF** Log into the Electronic Medical Record (EMR) using your username and secure password OR obtain the paper medical record from a secure location and assure it is kept away from public access	❏	❏	❏
15. Record the procedure, including the name of the medication and the patient's pulse before, during, and after the treatment	❏	❏	❏
16. When finished, log out of the EMR and/or replace the paper medical record in an appropriate and secure location	❏	❏	❏

CALCULATION

Total Possible Points: _____

Total Points Earned: _____ Multiplied by 100 = _____ Divided by Total Possible Points = _____ %

PASS   FAIL   COMMENTS:
  ❏   ❏

Student's signature _____ Date _____

Partner's signature _____ Date _____

Instructor's signature _____ Date _____

PSY PROCEDURE 31-3 Collect a Sputum Specimen

Name: _____ Date: _____ Time: _____ Grade: _____

EQUIPMENT/SUPPLIES: Physician order, patient's medical record, sterile specimen container, gloves, biohazard transport bag, laboratory request

STANDARDS: Given the needed equipment and a place to work, the student will perform this skill with _____ % accuracy in a total of _____ minutes. *(Your instructor will tell you what the percentage and time limits will be before you begin.)*

KEY: 4 = Satisfactory 0 = Unsatisfactory NA = This step is not counted

PROCEDURE STEPS	SELF	PARTNER	INSTRUCTOR
1. Wash your hands	❑	❑	❑
2. Assemble the equipment	❑	❑	❑
3. Greet and identify the patient. Identify yourself, including your title, and explain the procedure	❑	❑	❑
4. **AFF** Explain how to respond to a patient whose first language is not English	❑	❑	❑
_____ _____ _____ _____			
5. Provide the patient with a cup of water and instruct them to rinse their mouth with water	❑	❑	❑
6. Ask the patient to cough deeply, using the abdominal muscles as well as the accessory muscles to bring secretions from the lungs and not just the upper airway	❑	❑	❑
7. Instruct the patient to expectorate the specimen directly into the container without touching the inside of the container with the lips or tongue and without getting the specimen on the outside of the container	❑	❑	❑
8. When the specimen is in the container, apply gloves and after taking the container from the patient, cap the container immediately and place into a biohazard bag for transport to the laboratory with a laboratory requisition	❑	❑	❑
9. Once the specimen has been routed to the laboratory, remove your gloves and wash your hands	❑	❑	❑

(continues)

PSY PROCEDURE 31-3 **Collect a Sputum Specimen** (continued)

10. **AFF** Log into the Electronic Medical Record (EMR) using your username and secure password OR obtain the paper medical record from a secure location and assure it is kept away from public access	❏	❏	❏
11. Record the procedure, including the name of the medication and the patient's pulse before, during, and after the treatment	❏	❏	❏
12. When finished, log out of the EMR and/or replace the paper medical record in an appropriate and secure location	❏	❏	❏

CALCULATION

Total Possible Points: _____

Total Points Earned: _____ Multiplied by 100 = _____ Divided by Total Possible Points = _____ %

PASS **FAIL** **COMMENTS:**
❏ ❏

Student's signature _____ Date _____

Partner's signature _____ Date _____

Instructor's signature _____ Date _____

PSY PROCEDURE 31-4 | Perform a Pulmonary Function Test

Name: _____ Date: _____ Time: _____ Grade: _____

EQUIPMENT/SUPPLIES: Physician's order and patient's medical record, spirometer and appropriate cables, calibration syringe and log book, disposable mouthpiece, printer, nose clip

STANDARDS: Given the needed equipment and a place to work, the student will perform this skill with _____ % accuracy in a total of _____ minutes. *(Your instructor will tell you what the percentage and time limits will be before you begin.)*

KEY: 4 = Satisfactory   0 = Unsatisfactory   NA = This step is not counted

PROCEDURE STEPS	SELF	PARTNER	INSTRUCTOR
1. Wash your hands	❏	❏	❏
2. Assemble the equipment	❏	❏	❏
3. Greet and identify the patient. Identify yourself, including your title, and explain the procedure	❏	❏	❏
4. **AFF** Explain how to respond to a patient who has dementia	❏	❏	❏
5. Turn the PFT machine on, and if the spirometer has not been calibrated according to the office policy, calibrate the machine using the calibration syringe according to the manufacturer's instructions and record the calibration in the appropriate logbook	❏	❏	❏
6. With the machine on and calibrated, attach the appropriate cable, tubing, and mouthpiece for the type of machine being used	❏	❏	❏
7. Using the keyboard on the machine, input patient data into the machine including the patient's name or identification number, age, weight, height, sex, race, and smoking history	❏	❏	❏
8. Ask the patient to remove any restrictive clothing, such as a necktie, and instruct the patient in applying the nose clip	❏	❏	❏
9. Ask the patient to stand, breathe in deeply, and blow into the mouthpiece as hard as possible. They should continue to blow into the mouthpiece until the machine indicates that it is appropriate to stop blowing. A chair should be available in case the patient becomes dizzy or lightheaded	❏	❏	❏
10. Continue the procedure until three adequate readings or maneuvers are performed	❏	❏	❏
11. Properly care for the equipment and dispose of the mouthpiece into the biohazard container	❏	❏	❏
12. Wash your hands	❏	❏	❏

(continues)

PSY PROCEDURE 31-4 **Perform a Pulmonary Function Test** (continued)

13. **AFF** Log into the Electronic Medical Record (EMR) using your username and secure password OR obtain the paper medical record from a secure location and assure it is kept away from public access	❏	❏	❏
14. Record the procedure including the patient's response	❏	❏	❏
15. Print and/or scan the results and place in the medical record	❏	❏	❏
16. When finished, log out of the EMR and/or replace the paper medical record in an appropriate and a secure location	❏	❏	❏

CALCULATION

Total Possible Points: _____

Total Points Earned: _____ Multiplied by 100 = _____ Divided by Total Possible Points = _____ %

PASS **FAIL** **COMMENTS:**
❏ ❏

Student's signature _____ Date _____

Partner's signature _____ Date _____

Instructor's signature _____ Date _____

CHAPTER 32

Cardiology

LEARNING OUTCOMES

COG Cognitive Domain*

1. Spell key terms
2. *Identify the following related to body systems:*
   a. *Medical terms*
   b. *Abbreviations*
3. *Identify the structural organization of the human body*
4. *Identify major organs in each body system*
5. *Identify the anatomical location of major organs in each body system*
6. *Identify the normal function of each body system*
7. *Identify common pathology related to each body system including:*
   a. *Signs*
   b. *Symptoms*
   c. *Etiology*
   d. *Diagnostic measures*
   e. *Treatment modalities*
8. Describe the roles and responsibilities of the medical assistant during cardiovascular examinations and procedures
9. Discuss the information recorded on a basic 12-lead electrocardiogram
10. Explain the purpose of a Holter monitor

PSY Psychomotor Domain*

1. Perform electrocardiography (Procedure 32-1)
   a. *Instruct and prepare a patient for a procedure or treatment*
   b. *Assist provider with a patient exam*
   c. *Document patient care accurately in the medical record*
2. Apply a Holter monitor for a 24-hour test (Procedure 32-2)
   a. *Instruct and prepare a patient for a procedure or treatment*
   b. *Assist provider with a patient exam*
   c. *Document patient care accurately in the medical record*

AFF Affective Domain*

1. *Demonstrate critical thinking skills*
2. *Reassure patients*
3. *Demonstrate empathy for patients' concerns*
4. *Demonstrate active listening*
5. *Respect diversity*
6. *Recognize personal boundaries*
7. *Demonstrate tactfulness*
8. *Demonstrate self-awareness*
9. *Protect the integrity of the medical record*

MAERB Standards are Italicized.

ABHES Competencies

1. List all body systems and their structures and functions
2. Describe common diseases, symptoms, and etiology as they apply to each system
3. Identify diagnostic and treatment modalities as they relate to each body system
4. Apply medical terminology for each specialty
5. Follow documentation guidelines
6. Adapt care to address the developmental stages of life
7. Partner with healthcare teams to attain optimal patient health outcomes
8. Display effective interpersonal skills with patients and healthcare team members
9. Demonstrate cultural awareness
10. Assist provider with specialty examinations, including cardiac, respiratory, OB-GYN, neurologic, and gastroenterology
11. Perform specialty procedures, including but not limited to minor surgery, cardiac, respiratory, OB-GYN, neurologic, and gastroenterology
12. Make adaptations for patients with special needs (psychological or physical limitations)
13. Make adaptations to care for patients across their lifespan

Name: _____   Date: _____   Grade: _____

OOG MULTIPLE CHOICE

Circle the letter preceding the correct answer.

1. Chronic cases of myocarditis may lead to heart failure with:
   a. endocarditis.
   b. cardiomegaly.
   c. asthma.
   d. bronchitis.
   e. congestive heart failure.

2. To identify the causative agent, proper diagnosis of endocarditis requires a(n):
   a. chest radiograph.
   b. blood culture.
   c. electrocardiogram.
   d. x-ray.
   e. stool sample.

3. Arrhythmia may occur if the sinoatrial node initiates electrical impulses:
   a. too quietly or too loudly.
   b. too roughly or too smoothly.
   c. too fast or too slowly.
   d. always.
   e. 60 to 100 times a minute.

4. When a patient's heart conduction system cannot maintain normal sinus rhythm without assistance, an electrical source can be implanted to assist or replace the sinoatrial node. This device is called a(n):
   a. pacemaker.
   b. artifact.
   c. Holter monitor.
   d. aneurysm.
   e. lead.

5. Which condition may result from rheumatic heart disease?
   a. Valvular disease
   b. Cardiac arrhythmia
   c. Angina pectoris
   d. Mitral valve stenosis
   e. Endocarditis

6. One symptom of coronary artery disease is:
   a. bleeding around the heart.
   b. chronic head cold.
   c. swollen tongue.
   d. pressure or fullness in the chest.
   e. leg pain.

7. Patients who are considered hypertensive have a resting systolic blood pressure above _____ and a diastolic pressure above _____.
   a. 120 mm Hg; 70 mm Hg
   b. 130 mm Hg; 80 mm Hg
   c. 140 mm Hg; 90 mm Hg
   d. 150 mm Hg; 100 mm Hg
   e. 160 mm Hg; 110 mm Hg

8. Who is predisposed to varicose veins?
   a. People who use their brains more than their bodies
   b. People who run or jog excessively
   c. People who sit or stand for long periods of time without moving
   d. People who are obese over many years
   e. People who play a musical instrument

9. Another term for *thrombi* is:
   a. heart attack.
   b. blood clots.
   c. fever.
   d. racing heart.
   e. stroke.

10. Patients may refer to *anticoagulant medications* as:
    a. antipyretics.
    b. thrombolytics.
    c. sugar pills.
    d. thickening agents.
    e. blood thinners.

11. A common cause of cerebrovascular accident is:
    a. damage to the blood vessels in the heart.
    b. blockage of the cerebral artery by a thrombus.
    c. weakness or paralysis.
    d. pulmonary embolism.
    e. pleuritic chest pain.

12. Another term for *transient ischemic attack* is:
    a. peripheral vascular occlusion.
    b. mini-stroke.
    c. heart attack.
    d. brain damage.
    e. slurred speech.

13. Deficiencies in hemoglobin or in the numbers of red blood cells result in:
  a. tachycardia.
  b. thrombus.
  c. stroke.
  d. anemia.
  e. aneurysm.

14. During the physician's examination, what is used to evaluate the efficiency of the circulatory pathways and peripheral pulses?
  a. Palpation
  b. Blood pressure
  c. Weight
  d. Height
  e. Sign of fever

15. Electrocardiograms are not used to detect:
  a. ischemia.
  b. delays in impulse conduction.
  c. hypertrophy of the cardiac chambers.
  d. arrhythmias.
  e. heart murmurs.

16. How many leads does the standard ECG have?
  a. 2
  b. 10
  c. 12
  d. 18
  e. 20

17. A patient must keep a daily diary of activities when:
  a. wearing a Holter monitor.
  b. preparing for a cardiac examination.
  c. having an ECG.
  d. taking anticoagulants.
  e. completing a cardiac stress test.

18. Many patients with CHF have an enlarged:
  a. chest.
  b. throat.
  c. lung.
  d. heart.
  e. brain.

19. A person who can read and perform ECGs is called a(n):
  a. medical assistant.
  b. phlebotomist.
  c. ultrasonographer.
  d. sound technician.
  e. neurologist.

20. If atherosclerotic plaques are found during a catheterization, which procedure may be performed?
  a. Bypass graft
  b. Angioplasty
  c. Echocardiogram
  d. ECG
  e. Ultrasonograph

ⓒⓞⓖ MATCHING

Place the letter preceding the definition on the line next to the term.

Key Terms

21. _____ aneurysm
22. _____ angina pectoris
23. _____ artifact
24. _____ atherosclerosis
25. _____ bradycardia
26. _____ cardiomegaly
27. _____ cardiomyopathy
28. _____ cerebrovascular accident (CVA)
29. _____ congestive heart failure
30. _____ electrocardiography
31. _____ coronary artery bypass graft
32. _____ endocarditis
33. _____ leads
34. _____ myocardial infarction (MI)
35. _____ myocarditis
36. _____ palpitations
37. _____ percutaneous transluminal coronary angioplasty (PTCA)
38. _____ pericarditis
39. _____ tachycardia
40. _____ transient ischemic attack (TIA)

Definitions

a. a heart rate of less than 60 beats per minute
b. any disease affecting the myocardium
c. a surgical procedure that increases the blood flow to the heart by bypassing the occluded or blocked vessel with a graft
d. any activity recorded in an electrocardiogram caused by extraneous activity such as patient movement, loose lead, or electrical interference
e. a procedure that improves blood flow through a coronary artery by pressing the plaque against the wall of an artery with a balloon on a catheter, allowing for more blood flow
f. an inflammation of the inner lining of the heart
g. a death of cardiac muscle due to lack of blood flow to the muscle; also known as a heart attack
h. a local dilation in a blood vessel wall
i. a heart rate of more than 100 beats per minute
j. an acute episode of cerebrovascular insufficiency, usually a result of narrowing of an artery by atherosclerotic plaques, emboli, or vasospasm; usually passes quickly, but should be considered a warning for predisposition to cerebrovascular accidents
k. electrodes or electrical connections attached to the body to record electrical impulses in the body, especially the heart or brain
l. paroxysmal chest pain usually caused by a decrease in blood flow to the heart muscle due to coronary occlusion
m. ischemia of the brain due to an occlusion of the blood vessels supplying blood to the brain, resulting in varying degrees of debilitation
n. a buildup of fatty plaque on the interior lining of arteries
o. the feeling of an increased heart rate or pounding heart that may be felt during an emotional response or a cardiac disorder
p. a condition in which the heart cannot pump effectively
q. an inflammation of the sac that covers the heart
r. a procedure that produces a record of the electrical activity of the heart
s. an enlarged heart muscle
t. an inflammation of the myocardial layer of the heart

ⓒⓞⓖ MATCHING

Place the letter preceding the description on the line preceding the cardiac condition.

Conditions

41. _____ congestive heart failure
42. _____ myocardial infarction
43. _____ ventricular tachycardia
44. _____ defibrillation
45. _____ arrhythmia

Descriptions

a. electrical signals originate from cells in the ventricles very rapidly
b. a shock administered to restore normal cardiac electrical activity
c. symptoms may be similar to those felt during angina pectoris
d. occurs if the SA node initiates electrical impulses too quickly or too slowly or the electrical signal originates from somewhere other than the SA node
e. failure of the left ventricle leads to pulmonary congestion

COG **MATCHING**

_____ Grade: _____

Place the letter preceding the description on the line preceding the cardiac procedure.

Procedures
46. _____ electrocardiogram
47. _____ chest radiography
48. _____ cardiac stress test
49. _____ echocardiography
50. _____ cardiac catheterization

Descriptions
a. provides valuable information about the anatomical location and gross structures of the heart, great vessels, and lungs
b. uses sound waves generated by a small device called a transducer
c. a graphic record of the electrical current as it progresses through the heart
d. common invasive procedure used to help diagnose or treat conditions affecting coronary arterial circulation
e. measures the response of the cardiac muscle to increased demands for oxygen

COG **IDENTIFICATION**

_____ Grade: _____

51. Cardiac inflammation, or carditis, is a disorder of the heart that is usually the result of infection. In the chart below are descriptions of the three types of carditis. Read the descriptions and fill in the missing boxes with the correct type of carditis.

Disorder	Causes	Signs and Symptoms	Treatment
a. _____	a pathogen, neoplasm, or autoimmune disorder, such as lupus erythematosus or rheumatoid arthritis	sharp pain in the same locations as myocardial infarction	relieving the symptoms and, if possible, correcting the underlying cause, including administering an antibiotic for bacterial infection
b. _____	radiation, chemicals, and bacterial, viral, or parasitic infection	early signs: fever, fatigue, and mild chest pain chronic: cardiomegaly, arrhythmias, valvulitis	supportive care and medication as ordered by the physician to kill the responsible pathogen
c. _____	infection or inflammation of the inner lining of the heart, the endocardium	reflux, or backflow, of the valves or blood	directed at eliminating the infecting organism

Identify and circle the letter preceding the best answer.

52. Valvular disease is:

a. inflammatory lesions of the connective tissues, particularly in the heart joints, and subcutaneous tissues.

b. an acquired or congenital abnormality of any of the four cardiac valves.

c. a collection of fatty plaques made of calcium and cholesterol inside the walls of blood vessels.

d. a disordered blood flow within the valvular walls of the heart.

53. Atherosclerosis can sometimes result in:

a. rheumatic heart disease.

b. valvular disease.

c. coronary artery disease.

d. congestive heart failure.

54. Cerebrovascular accident (CVA) is sometimes called:

    a. heart attack.

    b. paralysis.

    c. blood clot.

    d. stroke.

55. Which of the following is a question you should ask the patient before a cardiovascular examination?

    a. Are you currently pregnant?

    b. How long have you had the pain/discomfort?

    c. How often do you exercise?

    d. What do you like to do in your free time?

56. A Holter monitor is used for:

    a. the diagnosis of intermittent cardiac arrhythmias and dysfunctions.

    b. obtaining a good-quality ECG without avoidable artifacts.

    c. obtaining basic information about the anatomical location and gross structures of the heart, great vessels, and lungs.

    d. measuring the response of the cardiac muscle to increased demands for oxygen.

57. Read the risk factors for developing thrombi below and indicate whether the risk factor is primary (P), or inherited, versus secondary (S), or acquired.

    a. _____ hemolytic anemia

    b. _____ long-term immobility

    c. _____ chronic pulmonary disease

    d. _____ thrombophlebitis

    e. _____ sickle cell disease

    f. _____ varicosities

    g. _____ defibrillation after cardiac arrest

58. Identify whether each description describes lead I, lead II, or lead III:

    a. _____ measures the difference in electrical potential between the right arm (RA) and the left leg (LL).

    b. _____ measures the difference in electrical potential between the right arm (RA) and the left arm (LA).

    c. _____ measures the difference in electrical potential between the left arm (LA) and the left leg (LL).

COG SHORT ANSWER _____ Grade: _____

59. List five symptoms of the various heart disorders.

_____

_____

_____

_____

60. List the four causes of congestive heart failure.

_____

_____

_____

_____

61. Explain how a pacemaker helps the heart maintain normal sinus rhythm.

_____

_____

_____

_____

62. List six potential causes of anemia.

_____

_____

_____

_____

63. Explain angiography, one of the procedures used to diagnose atherosclerosis.

_____

_____

_____

64. Explain why a physician often requires several blood pressure readings before making the diagnosis of hypertension.

_____

_____

_____

_____

_____

_____

_____

65. List the six elements that are taken into consideration during the ECG.

_____

_____

_____

_____

66. Explain the role of the medical assistant during an ECG.

_____

_____

_____

_____

COG TRUE OR FALSE?

Grade: _____

Indicate whether the statements are true or false by placing the letter T (true) or F (false) on the line preceding the statement.

67. _____ Congestive heart failure (CHF) is a condition in which the heart cannot pump effectively.

68. _____ Ventricular fibrillation is a medical emergency that occurs when the heart is contracting rather than quivering in an organized fashion.

69. _____ Diagnosis of atherosclerosis is often made by electrocardiography.

70. _____ Patients who have cerebrovascular accidents usually have varying degrees of weakness or paralysis of one side of the body.

COG AFF CASE STUDIES FOR CRITICAL THINKING

Grade: _____

71. You are interviewing a patient prior to a physical examination of the cardiovascular system. This is his first time in a medical office after many years' absence, and he is considerably anxious. What do you say to him to calm him down? How would you explain the procedure?

_____

_____

_____

_____

72. A patient comes into the office complaining of chest pain, nausea, and vomiting. Will he likely be admitted to the hospital right away? Why or why not?

_____

_____

_____

_____

73. A patient is given an artificial pacemaker. She would like to know how the device works and what changes she can expect from it. What do you tell her?

_____

_____

_____

_____

74. Why is it important that a patient continue taking her prescribed antihypertensive medication, even if her blood pressure has reached a manageable level?

_____

_____

_____

_____

75. Many cardiac conditions are preventable with proper diet and exercise. It's important to stress prevention over cure, because in most instances, there is no quick "cure." How will you send this message to patients? What kinds of tools will you use?

_____

_____

_____

_____

PSY PROCEDURE 32-1 Perform a 12-Lead Electrocardiogram

Name: _____ Date: _____ Time: _____ Grade: _____

EQUIPMENT/SUPPLIES: Physician order, ECG machine with cable and lead wires, ECG paper, disposable electrodes that contain coupling gel, patient gown and drape, skin preparation materials including a razor and antiseptic wipes

STANDARDS: Given the needed equipment and a place to work, the student will perform this skill with _____ % accuracy in a total of _____ minutes. *(Your instructor will tell you what the percentage and time limits will be before you begin.)*

KEY: 4 = Satisfactory 0 = Unsatisfactory NA = This step is not counted

PROCEDURE STEPS	SELF	PARTNER	INSTRUCTOR
1. Wash your hands	❏	❏	❏
2. Assemble the equipment	❏	❏	❏
3. Greet and identify the patient. Identify yourself, including your title, and explain the procedure	❏	❏	❏
4. Turn the ECG machine on and enter appropriate data into it. Include the patient's name and/or identification number, age, sex, height, weight, blood pressure, and medications	❏	❏	❏
5. Instruct the patient to disrobe above the waist **a.** Provide a gown for privacy **b.** Female patients should also be instructed to remove any nylons or tights	❏	❏	❏
6. Position patient comfortably in a supine position **a.** Provide pillows as needed for comfort **b.** Drape the patient for warmth and privacy	❏	❏	❏
7. Prepare the skin as needed **a.** Wipe away skin oil and lotions with the antiseptic wipes **b.** Shave hair that will interfere with good contact between skin and electrodes	❏	❏	❏
8. Apply the electrodes: **a.** Arms and legs: snugly against the fleshy, muscular parts of upper arms and lower legs according to the manufacturer's directions **b.** Chest: V_1 through V_6	❏	❏	❏
9. Connect the lead wires securely according to the color codes **a.** Untangle the wires before applying them to prevent electrical artifacts **b.** Each lead must lie unencumbered along the contours of the patient's body to decrease the incidence of artifacts **c.** Double check the placement	❏	❏	❏
10. Determine the sensitivity and paper speed settings on the ECG machine	❏	❏	❏
11. Depress the automatic button on the ECG machine to obtain the 12-lead ECG	❏	❏	❏

PSY PROCEDURE 32-1 **Perform a 12-Lead Electrocardiogram** (continued)

12. When the tracing is printed, check the ECG for artifacts and standardization mark	❏	❏	❏

13. If the tracing is adequate, turn off the machine
    a. Remove the electrodes from the patient's skin
    b. Assist the patient to a sitting position and help them with dressing, if needed
	❏	❏	❏

14. **AFF** Explain how to respond to a patient who has dementia	❏	❏	❏

_____

_____

_____

_____

15. For a single-channel machine, roll the ECG strip
    a. Do not secure the roll with clips
    b. This ECG will need to be mounted on an 8 × 11-inch paper or form
	❏	❏	❏

16. Discard disposable electrodes appropriately and put away the EKG machine. Wash your hands	❏	❏	❏
17. **AFF** Log into the Electronic Medical Record (EMR) using your username and secure password OR obtain the paper medical record from a secure location and assure it is kept away from public access	❏	❏	❏
18. Record the procedure	❏	❏	❏
19. Place the printed results in the medical record or scan into the electronic medical record, if appropriate	❏	❏	❏
20. Let the physician know that the ECG has been completed and is ready for review	❏	❏	❏
21. When finished, log out of the EMR and/or replace the paper medical record in an appropriate and secure location	❏	❏	❏

CALCULATION

Total Possible Points: _____

Total Points Earned: _____ Multiplied by 100 = _____ Divided by Total Possible Points = _____ %

PASS   FAIL   COMMENTS:
   ❏   ❏

Student's signature _____ Date _____

Partner's signature _____ Date _____

Instructor's signature _____ Date _____

PSY PROCEDURE 32-2 | **Apply a Holter Monitor for a 24-Hour Test**

Name: _____ Date: _____ Time: _____ Grade: _____

EQUIPMENT/SUPPLIES: Physician's order, Holter monitor with appropriate lead wires, fresh batteries, carrying case with strap, disposable electrodes that contain coupling gel, adhesive tape, patient gown and drape, skin preparation materials including a razor and antiseptic wipes, patient diary

STANDARDS: Given the needed equipment and a place to work, the student will perform this skill with _____ % accuracy in a total of _____ minutes. *(Your instructor will tell you what the percentage and time limits will be before you begin.)*

KEY: 4 = Satisfactory   0 = Unsatisfactory   NA = This step is not counted

PROCEDURE STEPS	SELF	PARTNER	INSTRUCTOR
1. Wash your hands	❏	❏	❏
2. Assemble the equipment	❏	❏	❏
3. Greet and identify the patient. Identify yourself, including your title, and explain the procedure	❏	❏	❏
4. Explain the importance of carrying out all normal activities during the monitoring and the reason for the incident diary. Emphasize the need to use the diary at all times during the test	❏	❏	❏
5. Ask the patient to remove all clothing from the waist up; gown and drape appropriately for privacy	❏	❏	❏
6. Prepare the patient's skin for electrode attachment 　**a.** Provide privacy and have the patient in a sitting position 　**b.** Shave the skin, if necessary, and cleanse with antiseptic wipes	❏	❏	❏
7. Apply the Holter electrodes at the specified sites: 　**a.** The right manubrium border 　**b.** The left manubrium border 　**c.** The right sternal border at the fifth-rib level 　**d.** The fifth rib at the anterior axillary line 　**e.** The right lower rib cage over the cartilage as a ground lead	❏	❏	❏
8. To do this, expose the adhesive backing of the electrodes and follow the manufacturer's instructions to attach each firmly. Check the security of the attachments	❏	❏	❏
9. Position electrode connectors downward toward the patient's feet	❏	❏	❏
10. Attach the lead wires and secure with adhesive tape	❏	❏	❏
11. Connect the cable and run a baseline ECG by hooking the Holter monitor to the ECG machine with the cable hookup	❏	❏	❏
12. Assist the patient to carefully redress with the cable extending through the garment opening. *Note:* Instruct the patient that clothing that buttons down the front is more convenient	❏	❏	❏

PSY PROCEDURE 32-2   **Apply a Holter Monitor for a 24-Hour Test** (continued)

13. Plug the cable into the recorder and mark the diary
  a. If needed, explain the purpose of the diary to the patient again
  b. Give instructions for a return appointment to evaluate the recording and the diary
	❏	❏	❏

14. Wash your hands	❏	❏	❏
15. **AFF** Log into the Electronic Medical Record (EMR) using your username and secure password OR obtain the paper medical record from a secure location and assure it is kept away from public access	❏	❏	❏
16. Record the procedure	❏	❏	❏
17. When finished, log out of the EMR and/or replace the paper medical record in an appropriate and secure location	❏	❏	❏

CALCULATION

Total Possible Points: _____

Total Points Earned: _____ Multiplied by 100 = _____ Divided by Total Possible Points = _____ %

PASS   FAIL   COMMENTS:
  ❏   ❏

Student's signature _____ Date _____

Partner's signature _____ Date _____

Instructor's signature _____ Date _____

CHAPTER 33

Gastroenterology

LEARNING OUTCOMES

COG Cognitive Domain*

1. Spell key terms
2. *Identify the following related to body systems:*
   a. *Medical terms*
   b. *Abbreviations*
3. *Identify structural organization of the human body*
4. *Identify major organs in each body system*
5. *Identify the anatomical location of major organs in each body system*
6. *Identify the normal function of each body system*
7. *Identify common pathology related to each body system including:*
   a. *Signs*
   b. *Symptoms*
   c. *Etiology*
   d. *Diagnostic measures*
   e. *Treatment modalities*
8. Describe the roles and responsibilities of the medical assistant in diagnosing and treating disorders of the gastrointestinal system

PSY Psychomotor Domain*

1. Assist with colon procedures (Procedure 33-1)
   a. *Instruct and prepare a patient for a procedure or treatment*
   b. *Assist provider with a patient exam*
   c. *Document patient care accurately in the medical record*

2. Test stool specimen for occult blood: Guaiac method (Procedure 33-2)
   a. *Collect specimens and perform: CLIA waived microbiology test*
   b. Differentiate between normal and abnormal results
   c. *Document patient care accurately in the medical record*

AFF Affective Domain*

1. *Demonstrate critical thinking skills*
2. *Reassure patients*
3. *Demonstrate empathy for patients' concerns*
4. *Demonstrate active listening*
5. *Respect diversity*
6. *Recognize personal boundaries*
7. *Demonstrate tactfulness*
8. *Demonstrate self-awareness*
9. Protect the integrity of the medical record

*MAERB Standards are Italicized.

ABHES Competencies

1. List all body systems and their structures and functions
2. Describe common diseases, symptoms, and etiology as they apply to each system
3. Identify diagnostic and treatment modalities as they relate to each body system

4. Apply medical terminology for each specialty
5. Follow documentation guidelines
6. Adapt care to address the developmental stages of life
7. Partner with healthcare teams to attain optimal patient health outcomes
8. Display effective interpersonal skills with patients and healthcare team members
9. Demonstrate cultural awareness
10. Assist provider with specialty examination, including cardiac, respiratory, OB-GYN, neurologic, and gastroenterology
11. Perform specialty procedures, including but not limited to minor surgery, cardiac, respiratory, OB-GYN, neurologic, and gastroenterology
12. Perform selected CLIA-waived tests that assist with diagnosis and treatment: Microbiology testing
13. Instruct patients on the collection of fecal specimen
14. Make adaptations for patients with special needs (psychological or physical limitations)
15. Make adaptations to care for patients across their lifespan

Name: _____   Date: _____   Grade: _____

⬤OG MULTIPLE CHOICE

Circle the letter preceding the correct answer.

1. Which of the following can trigger an outbreak of the herpes simplex virus?
   a. Food allergy
   b. Illness
   c. Lack of sleep
   d. Medication
   e. Poor diet

2. What commonly causes leukoplakia to develop?
   a. Hereditary genes
   b. Excessive alcohol intake
   c. Lack of exercise
   d. Tobacco irritation
   e. Obesity

3. Why should a patient complaining of heartburn be assessed immediately?
   a. The symptoms of gastroesophageal reflux disease may be similar to the chest pain of a patient with cardiac problems
   b. A patient with heartburn is more likely to develop a serious heart condition
   c. Heartburn is a symptom of a weak lower esophageal sphincter
   d. It is important to assess any gastrointestinal disorder immediately because they are usually serious
   e. Heartburn may be symptomatic of Barrett esophagus, which requires immediate surgery

4. Abnormal contact between the upper teeth and lower teeth is:
   a. malocclusion.
   b. dental caries.
   c. stomatitis.
   d. candidiasis.
   e. gingivitis.

5. If a patient is suffering from peptic ulcers, the symptoms will be most severe when the patient:
   a. is hungry.
   b. has a bowel movement.
   c. lies on his back.
   d. chews his food.
   e. is digesting a meal.

6. Gastroenteritis could become life threatening if a patient:
   a. is pregnant.
   b. suffers from diabetes mellitus.
   c. needs a heart operation.
   d. consumes excess alcohol.
   e. does not receive treatment immediately.

7. The study of morbid obesity is called:
   a. orthodontistry.
   b. gerontology.
   c. bariatrics.
   d. gastroenterology.
   e. pediatrics.

8. What is the minimum body mass index that a patient must have to be considered for gastric bypass surgery?
   a. 25
   b. 30
   c. 35
   d. 40
   e. 45

9. Crohn's disease becomes life threatening when:
   a. the bowel walls become inflamed and the lymph nodes enlarge.
   b. the fluid from the intestinal contents cannot be absorbed.
   c. edema of the bowel wall takes place.
   d. scarring narrows the colon and obstructs the bowel.
   e. patients have periods of constipation, anorexia, and fever.

10. How does irritable bowel syndrome differ from Crohn's disease?
    a. It does not involve weight loss.
    b. It is easily treatable.
    c. It is thought to be genetic.
    d. It requires a colectomy.
    e. It causes scarring.

Scenario for Questions 11 and 12: A patient is diagnosed with diverticulitis.

11. Which of the following treatments would the physician most likely recommend?
    a. Antibiotics
    b. Bed rest
    c. Antifungal agent
    d. Bland food
    e. Drinking less water

12. What advice might the physician have you give to the patient to help maintain good bowel habits in future?
    a. Never eat spicy foods
    b. Get some form of daily exercise
    c. Try to force a bowel movement at least once a day
    d. Use laxatives when suffering from constipation
    e. Cut out food products that contain wheat

13. How can a patient decrease their risk of developing a hernia?
    a. Avoid lifting heavy objects
    b. Switch from processed to organic foods
    c. Maintain good bowel habits
    d. Have regular medical checkups
    e. Walk at least a mile every day

14. What is the most effective treatment for appendicitis?
    a. Antibiotics
    b. Ileostomy
    c. Appendectomy
    d. Cryosurgery
    e. Radiation

15. Which of these factors increases the production of intestinal gas?
    a. Excess water
    b. Spicy or fatty foods
    c. Peristalsis
    d. Fast metabolism
    e. Lack of exercise

16. The most likely method of contracting hepatitis B is:
    a. contaminated food.
    b. poor hygiene.
    c. contaminated blood.
    d. stagnant water.
    e. weak immune system.

17. For which of the following procedures would the patient usually be put under anesthesia?
    a. Anoscopy
    b. Sigmoidoscopy
    c. Nuclear imaging
    d. Ultrasonography
    e. Endoscopic retrograde cholangiopancreatography

18. What is the caustic chemical secreted by the lining of the stomach that may cause erosion if too much of it is secreted?
    a. Pepsin
    b. Hydrochloric acid
    c. Insulin
    d. Oral mucosa
    e. Melena

19. How does lithotripsy break down gallstones to make them easy to pass?
    a. Lasers
    b. Sound waves
    c. Acidic liquid
    d. Heat
    e. Air pressure

20. Which piece of advice could best be given to a patient with a malabsorption syndrome by the physician?
    a. Drink more water
    b. Eat less processed food
    c. Take vitamin supplements
    d. Cut out spicy foods
    e. Exercise more often

21. Which of these groups of people are at the highest risk of developing esophageal cancer?
    a. Teenagers
    b. Pregnant women
    c. Young children
    d. Elderly women
    e. Elderly men

22. A male patient comes to the physician's office complaining of an acute pain in his upper abdomen and back. He also suffers from indigestion and nausea, particularly when he tries to eat foods that have a high fat content. Which of the following gastrointestinal disorders does the patient probably have?
    a. Cholelithiasis
    b. Peptic ulcers
    c. Gastritis
    d. Leukoplakia
    e. Caries

COG **MATCHING**

Grade: _____

Place the letter preceding the definition on the line next to the term.

Key Terms

23. _____ anorexia
24. _____ ascites
25. _____ dysphagia
26. _____ guaiac
27. _____ hematemesis
28. _____ hepatomegaly
29. _____ hepatotoxin
30. _____ insufflator
31. _____ leukoplakia
32. _____ malocclusion
33. _____ melena
34. _____ metabolism
35. _____ obturator
36. _____ peristalsis
37. _____ sclerotherapy
38. _____ stomatitis
39. _____ turgor

Definitions

a. an enlarged liver
b. a substance used in a laboratory test for occult blood in the stool
c. a device for blowing air, gas, or powder into a body cavity
d. the sum of chemical processes that results in growth, energy production, elimination of waste, and body functions performed as digested nutrients are distributed
e. black, tarry stools caused by digested blood from the gastrointestinal tract
f. the contraction and relaxation of involuntary muscles of the alimentary canal, producing wavelike movements of products through the digestive system
g. difficulty speaking
h. loss of appetite
i. a substance that can damage the liver
j. an accumulation of serous fluid in the peritoneal cavity
k. the use of chemical agents to treat esophageal varices to produce fibrosis and hardening of the tissue
l. an inflammation of the mucous membranes of the mouth
m. an abnormal contact between the teeth in the upper and lower jaws
n. the normal tension in a cell or the skin
o. vomiting blood or bloody vomitus
p. the smooth, rounded, removable inner portion of a hollow tube, such as an anoscope, that allows for easier insertion
q. white, thickened patches on the oral mucosa or tongue that are often precancerous

COG **MATCHING**

Grade: _____

Place the letter preceding the description on the line next to the name of the gastrointestinal disorder.

Disorders

40. _____ esophageal varices
41. _____ cholecystitis
42. _____ peptic ulcers
43. _____ stomatitis
44. _____ gastroesophageal reflux disease (GERD)
45. _____ diverticulosis
46. _____ hiatal hernia

Descriptions

a. a chronic disorder characterized by discomfort in the chest due to the backflow of gastric contents into the esophagus
b. a condition that occurs when part of the stomach protrudes up through the diaphragm
c. varicose veins of the esophagus resulting from pressure within the esophageal veins
d. an acute or chronic inflammation of the gall bladder
e. erosions or sores in the GI tract left by sloughed tissue
f. a disorder that usually occurs in the sigmoid colon, attributed to a diet deficient in roughage
g. an inflammation of the oral mucosa, caused by a virus, bacteria, or fungus

◦◦ᴳ MATCHING

Grade: _____

Place the letter preceding the description on the line next to the examination method.

Examination Methods

47. _____ endoscopic studies
48. _____ nuclear imaging
49. _____ ultrasonography
50. _____ radiology studies
51. _____ sigmoidoscopy
52. _____ endoscopic retrograde
            cholangiopancreatography
            (ERCP)
53. _____ anoscopy

Descriptions

a. instilling barium into the GI tract orally or rectally to outline the organs and identify abnormalities

b. injecting radionuclides into the body and taking images using a nuclear scanning device to detect abnormalities

c. using high-frequency sound waves to diagnose disorders of internal structures

d. passing soft, flexible tubes into the stomach, small intestine, or colon for direct visualization of the organs

e. a method of injecting dye into the ducts of the gallbladder and pancreas; used to visualize the esophagus, stomach, proximal duodenum, and pancreas with a flexible endoscope

f. the insertion of a metal or plastic anoscope into the rectal canal to inspect the anus and rectum and swab for cultures

g. a visual examination of the sigmoid colon

◦◦ᴳ IDENTIFICATION

Grade: _____

54. A patient comes into the office with abdominal pain and indigestion. The physician diagnoses the patient with a hiatal hernia. Which of the following diet modifications and treatments would the physician most likely suggest to the patient? Circle the correct answers. There may be more than one.

  a. Eat small, frequent meals

  b. Exercise vigorously three times a week

  c. Elevate the head of the bed when sleeping

  d. Do not eat for 2 hours before bedtime

  e. Drink less water

  f. Lose weight

55. As a medical assistant, you may be called on to assist with colon procedures in the medical office. Place a check mark on the line next to the task(s) that the medical assistant would be responsible for performing in the medical office.

  a. _____ Instruct the patient in the procedure of stool sample collection

  b. _____ Help to educate the patient about diet and the prevention of gastric disorders

  c. _____ Prescribe pain medication and antibiotics

  d. _____ Schedule radiographic and ultrasound procedures in an outpatient facility

  e. _____ Test the stool specimen when it is returned to the office

  f. _____ Compile detailed dietary regimens for obese patients

  g. _____ Assist the physician in performing colon examinations

  h. _____ Diagnose minor gastrointestinal disorders

56. Which of the following factors increase a person's risk of developing pancreatic cancer? Circle all that apply.

   a. Being female

   b. Drinking alcohol

   c. Smoking

   d. Being of African American descent

   e. Being male

   f. Being of Caucasian descent

   g. Eating high-fat foods

   h. A history of working with industrial chemicals

57. Some gastrointestinal disorders require specialist knowledge and equipment outside of the physician's office. In the table below, place a check mark in the appropriate box to indicate whether a procedure could be carried out in the physician's office or would likely require an outpatient facility.

Procedure	Physician's Office	Outpatient Facility
a. Ultrasonography		
b. Anoscopy		
c. Endoscopic retrograde cholangiopancreatography		
d. Nuclear imaging		
e. Sigmoidoscopy examination		

COG SHORT ANSWER

Grade: _____

58. Identify the part of the digestive system where the following gastrointestinal disorders occur.

   a. Appendicitis _____

   b. Hepatitis _____

   c. Cholelithiasis _____

   d. Crohn's disease _____

   e. Peptic ulcers _____

   f. Ulcerative colitis _____

   g. Diverticulosis _____

59. List three symptoms that could indicate a patient is suffering from gastric cancer.

_____

_____

_____

_____

60. A 40-year-old woman comes to the physician's office complaining of severe stomach cramps and vomiting. To help the physician assess her condition and make a diagnosis, the medical assistant should obtain some personal information. List four things that the physician will ask the patient before continuing with the exam.

_____

_____

_____

_____

61. A 25-year-old woman comes to the physician's office complaining of fatigue and joint pain. She looks jaundiced, and when the physician asks her for her medical history, she says that she recently returned from a 3-month trip to Ghana. Which two tests will the physician most likely recommend?

_____

_____

_____

_____

62. As a medical assistant, part of your job may be to educate patients about the care of teeth and gums. List three things that you could tell a patient to do that might help to prevent dental caries.

_____

_____

_____

_____

63. Which is the more widely accepted instrument to use during an endoscopic study: a rigid sigmoidoscope or a flexible fiberoptic sigmoidoscope? Explain your answer.

_____

_____

_____

_____

COG TRUE OR FALSE?

Grade: _____

Indicate whether the statements are true or false by placing the letter T (true) or F (false) on the line preceding the statement.

64. _____ Oral cancers are more common among people who smoke.

65. _____ Cancer of the esophagus is common and can easily be treated.

66. _____ A sign that a patient has a problem with malabsorption of fats includes stools that are loose.

67. _____ Irritable bowel syndrome usually results in chronic weight loss.

COG AFF CASE STUDIES FOR CRITICAL THINKING

Grade: _____

68. A 55-year-old woman comes to the physician's office and asks about gastric bypass surgery. She says that she has tried every diet available and is unable to lose weight. She suffers from shortness of breath and an inability to walk for long distances. You take the woman's vital signs and measure her height and weight. She appears to be in good health but is at least 60 pounds over the ideal weight for her height. The physician later confirms these facts. Is the patient likely to be a candidate for gastric bypass surgery? Explain your answer.

_____

_____

_____

_____

69. The physician tells a patient that he would like to schedule an endoscopic retrograde cholangiopancreatography in a local outpatient facility. After the physician leaves the room, you notice that the patient looks confused and worried. How would you explain the procedure to the patient to reassure him?

_____

_____

_____

_____

70. Mr. Thompson, a 50-year-old patient, is scheduled to have an endoscopic examination on Wednesday morning. You have given him all of the necessary information to prepare for the examination, including taking a laxative the night before and eating only a light meal on Tuesday evening, with no breakfast on Wednesday morning. Mr. Thompson calls you an hour before his appointment to tell you that he forgot to take the laxative the previous evening and has eaten breakfast. Explain what you would do.

_____

_____

_____

_____

71. A 15-year-old female patient comes into the physician's office with severe abdominal pains. She is extremely underweight for her height, and you suspect she might be anorexic. When the physician leaves the room, she confesses that she has been using laxatives every day to keep her weight down. Explain what you would do next.

_____

_____

_____

_____

72. A 50-year-old male patient has been diagnosed with pancreatic cancer. The patient is clearly devastated and tells you he has heard that people who develop pancreatic cancer have little chance of survival. What do you say to the patient?

_____

_____

_____

_____

PSY PROCEDURE 33-1 **Assisting with Colon Procedures**

Name: _____ Date: _____ Time: _____ Grade: _____

EQUIPMENT/SUPPLIES: Appropriate instrument (flexible or rigid sigmoidoscope, anoscope, or proctoscope); water-soluble lubricant; patient gown and drape; cotton swabs; suction (if not part of the scope); biopsy forceps; specimen container with preservative; completed laboratory requisition form; personal wipes or tissues; equipment for assessing vital signs; examination gloves

STANDARDS: Given the needed equipment and a place to work, the student will perform this skill with _____ % accuracy in a total of _____ minutes. *(Your instructor will tell you what the percentage and time limits will be before you begin.)*

KEY: 4 = Satisfactory   0 = Unsatisfactory   NA = This step is not counted

PROCEDURE STEPS	SELF	PARTNER	INSTRUCTOR
1. Wash your hands	❑	❑	❑
2. Assemble the equipment and supplies 　**a.** Place the name of the patient on the label on the outside of the specimen container 　**b.** Complete the laboratory requisition	❑	❑	❑
3. Check the illumination of the light source if using a flexible sigmoidoscope. Turn off the power after checking for working order	❑	❑	❑
4. Greet and identify the patient and explain the procedure. Identify yourself, including your title 　**a.** Inform patient that a sensation of pressure may be felt 　**b.** Tell the patient that the pressure is from the instrument 　**c.** Gas pressure may be felt when air is insufflated during the sigmoidoscopy	❑	❑	❑
5. Instruct the patient to empty their urinary bladder	❑	❑	❑
6. Assess the vital signs and record in the medical record	❑	❑	❑
7. Have the patient undress from the waist down and gown and drape appropriately	❑	❑	❑
8. Assist the patient onto the examination table 　**a.** If the instrument is an anoscope or a fiberoptic device, the Sims position or a side-lying position is most comfortable 　**b.** If a rigid instrument is used, position patient when doctor is ready: knee-chest position or on a proctologic table 　**c.** Drape the patient	❑	❑	❑
9. Assist the physician with lubricant, instruments, power, swabs, suction, etc	❑	❑	❑
10. Monitor the patient's response and offer reassurance 　**a.** Instruct the patient to breathe slowly through pursed lips 　**b.** Encourage relaxing as much as possible	❑	❑	❑

PSY PROCEDURE 33-1 **Assisting with Colon Procedures** (continued)

11. When the physician is finished:
   a. Assist the patient into a comfortable position and allow a rest period
   b. Offer personal cleaning wipes or tissues
   c. Take the patient's vital signs before allowing them to stand
   d. Assist the patient from the table and with dressing as needed
   e. Give the patient any instructions regarding postprocedure care
	❑	❑	❑

12. Clean the room and route the specimen to the laboratory with the requisition	❑	❑	❑
13. Disinfect or dispose of the supplies and equipment as appropriate	❑	❑	❑
14. Wash your hands	❑	❑	❑
15. **AFF** Log into the Electronic Medical Record (EMR) using your username and secure password OR obtain the paper medical record from a secure location and assure it is kept away from public access. Document your part in preparing specimens obtained and patient instructions after the procedure	❑	❑	❑
16. When finished, log out of the EMR and/or replace the paper medical record in an appropriate and secure location	❑	❑	❑

CALCULATION

Total Possible Points: _____

Total Points Earned: _____ Multiplied by 100 = _____ Divided by Total Possible Points = _____ %

PASS   **FAIL**   **COMMENTS:**
  ❑   ❑

Student's signature _____ Date _____

Partner's signature _____ Date _____

Instructor's signature _____ Date _____

PROCEDURE 33-2 Test Stool Specimen for Occult Blood: Guaiac Method

PSY

Name: _____ **Date:** _____ **Time:** _____ **Grade:** _____

EQUIPMENT/SUPPLIES: Gloves, labeled specimen pack or packs (the patient may bring in up to three samples per the office policy), test developer or reagent drops, biohazardous waste container.

STANDARDS: Given the needed equipment and a place to work, the student will perform this skill with _____ % accuracy in a total of _____ minutes. (*Your instructor will tell you what the percentage and time limits will be before you begin.*)

KEY: 4 = Satisfactory 0 = Unsatisfactory NA = This step is not counted

PROCEDURE STEPS	SELF	PARTNER	INSTRUCTOR
1. Wash your hands	❏	❏	❏
2. Assemble the equipment and supplies and put on gloves	❏	❏	❏
3. Verify that the stool sample collected by the patient is appropriately labeled and that the physician has ordered a stool sample test for occult blood	❏	❏	❏
4. Check the expiration date on the developer or reagent solution	❏	❏	❏
5. Open the test window on the back of each test pack. Apply one drop of the developer solution to each window according to the manufacturer's instructions	❏	❏	❏
6. Read the color change within the specified time period, usually 60 seconds	❏	❏	❏
7. Apply one drop of developer as directed on the control section or window of each test pack. Note whether the control results are positive or negative	❏	❏	❏
8. Explain the procedure to follow if the control is positive or negative	❏	❏	❏
9. Properly dispose of the test pack or packs and your gloves in a biohazardous waste container	❏	❏	❏
10. Wash your hands	❏	❏	❏
11. **AFF** Log into the Electronic Medical Record (EMR) using your username and secure password OR obtain the paper medical record from a secure location and assure it is kept away from public access. Document your part in preparing specimens obtained and patient instructions after the procedure	❏	❏	❏
12. When finished, log out of the EMR and/or replace the paper medical record in an appropriate and secure location	❏	❏	❏

PSY PROCEDURE 33-2 · **Test Stool Specimen for Occult Blood: Guaiac Method** (continued)

CALCULATION

Total Possible Points: _____

Total Points Earned: _____ Multiplied by 100 = _____ Divided by Total Possible Points = _____ %

PASS   **FAIL**   **COMMENTS:**
  ❑   ❑

Student's signature _____   Date _____

Partner's signature _____   Date _____

Instructor's signature _____   Date _____

CHAPTER 34

Neurology

LEARNING OUTCOMES

COG Cognitive Domain*

1. Spell key terms
2. Identify the following related to body systems:
   a. Medical terms
   b. Abbreviations
3. Identify structural organization of the human body
4. Identify major organs in each body system
5. Identify the anatomical location of major organs in each body system
6. Identify the normal function of each body system
7. Identify common pathology related to each body system including:
   a. Signs
   b. Symptoms
   c. Etiology
   d. Diagnostic measures
   e. Treatment modalities

PSY Psychomotor Domain*

1. Assist with a lumbar puncture (Procedure 34-1)
   a. Instruct and prepare a patient for a procedure or treatment
   b. Assist provider with a patient exam

c. Document patient care accurately in the medical record

AFF Affective Domain*

1. Demonstrate critical thinking skills
2. Reassure patients
3. Demonstrate empathy for patients' concerns
4. Demonstrate active listening
5. Respect diversity
6. Recognize personal boundaries
7. Demonstrate tactfulness
8. Demonstrate self-awareness
9. Protect the integrity of the medical record

*MAERB Standards are Italicized.

ABHES Competencies

1. List all body systems and their structures and functions
2. Describe common diseases, symptoms, and etiology as they apply to each system
3. Identify diagnostic and treatment modalities as they relate to each body system
4. Apply medical terminology for each specialty

5. Follow documentation guidelines
6. Adapt care to address the developmental stages of life
7. Partner with healthcare teams to attain optimal patient health outcomes
8. Display effective interpersonal skills with patients and healthcare team members
9. Demonstrate cultural awareness
10. Assist provider with specialty examinations, including cardiac, respiratory, OB-GYN, neurologic, and gastroenterology
11. Perform specialty procedures, including but not limited to minor surgery, cardiac, respiratory, OB-GYN, neurologic, and gastroenterology
12. Make adaptations for patients with special needs (psychological or physical limitations)
13. Make adaptations to care for patients across their lifespan

Name: _____ Date: _____ Grade: _____

⬛OG MULTIPLE CHOICE

Circle the letter preceding the correct answer.

1. Initial symptoms of tetanus include:
   a. muscle spasms and stiff neck.
   b. paralysis and stiff neck.
   c. drooling and thick saliva.
   d. seizures and dysphagia.
   e. muscle spasms and clenched teeth.

2. What is another name for grand mal seizures?
   a. Absence seizures
   b. Tonic–clonic seizures
   c. Partial seizures
   d. Nervous seizures
   e. Flashing seizures

3. Febrile seizures occur in:
   a. teenagers.
   b. middle-aged men.
   c. young children.
   d. older adult women.
   e. people of all ages.

4. There may be no signs of external deformity with:
   a. meningocele.
   b. myelomeningocele.
   c. spina bifida occulta.
   d. amyotrophic lateral sclerosis.
   e. poliomyelitis.

5. To diagnose meningitis, the physician may order a(n):
   a. urine sample.
   b. x-ray.
   c. MRI.
   d. throat culture.
   e. complete blood count.

6. Hydrophobia often occurs after the onset of:
   a. rabies.
   b. tetanus.
   c. encephalitis.
   d. cerebral palsy.
   e. meningitis.

7. A herpes zoster breakout typically develops on:
   a. the legs and arms.
   b. the genitals and mouth.
   c. the stomach and chest.
   d. the face, back, and chest.
   e. the face and neck.

8. A disease closely related to poliomyelitis is:
   a. encephalitis.
   b. meningitis.
   c. Parkinson's disease.
   d. PPMA syndrome.
   e. chicken pox.

9. Treatment for brain tumors may include:
   a. physical therapy and drug therapy.
   b. surgery and radiation therapy.
   c. surgery only.
   d. radiation therapy only.
   e. physical therapy and occupational therapy.

10. CSF removed and sent to the laboratory for a suspected diagnosis of meningitis may be tested for:
    a. glucose and white blood cells.
    b. cholesterol and white blood cell count.
    c. red blood cells and viruses
    d. glucose and bacteria.
    e. glucose and fatty acids.

11. You should encourage slow, deep breathing for:
    a. electrical tests.
    b. a lumbar puncture.
    c. radiologic tests.
    d. physical tests.
    e. the Romberg test.

12. Contrast medium helps distinguish between the soft tissues of the nervous system and:
    a. bones.
    b. tendons.
    c. tumors.
    d. muscles.
    e. arteries.

13. When assisting with a Queckenstedt test, you will be directed to:
    a. assist the patient into a side-curled position.
    b. support a forward-bending sitting position.
    c. maintain sterility of instruments.
    d. press against the patient's jugular vein.
    e. encourage the patient in slow, deep breathing.

14. AFP is generally performed:
    a. during the second trimester of pregnancy.
    b. during the first trimester of pregnancy.
    c. during the third trimester of pregnancy.
    d. before a woman gets pregnant.
    e. after the baby is born.

15. Which of the following is true of Lou Gehrig disease?
    a. It is officially known as multiple sclerosis.
    b. It is highly contagious.
    c. It is caused by a spinal cord injury.
    d. It is found most often in children.
    e. It is a terminal disease.

16. During the second phase of a grand mal seizure, the patient experiences:
    a. a tingling in extremities.
    b. a sensitivity to light.
    c. a complete loss of consciousness.
    d. an increased awareness of smell.
    e. a sense of drowsiness.

17. Which of the following is a cause of febrile seizures?
    a. Spinal cord damage
    b. Elevated body temperature
    c. Hypothermia
    d. Reye syndrome
    e. Neural tube defects

18. Paraplegia is:
    a. paralysis of all limbs.
    b. paralysis of the high thoracic vertebrae.
    c. paralysis on one side of the body, opposite the side of spinal cord involvement.
    d. paralysis of any part of the body above the point of spinal cord involvement.
    e. paralysis of any part of the body below the point of spinal cord involvement.

19. Which of the following is an infectious disorder of the nervous system?
    a. Tumors
    b. ALS
    c. Multiple sclerosis
    d. Encephalitis
    e. Febrile seizures

20. Parkinson's disease is a:
    a. convulsive disorder.
    b. degenerative disorder.
    c. developmental disorder.
    d. neoplastic disorder.
    e. traumatic disorder.

cog MATCHING

Grade: _____

Place the letter preceding the definition on the line next to the term.

Key Terms

21. _____ cephalalgia
22. _____ concussion
23. _____ contusion
24. _____ convulsion
25. _____ dysphagia
26. _____ dysphasia
27. _____ electroencephalogram
       (EEG)
28. _____ herpes zoster
29. _____ meningocele
30. _____ migraine
31. _____ myelogram
32. _____ myelomeningocele
33. _____ Queckenstedt test
34. _____ Romberg test
35. _____ seizure
36. _____ spina bifida occulta

Definitions

a. tracing of the electrical activity of the brain
b. a headache
c. meninges protruding through the spinal column
d. the protrusion of the spinal cord through the spinal defect
e. an invasive radiologic test in which dye is injected into the spinal fluid
f. a test to determine presence of obstruction in the CSF flow performed during a lumbar puncture
g. an injury to the brain due to trauma
h. difficulty speaking
i. sudden, involuntary muscle contraction of a voluntary muscle group
j. an infection caused by reactivation of varicella zoster virus, which causes chicken pox
k. a collection of blood tissues after an injury; a bruise
l. a type of severe headache, usually unilateral; may appear in clusters
m. a congenital defect in the spinal column caused by lack of union of the vertebrae
n. an abnormal discharge of electrical activity in the brain, resulting in involuntary contractions of voluntary muscles
o. a test for the inability to maintain body balance when eyes are closed and feet are together; indication of spinal cord disease
p. inability to swallow or difficulty in swallowing

cog MATCHING

Grade: _____

Place the letter preceding the examination method on the line next to the cranial nerve.

Cranial Nerves

37. _____ Olfactory (I)
38. _____ Trochlear (IV)
39. _____ Facial (VII)
40. _____ Glossopharyngeal (IX)
41. _____ Vagus (X)

Examination Methods

a. Ask patient to raise eyebrows, smile, show teeth, puff out cheeks.
b. Test for downward, inward eye movement.
c. Test each nostril for smell reception, interpretation.
d. Ask patient to say "ah," yawn to observe upward movement of palate; elicit gag response, note ability to swallow.
e. Ask patient to swallow and speak; note hoarseness.

cog MATCHING

Grade: _____

Place the letter preceding the response on the line next to the reflex. Responses may be used more than once.

Reflexes

42. _____ Brachioradialis
43. _____ Biceps
44. _____ Triceps
45. _____ Patellar
46. _____ Achilles
47. _____ Corneal

Responses

a. Closure of eyelid
b. Extension of elbow
c. Flexion of elbow
d. Plantar flexion of foot
e. Extension of leg

⬤⬤⬤ IDENTIFICATION

Grade: _____

Indicate whether the following disorders are infectious (I), degenerative (DG), convulsive (C), developmental (DV), traumatic (T), neoplastic (N), or a type of headache (H) by placing the identifying letter(s) on the line preceding the disorder.

48. _____ Amyotrophic lateral sclerosis

49. _____ Focal or Jacksonian

50. _____ Hydrocephalus

51. _____ Meningitis

52. _____ Neural tube defects

53. _____ Poliomyelitis

54. _____ Brain astrocytoma

55. _____ Herpes zoster

56. _____ Cerebral palsy

57. _____ Tetanus

58. _____ Febrile seizures

59. _____ Multiple sclerosis

60. _____ Spinal cord injury

61. Identify whether the disorders listed below affect children, women, men, or older adults. Place a check mark on the line under the appropriate groups.

Disorder	Children	Women	Men	Older Adults
a. Parkinson's disease				
b. Amyotrophic lateral sclerosis				
c. Multiple sclerosis				
d. Reye syndrome				
e. Febrile seizures				

62. Indicate whether the following symptoms occur at the onset of a migraine or after the migraine begins. Place a check mark on the line under the word "onset" or "after."

Symptoms	Onset	After Migraine Begins
a. experience of flashing lights		
b. photophobia		
c. nausea		
d. experience of wavy lines		
e. diplopia		

COG SHORT ANSWER

Grade: _____

63. Explain the difference between dysphagia and dysphasia.

_____

_____

_____

_____

64. Name three viral infections that lead to encephalitis.

_____

_____

_____

_____

65. What kind of outbreak might be caused by a varicella infection? What generally triggers this outbreak?

_____

_____

_____

_____

66. Which age group is most susceptible to traumatic brain injuries? Why? Which age group is most susceptible to spinal cord injuries? Why?

_____

_____

_____

_____

67. Name seven common diagnostic tests for the nervous system.

_____

_____

_____

_____

68. Explain the difference between the Romberg test and the Queckenstedt test and how or if you would assist the physician in each procedure.

_____

_____

_____

_____

69. List three responsibilities that you may have when working with patients with neurologic disorders.

_____

_____

_____

_____

70. Below are some of the steps involved in assisting the physician with a lumbar puncture. Explain the reasons for performing each task listed.

a. Check that the consent form is signed and in the chart. Warn the patient not to move during the procedure. Tell the patient that the area will be numb but pressure may still be felt after the local anesthetic is administered.

_____

_____

_____

_____

b. Throughout the procedure, observe the patient closely for signs such as dyspnea or cyanosis. Monitor the pulse at intervals and record the vital signs after the procedure. Note the patient's mental alertness and any leakage at the site, nausea, or vomiting. Assess lower limb mobility. Assist the physician as necessary.

_____

_____

_____

_____

c. If the Queckenstedt test is to be performed, you may be required to press against the patient's jugular veins in the neck (right, left, or both) while the physician monitors the pressure of CSF.

_____

_____

_____

COG TRUE OR FALSE?

Grade: _____

Indicate whether the statements are true or false by placing the letter T (true) or F (false) on the line preceding the statement.

71. _____ Ice, alcohol, and sponge baths are preferable to cool compresses in returning a child's body temperature to normal.

72. _____ If a patient is bitten by an animal, a copy of the animal's rabies tag and certificate should be placed in the patient's chart.

73. _____ Multiple sclerosis is a contagious disease.

74. _____ A lumbar puncture is more commonly performed in outpatient clinics than in the medical office.

75. _____ Herpes zoster may develop in patients who had a previous varicella infection.

COG AFF CASE STUDIES FOR CRITICAL THINKING

Grade: _____

76. A patient comes in for treatment because of a severe dog bite. The patient has already cleaned the wound himself and the physician attends to the wound immediately. Your patient then receives antibiotic and vaccine therapy. What is the next course of action and what may you be responsible for?

_____

_____

_____

_____

77. A patient in your clinic has been treated for epilepsy and is now seizure free. This patient has decided that she is going to stop her medication regimen. She has also expressed her excitement about being able to drive again soon. How might you advise this patient before she makes her decisions?

_____

_____

_____

_____

78. There is a patient who has recently started coming to your clinic for treatment for herpes zoster. She doesn't understand why she has shingles. She is a single mom who has been supporting her children and taking care of one child with severe Down syndrome. What would you explain as the likely cause for the herpes zoster outbreak? What kind of advice might you offer this patient toward improving her health?

_____

_____

_____

_____

79. A 40-year-old patient has been suffering from severe migraines for the last year. He is concerned about his condition because he is a truck driver. He is worried that it is just a matter of time before a migraine sets in while he is driving. Taking rests while he is on the road is a near impossibility. He is usually very tired, and he drinks a lot of coffee to keep himself awake on his long rides. How might you advise and educate this patient?

_____

_____

_____

_____

80. A patient comes in to the office and complains of headaches, blurred vision, and memory loss. What would your immediate concern be? What type of tests may need to be performed to learn more about this patient's symptoms?

_____

_____

_____

_____

PSY PROCEDURE 34-1 Assist with a Lumbar Puncture

Name: _____ Date: _____ Time: _____ Grade: _____

EQUIPMENT/SUPPLIES: Sterile gloves, examination gloves, 3- to 5-inch lumbar needle with a stylet (physician will specify gauge and length), sterile gauze sponges, specimen containers, local anesthetic and syringe, needle, adhesive bandages, fenestrated drape, sterile drape, antiseptic, skin preparation supplies (razor), biohazard sharps container, biohazard waste container

STANDARDS: Given the needed equipment and a place to work, the student will perform this skill with _____ % accuracy in a total of _____ minutes. *(Your instructor will tell you what the percentage and time limits will be before you begin.)*

KEY: 4 = Satisfactory   0 = Unsatisfactory   NA = This step is not counted

PROCEDURE STEPS	SELF	PARTNER	INSTRUCTOR
1. Wash your hands	❑	❑	❑
2. Assemble the equipment	❑	❑	❑
3. Identify yourself, including your title	❑	❑	❑
4. Identify the patient and explain the procedure	❑	❑	❑
5. Check that the consent form is signed and available in the chart	❑	❑	❑
6. Explain the importance of not moving during the procedure and explain that the area will be numbed but pressure may still be felt	❑	❑	❑
7. Have the patient void	❑	❑	❑
8. Direct the patient to disrobe and put on a gown with the opening in the back	❑	❑	❑
9. Prepare the skin unless this is to be done as part of the sterile preparation	❑	❑	❑
10. Assist as needed with administration of the anesthetic	❑	❑	❑

11. Assist the patient into the appropriate position
  a. For the side-lying position:
    (1) Stand in front of the patient and help by holding the patient's knees and top shoulder
    (2) Ask the patient to move, so the back is close to the edge of the table
  b. For the forward leaning, supported position:
    (1) Stand in front of the patient and rest your hands on the patient's shoulders
    (2) Ask the patient to breathe slowly and deeply
	❑	❑	❑

12. Throughout the procedure, observe the patient closely for signs of dyspnea or cyanosis
  a. Monitor the pulse at intervals and record the vital signs after the procedure
  b. Assess lower-limb mobility
	❑	❑	❑

PSY PROCEDURE 34-1 **Assist with a Lumbar Puncture** (continued)

13. When the physician has the needle securely in place, if specimens are to be taken: **a.** Put on gloves to receive the potentially hazardous body fluid **b.** Label the tubes in sequence as you receive them **c.** Label with the patient's identification and place them in biohazard bags	❏	❏	❏
14. If the Queckenstedt test is to be performed, you may be required to press against the patient's jugular veins in the neck, either right, left, or both, while the physician monitors the CSF pressure	❏	❏	❏
15. At the completion of the procedure: **a.** Cover the site with an adhesive bandage and assist the patient to a flat position **b.** The physician will determine when the patient is ready to leave	❏	❏	❏
16. Route the specimens as required	❏	❏	❏
17. Clean the examination room and care for or dispose of the equipment as needed	❏	❏	❏
18. Wash your hands	❏	❏	❏
19. **AFF** Log into the Electronic Medical Record (EMR) using your username and secure password OR obtain the paper medical record from a secure location and assure it is kept away from public access	❏	❏	❏
20. Document your part in preparing specimens obtained and patient instructions after the procedure	❏	❏	❏
21. When finished, log out of the EMR and/or replace the paper medical record in an appropriate and secure location	❏	❏	❏

CALCULATION

Total Possible Points: _____

Total Points Earned: _____ Multiplied by 100 = _____ Divided by Total Possible Points = _____ %

PASS   FAIL   COMMENTS:
   ❏   ❏

Student's signature _____ Date _____

Partner's signature _____ Date _____

Instructor's signature _____ Date _____

CHAPTER 35

Urology

LEARNING OUTCOMES

COG Cognitive Domain*

1. Spell key terms
2. *Identify the following related to body systems:*
   a. *Medical terms*
   b. *Abbreviations*
3. *Identify structural organization of the human body*
4. *Identify major organs in each body system*
5. *Identify the anatomical location of major organs in each body system*
6. *Identify the normal function of each body system*
7. *Identify common pathology related to each body system including:*
   a. *Signs*
   b. *Symptoms*
   c. *Etiology*
   d. *Diagnostic measures*
   e. *Treatment modalities*
8. Discuss the role of the medical assistant in diagnosing and treating disorders of the urinary system and the male reproductive system

PSY Psychomotor Domain*

1. Perform a female urinary catheterization (Procedure 35-1)
   a. *Instruct and prepare a patient for a procedure or treatment*
   b. *Assist the provider with a patient exam*
   c. *Document patient care accurately in the medical record*

2. Perform a male urinary catheterization (Procedure 35-2)
   a. *Instruct and prepare a patient for a procedure or treatment*
   b. *Assist provider with a patient exam*
   c. *Document patient care accurately in the medical record*
3. Instruct a male patient on the testicular self-examination (Procedure 35-3)
   a. *Instruct and prepare a patient for a procedure or treatment*
   b. *Assist the provider with a patient exam*
   c. *Document patient care accurately in the medical record*

AFF Affective Domain*

1. *Demonstrate critical thinking skills*
2. *Reassure patients*
3. *Demonstrate empathy for patients' concerns*
4. *Demonstrate active listening*
5. *Respect diversity*
6. *Recognize personal boundaries*
7. *Demonstrate tactfulness*
8. *Demonstrate self-awareness*
9. Protect the integrity of the medical record

MAERB Standards are Italicized.

ABHES Competencies

1. List all body systems and their structures and functions

2. Describe common diseases, symptoms, and etiology as they apply to each system
3. Identify diagnostic and treatment modalities as they relate to each body system
4. Apply medical terminology for each specialty
5. Follow documentation guidelines
6. Adapt care to address the developmental stages of life
7. Partner with healthcare teams to attain optimal patient health outcomes
8. Display effective interpersonal skills with patients and healthcare team members
9. Demonstrate cultural awareness
10. Assist provider with specialty examinations, including cardiac, respiratory, OB-GYN, neurologic, and gastroenterology
11. Perform specialty procedures, including but not limited to minor surgery, cardiac, respiratory, OB-GYN, neurologic, and gastroenterology
12. Make adaptations for patients with special needs (psychological or physical limitations)
13. Make adaptations to care for patients across their lifespan

Name: _____ Date: _____ Grade: _____

COG MULTIPLE CHOICE

Circle the letter preceding the correct answer.

1. Cystoscopy is:
   a. an inflammation of the urinary bladder.
   b. the direct visualization of the bladder and urethra.
   c. a procedure used to help patients pass calculi.
   d. the treatment used for men with an inguinal hernia.
   e. the use of a small camera inserted into the rectum.

2. Which of the following might contribute to psychogenic impotence?
   a. Disease in any other body system
   b. Injury to pelvic organs
   c. Medication
   d. Exhaustion
   e. Cardiovascular problems

3. Before scheduling a patient for an IVP or a retrograde pyelogram, you must check for a(n):
   a. protein allergy.
   b. lubricant allergy.
   c. iodine allergy.
   d. rubber allergy.
   e. latex allergy.

4. A procedure that cleanses the blood of waste products and excess fluid is:
   a. oliguria.
   b. lithotripsy.
   c. proteinuria.
   d. cystoscopy.
   e. dialysis.

5. Young girls are prone to urethritis because they:
   a. forget to practice good hand-washing technique.
   b. have a short urethra.
   c. don't take enough baths.
   d. urinate too frequently.
   e. wipe from front to back.

6. Which of the following instructions would be helpful for a patient trying to pass a stone?
   a. Eat a large amount of fiber
   b. Get plenty of bed rest and relaxation
   c. Drink lots of water
   d. Go to the hospital when the stone passes
   e. Do not consume anything until the stone has passed

7. Orchiopexy is surgery to correct:
   a. undescended testes.
   b. enlarged prostate.
   c. inguinal hernia.
   d. impotence.
   e. hydrocele.

8. One common urinary disorder in females is:
   a. benign prostatic hyperplasia.
   b. nocturia.
   c. hydrocele.
   d. cryptorchidism.
   e. urinary tract infection.

Scenario for questions 9 and 10: An elderly patient comes in for a routine checkup, and the physician discovers his prostate gland is very enlarged.

9. What is a blood test you can run to look for prostate cancer?
   a. PSA test
   b. Proteinuria
   c. Snellen test
   d. Digital rectal exam
   e. Dialysis

10. A urinary condition that might indicate an enlarged prostate gland is:
   a. proteinuria.
   b. oliguria.
   c. nocturia.
   d. hematuria.
   e. pyuria.

11. Seventy-five percent of men with prostate cancer are over age:
   a. 15 years.
   b. 30 years.
   c. 34 years.
   d. 50 years.
   e. 75 years.

12. What kind of juice is recommended to patients to acidify urine?
   a. Tomato juice
   b. Orange juice
   c. Grape juice
   d. Cranberry juice
   e. Grapefruit juice

13. A patient should be given a catheter when:
    a. the patient suffers from nocturia.
    b. the patient has a urinary tract infection.
    c. the patient's urine has high PSA levels.
    d. the patient has calculi.
    e. the patient has dysuria.

14. Which of the following instruments is used to view the bladder and urethra?
    a. Catheter
    b. Cystoscope
    c. Dialysis machine
    d. Ultrasound
    e. Pyelogram

15. Which of the following patients is most likely to develop a urinary tract infection?
    a. A young boy who frequently urinates
    b. A teenaged girl who takes bubble baths
    c. An elderly woman who only wears loose-fitting dresses
    d. An adult woman who showers immediately after sexual intercourse
    e. A middle-aged man who does not wash his hands very often

16. Which of the following is the initial step in catheterization of a patient?
    a. Wash your hands.
    b. Open the catheterization kit.
    c. Put on sterile gloves.
    d. Use antiseptic swabs to clean area.
    e. Assist patient to assume position.

17. What is a symptom of hydronephrosis?
    a. Proteinuria
    b. Chills
    c. Swollen prostate
    d. Back pain
    e. High PSA levels

18. Which of the following is true for catheterizing both men and women?
    a. Tray may be placed on the patient's lap for easy access to tools
    b. The patient's position is on their back, legs apart.
    c. Catheter is inserted 5 inches
    d. Nondominant hand is contaminated
    e. Coudé catheter may be used

19. Which of the following is a cause of organic impotence?
    a. Exhaustion
    b. Anxiety
    c. Depression
    d. Stress
    e. Endocrine imbalance

20. Ultrasonography can be used to treat which of the following?
    a. Renal failure
    b. Hydronephrosis
    c. Calculi
    d. Urinary tract infection
    e. Inguinal hernia

OOG MATCHING

Grade: _____

Place the letter preceding the definition on the line next to the term.

Key Terms

21. _____ anuria
22. _____ blood urea nitrogen
23. _____ catheterization
24. _____ cystoscopy
25. _____ dialysis
26. _____ dysuria
27. _____ enuresis
28. _____ hematuria
29. _____ impotence
30. _____ incontinence
31. _____ intravenous pyelogram (IVP)
32. _____ lithotripsy
33. _____ nephrostomy
34. _____ nocturia
35. _____ oliguria
36. _____ prostate-specific antigen
37. _____ proteinuria
38. _____ psychogenic
39. _____ pyuria
40. _____ retrograde pyelogram
41. _____ specific gravity
42. _____ ureterostomy
43. _____ urinalysis
44. _____ urinary frequency

Definitions

a. an inability to achieve or maintain an erection
b. painful or difficult urination
c. crushing a stone with sound waves
d. the removal of waste in blood not filtered by the kidneys by passing fluid through a semipermeable barrier that allows normal electrolytes to remain, either with a machine with circulatory access or by passing a balanced fluid through the peritoneal cavity
e. excessive urination at night
f. a blood test to determine the amount of nitrogen in blood or urea, a waste product normally excreted in urine
g. of psychological origin
h. a normal protein produced by the prostate that usually elevates in the presence of prostate cancer
i. the density of a liquid, such as urine, compared with water
j. radiography using contrast medium to evaluate kidney function
k. direct visualization of the urinary bladder through a cystoscope inserted through the urethra
l. an examination of the physical, chemical, and microscopic properties of urine
m. failure of kidneys to produce urine
n. blood in the urine
o. the presence of large quantities of protein in the urine; usually a sign of renal dysfunction
p. scant urine production
q. the urge to urinate occurring more often than is required for normal bladder elimination
r. a surgical opening to the outside of the body from the ureter to facilitate drainage of urine from an obstructed kidney
s. pus in the urine
t. bedwetting
u. the placement of a catheter in the kidney pelvis to drain urine from an obstructed kidney
v. the inability to control elimination of urine, feces, or both
w. a procedure for introducing a flexible tube into the body
x. an x-ray of the urinary tract using contrast medium injected through the bladder and ureters; useful in diagnosing obstructions

OOG SHORT ANSWER

Grade: _____

45. What is the difference between hemodialysis and peritoneal dialysis?

_____

_____

_____

_____

46. What are calculi?

_____
_____
_____
_____

47. List five microorganisms that may cause epididymitis.

_____
_____
_____
_____

a. _____

b. _____

c. _____

d. _____

e. _____

48. What are the symptoms of a possible tumor in the urinary system?

_____
_____
_____
_____

49. Are stones more likely to form when urine is alkaline or acidic?

_____
_____
_____
_____

50. Why is a woman more likely to have cystitis than a man?

_____
_____
_____
_____

51. Why are infections in the male urinary tract likely to spread to the reproductive system?

_____
_____
_____
_____

52. What are the three characteristics of the prostate that the physician is checking when performing a digital rectal examination?

_____

_____

_____

_____

53. An older adult male patient with prostatic hypertrophy must be given a catheter in order to obtain a urine sample. What is the best type of catheter to use, and why?

_____

_____

_____

_____

54. List three suggestions to help patients avoid urinary tract infections.

_____

_____

_____

_____

55. What is the difference between an intravenous pyelogram and a retrograde pyelogram? What might the medical assistant be responsible for with regard to the physician order for an intravenous pyelogram and retrograde pyelogram?

_____

_____

_____

_____

COG TRUE OR FALSE?

Grade: _____

Indicate whether the statements are true or false by placing the letter T (true) or F (false) on the line preceding the statement.

56. _____ Orchiopexy refers to either one or both undescended testes.

57. _____ A nephrologist is a physician who specializes in the physical characteristics of the urinary system.

58. _____ No other form of birth control is needed after a man receives a vasectomy.

59. _____ Your office is obligated to notify a patient if a procedure or medication is still in clinical trials, but likely to be approved.

60. A middle-aged patient in good shape comes in complaining of some pain in his groin. The physician suspects he might have an inguinal hernia. What is the procedure to diagnosis this, and how is it corrected?

_____

_____

_____

_____

61. An older adult patient has been diagnosed with renal failure and will need to undergo dialysis. However, he is not sure if hemodialysis or peritoneal dialysis would be better for his lifestyle. What information can you tell him about the two different processes, including the advantages and disadvantages of each?

_____

_____

_____

_____

62. The physician asks you to give information to one of the patients about passing small calculi. What would you tell the patient about calculi, and what suggestions would you give to help the patient pass the stones?

_____

_____

_____

_____

63. A man in his early 20s has come in for his physical, and the physician has instructed you to teach him about testicular disease. You will also need to teach him how to perform a self-examination. However, the man is shy and embarrassed about the procedure. What can you say to him to help him overcome his discomfort?

_____

_____

_____

_____

64. An older adult woman has chronic renal failure, and the physician decides that she will need a catheter for peritoneal dialysis. The woman is upset that she needs this, because she believes that it will limit her movement and ability to participate in activities she likes. What can you tell her about catheters and how her lifestyle will change that might put her more at ease?

_____

_____

_____

_____

PSY PROCEDURE 35-1 Perform a Female Urinary Catheterization

Name: _____ **Date:** _____ **Time:** _____ **Grade:** _____

EQUIPMENT/SUPPLIES: Straight catheterization tray that includes a No. 14 or No. 16 French catheter, a sterile tray, sterile gloves, antiseptic, a specimen cup with a lid, lubricant, and a sterile drape; an examination light; an anatomically correct female torso model for performing the catheterization; a biohazard container

STANDARDS: Given the needed equipment and a place to work, the student will perform this skill with _____ % accuracy in a total of _____ minutes. *(Your instructor will tell you what the percentage and time limits will be before you begin.)*

KEY: 4 = Satisfactory 0 = Unsatisfactory NA = This step is not counted

PROCEDURE STEPS	SELF	PARTNER	INSTRUCTOR
1. Wash your hands	❑	❑	❑
2. Greet the patient and identify yourself, including your title	❑	❑	❑
3. Identify the patient and explain the procedure 　**a.** Have the patient disrobe from the waist down 　**b.** Provide adequate gowning and draping materials	❑	❑	❑
4. Place the patient in the dorsal recumbent or lithotomy position 　**a.** Drape carefully to prevent unnecessary exposure 　**b.** Open the tray and place it between the patient's legs 　**c.** Adjust examination light to allow adequate visualization of the perineum	❑	❑	❑
5. Remove the sterile glove package and put on the sterile gloves	❑	❑	❑
6. Remove sterile drape and place it under the patient's buttocks	❑	❑	❑
7. Open the antiseptic swabs and place them upright inside the catheter tray	❑	❑	❑
8. Open the lubricant and squeeze a generous amount onto the tip of the catheter.	❑	❑	❑
9. Remove the sterile urine specimen cup and lid and place them to the side of the tray	❑	❑	❑
10. Using your nondominant hand, carefully expose the urinary meatus	❑	❑	❑
11. Using your sterile, dominant hand, use antiseptic swabs to cleanse the urinary meatus by starting at the top and moving the swab down each side of the urinary meatus and down the middle, using a new swab for each side and the middle. Do not contaminate the glove on this hand	❑	❑	❑
12. Pick up the catheter with the sterile, dominant hand and: 　**a.** Carefully insert the lubricated tip into the urinary meatus approximately 3 inches 　**b.** Leave the other end of the catheter in the tray	❑	❑	❑

PSY PROCEDURE 35-1 **Perform a Female Urinary Catheterization** (continued)

13. Once the urine begins to flow into the catheter tray, hold the catheter in position with your nondominant hand	❑	❑	❑
14. Use your dominant hand to direct the flow of urine into the specimen cup	❑	❑	❑
15. Remove catheter when urine flow slows or stops or 1,000 mL has been obtained	❑	❑	❑
16. Wipe the perineum carefully with the drape that was placed under the buttocks	❑	❑	❑

17. Dispose of urine appropriately and discard supplies in a biohazard container
  a. Label the specimen container and complete the necessary laboratory requisition
  b. Process the specimen according to the guidelines of the laboratory
	❑	❑	❑

18. Remove your gloves and wash your hands	❑	❑	❑
19. Instruct patient to dress and give any follow-up information	❑	❑	❑
20. **AFF** Log into the Electronic Medical Record (EMR) using your username and secure password OR obtain the paper medical record from a secure location and assure it is kept away from public access	❑	❑	❑
21. Document the procedure in the patient's medical record	❑	❑	❑
22. When finished, log out of the EMR and/or replace the paper medical record in an appropriate and secure location	❑	❑	❑

CALCULATION

Total Possible Points: _____

Total Points Earned: _____ Multiplied by 100 = _____ Divided by Total Possible Points = _____ %

PASS   FAIL   COMMENTS:
  ❑   ❑

Student's signature _____ Date _____

Partner's signature _____ Date _____

Instructor's signature _____ Date _____

PSY PROCEDURE 35-2 **Perform a Male Urinary Catheterization**

Name: _____ **Date:** _____ **Time:** _____ **Grade:** _____

EQUIPMENT/SUPPLIES: Straight catheterization tray that includes a No. 14 or No. 16 French catheter, a sterile tray, sterile gloves, antiseptic, a specimen cup with a lid, lubricant, and a sterile drape; an examination light; an anatomically correct male torso model for performing the catheterization; a biohazard container

STANDARDS: Given the needed equipment and a place to work, the student will perform this skill with _____ % accuracy in a total of _____ minutes. *(Your instructor will tell you what the percentage and time limits will be before you begin.)*

KEY: 4 = Satisfactory 0 = Unsatisfactory NA = This step is not counted

PROCEDURE STEPS	SELF	PARTNER	INSTRUCTOR
1. Wash your hands	❑	❑	❑
2. Greet the patient and identify yourself, including your title	❑	❑	❑

3. Identify the patient
  a. Explain the procedure and have the patient disrobe from the waist down
  b. Provide adequate gowning and draping materials
	❑	❑	❑

4. Place the patient in the supine position
  a. Drape carefully to prevent unnecessary exposure
  b. Open the tray and place it to the side or on the patient's thighs
  c. Adjust examination light to allow adequate visualization of the perineum
	❑	❑	❑

5. Remove the sterile glove package and put on the sterile gloves	❑	❑	❑
6. Carefully remove the sterile drape and place it under the glans penis	❑	❑	❑
7. Open the antiseptic swabs and place them upright inside the catheter tray	❑	❑	❑
8. Open lubricant and squeeze a generous amount onto the tip of the catheter	❑	❑	❑
9. Remove sterile urine specimen cup and lid and place them to the side of the tray	❑	❑	❑
10. Using your nondominant hand, pick up the penis to expose the urinary meatus	❑	❑	❑
11. Using your sterile, dominant hand, use antiseptic swabs to cleanse the urinary meatus by starting at the top and moving the swab around each side of the urinary meatus and down the middle, using a new swab for each side and the middle. Do not contaminate the glove on this hand	❑	❑	❑

12. Using your sterile, dominant hand, pick up the catheter
  a. Carefully insert the lubricated tip into the meatus approximately 4 to 6 inches
  b. The other end of the catheter should be left in the tray
	❑	❑	❑

PSY PROCEDURE 35-2 **Perform a Male Urinary Catheterization** (continued)

13. Once the urine begins to flow into the catheter tray, hold the catheter in position	❑	❑	❑
14. Use your dominant hand to direct the flow of urine into the specimen cup	❑	❑	❑
15. Remove the catheter when urine flow slows or stops or 1,000 mL has been obtained	❑	❑	❑
16. Wipe the glans penis carefully with the drape that was placed under the buttocks	❑	❑	❑
17. Dispose of urine appropriately and discard supplies in a biohazard container	❑	❑	❑
18. Label the specimen container and complete the necessary laboratory requisition	❑	❑	❑
19. Process the specimen according to the guidelines of the laboratory	❑	❑	❑
20. Remove your gloves and wash your hands	❑	❑	❑
21. Instruct patient to dress and give any follow-up information	❑	❑	❑
22. **AFF** Log into the Electronic Medical Record (EMR) using your username and secure password OR obtain the paper medical record from a secure location and assure it is kept away from public access	❑	❑	❑
23. Document the procedure in the patient's medical record	❑	❑	❑
24. When finished, log out of the EMR and/or replace the paper medical record in an appropriate and secure location	❑	❑	❑

CALCULATION

Total Possible Points: _____

Total Points Earned: _____ Multiplied by 100 = _____ Divided by Total Possible Points = _____ %

PASS   FAIL   COMMENTS:
  ❑   ❑

Student's signature _____ Date _____

Partner's signature _____ Date _____

Instructor's signature _____ Date _____

PSY PROCEDURE 35-3	**Instruct a Male Patient on the Self-Testicular Examination**

Name: _____ **Date:** _____ **Time:** _____ **Grade:** _____

EQUIPMENT/SUPPLIES: A patient instruction sheet if available; a testicular examination model or pictures

STANDARDS: Given the needed equipment and a place to work, the student will perform this skill with _____ % accuracy in a total of _____ minutes. *(Your instructor will tell you what the percentage and time limits will be before you begin.)*

KEY: 4 = Satisfactory   0 = Unsatisfactory   NA = This step is not counted

PROCEDURE STEPS	SELF	PARTNER	INSTRUCTOR
1. Wash your hands	❑	❑	❑
2. Greet the patient and identify yourself, including your title	❑	❑	❑
3. Identify the patient and explain the procedure	❑	❑	❑

4. Using the testicular model or pictures, explain the procedure
  a. Tell the patient to examine each testicle by gently rolling between the fingers and the thumb with both hands
  b. Check for lumps or thickenings
	❑	❑	❑

5. Explain that the epididymis is located on top of each testicle
  a. Palpate to avoid incorrectly identifying it as an abnormal growth or lump
  b. Instruct patient to report abnormal lumps or thickenings to the physician
	❑	❑	❑

6. Allow the patient to ask questions related to the testicular self-examination	❑	❑	❑
7. **AFF** Log into the Electronic Medical Record (EMR) using your username and secure password OR obtain the paper medical record from a secure location and assure it is kept away from public access	❑	❑	❑
8. Document the procedure in the patient's medical record	❑	❑	❑
9. When finished, log out of the EMR and/or replace the paper medical record in an appropriate and secure location	❑	❑	❑

CALCULATION

Total Possible Points: _____

Total Points Earned: _____ Multiplied by 100 = _____ Divided by Total Possible Points = _____ %

PASS   FAIL   COMMENTS:
  ❑   ❑

Student's signature _____ Date _____

Partner's signature _____ Date _____

Instructor's signature _____ Date _____

CHAPTER 36

Obstetrics and Gynecology

LEARNING OUTCOMES

COG Cognitive Domain*

1. Spell key terms
2. *Identify the following related to body systems:*
   a. *Medical terms*
   b. *Abbreviations*
3. *Identify structural organization of the human body*
4. *Identify major organs in each body system*
5. *Identify the anatomical location of major organs in each body system*
6. *Identify the normal function of each body system*
7. *Identify common pathology related to each body system including:*
   a. *Signs*
   b. *Symptoms*
   c. *Etiology*
   d. *Diagnostic measures*
   e. *Treatment modalities*
8. Identify your role in the care of gynecologic and obstetric patients
9. Describe the components of prenatal and postpartum patient care
10. Identify the various methods of contraception
11. Describe menopause

PSY Psychomotor Domain*

1. Instruct the patient on the breast self-examination (Procedure 36-1)
   a. *Instruct and prepare a patient for a procedure or treatment*

b. *Assist provider with a patient exam*
   c. *Document patient care accurately in the medical record*
2. Assist with the pelvic examination and Pap smear (Procedure 36-2)
   a. *Instruct and prepare a patient for a procedure or treatment*
   b. *Assist provider with a patient exam*
   c. *Document patient care accurately in the medical record*
3. Assist with colposcopy and cervical biopsy (Procedure 36-3)
   a. *Instruct and prepare a patient for a procedure or treatment*
   b. *Assist provider with a patient exam*
   c. *Document patient care accurately in the medical record*

AFF Affective Domain*

1. *Demonstrate critical thinking skills*
2. *Reassure patients*
3. *Demonstrate empathy for patients' concerns*
4. *Demonstrate active listening*
5. *Respect diversity*
6. *Recognize personal boundaries*
7. *Demonstrate tactfulness*
8. *Demonstrate self-awareness*
9. Protect the integrity of the medical record

MAERB Standards are Italicized.

ABHES Competencies

1. List all body systems and their structures and functions
2. Describe common diseases, symptoms, and etiology as they apply to each system
3. Identify diagnostic and treatment modalities as they relate to each body system
4. Apply medical terminology for each specialty
5. Follow documentation guidelines
6. Adapt care to address the developmental stages of life
7. Partner with healthcare teams to attain optimal patient health outcomes
8. Display effective interpersonal skills with patients and healthcare team members
9. Demonstrate cultural awareness
10. Assist provider with specialty examinations, including cardiac, respiratory, OB-GYN, neurologic, and gastroenterology
11. Perform specialty procedures, including but not limited, to minor surgery, cardiac, respiratory, OB-GYN, neurologic, and gastroenterology
12. Make adaptations for patients with special needs (psychological or physical limitations)
13. Make adaptations to care for patients across their lifespan

Name: _____   Date: _____   Grade: _____

COG MULTIPLE CHOICE

Circle the letter preceding the correct answer.

1. Within 24 hours before a gynecologic examination, a patient should avoid:
   a. showering.
   b. using vaginal medication.
   c. taking a home pregnancy test.
   d. performing a breast self-examination.
   e. taking a medication containing aspirin.

2. A cesarean section is used to:
   a. diagnose gynecologic cancers.
   b. screen the fetus for defects in the neural tube.
   c. analyze fluid from the amniotic sac for nervous system disorders.
   d. deliver an infant when vaginal delivery is not possible or advisable.
   e. stabilize an infant that was delivered before the 37th week of pregnancy.

3. Morning sickness that has escalated to a serious condition is known as:
   a. eclampsia.
   b. proteinuria.
   c. abruptio placentae.
   d. hyperemesis gravidarum.
   e. endometriosis.

4. A pessary may be used to treat:
   a. leiomyomas.
   b. ovarian cysts.
   c. endometriosis.
   d. uterine prolapse.
   e. ectopic pregnancy.

5. The most common sexually transmitted disease in the United States is:
   a. syphilis.
   b. gonorrhea.
   c. chlamydia.
   d. herpes genitalis.
   e. AIDS.

6. Which of the following methods of contraception works hormonally and is worn on the skin for 3 out of 4 weeks to prevent ovulation?
   a. Pill
   b. Ring
   c. Patch
   d. Condom
   e. Spermicide

7. Which of the following is a presumptive sign of pregnancy?
   a. Goodell sign
   b. Fetal heart tone
   c. Nausea and vomiting
   d. HCG in urine and blood
   e. Visualization of the fetus

8. A contraction stress test (CST) should be performed in the:
   a. hospital.
   b. patient's home.
   c. obstetrician's office.
   d. gynecologist's office.
   e. laboratory.

9. A hysterosalpingography is used to determine:
   a. the location and severity of cervical lesions.
   b. whether the patient will abort or miscarry a fetus.
   c. the presence of abnormal cells associated with cervical cancer.
   d. the position of the uterus and the patency of the fallopian tubes.
   e. the size of the pelvic anatomy for a vaginal delivery.

Scenario for Questions 10 and 11: Your patient is a pregnant 32-year-old woman in her 22nd week of gestation. She is complaining of edema, headaches, blurred vision, and vomiting. After laboratory results confirm proteinuria, the physician concludes that the patient has preeclampsia.

10. Which of the following would the physician advise the patient to increase in her diet?
   a. Protein
   b. Sodium
   c. Calcium
   d. Folic acid
   e. Iron

11. What more severe condition could result if her present condition does not improve?
   a. Epilepsy
   b. Eclampsia
   c. Posteclampsia
   d. Premature labor
   e. Hyperemesis gravidarum

12. An undiagnosed ectopic pregnancy could lead to:
    a. polymenorrhea.
    b. salpingo-oophorectomy.
    c. herniation of the ovaries.
    d. displacement of the uterus.
    e. rupture of the fallopian tube.

13. How should the lochia appear immediately and for up to 6 days after delivery?
    a. White
    b. Red
    c. Green
    d. Yellow
    e. Clear

14. The onset of eclampsia is marked by:
    a. seizures.
    b. vomiting.
    c. hypertension.
    d. premature labor.
    e. contractions.

15. A woman who is pregnant for the first time is:
    a. nulligravida.
    b. primigravida.
    c. nullipara.
    d. primipara.
    e. multipara.

16. If animal research indicates no fetal risk concerning the use of a medication, but no human studies have been completed, the medication can be found in which category of drugs?
    a. Category A
    b. Category B
    c. Category C
    d. Category D
    e. Category X

17. The onset of first menses is called:
    a. menarche.
    b. menses.
    c. menorrhagia.
    d. metrorrhagia.
    e. polymenorrhea.

18. Surgery to occlude the vagina is called:
    a. colporrhaphy.
    b. laparoscopy.
    c. ultrasound.
    d. pessary.
    e. colpocleisis.

19. The height of the fundus is determined at each visit by:
    a. ultrasound.
    b. blood work.
    c. urinalysis.
    d. fetal heart monitor.
    e. palpation.

20. Elevated AFP levels in a pregnant woman may indicate:
    a. fetal nervous system deformities.
    b. preeclampsia.
    c. hyperemesis gravidarum.
    d. placenta previa.
    e. uterine contractions.

COG MATCHING

Grade: _____

Place the letter preceding the definition on the line next to the term.

Key Terms	Definitions
21. _____ abortion	**a.** a woman who has never given birth to a viable fetus
22. _____ amenorrhea	**b.** softening of the cervix early in pregnancy
23. _____ amniocentesis	**c.** the presence of large amounts of protein in the urine; usually a sign of renal dysfunction
24. _____ Braxton-Hicks	
25. _____ Chadwick sign	**d.** herniation of the rectum into the vaginal area
26. _____ colpocleisis	**e.** surgical puncture and aspiration of fluid from the vaginal cul-de-sac for diagnosis or therapy
27. _____ culdocentesis	
28. _____ cystocele	**f.** when inserted into the vagina, device that supports the uterus
29. _____ dysmenorrheal	**g.** sign of early pregnancy in which the vaginal, cervical, and vulvar tissues develop a bluish violet color
30. _____ dyspareunia	
31. _____ Goodell sign	**h.** herniation of the urinary bladder into the vagina
32. _____ hirsutism	**i.** period of time (about 6 weeks) from childbirth until reproductive structures return to normal
33. _____ human chorionic gonadotropin (HCG)	**j.** hormone secreted by the placenta and found in the urine and blood of a pregnant female
34. _____ hysterosalpingogram	**k.** irregular uterine bleeding
35. _____ menorrhagia	**l.** puncture of the amniotic sac to remove fluid for testing
36. _____ menarche	**m.** termination of pregnancy or products of conception prior to fetal viability and/or 20 weeks' gestation
37. _____ metrorrhagia	
38. _____ multipara	**n.** condition of not menstruating
39. _____ nullipara	**o.** painful coitus or sexual intercourse
40. _____ pessary	**p.** a woman who has given birth to one viable infant
41. _____ polymenorrhea	**q.** abnormally frequent menstrual periods
42. _____ primipara	**r.** surgery to occlude the vagina
43. _____ proteinuria	**s.** a woman who has given birth to more than one fetus
44. _____ puerperium	**t.** surgical excision of both the fallopian tube and the ovary
45. _____ rectocele	**u.** sporadic uterine contractions during pregnancy
46. _____ salpingo-oophorectomy	**v.** painful menstruation
	w. abnormal or excessive hair growth in women
	x. radiograph of the uterus and fallopian tubes after injection with a contrast medium
	y. onset of first menstruation
	z. excessive bleeding during menstruation

COG MATCHING

Grade: _____

Place the letter preceding the description on the line next to the stage of lochia it describes.

STDs	Microorganisms
47. _____ AIDS	**a.** Herpes simplex virus 2 (HSV2)
48. _____ Syphilis	**b.** Human papilloma virus (HPV)
49. _____ Chlamydia	**c.** *Treponema pallidum*
50. _____ Condylomata acuminata	**d.** *Chlamydia trachomatis*
51. _____ Gonorrhea	**e.** Human immunodeficiency virus (HIV)
52. _____ Herpes genitalis	**f.** *Neisseria gonorrhoeae*

OOG MATCHING

Grade: _____

Match each of the following stages of lochia with the correct description.

Lochia Stages
53. _____ Lochia rubra
54. _____ Lochia serosa
55. _____ Lochia alba

Descriptions
a. Thin, brownish discharge lasting approximately 3 to 4 days after the previous stage
b. Blood-tinged discharge within 6 days of delivery
c. White discharge that has no evidence of blood that can last up to week 6

PSY IDENTIFICATION

Grade: _____

56. Identify which of the following tasks may be the responsibility of the medical assistant in the care of the gynecologic and obstetric patient by placing a check mark on the line preceding the task.

a. _____ Give the patient instructions prior to her pelvic examination, such as refraining from douching, intercourse, and applying vaginal medication for 24 hours before her exam

b. _____ Warm the speculum prior to the pelvic exam

c. _____ Perform a breast examination

d. _____ Instruct the patient to change into an examining gown

e. _____ Inform the patient of the effectiveness of different birth control methods

f. _____ Confirm whether a patient is gravid

g. _____ Decide whether a patient should go to the medical office or go to the hospital after displaying signs and/or symptoms of labor

h. _____ Determine if the patient's medical history includes any over-the-counter medications known to be harmful to a developing fetus

57. Identify the obstetric disorder associated with the following signs and symptoms by writing the name of the disorder on the line following the signs and symptoms.

a. Nausea and vomiting (morning sickness) that has escalated to an unrelenting level, resulting in dehydration, electrolyte imbalance, and weight loss _____

b. The premature separation or detachment of the placenta from the uterus

_____

c. Hypertension that is directly related to pregnancy and can be classified as either preeclampsia or eclampsia _____

d. The loss of pregnancy before the fetus is viable; preceded by vaginal bleeding, uterine cramps, and lower back pain _____

e. A fertilized ovum that has implanted somewhere other than the uterine cavity, such as the fallopian tubes, the abdomen, the ovaries, or the cervical os, causing breast enlargement or tenderness, nausea, pelvic pain, syncope, abdominal symptoms, painful sexual intercourse, and irregular menstrual bleeding _____

58. During the first prenatal visit, you will be responsible for instructing the patient to contact the physician if she experiences certain alarming signs or symptoms. Below, eliminate the signs or symptoms that should not be included in the list by placing a check mark on the line next to the sign or symptom that should *not* be included.

a. _____ Vaginal bleeding or spotting

b. _____ Persistent vomiting

c. _____ Weight gain

d. _____ Increased appetite

e. _____ Fever or chills

f. _____ Dysuria

g. _____ Frequent urination

h. _____ Unusual food cravings

i. _____ Abdominal or uterine cramping

j. _____ Leaking amniotic fluid

k. _____ Alteration in fetal movement

l. _____ Depressed mood

m. _____ Dizziness or blurred vision

59. Review the list of contraceptive methods. Then place a check mark on the line under the column to identify the type of contraceptive that describes the method.

Methods	Surgical	Hormonal	Barrier	Other
a. The pill				
b. Vasectomy				
c. Male condom				
d. Spermicide				
e. Injection				
f. The patch				
g. Emergency contraception				
h. Female condom				
i. The ring				
j. Diaphragm/spermicide				
k. Fertility awareness				
l. IUD				

COG SHORT ANSWER

_____ Grade: _____

60. Some ovarian cysts are functional, whereas others are problematic. Give an example of each.

_____

61. How is premenstrual dysphoric disorder (PMDD) diagnosed and treated?

_____

62. What is the difference between HIV and AIDS?

_____

63. A pregnant patient is listed as gr iv, pret 0, ab 2, p i. What does this listing describe?

_____

64. What is a cesarean section? List the reasons that this procedure would be necessary.

_____

65. Which muscles are strengthened by Kegel exercises? How can these exercises benefit a patient?

_____

66. A patient has just learned she is pregnant. What will you tell her to expect during her first prenatal visit? How often will you schedule the patient's subsequent prenatal visits?

_____

67. After a patient's AFP (alpha-fetoprotein) levels were found to be abnormal, the physician has ordered an amniocentesis and a fetal ultrasonography. Describe the responsibilities of the medical assistant regarding these procedures performed in the medical office.

_____

68. What signs differentiate true labor from false labor?

_____

_____

69. What should a patient nearing the age range of 45 to 50 years be told to expect during menopause?

_____

COG COMPLETION

Grade: _____

70. Complete this chart, which shows common gynecologic disorders, their signs and symptoms, and possible treatments.

Disorder	Signs and Symptoms	Treatment
Dysfunctional uterine bleeding	**a.**	Hormone therapy, contraceptives, curettage, hysterectomy
Premenstrual syndrome	Severe physical, psychological, and behavioral signs and symptoms during the 7 to 10 days before menses	**b.**
Endometriosis	**c.**	Hormone and drug therapy, laparoscopic excision, hysterectomy, bilateral salpingo-oophorectomy
Uterine prolapse and displacement	Pelvic pressure, dyspareunia, urinary problems, constipation	**d.**
Leiomyomas	**e.**	Monitoring, myomectomy, hysterectomy
f.	Anovulation, irregular menses or amenorrhea, hirsutism	Hormone therapy, oral contraceptives
Infertility	Inability to conceive	**g.**

71. Complete this chart, which shows common diagnostic and therapeutic procedures and their purposes.

Procedure	Description	Purpose
Pelvic examination	**a.**	To identify or diagnose any abnormal conditions
Breast examination	Examination of the breast and surrounding tissue; performed with the hands	**b.**
Papanicolaou (Pap) test	**c.**	To detect signs of cervical cancer
Colposcopy	Visual examination of the vaginal and cervical surfaces using a stereoscopic microscope called a *colposcope*	**d.**
e.	Injection of a contrast medium into the uterus and fallopian tubes followed by a radiograph, using a hysterosalpingogram	To determine the configuration of the uterus and the patency of the fallopian tubes for patients with infertility
Dilation and curettage	**f.**	To remove uterine tissue for diagnostic testing, to remove endocrine tissue, to prevent or treat menorrhagia, or to remove retained products of conception after a spontaneous abortion or miscarriage

OOG TRUE OR FALSE?

Grade: _____

Indicate whether the statements are true or false by placing the letter T (true) or F (false) on the line preceding the statement.

72. _____ A woman's first Pap test and pelvic examination should be performed about 3 years after her first sexual intercourse or by age 21 years, whichever comes first, as recommended by the American College of Obstetricians and Gynecologists (ACOG)

73. _____ A pelvic examination is performed for a pregnant patient during each prenatal visit to the obstetrician's office

74. _____ The presence of Braxton-Hicks contractions is a conclusive sign of pregnancy and leads to a formal diagnosis of pregnancy

75. _____ The date on which the patient last had sexual intercourse is used to calculate the expected date of delivery

OOG AFF CASE STUDIES FOR CRITICAL THINKING

Grade: _____

76. A patient at your medical office tested positive for a sexually transmitted disease (STD). What will be your responsibilities in connection with this diagnosis?

_____

_____

_____

_____

77. While working at a gynecological/obstetrics office, you receive a frantic phone call from a pregnant patient who is experiencing vaginal bleeding, uterine cramps, and lower back pain. You put the patient on hold in order to consult the physician, but you learn that the physician has just been called to the hospital for a delivery. How would you handle this call?

_____

_____

_____

_____

78. Your 34-year-old patient is concerned about gynecological cancers because there are cases of breast cancer and cervical cancer in her family history. What can you recommend the patient do to ensure early detection of any gynecologic problems? Describe these procedures to her in a way that will ease her anxieties.

_____

_____

_____

_____

79. A 20-year-old female patient has made an appointment with the physician because she believes that she has PMDD, which she blames for her failing grades and damaged personal relationships. When you meet with the patient to assess her medical history, she asks you to write a note to her professors excusing her from any missed assignments. What should you do next?

_____

_____

_____

_____

PSY PROCEDURE 36-1 | **Instruct the Patient on the Breast Self-Examination**

Name: _____ Date: _____ Time: _____ Grade: _____

EQUIPMENT/SUPPLIES: Patient education instruction sheet, if available; breast examination model, if available

STANDARDS: Given the needed equipment and a place to work, the student will perform this skill with _____ % accuracy in a total of _____ minutes. *(Your instructor will tell you what the percentage and time limits will be before you begin.)*

KEY: 4 = Satisfactory | 0 = Unsatisfactory | NA = This step is not counted

PROCEDURE STEPS	SELF	PARTNER	INSTRUCTOR
1. Wash your hands	❑	❑	❑
2. Greet the patient and identify yourself, including your title. Identify the patient	❑	❑	❑
3. Explain the purpose and frequency of examining the breasts	❑	❑	❑
4. Describe three positions necessary for the patient to examine the breasts: in front of a mirror, in the shower, and while lying down	❑	❑	❑
5. In front of a mirror: **a.** Disrobe and inspect the breasts with her arms at sides and with arms raised above her head **b.** Look for any changes in contour, swelling, dimpling of the skin, or changes in the nipple	❑	❑	❑
6. In the shower: **a.** Feel each breast with hands over wet skin using the flat part of the first three fingers **b.** Check for any lumps, hard knots, or thickenings **c.** Use right hand to lightly press over all areas of left breast **d.** Use left hand to examine right breast	❑	❑	❑
7. Lying down: **a.** Place a pillow or folded towel under the right shoulder, and place the right hand behind head to examine the right breast **b.** With left hand, use flat part of the fingers to palpate the breast tissue **c.** Begin at the outermost top of the right breast **d.** Work in a small circular motion around the breast in a clockwise rotation	❑	❑	❑
8. Encourage patient to palpate the breast carefully moving her fingers inward toward the nipple and palpating every part of the breast, including the nipple.	❑	❑	❑
9. Repeat the procedure for the left breast. Place a pillow or folded towel under the left shoulder with the left hand behind the head	❑	❑	❑
10. Gently squeeze each nipple between the thumb and index finger **a.** Report any clear or bloody discharge to the physician **b.** Promptly report any abnormalities found in the breast self-examination to the physician	❑	❑	❑

(continues)

PSY PROCEDURE 36-1	**Instruct the Patient on the Breast Self-Examination** (continued)		
11. **AFF** Explain how to respond to a patient who is visually impaired	❑	❑	❑
_____ _____ _____ _____			
12. **AFF** Log into the Electronic Medical Record (EMR) using your username and secure password OR obtain the paper medical record from a secure location and assure it is kept away from public access	❑	❑	❑
13. Document the patient education	❑	❑	❑
14. When finished, log out of the EMR and/or replace the paper medical record in an appropriate and secure location	❑	❑	❑

CALCULATION

Total Possible Points: _____

Total Points Earned: _____ Multiplied by 100 = _____ Divided by Total Possible Points = _____ %

PASS **FAIL** **COMMENTS:**
❑ ❑

Student's signature _____ Date _____

Partner's signature _____ Date _____

Instructor's signature _____ Date _____

PSY PROCEDURE 36-2 | **Assist with the Pelvic Examination and Pap Smear**

Name: _____ Date: _____ Time: _____ Grade: _____

EQUIPMENT/SUPPLIES: Gown and drape; appropriate size vaginal speculum; cotton-tipped applicators; water-soluble lubricant; examination gloves; examination light; tissues; materials for Pap smear: cervical brush, liquid-based preservative (SurePath® or ThinPrep®), laboratory request form, identification labels, and other materials that may be required by laboratory; biohazard transport bag, and biohazard waste container

STANDARDS: Given the needed equipment and a place to work, the student will perform this skill with _____ % accuracy in a total of _____ minutes. *(Your instructor will tell you what the percentage and time limits will be before you begin.)*

KEY: 4 = Satisfactory 0 = Unsatisfactory NA = This step is not counted

PROCEDURE STEPS	SELF	PARTNER	INSTRUCTOR
1. Wash your hands	❑	❑	❑
2. Assemble the equipment and supplies **a.** Warm vaginal speculum by running under warm water **b.** Do not use lubricant on the vaginal speculum before insertion	❑	❑	❑
3. Label the outside of the liquid-based preservative container	❑	❑	❑
4. Greet and identify yourself, including your title	❑	❑	❑
5. Identify the patient and explain the procedure	❑	❑	❑
6. Ask the patient to empty her bladder and, if necessary, collect a urine specimen	❑	❑	❑
7. Provide a gown and drape, and ask the patient to disrobe from the waist down	❑	❑	❑
8. Position patient in the dorsal lithotomy position—buttocks at bottom edge of table	❑	❑	❑
9. Adjust drape to cover patient's abdomen and knees but expose the genitalia	❑	❑	❑
10. Adjust light over the genitalia for maximum visibility	❑	❑	❑
11. Assist physician with the examination as needed	❑	❑	❑
12. Put on examination gloves. Hold cytology liquid container for physician or insert brush as directed and mix with cytology liquid	❑	❑	❑
13. Have a basin or other container ready to receive the now-contaminated speculum	❑	❑	❑
14. Apply lubricant across the physician's two fingers	❑	❑	❑
15. Encourage the patient to relax during the bimanual examination as needed	❑	❑	❑
16. After the examination, assist the patient in sliding up to the top of the examination table and remove both feet at the same time from the stirrups	❑	❑	❑

(continues)

PSY PROCEDURE 36-2 **Assist with the Pelvic Examination and Pap Smear** (continued)

17. Offer the patient tissues to remove excess lubricant
   a. Assist her to a sitting position, if necessary
   b. Watch for signs of vertigo
   c. Ask the patient to get dressed and assist, as needed
   d. Provide for privacy as the patient dresses
	❑	❑	❑

18. Reinforce any physician instructions regarding follow-up appointments needed **a.** Advise patient on the procedure for obtaining results from the Pap smear	❑	❑	❑
19. **AFF** Explain how to respond to a patient who has dementia	❑	❑	❑
_____			
20. Properly care for or dispose of equipment and clean the examination room. Prepare the specimen for transport to the laboratory	❑	❑	❑
21. Remove your gloves and wash your hands	❑	❑	❑
22. **AFF** Log into the Electronic Medical Record (EMR) using your username and secure password OR obtain the paper medical record from a secure location and assure it is kept away from public access	❑	❑	❑
23. Document your responsibilities during the procedure	❑	❑	❑
24. When finished, log out of the EMR and/or replace the paper medical record in an appropriate and secure location	❑	❑	❑

CALCULATION

Total Possible Points: _____

Total Points Earned: _____ Multiplied by 100 = _____ Divided by Total Possible Points = _____ %

PASS   **FAIL**   **COMMENTS:**
 ❑   ❑

Student's signature _____ Date _____

Partner's signature _____ Date _____

Instructor's signature _____ Date _____

PSY PROCEDURE 36-3 | **Assist with Colposcopy and Cervical Biopsy**

Name: _____ Date: _____ Time: _____ Grade: _____

EQUIPMENT/SUPPLIES: Patient gown and drape, vaginal speculum, colposcope, specimen container with preservative (10% formalin), sterile gloves, appropriate size sterile cotton-tipped applicators, sterile normal saline solution, sterile 3% acetic acid, sterile povidone–iodine (Betadine), silver nitrate sticks or ferric subsulfate (Monsel solution), sterile biopsy forceps or punch biopsy instrument, sterile uterine curette, sterile uterine dressing forceps, sterile 4 × 4 gauze pad, sterile towel, sterile endocervical curette, sterile uterine tenaculum, sanitary napkin, examination gloves, examination light, tissues, biohazard container

STANDARDS: Given the needed equipment and a place to work, the student will perform this skill with _____ % accuracy in a total of _____ minutes. (*Your instructor will tell you what the percentage and time limits will be before you begin.*)

KEY: 4 = Satisfactory 0 = Unsatisfactory NA = This step is not counted

PROCEDURE STEPS	SELF	PARTNER	INSTRUCTOR
1. Wash your hands	❏	❏	❏
2. Verify that the patient has signed the consent form	❏	❏	❏
3. Assemble the equipment and supplies	❏	❏	❏
4. Check the light on the colposcope	❏	❏	❏
5. Set up the sterile field without contaminating it	❏	❏	❏
6. Pour sterile normal saline and acetic acid into their respective sterile containers	❏	❏	❏
7. Cover the field with a sterile drape	❏	❏	❏
8. Greet and identify yourself, including your title	❏	❏	❏
9. Identify the patient and explain the procedure	❏	❏	❏
10. When the physician is ready to proceed with the procedure: **a.** Assist the patient into the dorsal lithotomy position **b.** Put on sterile gloves after positioning the patient, if necessary	❏	❏	❏
11. Hand the physician: **a.** The applicator immersed in normal saline **b.** Followed by the applicator immersed in acetic acid **c.** The applicator with the antiseptic solution (Betadine)	❏	❏	❏
12. If you did not apply sterile gloves to assist the physician: **a.** Apply clean examination gloves **b.** Accept the biopsy specimen into a container of 10% formalin preservative	❏	❏	❏
13. Provide the physician with Monsel solution or silver nitrate sticks	❏	❏	❏

(continues)

PSY PROCEDURE 36-3   **Assist with Colposcopy and Cervical Biopsy** (continued)

14. When the physician is finished with the procedure:
   a. Assist the patient from the stirrups and into a sitting position
   b. Explain to the patient that a small amount of bleeding may occur
   c. Have a sanitary napkin available for the patient
   d. Ask the patient to get dressed and assist as needed
   e. Provide for privacy as the patient dresses
   f. Reinforce any physician instructions regarding follow-up appointments
   g. Advise the patient on how to obtain the biopsy results
	❏	❏	❏

15. **AFF** Explain how to respond to a patient who does not speak English or speaks English as a second language	❏	❏	❏

16. Label the specimen container with the patient's name and date
   a. Prepare the laboratory request
   b. Transport the specimen and form to the laboratory
	❏	❏	❏

17. Properly care for, or dispose of, equipment and clean the examination room	❏	❏	❏
18. Wash your hands	❏	❏	❏
19. **AFF** Log into the Electronic Medical Record (EMR) using your username and secure password OR obtain the paper medical record from a secure location and assure it is kept away from public access	❏	❏	❏
20. Document your responsibilities during the procedure	❏	❏	❏
21. When finished, log out of the EMR and/or replace the paper medical record in an appropriate and secure location	❏	❏	❏

CALCULATION

Total Possible Points: _____

Total Points Earned: _____ Multiplied by 100 = _____ Divided by Total Possible Points = _____ %

PASS   **FAIL**   **COMMENTS:**
❏   ❏

Student's signature _____ Date _____

Partner's signature _____ Date _____

Instructor's signature _____ Date _____

CHAPTER 37

Endocrinology

LEARNING OUTCOMES

COG Cognitive Domain*

1. Spell key terms
2. *Identify the following related to body systems:*
   a. *Medical terms*
   b. *Abbreviations*
3. *Identify structural organization of the human body*
4. *Identify major organs in each body system*
5. *Identify the anatomical location of major organs in each body system*
6. *Identify the normal function of each body system*
7. *Identify common pathology related to each body system including:*
   a. *Signs*
   b. *Symptoms*
   c. *Etiology*
   d. *Diagnostic measures*
   e. *Treatment modalities*
8. Explain your role in working with patients with endocrine system disorders

PSY Psychomotor Domain*

1. Manage a patient with a diabetic emergency (Procedure 37-1)
   a. *Instruct and prepare a patient for a procedure or treatment*

b. *Assist provider with a patient exam*
c. *Document patient care accurately in the medical record*

AFF Affective Domain*

1. *Demonstrate critical thinking skills*
2. *Reassure patients*
3. *Demonstrate empathy for patients' concerns*
4. *Demonstrate active listening*
5. *Respect diversity*
6. *Recognize personal boundaries*
7. *Demonstrate tactfulness*
8. *Demonstrate self-awareness*
9. Protect the integrity of the medical record

MAERB Standards are Italicized.

ABHES Competencies

1. List all body systems and their structures and functions
2. Describe common diseases, symptoms, and etiology as they apply to each system
3. Identify diagnostic and treatment modalities as they relate to each body system

4. Apply medical terminology for each specialty
5. Follow documentation guidelines
6. Adapt care to address the developmental stages of life
7. Partner with healthcare teams to attain optimal patient health outcomes
8. Display effective interpersonal skills with patients and healthcare team members
9. Demonstrate cultural awareness
10. Assist provider with specialty examinations, including cardiac, respiratory, OB-GYN, neurologic, and gastroenterology
11. Perform specialty procedures, including but not limited to minor surgery, cardiac, respiratory, OB-GYN, neurologic, and gastroenterology
12. Make adaptations for patients with special needs (psychological or physical limitations)
13. Make adaptations to care for patients across their lifespan

Name: _____   Date: _____   Grade: _____

OCG MULTIPLE CHOICE

Circle the letter preceding the correct answer:

1. A patient with hypothyroidism must take hormone replacements:
   a. for as many years as they have had the disease.
   b. until the conclusion of puberty.
   c. for their entire life.
   d. until middle age.
   e. for 10 years.

2. Diabetics may need supplemental insulin to:
   a. test blood glucose levels.
   b. reverse vascular changes.
   c. reduce the presence of ketones.
   d. restore pancreatic function.
   e. control blood glucose levels.

3. One symptom of ketoacidosis is:
   a. shallow respirations.
   b. low blood glucose levels.
   c. overhydration.
   d. abdominal pain.
   e. pale, moist skin.

4. Diabetes mellitus affects metabolism of which type of molecule?
   a. Neurotransmitters
   b. Carbohydrates
   c. Hormones
   d. Vitamins
   e. Lipids

5. One symptom of type 1 diabetes mellitus is:
   a. polyuria.
   b. exophthalmia.
   c. anorexia.
   d. weight gain.
   e. a goiter.

6. Hyperpigmentation of the skin might be an indication of:
   a. Cushing's syndrome.
   b. Hashimoto's thyroiditis.
   c. Graves' disease.
   d. Addison's disease.
   e. diabetes insipidus.

7. To control gestational diabetes, a blood glucose specimen should be taken from a pregnant woman between:
   a. 28 and 32 weeks of gestation.
   b. 24 and 28 weeks of gestation.
   c. 20 and 24 weeks of gestation.
   d. 16 and 20 weeks of gestation.
   e. 12 and 16 weeks of gestation.

8. Cushing's syndrome sufferers may experience accelerated:
   a. Addison's disease.
   b. endocarditis.
   c. osteoporosis.
   d. arthritis.
   e. dementia.

9. Acromegaly results primarily in:
   a. an increase in bone width.
   b. muscular atrophy.
   c. an increase in bone length.
   d. muscular hypertrophy.
   e. an increase in bone density.

10. Growth can be stimulated for children with dwarfism by:
    a. repairs in the pituitary gland.
    b. administration of growth hormone.
    c. psychotherapy.
    d. increased physical activity.
    e. a high-protein diet.

11. Diabetes insipidus results from a deficiency of:
    a. adrenocorticotropic hormone.
    b. anterior pituitary hormones.
    c. human growth hormone.
    d. antidiuretic hormone.
    e. thyroid hormones.

12. Insulin shock is a result of:
    a. Cushing's syndrome.
    b. Addison's disease.
    c. Graves' disease.
    d. hyperglycemia.
    e. hypoglycemia.

13. Diabetes mellitus patients need to care for their feet because:
- **a.** they regularly develop ingrown toenails.
- **b.** their peripheral circulation may be poor.
- **c.** they suffer severe joint pain.
- **d.** they have weak calves.
- **e.** foot pain occurs.

14. Exophthalmia is a protrusion of the:
- **a.** thyroid gland.
- **b.** pancreas.
- **c.** gall bladder.
- **d.** eyes.
- **e.** liver.

15. Patients taking corticosteroids may be at risk for:
- **a.** Cushing's disease.
- **b.** Addison's disease.
- **c.** type 2 diabetes mellitus.
- **d.** Graves' disease.
- **e.** Hashimoto's thyroiditis.

16. The A1C test determines how well blood glucose has been controlled during the previous:
- **a.** 2 to 3 hours.
- **b.** 2 to 3 days.
- **c.** 2 to 3 weeks.
- **d.** 2 to 3 months.
- **e.** 2 to 3 years.

17. Gigantism is a disorder of the:
- **a.** adrenal glands.
- **b.** pancreas.
- **c.** liver.
- **d.** thyroid.
- **e.** pituitary gland.

18. A thyroid scan relies on a radioactive isotope of what element?
- **a.** Iodine
- **b.** Barium
- **c.** Indium
- **d.** Bismuth
- **e.** Iridium

19. Addison's disease is a disorder of the:
- **a.** pituitary gland.
- **b.** pancreas.
- **c.** thyroid.
- **d.** adrenal gland.
- **e.** salivary glands.

20. Both Graves' disease and goiters are examples of:
- **a.** hypothyroidism.
- **b.** hypoglycemia.
- **c.** hyperthyroidism.
- **d.** hyperglycemia.
- **e.** hypertension.

COG MATCHING

Grade: _____

Place the letter preceding the definition on the line next to the term.

Key Terms

21. _____ acromegaly
22. _____ Addison's disease
23. _____ Cushing's syndrome
24. _____ diabetes insipidus
25. _____ dwarfism
26. _____ endocrinologist
27. _____ exophthalmia
28. _____ gigantism
29. _____ glycosuria
30. _____ goiter
31. _____ Graves' disease
32. _____ Hashimoto's thyroiditis
33. _____ hormones
34. _____ hyperglycemia
35. _____ hyperplasia
36. _____ hypoglycemia
37. _____ insulin-dependent diabetes mellitus
38. _____ ketoacidosis
39. _____ ketones
40. _____ non–insulin-dependent diabetes mellitus
41. _____ polydipsia
42. _____ polyphagia
43. _____ polyuria
44. _____ pruritus
45. _____ radioimmunoassay
46. _____ thyrotoxicosis

Definitions

a. an enlargement of the thyroid gland
b. a substance that is produced by an endocrine gland and travels through the blood to a distant organ or gland where it acts to modify the structure or function of that gland or organ
c. an adrenal gland disorder that results in an increased production of ACTH from the pituitary glands
d. excess quantities of thyroid hormone in tissues
e. excessive proliferation of normal cells in the normal tissue arrangement of an organism
f. the end products of fat metabolism
g. itching
h. pronounced hyperthyroidism with signs of enlarged thyroid and exophthalmos
i. a type of diabetes in which patients do not require insulin to control blood sugar
j. a deficiency in insulin production that leads to an inability to metabolize carbohydrates
k. partial or complete failure of the adrenal cortex functions, causing general physical deterioration
l. the presence of glucose in the urine
m. a disease of the immune system in which the tissue of the thyroid gland is replaced with fibrous tissue
n. excessive thirst
o. abnormal underdevelopment of the body with extreme shortness but normal proportion; achondroplastic dwarfism is an inherited growth disorder characterized by shortened limbs and a large head but almost normal trunk proportions
p. acidosis accompanied by an accumulation of ketones in the body
q. excessive size and stature caused most frequently by hypersecretion of the human growth hormone
r. deficiency of sugar in the blood
s. an unusual protrusion of the eyeballs as a result of a thyroid disorder
t. a disorder of metabolism characterized by polyuria and polydipsia; caused by a deficiency in ADH or an inability of the kidneys to respond to ADH
u. excessive excretion and elimination of urine
v. hyperfunction of the anterior pituitary gland near the end of puberty that results in increased bone width.
w. the introduction of radioactive substances in the body to determine the concentration of a substance in the serum, usually the concentration of antigens, antibodies, or proteins
x. a doctor who diagnoses and treats disorders of the endocrine system and its hormone-secreting glands
y. abnormal hunger
z. an increase in blood sugar, as in diabetes mellitus

⬤OG IDENTIFICATION

Grade: _____

47. Read the following list of symptoms. Are these symptoms representative of hyperglycemia or hypoglycemia? Place the prefix "hyper" on the line preceding the symptoms for hyperglycemia and "hypo" for hypoglycemia.

a. _____ Pale complexion

b. _____ Deep respirations

c. _____ Moist skin

d. _____ Shallow respirations

e. _____ Abdominal pain

f. _____ Rapid, bounding pulse

g. _____ Fruity breath

h. _____ Subnormal blood glucose levels

⬤OG SHORT ANSWER

Grade: _____

48. When does ketoacidosis occur?

_____

_____

_____

_____

49. A patient is stunned to learn that she has been diagnosed with type 2 diabetes mellitus. She is 43 years old and in excellent health. As a personal trainer and nutritionist, she has always taken good care of her body. What potential cause of type 2 diabetes mellitus might she be overlooking?

_____

_____

_____

_____

50. A patient complains that, lately, his appetite has been ferocious, but he is actually losing weight. He does not understand why this is happening. What do you tell him?

_____

_____

_____

_____

51. Why is it difficult for many sufferers of endocrine disorders to comply with physicians' orders?

_____

_____

_____

_____

52. A patient who has been diagnosed with type 2 diabetes mellitus explains that a friend told him the disease is sometimes called _non–insulin-dependent diabetes mellitus._ He asks if this means that he will not need to take insulin. Is he correct? Why, or why not?

_____

_____

_____

_____

53. Who might be at risk for gestational diabetes mellitus?

_____

_____

_____

_____

54. What is the cause of hypoglycemia?

_____

_____

_____

_____

55. How is Addison's disease treated?

_____

_____

_____

_____

56. A patient is diagnosed with dwarfism, and the patient's mother is extremely distressed, wondering if certain body parts will grow normally while others will not. She also wonders if her daughter could ever grow normally. What could you tell the mother?

_____

_____

_____

_____

57. What do the fasting glucose test and glucose tolerance test for diabetes mellitus have in common?

_____

_____

_____

_____

58. What is the purpose of the A1C blood test?

_____

_____

_____

_____

59. Cushing's syndrome and Addison's disease are both disorders of which gland?

_____

_____

_____

_____

60. Why is it important that patients with diseases of the endocrine system wear a medical alert bracelet or necklace?

_____

_____

_____

_____

COG TRUE OR FALSE?

Grade: _____

Indicate whether the statements are true or false by placing the letter T (true) or F (false) on the line preceding the statement.

61. _____ Endocrine glands are unlike other glands in the body because they are ductless.

62. _____ Hashimoto's thyroiditis is a disease of the endocrine system.

63. _____ Type 1 diabetes mellitus occurs only in children and young adults.

64. _____ Addison's disease has no effect on the pituitary gland.

COG **AFF** CASE STUDIES FOR CRITICAL THINKING

Grade: _____

65. A patient is worried that a thyroid function test requires the use of radioactive material. Explain, to the best of your ability, how the test works and why there is no need to be concerned about radiation. If necessary, do additional research on thyroid function tests to prepare your answer.

_____

_____

_____

_____

66. After an examination, a pregnant patient asks why the physician performed a test on her blood glucose level. She says she does not have diabetes. Explain why the physician chose to do the test.

_____

_____

_____

_____

67. Young children are sometimes afflicted with diabetes mellitus. This can be difficult for both the child and the family. What is your perspective of the medical assistant's role in this situation?

_____

_____

_____

_____

68. A patient with hyperthyroidism says she would prefer not to be treated because she has few negative symptoms, and the increased metabolic rate helps keep her thin. How would you respond to this?

_____

_____

_____

_____

PSY PROCEDURE 37-1 | Manage a Patient with a Diabetic Emergency

Name: _____ Date: _____ Time: _____ Grade: _____

EQUIPMENT/SUPPLIES: Gloves, blood glucose monitor and strips, fruit juice or oral glucose tablets

STANDARDS: Given the needed equipment and a place to work, the student will perform this skill with _____ % accuracy in a total of _____ minutes. *(Your instructor will tell you what the percentage and time limits will be before you begin.)*

KEY: 4 = Satisfactory   0 = Unsatisfactory   NA = This step is not counted

PROCEDURE STEPS	SELF	PARTNER	INSTRUCTOR
1. Wash your hands	❑	❑	❑
2. Recognize the signs and symptoms of hyperglycemia and hypoglycemia	❑	❑	❑
3. Greet the patient and identify yourself, including your title. Identify the patient	❑	❑	❑
4. Escort the patient into the examination room while making the observation that there is a problem	❑	❑	❑
5. Determine if the patient has been previously diagnosed with diabetes mellitus and acknowledge that the patient is a diabetic	❑	❑	❑
6. Ask the patient if they have eaten today or have taken any medication	❑	❑	❑
7. Notify the physician about the patient and perform a capillary stick for a blood glucose test as directed	❑	❑	❑

8. Notify the physician with the results of the blood glucose test and treat the patient as ordered by the physician
  a. Administer insulin subcutaneously to a patient with hyperglycemia
  b. Administer a quick-acting sugar, such as an oral glucose tablet or fruit juice, for a patient with hypoglycemia
	❑	❑	❑

9. **AFF** Explain how to respond to a patient who is developmentally challenged	❑	❑	❑

_____

_____

_____

_____

(continues)

PSY PROCEDURE 37-1	**Manage a Patient with a Diabetic Emergency** (continued)		
10. Be prepared to notify EMS as directed by the physician if the symptoms do not improve or they worsen	❏	❏	❏
11. **AFF** Log into the Electronic Medical Record (EMR) using your username and secure password OR obtain the paper medical record from a secure location and assure it is kept away from public access	❏	❏	❏
12. Document any observations and treatments given	❏	❏	❏

CALCULATION

Total Possible Points: _____

Total Points Earned: _____ Multiplied by 100 = _____ Divided by Total Possible Points = _____ %

PASS   FAIL   COMMENTS:
 ❏   ❏

Student's signature _____ Date _____

Partner's signature _____ Date _____

Instructor's signature _____ Date _____

CHAPTER 38

Pediatrics

LEARNING OUTCOMES

COG Cognitive Domain*

1. Spell key terms
2. *Identify the following related to body systems:*
   a. *Medical terms*
   b. *Abbreviations*
3. *Identify the structure and function of the human body across the life span*
4. *Identify normal and abnormal results as reported in*
   a. *Graphs*
   b. *Tables*
5. *Identify common pathology related to each body system including:*
   a. *Signs*
   b. *Symptoms*
   c. *Etiology*
   d. *Diagnostic measures*
   e. *Treatment modalities*
6. List safety precautions for the pediatric office
7. Explain the difference between a well-child and a sick-child visit
8. *Identify appropriate vaccinations based on an immunization schedule*
9. Describe the types of feelings a child might have during an office visit
10. List and explain how to record the anthropometric measurements obtained in a pediatric visit
11. Identify two injection sites to use on an infant and two to use on a child
12. Describe the role of the parent or caregiver during the office visit
13. List the names, symptoms, and treatments for common pediatric illnesses

PSY Psychomotor Domain*

1. Obtain an infant's length and weight (Procedure 38-1)
   a. Instruct and prepare a patient for a procedure or treatment
   b. Assist provider with a patient exam
   c. Document patient care accurately in the medical record
2. Obtain the head and chest circumference (Procedure 38-2)
   a. Instruct and prepare a patient for a procedure or treatment
   b. Assist provider with a patient exam
   c. Document patient care accurately in the medical record

AFF Affective Domain*

1. *Demonstrate critical thinking skills*
2. *Reassure patients*
3. *Demonstrate empathy for patients' concerns*
4. *Demonstrate active listening*
5. *Respect diversity*
6. *Recognize personal boundaries*
7. *Demonstrate tactfulness*
8. *Demonstrate self-awareness*
9. Protect the integrity of the medical record

MAERB Standards are Italicized.

ABHES Competencies

1. List all body systems and their structures and functions
2. Describe common diseases, symptoms, and etiology as they apply to each system
3. Identify diagnostic and treatment modalities as they relate to each body system
4. Apply medical terminology for each specialty
5. Follow documentation guidelines
6. Adapt care to address the developmental stages of life
7. Partner with healthcare teams to attain optimal patient health outcomes
8. Display effective interpersonal skills with patients and healthcare team members
9. Demonstrate cultural awareness
10. Assist provider with specialty examinations, including cardiac, respiratory, OB-GYN, neurologic, and gastroenterology
11. Perform specialty procedures, including but not limited to minor surgery, cardiac, respiratory, OB-GYN, neurologic, and gastroenterology
12. Make adaptations for patients with special needs (psychological or physical limitations)
13. Make adaptations to care for patients across their lifespan

© YASNARADA/Shutterstock

Name: _____   Date: _____   Grade: _____

COG MULTIPLE CHOICE

Circle the letter preceding the correct answer.

1. The top priority in a pediatric office is:
    a. organization.
    b. safety.
    c. efficiency.
    d. location.
    e. size.

2. In a pediatrician's waiting room, it is most important that the toys are:
    a. trendy.
    b. interesting to all age groups.
    c. large enough to share.
    d. washable.
    e. educational.

3. Which method of taking a temperature is most readily accepted by children of all ages?
    a. Tympanic
    b. Oral
    c. Rectal
    d. Axillary
    e. Touch

4. One symptom of meningitis is:
    a. dysuria.
    b. disorientation.
    c. coughing.
    d. stiff neck.
    e. chills.

5. Which of the following has been associated with Reye syndrome?
    a. Pyloric stenosis
    b. Aspirin
    c. Cerebral palsy
    d. Phenylalanine hydroxylase
    e. Otitis media

6. Which of the following is something that is routinely done at a child's wellness exam?
    a. Blood test
    b. Urine test
    c. Immunization
    d. Radiography
    e. Measurements

7. To minimize a child's anxiety during a visit, you should:
    a. avoid talking to the child.
    b. speak directly to the parent.
    c. be gentle but firm.
    d. ask the child to be quiet.
    e. spend as little time in the room as possible.

8. Which of the following statements is true?
    a. The reflexes present in a newborn disappear by age 3 months.
    b. A pediatrician is responsible for a child's physical and mental health.
    c. Disinfectants should be kept in patient rooms for easy access.
    d. Vaccination Information Statements may be provided upon request.
    e. The DDST measures all physical and mental aspects of a child.

9. One warning sign of child abuse is a child who:
    a. comes in with scraped knees.
    b. shrinks away as you approach.
    c. has a poor growth pattern.
    d. has a bloody nose.
    e. screams when you administer a shot.

10. What might make the examination more fun for a 4- or 5-year-old child?
    a. Allowing the child to crawl on the floor
    b. Answering all of the questions they ask
    c. Showing the child medical pictures
    d. Letting the child listen to their heartbeat
    e. Asking the parent to assist with the exam

Scenario for Questions 11 and 12: Mary is brought in for a well-child visit and begins to panic when she hears she will need to get a vaccination.

11. What should you do?
    a. Let another assistant give her the shot
    b. Ask the parent or caregiver to calm her down
    c. Show her the needle ahead of time
    d. Tell her gently that it won't hurt at all
    e. Hide the needle until you give her the shot

12. After you administer the medication, the girl becomes sullen and withdrawn. What is the best way to address this behavior?
    a. Leave and allow her mother to comfort her
    b. Praise and comfort her before you leave
    c. Ask her if the shot was really that bad
    d. Promise it won't hurt so much next time
    e. Laugh and say it was just a little shot

13. Which of the following disorders has symptoms that may become obvious only with the passage of time?
    a. Meningitis
    b. Croup
    c. Epiglottitis
    d. Cerebral palsy
    e. Pyloric stenosis

14. Children are more likely to develop ear infections than adults because they have:
    a. an immature nervous system.
    b. short and straight Eustachian tubes.
    c. decreased resistance to diseases.
    d. more exposure to bacteria.
    e. poor handwashing skills.

15. Which infant reflex is a result of the cheek being stroked?
    a. Rooting
    b. Moro
    c. Stepping
    d. Fencing
    e. Babinski

16. Children have lower blood pressure than adults because:
    a. they cannot sit still for long periods of time.
    b. they require a smaller cuff for measurements.
    c. their hearts do not pump as quickly as adults' hearts.
    d. their vessels are softer and less resistant.
    e. you must use a standard sphygmomanometer.

17. At what age does a child's respiratory rate slow to that of an adult's?
    a. 0 to 1 year
    b. 1 to 5 years
    c. 5 to 10 years
    d. 10 to 15 years
    e. 15 to 20 years

18. Which of the following can help a physician test an infant for pyloric stenosis?
    a. Blood tests
    b. Urine tests
    c. Parental history
    d. Percentile comparisons
    e. Weight

19. Which of the following disorders cannot be cured at this time?
    a. Meningitis
    b. Impetigo
    c. Tetanus
    d. Syphilis
    e. Cerebral palsy

20. A sharp barking cough is a symptom of:
    a. meningitis.
    b. croup.
    c. tetanus.
    d. encephalitis.
    e. impetigo.

OG MATCHING

Grade: _____

Place the letter preceding the definition on the line next to the term.

Key Terms

21. _____ aspiration
22. _____ autonomous
23. _____ congenital anomaly
24. _____ immunization
25. _____ neonatologist
26. _____ pediatrician
27. _____ pediatrics
28. _____ psychosocial
29. _____ restrain
30. _____ sick-child visit
31. _____ varicella zoster
32. _____ well-child visit

Definitions

a. to control or confine movement

b. a physician who specializes in the care and treatment of newborns

c. a viral infection manifested by the characteristic rash of successive crops of vesicles that scab before resolution; also called chicken pox

d. a physician who specializes in the care of infants, children, and adolescents

e. a visit to the medical office for the administration of immunizations and evaluation of growth and development

f. drawing in or out by suction, as in breathing objects into the respiratory tract or suctioning substances from a site

g. an abnormality, either structural or functional, present at birth

h. a pediatric visit for the treatment of illness or injury

i. a specialty of medicine that deals with the care of infants, children, and adolescents

j. existing or functioning independently

k. relating to mental and emotional aspects of social encounters

l. the act or process of rendering an individual immune to specific disease

OG MATCHING

Grade: _____

Place the letter preceding the pulse rate range on the line preceding the appropriate age.

Ages

33. _____ newborn
34. _____ 3 months to 2 years
35. _____ 2 years to 10 years
36. _____ 10 years and older

Pulse Rate Ranges

a. 80 to 150/minute
b. 60 to 100/minute
c. 100 to 180/minute
d. 65 to 130/minute

PSY IDENTIFICATION

Grade: _____

37. Review the most current pediatric immunization schedule on the CDC (Centers for Disease Control and Prevention website) to answer the following questions:

a. How many doses of the rotavirus vaccine are given? When?

_____

b. How many immunizations do children receive at 4 months? Which ones?

_____

c. When do children start receiving a yearly influenza vaccination?

_____

d. How many doses of the hepatitis B vaccine are administered?

_____

38. What are five different ways to check a child's temperature?

a. _____

b. _____

c. _____

d. _____

e. _____

39. What are the seven "rights" of drug administration?

a. _____

b. _____

c. _____

d. _____

e. _____

f. _____

g. _____

40. Identify six symptoms of meningitis:

_____

_____

COG SHORT ANSWER

Grade: _____

41. What does the Federal Child Abuse Prevention and Treatment Act mandate?

_____

_____

_____

_____

42. What is the VIS? Why do you give the parent or caregiver of a child a copy?

_____

_____

_____

_____

43. Why do sick-child visits occur frequently during early childhood?

_____

_____

_____

_____

44. What is the difference between a well-child and a sick-child visit?

_____

_____

_____

_____

45. List five feelings a child might have during an office visit.

_____

_____

_____

_____

46. What role does a parent or caregiver play in the child's exam?

_____

_____

_____

_____

47. How is a child's medication dosage calculated?

_____

_____

_____

_____

48. Why is epiglottitis considered more serious than croup?

_____

_____

_____

_____

49. If a child has been reported as being easily distracted, forgetful, extremely talkative, impulsive, and showing a dislike for school activities, does the child have attention deficit hyperactivity disorder (ADHD)?

_____

_____

_____

_____

50. A worried mother calls in because her newborn baby is vomiting. She wants to know if she should bring her baby into the office for an examination. What do you tell her?

_____

_____

_____

_____

COG COMPLETION

Grade: _____

51. Complete the chart below with information about childhood reflexes. Briefly describe each response and note the age it generally disappears.

Reflex	Response	Age When It Generally Disappears
a. Sucking, or rooting		
b. Moro, or startle		
c. Grasp		
d. Tonic neck, or fencing		
e. Placing, or stepping		
f. Babinski		

COG TRUE OR FALSE?

Grade: _____

Indicate whether the statements are true or false by placing the letter T (true) or F (false) on the line preceding the statement.

52. _____ Infant scales should always be placed on the floor next to the adult scale.

53. _____ It is a violation of HIPAA to have two separate waiting rooms for sick children and well children.

54. _____ There should be no toys in the waiting room because they may help spread germs.

55. _____ Children outgrow child-sized furniture too quickly, so it is not a worthwhile investment.

56. _____ Many childhood diseases are highly contagious and can be controlled by stringent handwashing measures.

57. _____ Immunization schedules change every 5 years.

58. _____ A child's heartbeat is much slower than an adult's heart rate.

59. _____ Asthma is a respiratory problem that usually develops after puberty.

60. _____ Minors do not need to be informed of what you're going to do.

OOG **AFF** **CASE STUDIES FOR CRITICAL THINKING** _____ Grade: _____

61. A mother calls in, saying her 15-month-old daughter has been fussy and tugging at her ear. There is no fever, but the girl has been tired and had a cold a few days before. What do you tell her to do?

_____

_____

_____

_____

62. A young boy, accompanied by his mother, greets you in the examination room and starts asking all kinds of questions about things you do. He enjoys helping you test his reflexes and reading the vision chart, but he firmly refuses to cooperate when you try to give him a shot. What can you or his mother do to get him settled down enough to give him the shot?

_____

_____

_____

_____

63. A 16-year-old boy has been diagnosed as obese, and his parents have come in to find out what they can do to help their son achieve a healthy weight. The physician wants the boy to exercise at a local gym and to return in 6 months to check his progress. What education can you provide that will help the boy and his parents start a healthier lifestyle?

_____

_____

_____

_____

64. A young child has come in with a broken arm. During the examination, you notice the child also has several scrapes and bruises on his legs and feet as well. His mother says he got them from playing outdoors. Do you report this as child abuse to the physician? If not, what do you do?

_____

_____

_____

_____

65. Spanking children for misbehaving is sometimes considered child abuse. However, the parents who spank their children say that they were spanked when they were young, and they believe it is the best way to safely punish bad behavior. They also say that children who are not spanked become spoiled and difficult to control. What do you think? Is it your duty to report spanking as child abuse?

_____

_____

_____

_____

PROCEDURE 38-1 | Obtain an Infant's Length and Weight

PSY

Name: _____ Date: _____ Time: _____ Grade: _____

EQUIPMENT/SUPPLIES: Examining table with clean paper, tape measure, infant scale, protective paper for the scale, appropriate growth chart

STANDARDS: Given the needed equipment and a place to work, the student will perform this skill with _____ % accuracy in a total of _____ minutes. *(Your instructor will tell you what the percentage and time limits will be before you begin.)*

KEY: 4 = Satisfactory   0 = Unsatisfactory   NA = This step is not counted

PROCEDURE STEPS	SELF	PARTNER	INSTRUCTOR
1. Wash your hands	❏	❏	❏
2. Greet the patient and caregiver and identify yourself, including your title.	❏	❏	❏
3. Explain the procedure to the parent or caregiver	❏	❏	❏
4. Ask the parent to remove the infant's clothing except for the diaper	❏	❏	❏
5. Place the child on a firm examination table covered with clean table paper	❏	❏	❏
6. Fully extend the child's body by holding the head in the midline	❏	❏	❏
7. Grasp the knees and press flat onto the table gently but firmly	❏	❏	❏
8. Make a mark on table paper with pen at the top of the head and heel of the feet	❏	❏	❏
9. Measure between marks in either inches or centimeters	❏	❏	❏
10. Record the child's length on the growth chart and in the patient's chart	❏	❏	❏
11. Either carry the infant or have the parent carry the infant to the scale	❏	❏	❏
12. Place a protective paper on the scale and balance the scale	❏	❏	❏
13. Remove the diaper just before laying the infant on the scale	❏	❏	❏
14. Place the child gently on the scale. Keep one of your hands over or near the child on the scale at all times	❏	❏	❏
15. Balance the scale quickly but carefully	❏	❏	❏
16. Pick the infant up and instruct the parent to replace the diaper, if removed	❏	❏	❏

(continues)

PSY PROCEDURE 38-1 **Obtain an Infant's Length and Weight** (continued)

17. Wash your hands	❑	❑	❑
18. **AFF** Log into the Electronic Medical Record (EMR) using your username and secure password OR obtain the paper medical record from a secure location and assure it is kept away from public access	❑	❑	❑
19. Record the infant's weight on the growth chart and in the patient medical record	❑	❑	❑
20. When finished, log out of the EMR and/or replace the paper medical record in an appropriate and secure location	❑	❑	❑

CALCULATION

Total Possible Points: _____

Total Points Earned: _____ Multiplied by 100 = _____ Divided by Total Possible Points = _____ %

PASS   **FAIL**   **COMMENTS:**
❑   ❑

Student's signature _____   Date _____

Partner's signature _____   Date _____

Instructor's signature _____   Date _____

PSY PROCEDURE 38-2 **Obtain the Head and Chest Circumference**

Name: _____ Date: _____ Time: _____ Grade: _____

EQUIPMENT/SUPPLIES: Paper or cloth measuring tape, growth chart

STANDARDS: Given the needed equipment and a place to work, the student will perform this skill with _____ % accuracy in a total of _____ minutes. *(Your instructor will tell you what the percentage and time limits will be before you begin.)*

KEY: 4 = Satisfactory 0 = Unsatisfactory NA = This step is not counted

PROCEDURE STEPS	SELF	PARTNER	INSTRUCTOR
1. Wash your hands	❑	❑	❑
2. Place the infant in the supine position on the examination table, or ask the parent to hold the infant	❑	❑	❑
3. Measure around the head above the eyebrow and posteriorly at the largest part of the occiput	❑	❑	❑
4. Record the child's head circumference on the growth chart	❑	❑	❑
5. With the infant's clothing removed from the chest, measure around the chest at the nipple line, keeping the measuring tape at the same level anteriorly and posteriorly	❑	❑	❑
6. Wash your hands	❑	❑	❑
7. **AFF** Log into the Electronic Medical Record (EMR) using your username and secure password OR obtain the paper medical record from a secure location and assure it is kept away from public access	❑	❑	❑
8. Record the child's chest circumference on the growth chart	❑	❑	❑
9. When finished, log out of the EMR and/or replace the paper medical record in an appropriate and secure location	❑	❑	❑

CALCULATION

Total Possible Points: _____

Total Points Earned: _____ Multiplied by 100 = _____ Divided by Total Possible Points = _____ %

PASS FAIL COMMENTS:
❑ ❑

Student's signature _____ Date _____

Partner's signature _____ Date _____

Instructor's signature _____ Date _____

CHAPTER 39

Geriatrics

LEARNING OBJECTIVES

Cognitive Domain*

1. Spell key terms
2. *Identify the following related to body systems:*
   a. *Medical terms*
   b. *Abbreviations*
3. *Identify common pathology related to each body system including:*
   a. *Signs*
   b. *Symptoms*
   c. *Etiology*
   d. *Diagnostic measures*
   e. *Treatment modalities*
4. Explain how aging affects thought processes
5. Describe methods to increase compliance with health maintenance programs among older adults
6. Discuss communication problems that may occur with the older adult and list steps to maintain open communication
7. Recognize and describe the coping mechanisms used by the older adult to deal with multiple losses
8. Name the risk factors and signs of elder abuse

9. Explain the types of long-term care facilities available
10. Describe the effects of aging on the way the body processes medication
11. Discuss the responsibility of medical assistants with regard to teaching older adult patients

Affective Domain*

1. *Demonstrate critical thinking skills*
2. *Reassure patients*
3. *Demonstrate empathy for patients' concerns*
4. *Demonstrate active listening*
5. *Respect diversity*
6. *Recognize personal boundaries*
7. *Demonstrate tactfulness*
8. *Demonstrate self-awareness*

*MAERB Standards are Italicized.

ABHES Competencies

1. List all body systems and their structures and functions
2. Describe common diseases, symptoms, and etiology as they apply to each system

3. Identify diagnostic and treatment modalities as they relate to each body system
4. Apply medical terminology for each specialty
5. Follow documentation guidelines
6. Adapt care to address the developmental stages of life
7. Partner with healthcare teams to attain optimal patient health outcomes
8. Display effective interpersonal skills with patients and healthcare team members
9. Demonstrate cultural awareness
10. Assist the provider with specialty examinations, including cardiac, respiratory, OB-GYN, neurologic, and gastroenterology
11. Perform specialty procedures, including but not limited to minor surgery, cardiac, respiratory, OB-GYN, neurologic, and gastroenterology
12. Make adaptations for patients with special needs (psychological or physical limitations)
13. Make adaptations to care for patients across their lifespan

Name: _____ Date: _____ Grade: _____

COG MULTIPLE CHOICE

Circle the letter preceding the correct answer.

1. Which of the following statements is true about older adult patients who require long-term medication?
   a. If older adult patients take their medication every day, they are unlikely to forget a dose
   b. Compliance over a long period of time can become problematic in older adult patients
   c. With a chronic illness, an older adult patient can neglect to take their medication for a few weeks with no side effects
   d. Patients who take their medications for a long period of time will eventually notice a significant improvement
   e. Older adult patients will eventually become immune to long-term medication

2. Which of these conditions can sometimes be improved by taking the herbal supplement gingko?
   a. Arthritis
   b. Parkinson's disease
   c. Loss of appetite
   d. Poor concentration
   e. Alzheimer's disease

3. The purpose of an advance directive is to:
   a. divide a person's possessions in the event of death.
   b. inform the physician of any allergies that an individual has to specific medications.
   c. outline a person's wishes about end-of-life care.
   d. transfer a patient's medical records between physicians' offices.
   e. order a physician not to resuscitate a patient under any circumstances.

4. Which of these is a task performed by a home health aide?
   a. Light housecleaning
   b. Refilling prescriptions
   c. Reorganizing bulky furniture
   d. Writing daily task lists and reminders
   e. Keeping the older adult occupied

5. Which of these is a good place to find information about respite care for older adult relatives?
   a. Local newspaper
   b. Television advertisement
   c. Community senior citizen program
   d. Local business directory
   e. Library bulletin board

6. What is an example of passive neglect of an older adult patient?
   a. Withholding medication from the patient
   b. Locking the patient in a room
   c. Overmedicating the patient to make them easier to care for
   d. Isolating the patient from friends and family
   e. Forgetting to give the patient regular baths

7. Which of the following statements is true about the aging process?
   a. Longevity is based entirely on environmental factors
   b. People who have dangerous occupations will not live as long as people who do not
   c. Longevity is hereditary, so it does not make a difference how you live your life
   d. Longevity is largely hereditary, but environmental factors play a significant role
   e. An obese, physically inactive smoker will have a shorter lifespan than a healthy nonsmoker

8. What is the best way to deal with a patient who is hearing impaired?
   a. Raise your voice until the patient can hear you
   b. Give written instructions whenever possible
   c. Talk to the patient with your back to the light
   d. Talk directly into the patient's ear
   e. Find a coworker who is able to communicate using sign language

Scenario for Questions 9 to 11: A 55-year-old patient comes into the physician's office and tells you that he thinks he is suffering from Parkinson's disease.

9. The physician would diagnose the patient by:
   a. taking a blood test.
   b. performing dexterity tasks.
   c. excluding other causes.
   d. performing an MRI scan.
   e. testing his reflexes.

10. How would you explain deep brain stimulation to the patient?
    a. It increases the levels of dopamine in the brain
    b. It lowers a person's acetylcholine levels
    c. It blocks the impulses that cause tremors
    d. It controls a person's stress and anxiety levels
    e. It acts as a muscle relaxant and prevents rigidity

11. What would you tell the patient about Levodopa?
    a. It has no serious side effects
    b. It remains effective for the entire length of the disease
    c. It can cause headaches and migraines
    d. It should not be taken with alcohol
    e. It may aggravate stomach ulcers

12. When older adult patients are beginning a new exercise regimen, it is a good idea for them to:
    a. rest when they get tired.
    b. start with a brisk 30-minute jog.
    c. keep to the same weekly routine.
    d. exercise alone so they are not distracted.
    e. work through any initial pain or discomfort.

13. Which of the following statements is true about the nutritional requirements of older adult patients?
    a. Older adult patients need less food and water than younger patients because older adults are not as active
    b. It is easier for older adult patients to maintain good nutrition because they have more time to prepare meals
    c. Vitamin and mineral requirements are lower in older adult patients than in younger patients
    d. Older adult patients should eat smaller, more frequent meals to aid digestion
    e. Older adult patients can replace meals with liquid dietary supplements without damaging their health

14. A caregiver can help increase safety in the home of an older adult patient by:
    a. installing handrails in the bathtub and near the commode.
    b. placing childproof locks on the kitchen cupboards.
    c. encouraging the patient to exercise regularly.
    d. covering highly polished floors with scatter rugs.
    e. keeping the patient's medicine in a locked bathroom cabinet.

15. What action should you take if you suspect older adult abuse?
    a. Try to separate the caregiver from the patient for the examination
    b. Tell the caregiver you will be reporting them to the authorities
    c. Question the patient about suspicious injuries until she tells you the truth
    d. Call the police while the patient is in the examination room
    e. Wait to inform the physician of your suspicions until you are sure they are correct

16. What does the acronym HOH mean in a patient chart?
    a. Has ordinary hearing
    b. Head of household
    c. Has own home
    d. Hard on health
    e. Hard of hearing

17. Another name for the herbal supplement gingko is:
    a. folic acid.
    b. kew tree.
    c. aloe vera.
    d. green tea.
    e. milk thistle.

18. What is the best advice to give a patient who is having difficulty swallowing medication?
    a. Grind the medication into powder
    b. Ask the pharmacist for smaller pills
    c. Put the medication on the back of the tongue and drink water with a straw
    d. Lie down and swallow the medication with a lot of water
    e. Dissolve the medication in a hot drink

19. A physician who specializes in disorders that affect the aging population is called a(n):
    a. gastroenterologist.
    b. gerontologist.
    c. oncologist.
    d. otorhinolaryngologist.
    e. rheumatologist.

20. An eye condition that causes increased intraocular pressure and intolerance to light is:
    a. cataracts.
    b. kyphosis.
    c. bradykinesia.
    d. osteoporosis.
    e. glaucoma.

COG MATCHING

Grade: _____

Place the letter preceding the definition on the line next to the term.

Key Terms

21. _____ activities of daily living (ADL)
22. _____ biotransform
23. _____ bradykinesia
24. _____ cataracts
25. _____ cerebrovascular accident (CVA)
26. _____ compliance
27. _____ degenerative joint disease (DJD)
28. _____ dementia
29. _____ dysphagia
30. _____ gerontologist
31. _____ glaucoma
32. _____ Kegel exercises
33. _____ keratosis (senile)
34. _____ kyphosis (dowager's hump)
35. _____ lentigines
36. _____ osteoporosis
37. _____ potentiation
38. _____ presbycusis
39. _____ presbyopia
40. _____ senility
41. _____ syncope
42. _____ transient ischemic attack (TIA)
43. _____ vertigo

Definitions

a. a specialist who studies aging
b. general mental deterioration associated with old age
c. to convert the molecules of a substance from one form to another, as in medications within the body
d. a sensation of whirling of oneself or the environment, dizziness
e. abnormally slow voluntary movements
f. a sudden fall in blood pressure or cerebral hypoxia resulting in loss of consciousness
g. progressive organic mental deterioration with loss of intellectual function
h. a skin condition characterized by overgrowth and thickening
i. difficulty speaking
j. an abnormal porosity of the bone, most often found in the older adult, predisposing the affected bony tissue to fracture
k. an acute episode of cerebrovascular insufficiency, usually a result of narrowing of an artery by atherosclerotic plaques, emboli, or vasospasm; usually passes quickly but should be considered a warning for predisposition to cerebrovascular accidents
l. a progressive loss of transparency of the lens of the eye, resulting in opacity and loss of sight
m. describes the actions of two drugs taken together in which the combined effects are greater than the sum of the independent effects
n. a vision change (farsightedness) associated with aging
o. isometric exercises in which the muscles of the pelvic floor are voluntarily contracted and relaxed while urinating
p. brown skin macules occurring after prolonged exposure to the sun; freckles
q. a loss of hearing associated with aging
r. an abnormally deep dorsal curvature of the thoracic spine; also known as humpback or hunchback
s. activities usually performed in the course of the day, i.e., bathing, dressing, feeding oneself
t. also known as *osteoarthritis*; arthritis characterized by degeneration of the bony structure of the joints, usually noninflammatory
u. willingness of a patient to follow a prescribed course of treatment
v. ischemia of the brain due to an occlusion of the blood vessels supplying the brain, resulting in varying degrees of debilitation
w. an abnormal increase in the fluid of the eye, usually as a result of obstructed outflow, resulting in degeneration of the intraocular components and blindness

COG MATCHING

Grade: _____

Place the letter preceding the description of the facility on the line preceding the type of facility.

Facilities

44. _____ Group homes or assisted living facilities
45. _____ Long-term care facilities
46. _____ Skilled-nursing facilities

Descriptions

a. Facilities for those who need help with most areas of personal care and moderate medical supervision
b. Facilities for those who are gravely or terminally ill and need constant supervision
c. Facilities for those who can tend to their own activities of daily living but need companionship and light supervision for safety

COG IDENTIFICATION

Grade: _____

47. Some older adult patients suffer from memory loss, which may make it difficult for them to remember to take their medications. As a medical assistant, it is important to give these patients tools to help them remember and maintain their medication regimens. Identify and list five ways you can help older adult patients remember their medication regimens.

_____

_____

_____

_____

48. Which of the following are common reasons for older adult patients not taking their medications correctly? Place a check mark on the line next to all that apply.

a. _____ Financial difficulties

b. _____ To attract attention

c. _____ Forgetfulness

d. _____ Tiring of the constraints of taking long-term medication

e. _____ Deliberate defiance

49. Mrs. Kim is 89 years old and suffers from memory lapses. It is apparent that she is both frustrated and lonely. Identify and list three ways that you can maintain good communication with her and help her express her feelings.

_____

_____

_____

_____

50. Mrs. Driscoll is 84 years old with poor eyesight and suffers from forgetfulness. She needs to take two different types of medication three times a day. Identify and list four ways that you could help ensure that Mrs. Driscoll adheres to her medication regimen.

_____

_____

_____

_____

51. Patients who react negatively to moving to a long-term care facility can show signs of grief. Identify and list five symptoms that could indicate that a patient is suffering from a sense of loss.

_____

_____

_____

_____

52. Sometimes an older adult patient will turn to alcohol as a way of coping. The effects of drinking alcohol can often be mistaken for other ailments. Identify and list three conditions that exhibit symptoms similar to the influence of alcohol.

_____

_____

_____

_____

53. Suicide is a risk for older adult patients, especially those who have recently lost a spouse to death or divorce. Which of the following warning signs indicate that an older adult patient is contemplating suicide? Place a check mark on the line next to all that apply.

a. _____ Giving away favored objects

b. _____ Increased interest in family affairs

c. _____ Secretive behavior

d. _____ Increased anger, hostility, or isolation

e. _____ Increased forgetfulness

f. _____ Increased alcohol or drug use

g. _____ Loss of interest in health matters

54. Which of the following indicate that a patient is suffering from older adult abuse? Place a check mark on the line preceding all that apply.

a. _____ Disturbed sleep patterns

b. _____ Signs of restraint on the wrists or ankles

c. _____ Large, deep pressure ulcers

d. _____ Incontinence

e. _____ Poor hygiene or poor nutrition

f. _____ Untreated injury or condition

g. _____ Dehydration not caused by disease

55. Which of the following are symptoms of Parkinson disease? Circle the letter preceding all that apply.

a. Muscle rigidity

b. Increased anger

c. Involuntary tremors

d. Difficulty walking

e. Loss of memory

f. Dysphagia and drooling

g. Expressionless face and infrequent blinking

56. Identify and list three reasons why an older adult patient can have difficulty maintaining good nutrition.

a. _____

b. _____

c. _____

COG SHORT ANSWER
_____ Grade: _____

57. You ask Mr. Walton if he is taking his blood pressure medication and he tells you that he is taking it every day. Later, the physician tells you that Mr. Walton has been taking three pills a day instead of just one. How could this situation be avoided with other older adult patients?

_____

_____

_____

_____

58. Mrs. Dawson is a widow who lives in a long-term care facility. Her family is worried that she has recently become withdrawn and uncommunicative. Before her husband died, Mrs. Dawson led an active life and took a large role in running the household. What could you say to Mrs. Dawson's family to help her cope with the loss of her spouse and her independence?

_____

_____

_____

_____

59. Mr. Gonzalez is an 85-year-old patient who lives alone. He is still fairly active and is able to carry out most activities of daily living by himself. However, members of his family have expressed some concerns that he is lonely and that they are not able to visit him as often as they would like. What options could you discuss with the family?

_____

_____

_____

_____

ᴄᴏɢ **COMPLETION**

Grade: _____

60. Older adult patients whose health and economic situation are unstable may experience feelings of grief and loss. These feelings can be about both specific and nonspecific aspects of their lives. Fill in the chart below, listing five specific and nonspecific losses older adult patients may find difficult to cope with.

Specific Losses	Nonspecific Losses
a.	
b.	
c.	
d.	
e.	

61. The passage below describes how medications affect the body of an older adult. However, some of the important terms are missing. Read the passage and fill in the correct words from the list below.

The _____ system no longer moves medications along as efficiently because it has slowed. The _____ system does not absorb dissolved medication from the _____ or the _____ and delivers it to the target tissue as quickly. The _____ does not _____ medication as quickly, causing medications to remain in the body longer than desirable and possibly add to the cumulative effect. Finally, the _____ receive less blood, so less medication is filtered and removed from the body. These decreases in body system function can result in possible _____ of medications in the older adult.

circulatory system	*gastrointestinal system*	*intestines*	*biotransform*	*kidneys*
toxic effects		*liver*	*peristalsis*	*injection site*

62. Complete the following table by indicating whether the following suggestions are appropriate for a patient with Parkinson's disease or for a patient with Alzheimer's disease. Place a check mark in the appropriate box.

Suggestion	Patient with Parkinson's Disease	Patient with Alzheimer's Disease
a. Speak calmly and without condescension		
b. Do not argue with the patient		
c. Tell the patient to take small bites and chew each mouthful carefully before swallowing		
d. Encourage the patient to use no-spill cups, plates with high sides, and special utensils		
e. Free the home from rugs and loose cords that may cause tripping		
f. Speak in short, simple, direct sentences and explain one action at a time		

g. Listen to the patient and stimulate his intelligence		
h. Remind the patient who you are and what you must do		

COG TRUE OR FALSE?

Grade: _____

Indicate whether the statements are true or false by placing the letter T (true) or F (false) on the line preceding the statement.

63. _____ Newspaper word puzzles are just a temporary distraction to help entertain older adults.

64. _____ Attempts to commit suicide by older adults are usually just a cry for help.

65. _____ If a patient has an advance directive on file somewhere other than the medical office, it should be noted in her medical record.

66. _____ Most older adult abuse is committed by workers in long-term care facilities.

COG AFF CASE STUDIES FOR CRITICAL THINKING

Grade: _____

67. Read the following case studies and think about what you know about the causes of older adult abuse. Circle the letter preceding the case study that describes the patient who falls in the highest risk category for abuse.

a. Mr. Simpson is an 89-year-old widower who lives alone. He is still fairly active and is able to carry out most daily activities by himself. He has a daughter and a son, who take turns visiting him every week and doing his shopping and laundry for him. Mr. Simpson takes medication for high blood pressure and angina.

b. Mrs. Lewis is an 83-year-old patient who lives in a long-term care facility. She suffers from mild senile dementia, which her family sometimes finds frustrating but is learning to cope with. Mrs. Lewis has a home health aide and private nurse to help her carry out activities of daily living. She sleeps for most of the day.

c. Mrs. Beddowes is a 90-year-old widow who lives with her son. She suffers from senile dementia, incontinence, and insomnia. Her family members cannot afford to place her in a long-term care facility, so they share the responsibility of taking care of her. However, most of the responsibility falls on her son, who helps Mrs. Beddowes carry out most activities of daily living.

d. Mr. Williams is an 81-year-old patient who lives in an assisted-living facility. He was recently widowed and is having difficulty coming to terms with his wife's death. Mr. Williams used to be extremely active but has recently become withdrawn and has started drinking heavily. He has two daughters who visit him regularly.

68. Your patient is a 90-year-old man with various age-associated health problems. He has been recently diagnosed with dementia, but during his recent visits to the physician's office, you have smelled alcohol on his breath. How would you handle this situation? What would you do?

_____

_____

_____

_____

69. Your patient is an 82-year-old woman who suffers from mild hearing loss. She recently lost her husband and has been making frequent appointments at the physician's office for minor complaints. You suspect that the patient is lonely and is visiting the office for company and human interaction. Explain what you would do.

_____

_____

_____

_____

70. Your patient is an 80-year-old woman who has recently lost a noticeable amount of weight. She tells you that she has not been very hungry lately and has not felt like eating very much. The physician has asked you to write a list of nutritional guidelines for her to follow and explain why they are important. What would you put in the guidelines?

_____

_____

_____

_____

71. Your patient is a 91-year-old man with Alzheimer's disease. After his appointment with the physician, you overhear his family trying to get him into the car. The patient has forgotten where he is and refuses to leave the physician's office. His daughter loses her temper and shouts at her father loudly until he complies. What would you do? Explain your actions.

_____

_____

_____

_____

72. You overhear a coworker asking a 77-year-old patient about her medical history. When the patient tells your coworker that she is taking gingko to improve her memory, your coworker tells her that she only needs to know about actual medications. What would you say to your coworker?

_____

_____

_____

_____

PART 4

The Clinical Laboratory

UNIT SIX

Fundamentals of Laboratory Procedures

CHAPTER 40

Introduction to the Physician Office Laboratory

LEARNING OUTCOMES

COG Cognitive Domain*

1. Spell key terms
2. *Identify the following related to body systems:*
   a. *Medical terms*
   b. *Abbreviations*
3. List the various types of clinical laboratories including the physician office laboratory
4. Explain the types of departments found in most large laboratories
5. Explain the significance of the Clinical Laboratory Improvement Amendments (CLIA) and how to maintain compliance in the physician office laboratory

6. *Identify CLIA waived tests associated with common diseases*
7. *Identify quality assurance practices in health care*
8. Identify equipment found in the physician's office laboratory and routine maintenance
9. List and describe the parts of a microscope
10. Discuss the role of the medical assistant in clinical laboratory testing
11. Define critical values
12. *Identify normal and abnormal results as reported in:*
    a. *Graphs*
    b. *Tables*

PSY Psychomotor Domain*

1. Care of the microscope (Procedure 40-1)
2. Screen test results (Procedure 40-2)
3. *Record laboratory results into the patient's record (Procedures 40-3 and 40-4)*

AFF Affective Domain*

1. *Demonstrate critical thinking skills*

*MAERB Standards are Italicized.

Name: _____   Date: _____   Grade: _____

⬛OG MULTIPLE CHOICE

1. Laboratory test results are evaluated to determine the relative health of body systems or organs by comparison with:
   a. panels.
   b. constituents.
   c. reference intervals.
   d. calibration ranges.
   e. quality control ranges.

2. A large facility in which thousands of tests of various types are performed each day is a:
   a. hospital laboratory.
   b. Physician Office Laboratory (POL).
   c. waived-testing laboratory.
   d. clinical chemistry laboratory.
   e. referral laboratory.

3. A Pap test specimen would be sent to which department for analysis?
   a. Histology
   b. Cytology
   c. Immunohematology
   d. Microbiology
   e. Clinical chemistry

4. Hematology includes the study of:
   a. etiology, diagnosis, and treatment of blood diseases.
   b. analysis of body fluids.
   c. the study of hormones.
   d. the study of the immune system and antibodies.
   e. the study of drugs.

5. Mycology is the study of:
   a. protozoa and worms.
   b. viruses.
   c. bacteria.
   d. tuberculosis.
   e. fungi and yeasts.

6. The test panel defined by the American Medical Association (AMA) for national standardization of nomenclature and testing used to test cholesterol, triglycerides, HDL, and LDL is the:
   a. comprehensive metabolic panel.
   b. basic metabolic panel.
   c. electrolyte panel.
   d. hepatic panel.
   e. lipid panel.

7. A laboratory must have a written quality assurance policy that:
   a. is communicated to all staff.
   b. is stored neared the site of use.
   c. includes all HazCom requirements.
   d. includes all MSDSs supplied by the manufacturers.
   e. is updated once a week.

8. The best source of normal values for the POL is:
   a. the *Physicians' Desk Reference*.
   b. the manufacturer's packaging insert.
   c. the ICD-9 CM.
   d. the Laboratory Procedure Manual.
   e. the CLIA certificate.

9. The presence of a panic value in test results indicates:
   a. an outbreak of a contagious virus.
   b. imminent death of the patient.
   c. general good health.
   d. a potentially life-threatening situation.
   e. negligence on the part of the laboratory.

10. Who provides quality control instructions for a given test?
    a. FDA
    b. CLSI
    c. Laboratory director
    d. Manufacturer
    e. OSHA

11. Urine dipsticks and pregnancy tests are examples of:
    a. waived tests.
    b. moderately complex tests.
    c. provider-performed microscopy.
    d. high-complexity tests.
    e. referral tests.

12. What CLIA-waived test may be ordered on a patient presenting with a sore throat?

   a. Hematocrit

   b. Urine dipstick

   c. Glucose meter measurement

   d. Rapid strep test

   e. CBC

13. You bring your lunch to work and need to refrigerate it. You would:

   a. store it in the laboratory refrigerator. It is nearest to you while you work.

   b. store it in the refrigerator in the break room. That refrigerator does not have a biohazard label.

   c. store it in the refrigerator with drugs and vaccines.

   d. store it in a drawer in the laboratory.

   e. store it in an empty drawer in the procedure room.

COG MATCHING

Grade: _____

Match the following key terms to their definitions.

Key Terms

14. _____ aliquots

15. _____ analytes

16. _____ antibodies

17. _____ antigen

18. _____ anticoagulant

19. _____ autoimmunity

20. _____ centrifugation

21. _____ centers for Medicare and Medicaid Services (CMS)

22. _____ coagulation

23. _____ cytogenetics

24. _____ cytology

25. _____ hematology

26. _____ histology

27. _____ immunodeficiency

28. _____ immunohematology

29. _____ immunology

30. _____ microbiology

Definitions

a. substance or constituent for which a laboratory conducts testing

b. anything that prevents or delays blood clotting

c. testing based on the reactions of antibodies in the presence of antigens

d. proteins formed in the body in response to foreign substances

e. substance that, when introduced into the body, causes the development of immune responses

f. disorder of the immune system in which parts of the immune system fail to provide an adequate response

g. disorders of the immune system in which the immune system attacks its own host's body

h. study of the microscopic structure of tissue; samples of tissue are prepared, stained, and evaluated under a microscope to determine whether disease is present

i. involves a wide variety of procedures used in donor selection, component preparation and use, and techniques used to detect antigen/antibody reactions that may adversely affect a patient receiving a transfusion

j. study of the microscopic structure of cells; individual cells in body fluids and other specimens are evaluated microscopically for the presence of disease such as cancer.

k. genetic structure of the cells obtained from tissue, blood, or body fluids, such as amniotic fluid, is examined or tested for chromosome deficiencies related to genetic disease.

l. the process of separating blood or other body fluid cells from liquid components

m. portions of the original specimen

n. require the use of test panels created by the AMA

o. the study of blood and blood-forming tissues

p. the study of the blood's ability to clot

q. the study of pathogen identification and antibiotic susceptibility determination

COG MATCHING

Match the following key terms to their definitions.

Key Terms

31. _____ aerosol
32. _____ calibration
33. _____ confirmatory test
34. _____ control
35. _____ critical values
36. _____ external control
37. _____ internal control
38. _____ qualitative test
39. _____ quantitative test
40. _____ reconstitution
41. _____ shifts
42. _____ therapeutic range
43. _____ trends

Definitions

a. an additional, more specific test performed to rule out or confirm a preliminary test result to provide a final result

b. a device or solution used to monitor the test for accuracy and precision

c. life-threatening test results

d. a method provided by the manufacturer to standardize a test or laboratory instrument

e. control built into the testing device

f. control that acts just like a patient specimen

g. particles suspended in gas or air

h. the test result range the physician wants for the patient

i. test has positive or negative results

j. tests are measured and reported in a number value

k. when QC results make an obvious change

l. when results increase or decrease over time

m. adding water to bring a material back to its liquid state

COG MATCHING

Match the following key terms to their definitions.

Key Terms

44. _____ oncology
45. _____ panels
46. _____ pathogen
47. _____ physician office laboratory (POL)
48. _____ plasma
49. _____ product insert
50. _____ quality assurance (QA)
51. _____ quality control (QC)
52. _____ reference intervals
53. _____ referral laboratory
54. _____ serum
55. _____ specimens
56. _____ surgical pathology
57. _____ toxicology
58. _____ unitized test device
59. _____ urinalysis
60. _____ whole blood

Definitions

a. acceptable ranges for a healthy population

b. designed to ensure thorough patient care

c. procedures to monitor and evaluate testing procedures, supplies, and equipment to ensure accuracy in laboratory performance

d. standard groups of laboratory tests organized to effectively evaluate disease processes or organ systems

e. contains instructions and critical details for performing a test

f. top layer of a whole blood specimen if the specimen was anticoagulated and not allowed to clot

g. the study and medical treatment of cancer

h. a limited testing laboratory in a medical office

i. a large facility in which thousands of tests of various types are performed each day

j. blood containing all of its cellular and liquid components

k. disease-causing microorganism

l. the liquid portion of the blood after the blood has been allowed to clot

m. examination of the physical, chemical, and microscopic properties of urine

n. the pathologist in this department gives a diagnosis of the presence or absence of disease in tissue that is surgically removed from a patient

o. used for a single test and discarded after testing

p. small portions of anything used to evaluate the nature of the whole

q. branch of chemistry that studies the amounts and identification of chemicals foreign to the body

COG IDENTIFICATION
Grade: _____

Each of the medical assistants below needs a laboratory test completed for a patient. Review the task that must be performed and then decide which laboratory department should handle each task.

61. Ericka needs to send in blood for a complete blood count. _____

62. Kwon needs results of the chemical properties of a patient's urine. _____

63. Darren has to send a patient to the lab for glucose testing. _____

64. Don has a mole removed and sent to the lab for analysis. _____

65. Rochelle collects a clean-catch urine for culture. _____

COG SHORT ANSWER
Grade: _____

66. Why does the laboratory need the patient's birth date and gender?

_____

_____

_____

_____

67. How does the laboratory use the date and time of collection?

_____

_____

_____

_____

68. List six good laboratory practices for POLs performing POC testing.

_____

_____

_____

_____

69. Identify the source of instrument maintenance and calibration instructions.

_____

_____

_____

_____

70. In the context of laboratory medical testing, what is the purpose of a control?

_____

_____

_____

_____

71. Explain the difference between qualitative and quantitative tests.

_____

_____

_____

_____

72. How do you identify whether patient values are inside or outside of the reference interval?

_____

_____

_____

_____

73. In reviewing patient results, how do you determine patient values requiring follow-up?

_____

_____

_____

_____

COG PSY AFF CASE STUDIES FOR CRITICAL THINKING

Grade: _____

74. The physician in the family practice office where you work asks you to perform a streptococcus test on a throat specimen. You know that the test is performed using a waived-testing kit; however, when you open the box, the package insert is missing. This insert is necessary to use as a guide to perform the test and contains the instructions. How do you obtain directions for performing the test?

_____

_____

_____

_____

75. A test is showing systematically low results; that is, in each case, the result is proportionately lower than expected. The results are precise but inaccurate. What must you do to ensure proper results?

_____

_____

_____

_____

76. You are performing a glucose test on your patient using a glucose meter. The patient's glucose result is below the level that the meter can detect. The glucose meter can detect values as low as 40 mg/dL. What kind of value is this and what steps should you take with the test results?

_____

_____

_____

_____

PSY PROCEDURE 40-1 **Care of the Microscope**

Name: _____ Date: _____ Time: _____ Grade: _____

EQUIPMENT/SUPPLIES: Lens paper, lens cleaner, gauze, mild soap solution, microscope, hand disinfectant, surface disinfectant

STANDARDS: Given the needed equipment and a place to work, the student will perform this skill with _____ % accuracy in a total of _____ minutes. *(Your instructor will tell you what the percentage and time limits will be before you begin practicing.)*

KEY: 4 = Satisfactory 0 = Unsatisfactory NA = This step is not counted

PROCEDURE STEPS	SELF	PARTNER	INSTRUCTOR
1. Wash your hands	❏	❏	❏
2. Assemble the equipment	❏	❏	❏
3. If you need to move the microscope, carry it in both hands, one holding the base and the other holding the arm	❏	❏	❏

4. Clean the optical areas
  a. Place a drop or two of lens cleaner on a piece of lens paper
  b. Wipe each eyepiece thoroughly with the lens paper. Do not touch the optical areas with your fingers. Wipe each eyepiece with lens paper and lens cleaner
  c. Wipe each objective lens, starting with the lowest power and continuing to the highest power (usually an oil immersion lens). If the lens paper appears to have dirt or oil on it, use a clean section of the lens paper or a new piece of lens paper with cleaner. Wipe each objective lens with lens paper and lens cleaner. Clean the oil objective last so you do not carry its oil to the other objective lenses
  d. Using a new piece of dry lens paper, wipe each eyepiece and objective lens so that no cleaner remains
  e. With a new piece of lens paper moistened with lens cleaner, clean the condenser and illuminator optics. Clean and dry the condenser and illuminator optics
	❏	❏	❏

5. Clean the areas other than the optics
  a. Moisten gauze with mild soap solution or use an alcohol wipe and wipe all areas other than the optics, including the stage, base, and adjustment knobs
  b. Moisten another gauze with water and rinse the washed areas
	❏	❏	❏

6. To store the cleaned microscope, ensure that the light source is turned off. Rotate the nosepiece so that the low-power objective is pointed down toward the stage. Cover the microscope with the plastic dust cover that came with it or a small trash bag	❏	❏	❏
7. Document microscope cleaning on the microscope maintenance log sheet (sample instrument log sheet)	❏	❏	❏

(continues)

PSY   PROCEDURE 40-1   **Care of the Microscope** (continued)

_____

_____

_____

_____

_____

CALCULATION

Total Possible Points: _____

Total Points Earned: _____ Multiplied by 100 = _____ Divided by Total Possible Points = _____ %

PASS   FAIL   COMMENTS:
❑   ❑

Student's signature _____ Date _____

Partner's signature _____ Date _____

Instructor's signature _____ Date _____

PSY PROCEDURE 40-2 **Screen and Follow-up Test Results**

Name: _____ Date: _____ Time: _____ Grade: _____

EQUIPMENT/SUPPLIES: Patient laboratory results, critical values list for office, patient medical record

STANDARDS: Given the needed equipment and a place to work, the student will perform this skill with _____ % accuracy in a total of _____ minutes. *(Your instructor will tell you what the percentage and time limits will be before you begin practicing.)*

KEY: 4 = Satisfactory   0 = Unsatisfactory   NA = This step is not counted

PROCEDURE STEPS	SELF	PARTNER	INSTRUCTOR
1. Review laboratory reports received from reference laboratory	❏	❏	❏
2. Note which reports may be placed directly on the patient's chart and which require immediate notification due to critical results	❏	❏	❏
3. Notify the physician of the result. Take any immediate instructions from the physician	❏	❏	❏
4. Follow instructions and document notification and follow-up	❏	❏	❏
5. Chart remaining reports appropriately	❏	❏	❏

CALCULATION

Total Possible Points: _____

Total Points Earned: _____ Multiplied by 100 = _____ Divided by Total Possible Points = _____ %

PASS   FAIL   COMMENTS:
❏   ❏

Student's signature _____ Date _____

Partner's signature _____ Date _____

Instructor's signature _____ Date _____

PSY PROCEDURE 40-3   Use a Laboratory Flow Sheet

Name: _____ Date: _____ Time: _____ Grade: _____

EQUIPMENT/SUPPLIES: Flow sheet for documenting a patient's anticoagulation therapy and test results; scenarios for patient Jacob Wisliki

STANDARDS: Patient Jacob Wisliki is on Coumadin (warfarin) therapy following a stroke. Dr. Wilson requests that you maintain a flow sheet on this patient and orders weekly INR (coagulation) testing.

The student will perform this skill with _____ % accuracy in a total of _____ minutes. *(Your instructor will tell you what the percentage and time limits will be before you begin practicing.)*

PATIENT SCENARIOS:

- Today is November 1, 2016. Mr. Wisliki's INR is 1.8, which is below Dr. Wilson's target range. Dr. Wilson increases Mr. Wisliki's dose to 2.5 mg qd and requests that Mr. Wisliki return in a week for another INR.

- Mr. Wisliki returns and his INR is 2.1, which is in Dr. Wilson's therapeutic range. Dr. Wilson would like to see the value higher so he increases Mr. Wisliki's Coumadin dose to 3.5 mg qd and asks the patient to have another INR performed in 1 week.

- The following week, Mr. Wisliki returns and his INR result is 3.5, which is higher than Dr. Wilson's therapeutic range. Dr. Wilson decreases Mr. Wisliki's dose to 3.0 mg qd and requests Mr. Wisliki to return in 1 week.

- Mr. Wisliki returns on schedule the following week and his INR is 3.1. Dr. Wilson is concerned that Mr. Wisliki's INR did not respond as usual to the decrease in the dose. Mr. Wisliki is instructed to avoid eating green leafy vegetables while on anticoagulant therapy and his dose is not changed. He is instructed to return in a week as ordered by Dr. Wilson.

- Mr. Wisliki is back for his weekly INR check, and today, it is 2.5. Dr. Wilson is pleased with this INR result and does not change the dose. You instruct Mr. Wisliki to return in a week as Dr. Wilson ordered.

- Mr. Wisliki is back for his INR, which is 2.5. Because his INR is stable, Dr. Wilson does not change his dose.

KEY: 4 = Satisfactory   0 = Unsatisfactory   NA = This step is not counted

PROCEDURE STEPS	SELF	PARTNER	INSTRUCTOR
1. Obtain the anticoagulant flow sheet and the scenarios and data for Jacob Wisliki	❑	❑	❑
2. Record the INR results, medication dosage change (new dose), and your name (first initial, last name) on the first line (date 11/01/2016) of the flow sheet	❑	❑	❑
3. Record the date, INR results, medication dosage change, and your name for the 2nd week of the scenario	❑	❑	❑
4. Record the date, INR results, medication dosage change, and your name for each of the following weeks (weeks # 2, 3, 4, 5, and 6)	❑	❑	❑
5. Each weekly entry is complete, legible, and accurate	❑	❑	❑
6. Explain that the flow sheet is maintained in the patient medical record	❑	❑	❑

PSY PROCEDURE 40-3 **Use a Laboratory Flow Sheet** (continued)

CALCULATION

Total Possible Points: _____

Total Points Earned: _____ Multiplied by 100 = _____ Divided by Total Possible Points = _____ %

PASS   FAIL   COMMENTS:
❏   ❏

Student's signature _____   Date _____

Partner's signature _____   Date _____

Instructor's signature _____   Date _____

PSY PROCEDURE 40-4 **Anticoagulant Flow Sheet**

Name: _____ Date: _____ Time: _____ Grade: _____

PATIENT'S NAME: Jacob Wisliki

DATE OF BIRTH: 03/20/1940

TARGET INTERNATIONAL NORMALIZED RATIO (INR): √ 2.0–3.0 ☐ 2.5–3.5 Other: _____

Date	Current Dose	INR	Medication	New Dose	Signature
11/01/2016	2 mg qd				

CHAPTER 41

Phlebotomy

LEARNING OUTCOMES

COG Cognitive Domain*

1. Spell and define the key terms
2. *Identify the following as related to body systems:*
   a. *medical terms*
   b. *abbreviations*
3. Identify equipment and supplies used to obtain a routine venous specimen and a routine capillary skin puncture
4. Describe the proper use of specimen collection equipment
5. List the major anticoagulants, their color codes, and the suggested order in which they are filled during a venipuncture
6. Describe the location and selection of the blood collection sites using capillaries and veins
7. Differentiate between the feel of a vein, tendon, and artery
8. Describe care for a puncture site after blood has been drawn
9. *Identify quality assurance practices in health care*

PSY Psychomotor Domain*

1. Obtain a blood specimen by evacuated tube or winged infusion set (Procedure 41-1)

a. *Perform the following procedures: a. electrocardiograph b. venipuncture c. capillary puncture d. pulmonary function testing*
b. *Instruct and prepare a patient for a procedure or treatment*
c. *Perform quality control measures*
d. *Document patient care accurately in the medical record*
2. Obtain a blood specimen by capillary puncture (Procedure 41-2)
   a. *Perform the following procedures: a. electrocardiography b. venipuncture c. capillary puncture d. pulmonary function testing*
   b. *Instruct and prepare a patient for a procedure or treatment*
   c. *Perform quality control measure*
   d. *Document patient care accurately in the medical record*

AFF Affective Domain*

1. *Demonstrate critical thinking skills*
2. *Reassure patients*
3. *Demonstrate empathy for patients' concerns*

4. *Demonstrate active listening*
5. *Respect diversity*
6. *Recognize personal boundaries*
7. *Demonstrate tactfulness*
8. *Demonstrate self-awareness*
9. Protect the integrity of the medical record

MAERB Standards are Italicized.

ABHES Competencies

1. Practice quality control
2. Dispose of biohazardous materials
3. Collect, label, and process specimens: 1). Perform venipuncture 2). Perform capillary puncture
4. Follow documentation guidelines
5. Adapt care to address the developmental stages of life
6. Display effective interpersonal skills with patients and health care team members
7. Demonstrate cultural awareness
8. Make adaptations for patients with special needs (psychological or physical limitations)
9. Make adaptations to care for patients across their lifespan

Name: _____ Date: _____ Grade: _____

◨ MULTIPLE CHOICE

Circle the letter preceding the correct answer.

1. When obtaining a blood specimen from a winged infusion set, you need all of the following except:
   a. evacuated tubes.
   b. tourniquet.
   c. gauze pads.
   d. syringe.
   e. permanent marker.

2. A source of error in venipuncture is:
   a. puncturing the wrong area of an infant's heel.
   b. inserting needle bevel side down.
   c. prolonged tourniquet application.
   d. pulling back on syringe plunger too forcefully.
   e. all of the above.

3. When your patient is feeling faint during venipuncture, you should do all of the following except:
   a. remove the tourniquet and withdraw the needle.
   b. divert attention from the procedure.
   c. have patient breathe deeply.
   d. loosen a tight collar or tie.
   e. apply a cold compress or washcloth.

4. To avoid hemoconcentration, the phlebotomist should:
   a. ensure the tourniquet is not too tight.
   b. have patient make a fist.
   c. use occluded veins.
   d. draw blood from the heel.
   e. use a needle with a small diameter.

5. If you accidentally puncture an artery, you should:
   a. hold pressure over the site for a full 5 minutes.
   b. use a cold compress to reduce pain.
   c. perform a capillary puncture.
   d. use a multisample needle instead.
   e. use a flatter angle when inserting the needle.

6. What is the difference between NPO and fasting?
   a. Fasting is no food, and NPO is no water.
   b. Fasting and NPO are basically the same.
   c. Fasting allows the patient to drink water, whereas NPO does not.
   d. NPO requires that the patient drink water, whereas fasting does not.
   e. Fasting is for surgery, and NPO is for getting true test results.

7. Aseptic techniques to prevent infection of the venipuncture site include:
   a. using sterile gloves.
   b. wearing a lab coat.
   c. using a gel separator.
   d. not opening bandages ahead of time.
   e. not speaking while you draw blood.

8. When collecting a blood sample from the fingers, you should use:
   a. the thumb.
   b. the second finger.
   c. the fifth finger.
   d. all fingers.
   e. the third and fourth fingers.

9. You should not draw blood using a small gauge needle because:
   a. there is a greater likelihood of it breaking off in the vein.
   b. blood cells will rupture, causing hemolysis of the specimen.
   c. the luer adaptor will not fit venipuncture cuffs.
   d. the small needles are awkward to hold and manipulate.
   e. the small needles do not allow you to collect enough blood.

10. Which of the following may trigger hematoma formation?
    a. Pressure is applied after venipuncture
    b. The needle is removed after the tourniquet is removed
    c. The needle penetrates all the way through the vein
    d. The needle is fully inserted into the vein
    e. The patient has not followed preparation instructions properly.

11. The most commonly used antiseptic for routine blood collection is:
    a. 70% isopropyl alcohol.
    b. povidone iodine.
    c. 0.5% chlorhexidine gluconate.
    d. benzalkonium chloride.
    e. sodium chloride.

12. Which tubes must be first in the order of the draw?
   a. Blood culture tubes
   b. Coagulation tubes
   c. Heparin tubes
   d. Serum separator tubes (SSTs)
   e. Plain tubes

13. Which of the following is true of ethylenediaminetetraacetic acid (EDTA) tubes?
   a. They cause the least interference in tests
   b. They should be filled after hematology tubes
   c. They are the same as PSTs
   d. They minimize the chance of microbial contamination
   e. They elevate sodium and potassium levels

14. What safety features are available for the holder used with the evacuated tube system?
   a. Shields that cover the needle, or devices that retract the needle into the holder
   b. A self-locking cover for recapping the needle
   c. A gripper to clamp the holder to the Vacutainer tube, preventing slippage
   d. Orange color as a reminder to discard in biohazard container
   e. A beveled point on only one end

15. What example explains the best advantage of using the evacuated tube system?
   a. Multiple tubes may be filled from a single venipuncture
   b. The tubes are color coded according to the tests to be done
   c. The vacuum draws the blood into the tubes
   d. It is a universal system, used in all phlebotomy laboratories around the country
   e. It is the least painful way to draw blood from a patient

⬛ MATCHING

Match each key term with the correct definition.

Key Terms

16. _____ antecubital space
17. _____ anticoagulant
18. _____ blood cultures
19. _____ breathing the syringe
20. _____ butterfly
21. _____ cultured
22. _____ evacuated tube
23. _____ fasting
24. _____ gel separator
25. _____ hemochromatosis
26. _____ hematocrit
27. _____ hematoma
28. _____ hemoconcentration
29. _____ hemolysis
30. _____ luer adapter

Definitions

a. blood collection tube additive used because it prevents clotting
b. forms a physical barrier between the cellular portion of a specimen and the serum or plasma portion after the specimen has been centrifuged
c. specimens drawn to culture the blood for pathogens
d. winged infusion set
e. grown in the laboratory
f. pull back the plunger to about halfway up the barrel, and then push it back
g. the inside of the elbow
h. the patient must eat nothing after midnight until the blood specimen is drawn, including chewing gum, breath mints, and coffee; the patient can have water
i. formation caused by blood leaking into the tissues during or after venipuncture
j. packed red blood cell volume
k. a condition that causes an elevated hematocrit
l. disorder that increases the amount of iron in the blood to dangerous levels
m. tubes that fill with a predetermined volume of blood because of the vacuum inside the tube (the vacuum is premeasured by the manufacturer to draw the precise amount of blood into the tube; the tube fills until the vacuum is exhausted)
n. rupturing of red blood cells, causing release of intracellular contents into the plasma
o. needle holder

⬛ MATCHING

Match each key term with the correct definition.

Key Terms

31. _____ lymphedema
32. _____ multisample needle
33. _____ order of draw
34. _____ palpate
35. _____ peak level
36. _____ polycythemia vera
37. _____ prophylaxis
38. _____ thrombosed
39. _____ trough level
40. _____ venipuncture

Definitions

a. protective treatment for the prevention of disease once exposure has occurred
b. the process of puncturing a vein with a needle for the purpose of obtaining a blood sample for analysis; also known as a phlebotomy procedure
c. system that facilitates collecting multiple tubes with a single venipuncture
d. tube filling sequence for both collection of evacuated tubes and filling evacuated tubes from a syringe
e. disease of having too many red blood cells; abnormally high hematocrit
f. veins that have been injured, lack resilience, and roll easily
g. lymphatic obstruction
h. the highest serum level of a drug in a patient based on a dosing schedule, which is usually measured about 60 minutes after the end of the infusion
i. drug level drawn immediately prior to a dose
j. using the tip of the index finger to evaluate veins by feeling to determine their suitability

COG **SHORT ANSWER**

Grade: _____

41. List four techniques you can use to avoid hemoconcentration in a blood specimen.

a. _____

b. _____

c. _____

d. _____

42. Name three issues that can be avoided by using the correct order of draw.

_____

_____

_____

_____

43. Describe six sites to avoid when performing a venipuncture.

_____

_____

_____

_____

44. What should you do if a hematoma begins to form during venipuncture?

_____

_____

_____

_____

45. Name eight sources of error in venipuncture procedure.

_____

_____

_____

_____

COG MATCHING

Grade: _____

Match each tube with its description.

Tubes
46. _____ Heparin tubes
47. _____ Tubes for coagulation testing
48. _____ EDTA tubes
49. _____ Tubes for blood cultures
50. _____ PST tubes
51. _____ Serum separator gel tubes
52. _____ Plain (nonadditive) tubes

Descriptions
a. Drawn first to minimize chance of microbial contamination
b. Prevents contamination by additives in other tubes
c. Must be the first additive tube in the order because all other additive tubes affect coagulation tests
d. Come after coagulation tests because silica particles activate clotting and affect coagulation tests; carryover of silica into subsequent tubes can be overridden by the anticoagulant in them
e. Affects coagulation tests and interferes in collection of serum specimens; causes the least interference in tests other than coagulation tests
f. Causes more carryover problems than any other additive; elevates sodium and potassium levels; chelates and decreases calcium and iron levels; elevates prothrombin time and partial thromboplastin time results
g. Causes the least interference in tests other than coagulation tests and contains a gel separator to separate plasma from the blood cells in the specimen

COG TRUE OR FALSE?

Grade: _____

Indicate whether the statements are true or false by placing the letter T (true) or F (false) on the line preceding the statement.

53. _____ Winged sets cause increased numbers of needlesticks to phlebotomists.

54. _____ For finger puncture sites, it is best to have the hand below the heart.

55. _____ Never believe patients when they say they faint during venipuncture.

56. _____ Warmers decrease blood flow before the skin is punctured.

57. _____ Excessive massaging of the puncture site is a source of error in skin puncture.

COG SHORT ANSWER

Grade: _____

58. List the use of each item of equipment listed that may be used during a routine venipuncture and/or a routine capillary skin puncture.

a. Evacuated collection tubes:

_____

_____

_____

_____

b. Multisample needles:

_____

_____

_____

_____

c. Winged infusion sets:

_____

_____

_____

_____

d. Holders/adapters:

_____

_____

_____

_____

e. Tourniquets:

_____

_____

_____

_____

f. Puncture devices:

_____

_____

_____

_____

g. Microhematocrit tubes:

_____

_____

_____

_____

h. Microcollection containers:

_____

_____

_____

_____

59. Supply the color code for each type of blood collection tube.

a. Blood cultures _____

b. Coagulation tests _____

c. Serum separator tubes _____

d. Ethylenediaminetetraacetic acid _____

e. Plain (nonadditive) tubes _____

f. Plasma tubes and plasma separator tubes _____

⬛COG IDENTIFICATION

Grade: _____

60. Fill in artery (A), tendon (T), or vein (V) by the feeling when palpating a vein.

a. _____ cordlike

b. _____ lacks resilience

c. _____ most elastic

d. _____ palpable

e. _____ pulsatile

f. _____ resilient

g. _____ trackable

COG **PLACE IN ORDER**

Grade: _____

61. Numbering from 1 to 25, place the steps for performing a venipuncture in the correct order.

_____ Greet and identify the patient. Explain the procedure. Ask for and answer any questions.

_____ Tap the tubes that contain additives to ensure that the additive is dislodged from the stopper and wall of the tube. Insert the tube into the adaptor until the needle slightly enters the stopper. Do not push the top of the tube stopper beyond the indentation mark. If the tube retracts slightly, leave it in the retracted position.

_____ Check the physician order and fill out a laboratory requisition form, if necessary.

_____ If a fasting specimen is required, ask the patient the last time they ate or drank anything other than water.

_____ Select a vein by palpating. Use your gloved index finger to trace the path of the vein and judge its depth.

_____ Wash your hands.

_____ Apply the tourniquet around the patient's arm 3 to 4 inches above the elbow.

_____ Cleanse the venipuncture site with an alcohol pad, starting in the center of the puncture site and work outward in a circular motion. Allow the site to dry or dry the site with sterile gauze. Do not touch the area after cleansing.

_____ With the bevel up, line up the needle with the vein approximately ¼ to ½ an inch below the site where the vein is to be entered. At a 15- to 30-degree angle, rapidly and smoothly insert the needle through the skin. Place two fingers on the flanges of the adapter, and with the thumb, push the tube onto the needle inside the adapter. Allow the tube to fill to capacity. Release the tourniquet and allow the patient to release their fist. When blood flow ceases, remove the tube from the adapter by gripping the tube with your nondominant hand and place your thumb against the flange during removal. Twist and gently pull out the tube. Steady the needle in the vein. Avoid pulling up or pressing down on the needle while it is in the vein. Insert any other necessary tubes into the adapter and allow each to fill to capacity.

_____ Assemble the equipment. Check the expiration date on the tubes.

_____ Record the procedure.

_____ Put on nonsterile latex or vinyl gloves. Use other personal protective equipment as defined by facility policy.

_____ Place a sterile gauze pad over the puncture site at the time of needle withdrawal. Do not apply any pressure to the site until the needle is completely removed. After the needle is removed, immediately activate the safety device and apply pressure or have the patient apply direct pressure for 3 to 5 minutes. Do not bend the arm at the elbow.

_____ Instruct the patient to sit with a well-supported arm.

_____ Label the tubes with patient information as defined in facility protocol.

_____ Release the tourniquet after palpating the vein if it has been left on for more than 1 minute. Have patient release their fist.

_____ Test, transfer, or store the blood specimen according to the medical office policy.

_____ Remove the needle cover. Hold the needle assembly in your dominant hand, thumb on top of the adaptor and fingers under it. Grasp the patient's arm with the other hand, using your thumb to draw the skin taut over the site. This anchors the vein about 1 to 2 inches below the puncture site and helps keep it in place during needle insertion.

_____ If the vacuum tubes contain an anticoagulant, they must be mixed immediately by gently inverting the tube 8 to 10 times. Do not shake the tube.

_____ If blood being drawn for culture will be used in diagnosing a septic condition, make sure the specimen is sterile. To do this, apply alcohol to the area for 2 full minutes. Then apply a 2% iodine solution in ever-widening circles. Never move the wipes back over areas that have been cleaned; use a new wipe for each sweep across the area.

_____ Thank the patient. Instruct the patient to leave the bandage in place for at least 15 minutes and not to carry a heavy object (such as a purse) or lift heavy objects with that arm for 1 hour.

_____ Properly care for or dispose of all equipment and supplies. Clean the work area. Remove personal protective equipment and wash your hands.

_____ Reapply the tourniquet if it was removed after palpation. Ask the patient to make a fist.

_____ Check the puncture site for bleeding. Apply a dressing, a clean 2 × 2 gauze pad folded in quarters, and hold in place by an adhesive bandage or 3-inch strip of tape.

_____ With the tourniquet released, remove the tube from the adapter before removing the needle from the arm.

62. Numbering from 1 to 16, place the steps for performing a capillary puncture in the correct order.

_____ Thank the patient. Instruct the patient to leave the bandage in place for at least 15 minutes.

_____ Greet and identify the patient. Explain the procedure. Ask for and answer any questions.

_____ Check the physician order and fill out a laboratory requisition form, if necessary.

_____ Select the puncture site. Use the appropriate puncture device for the site selected.

_____ Obtain the first drop of blood. Wipe away the first drop of blood with dry gauze. Apply pressure toward the site but do not milk the site.

_____ Wash your hands.

_____ Grasp the finger firmly between your nondominant index finger and thumb, or grasp the infant's heel firmly with your index finger wrapped around the foot and your thumb wrapped around the ankle. Cleanse the selected area with 70% isopropyl alcohol and allow to air dry.

_____ Record the procedure.

_____ Assemble the equipment.

_____ Hold the patient's finger or heel firmly and make a swift, firm puncture. Perform the puncture perpendicular to the whorls of the fingerprint or footprint. Dispose of the used puncture device in a sharps container.

_____ Test, transfer, or store the specimen according to the medical office policy.

_____ Put on gloves.

_____ Collect the specimen in the chosen container or slide. Touch only the tip of the collection device to the drop of blood. Blood flow is encouraged if the puncture site is held downward and gentle pressure is applied near the site. Cap microcollection tubes with the caps provided and mix the additives by gently tilting or inverting the tubes 8 to 10 times.

_____ Make sure the site chosen is warm and not cyanotic or edematous. Gently massage the finger from the base to the tip or massage the infant's heel.

_____ Properly care for or dispose of equipment and supplies. Clean the work area. Remove gloves and wash your hands.

_____ When collection is complete, apply clean gauze to the site with pressure. Hold pressure or have the patient hold pressure until bleeding stops. Label the containers with the proper information. Do not apply a dressing to a skin puncture of an infant under age 2 years. Never release a patient until the bleeding has stopped.

COG TRUE OR FALSE?

Grade: _____

Indicate whether the statements are true or false by placing the letter T (true) or F (false) on the line preceding the statement.

63. _____ After the needle is removed, activate the safety device as soon as possible.

64. _____ The phlebotomy equipment should be easily accessible by everyone in the medical office.

65. _____ A safety device locks the armrest in place in front of the patient to prevent falling from the chair if fainting occurs.

66. _____ Needle holders do not include a safety device, so needle safety devices are required.

67. _____ The Needlestick Safety and Prevention Act requires each phlebotomist to be responsible for their own safety.

68. _____ Quick activation of the safety device relieves the phlebotomist of concern for caution.

69. _____ Holder safety features may include a shield that covers the needle or a device that retracts the needle into the holder after it is withdrawn from the vein.

70. _____ Regardless of safety features, immediately dispose of used needles, lancets, and other sharp objects in a puncture-resistant, leak-proof disposable container called a sharps container.

COG FILL IN THE BLANK

Grade: _____

71. Postural changes (_____, _____, _____) are known to vary laboratory results of some analytes. The differences in these lab values have been attributed to shifts in _____ _____. Fluids tend to stay in the vascular compartment (bloodstream) when the patient is _____ or _____. This tends to _____ the blood. There is a _____ of fluids to the interstitial spaces upon standing or ambulation. The lab tests that are the most affected by this phenomenon are proteins (_____, _____, _____) and protein-bound substances, such as _____, _____, _____, _____ and _____.

72. The maximum time limit for leaving the tourniquet in place is _____ minutes. Extending the time limit can alter test results by causing _____ and _____. The _____ of fluid in hemoconcentrated blood results in a(n) _____ of cellular components in that blood. This _____ elevation results in _____ laboratory measurement of _____, _____, and some _____. _____ tourniquet placement may significantly increase total protein, aspartate aminotransferase (AST), total lipids, cholesterol, iron, and hematocrit.

73. The most common complication of venipuncture is _____ formation caused by blood leaking into the tissues during or after venipuncture.

74. Situations that may trigger hematoma formation include:

   a. The vein is _____ or too _____ for the needle.

   b. The needle _____ all the way through the _____.

   c. The needle is only _____ _____ into the vein.

   d. Excessive or _____ _____ is used to find the vein.

   e. The needle is removed while the _____ _____ _____ _____.

   f. _____ is not adequately applied after venipuncture.

75. _____ veins (lack resilience) feel like rope or cord and _____ easily.

76. Accidental puncture of an _____ is recognized by the blood's bright red color and the _____ of the specimen into the tube.

77. Permanent _____ damage may result from _____ site selection, movement of the _____ during needle insertion, inserting the needle too _____ or, _____ or excessive blind _____.

78. Make sure the needle fully _____ the _____ most wall of the vein. (Partial _____ allow blood to leak into the soft tissue surrounding the vein by way of the needle _____.)

79. If an insufficient amount or no blood is collected:

a. Change the _____ of the _____. Move it forward (it may not be in the _____). Or, move it backward (it may have _____ _____ _____).

b. Adjust the angle (the _____ may be against the vein _____).

c. Loosen the tourniquet; it may be _____ blood _____.

d. Try _____ tube. There may be no _____ in the _____ _____ _____.

e. _____ the vein. Veins sometimes _____ _____ from the _____ of the needle and puncture site.

f. The vein may have _____; _____ the tourniquet to increase _____ filling. If this is not successful, remove the _____, take care of the _____ site, and _____.

g. The _____ may have pulled _____ _____ _____ _____ when switching tubes. _____ equipment firmly and place against _____ the patient's arm, using the _____ for leverage when withdrawing and inserting _____.

AFF PSY CASE STUDIES FOR CRITICAL THINKING Grade: _____

80. You have a patient who says that he always becomes nervous at the sight of his own blood but has never fainted before. You ask the patient to lie down during the procedure. Your patient is fine with the needle insertion, but as soon as he sees the sight of his own blood, he passes out. What should you do?

_____

_____

_____

81. You are reviewing test results received from the referral laboratory. You notice that the HIV results on your neighbor, Alice Sihotang, are positive. Your friend Kaylene Oyakawa meets you for lunch. She tells you that all of your neighbors are worried about Alice because she looks so ill and has been losing weight. Kaylene says that she knows Alice is a patient at your medical office and asks you what is wrong with Alice. What do you say?

_____

_____

_____

82. After drawing blood with a winged set, you inadvertently stick yourself with the needle. How would you handle this situation?

_____

_____

_____

83. Your last patient of the day, a young child accompanied by her mother, accidentally knocks over your collection tubes that were within her reach as you were disposing of sharps. How would you handle this situation?

_____

_____

_____

84. The medical office has closed and you are completing preparation of specimens for the reference laboratory pickup. You find you have two requisitions without labeled specimens to accompany them. You have two unlabeled blood tubes. There is no way to identify the two specimens. What do you do?

_____

_____

_____

PSY PROCEDURE 41-1 | **Obtain a Blood Specimen by Evacuated Tube or Winged Infusion Set**

Name: _____ Date: _____ Time: _____ Grade: _____

EQUIPMENT/SUPPLIES: Multisample needle and adaptor or winged infusion set, evacuated tubes, tourniquet, sterile gauze pads, bandages, sharps container, 70% alcohol pad, permanent marker or pen, appropriate personal protective equipment (e.g., gloves, impervious gown, face shield)

STANDARDS: Given the needed equipment and a place to work, the student will perform this skill with _____ % accuracy in a total of _____ minutes. *(Your instructor will tell you what the percentage and time limits will be before you begin practicing.)*

KEY: 4 = Satisfactory 0 = Unsatisfactory NA = This step is not counted

PROCEDURE STEPS	SELF	PARTNER	INSTRUCTOR
1. Check the physician order and complete the requisition slip if appropriate	❑	❑	❑
2. Wash your hands and assemble the equipment	❑	❑	❑
3. Check the expiration date on the tubes. Discard expired supplies according to office policy and procedure	❑	❑	❑
4. **AFF** Greet and identify the patient and yourself, including your title. Explain the procedure	❑	❑	❑
5. **AFF** Demonstrate recognition of the patient's level of understanding communications. Apply active listening skills. Modify communication to the patient's level of understanding, or obtain assistance with language differences	❑	❑	❑
6. Ask the patient about any dietary restrictions and the use of medications that increase bleeding time. If a fasting or NPO specimen is required, ask the patient for the last time they ate or drank anything	❑	❑	❑
7. Put on nonsterile latex or vinyl gloves. Use other personal protective equipment as defined by office policy	❑	❑	❑
8. *For evacuated tube collection*: Break the seal of the needle cover and thread the sleeved needle into the adaptor, using the needle cover as a wrench *For winged infusion set collection*: Extend the tubing. Thread the sleeved needle into the adaptor *For both methods*: Tap the tubes that contain additives to ensure that the additive is dislodged from the stopper and wall of the tube. Insert the tube into the adaptor until the needle slightly enters the stopper. Do not push the top of the tube stopper beyond the indentation mark. If the tube retracts slightly, leave it in the retracted position	❑	❑	❑
9. Instruct the patient to sit with a well-supported arm	❑	❑	❑

PSY PROCEDURE 41-1 **Obtain a Blood Specimen by Evacuated Tube or Winged Infusion Set** (continued)

10. After reviewing veins in both arms, choose one arm and apply the tourniquet 3 to 4 inches above the elbow
  a. Apply the tourniquet snuggly, but not too tightly
  b. Secure the tourniquet by using the half-bow knot
  c. Make sure the tails of the tourniquet extend upward to avoid contaminating the venipuncture site
  d. Ask the patient to make a fist and hold it but not to pump their fist
	❑	❑	❑

11. Select a vein by palpating. Use your gloved index finger to trace the path of the vein and judge its depth	❑	❑	❑
12. Release tourniquet after palpating the vein if it has been left on for more than 1 minute. Have patient release their fist	❑	❑	❑
13. Cleanse the venipuncture site with an alcohol pad, starting in the center of the puncture site and working outward in a circular motion. Allow the site to dry or dry the site with sterile gauze. Do not touch the area after cleansing	❑	❑	❑
14. If blood is being drawn for a blood culture, make sure the area is cleansed using a 2% iodine solution for 2 full minutes	❑	❑	❑
15. Reapply the tourniquet if it was removed after palpation. Ask the patient to make a fist	❑	❑	❑
16. Remove the needle cover. Hold the needle assembly in your dominant hand, thumb on top of the adaptor and fingers under it. Grasp the patient's arm with the other hand, using your thumb to draw the skin taut over the site. This anchors the vein about 1 to 2 inches below the puncture site and helps keep it in place during the needle insertion	❑	❑	❑
17. With the bevel up, line up the needle with the vein approximately ¼ to ½ inch below the site where the vein is to be entered. At a 15- to 30-degree angle, rapidly and smoothly insert the needle through the skin. Use a lesser angle for winged infusion set collections. Place two fingers on the flanges of the adapter and with the thumb, push the tube onto the needle inside the adapter. Allow the tube to fill to capacity. Release the tourniquet and allow the patient to release their fist. When blood flow ceases, remove the tube from the adapter by gripping the tube with your nondominant hand and placing your thumb against the flange during removal. Twist and gently pull out the tube. Steady the needle in the vein. Avoid pulling up or pressing down on the needle while it is in the vein. Insert any other necessary tubes into the adapter and allow each to fill to capacity	❑	❑	❑
18. With the tourniquet released, remove the tube from the adapter before removing the needle from the arm	❑	❑	❑

(continues)

19. Place a sterile gauze pad over the puncture site at the time of needle withdrawal. Do not apply any pressure to the site until the needle is completely removed **a.** After the needle is removed, immediately activate the safety device and apply pressure or have the patient apply direct pressure for 3 to 5 minutes. Do not bend the arm at the elbow	❏	❏	❏
20. After the needle is removed, immediately activate the safety device and apply pressure, or have the patient apply direct pressure for 3 to 5 minutes. Do not bend the arm at the elbow	❏	❏	❏
21. If the vacuum tubes contain an anticoagulant, they must be mixed immediately by gently inverting the tube 8 to 10 times. Do not shake the tube	❏	❏	❏
22. Label the tubes with patient information as defined by the office or laboratory protocol	❏	❏	❏
23. Check the puncture site for bleeding. Apply a dressing, a clean 2 × 2 gauze pad folded in quarters, and hold in place by an adhesive bandage or 3-inch strip of tape	❏	❏	❏
24. **AFF** Thank the patient. Instruct the patient to leave the bandage in place for at least 15 minutes and not to carry a heavy object (such as a purse) or lift heavy objects with that arm for 1 hour	❏	❏	❏
25. Properly care for or dispose of all equipment and supplies. Clean the work area. Remove personal protective equipment and wash your hands	❏	❏	❏
26. Test, transfer, or store the blood specimen according to the medical office policy	❏	❏	❏
27. Log into the Electronic Medical Record (EMR) using your username and secure password OR obtain the paper medical record from a secure location and assure it is kept away from public access. Record the procedure, noting the date, time, site of the venipuncture, test results for CLIA-waived POC procedures or the name of the lab where the specimen was sent, and your name	❏	❏	❏
28. When finished, log out of the EMR and/or replace the paper medical record in an appropriate and secure location	❏	❏	❏
29. **AFF** Explain how to respond to a patient who is deaf, hearing impaired, visually impaired, developmentally challenged, or speaks English as a second language (ESL) or who has dementia, cultural or religious concerns, or generational differences	❏	❏	❏

PSY PROCEDURE 41-1 **Obtain a Blood Specimen by Evacuated Tube or Winged Infusion Set** (continued)

_____

_____

_____

_____

CALCULATION

Total Possible Points: _____

Total Points Earned: _____ Multiplied by 100 = _____ Divided by Total Possible Points = _____ %

PASS   FAIL   COMMENTS:
❏   ❏

Student's signature _____ Date _____

Partner's signature _____ Date _____

Instructor's signature _____ Date _____

PSY PROCEDURE 41-2 Obtain a Blood Specimen by Capillary Puncture

Name: _____ **Date:** _____ **Time:** _____ **Grade:** _____

EQUIPMENT/SUPPLIES: Skin puncture device, 70% alcohol pads, 2 × 2 gauze pads, microcollection tubes or containers, heel warming device if needed, small band aids, pen or permanent marker and personal protective equipment (e.g., gloves, impervious gown, face shield)

STANDARDS: Given the needed equipment and a place to work, the student will perform this skill with _____ % accuracy in a total of _____ minutes. *(Your instructor will tell you what the percentage and time limits will be before you begin.)*

KEY: 4 = Satisfactory 0 = Unsatisfactory NA = This step is not counted

PROCEDURE STEPS	SELF	PARTNER	INSTRUCTOR
1. Check the physician order and complete the requisition slip, if appropriate	❑	❑	❑
2. Wash your hands	❑	❑	❑
3. Assemble the equipment	❑	❑	❑
4. **AFF** Greet and identify the patient and yourself, including your title. Explain the procedure	❑	❑	❑
5. **AFF** Evaluate your patient for their ability to understand your instructions. When indicated, whether the problem is deafness, hearing impairment, visual impairment, a developmental challenge, English as a second language (ESL), dementia, cultural or religious concerns, or generational differences, you are responsible for helping the patient understand the procedure before beginning the phlebotomy. This may include obtaining help from the person who brought the patient to the office or from a translator	❑	❑	❑
6. Put on gloves	❑	❑	❑
7. Ask the patient or caregiver of an infant or small child about any dietary restrictions and the use of medications that increase bleeding time as appropriate. If a fasting or NPO specimen is required, ask the patient about the last time they ate or drank anything	❑	❑	❑
8. Select the puncture site (the lateral portion of the tip of the middle or ring finger of the nondominant hand or lateral curved surface of the heel of an infant). The puncture should be made in the fleshy central portion of the second or third finger, slightly to the side of center, and perpendicular to the grooves of the fingerprint. Perform heel puncture only on the plantar surface of the heel, medial to an imaginary line extending from the middle of the great toe to the heel, and lateral to an imaginary line drawn from between the fourth and fifth toes to the heel. Use the appropriate puncture device for the site selected	❑	❑	❑

PSY PROCEDURE 41-2 **Obtain a Blood Specimen by Capillary Puncture** (continued)

9. Make sure the site chosen is warm and not cyanotic or edematous. Gently massage the finger from the base to the tip or massage the infant's heel	❏	❏	❏
10. Grasp the finger firmly between your nondominant index finger and thumb, or grasp the infant's heel firmly with your index finger wrapped around the foot and your thumb wrapped around the ankle. Cleanse the selected area with 70% isopropyl alcohol and allow to air dry	❏	❏	❏
11. Hold the patient's finger or heel firmly and make a swift, firm puncture. Perform the puncture perpendicular to the whorls of the fingerprint or footprint. Dispose of the used puncture device in a sharps container	❏	❏	❏

12. Obtain the first drop of blood
  a. Wipe away the first drop of blood with dry gauze
  b. Apply pressure toward the site but do not milk the site
	❏	❏	❏

13. Collect the specimen in the chosen container or slide. Touch only the tip of the collection device to the drop of blood. Blood flow is encouraged if the puncture site is held downward, and gentle pressure is applied near the site. Cap micro-collection tubes with the caps provided and mix the additives by gently tilting or inverting the tubes 8 to 10 times	❏	❏	❏
14. When the collection is complete, apply clean gauze to the site with pressure. Hold pressure or have the patient or caregiver hold pressure until the bleeding stops. Label the containers with the proper information. Do not apply a dressing to a skin puncture of an infant under age 2 years. Never release a patient until the bleeding has stopped	❏	❏	❏
15. **AFF** Thank the patient. Instruct the patient to leave the bandage in place for at least 15 minutes, if appropriate	❏	❏	❏
16. Properly care for or dispose of equipment and supplies. Clean the work area. Remove gloves and wash your hands	❏	❏	❏
17. Test, transfer, or store the specimen according to the medical office policy	❏	❏	❏
18. Log into the Electronic Medical Record (EMR) using your username and secure password OR obtain the paper medical record from a secure location and assure it is kept away from public access. Record the procedure, noting the date, time, site of the capillary puncture, test results for CLIA-waived POC procedures or the name of the lab where the specimen was sent and your name	❏	❏	❏

(continues)

PSY PROCEDURE 41-2 | **Obtain a Blood Specimen by Capillary Puncture** (continued)

19. When finished, log out of the EMR and/or replace the paper medical record in an appropriate and secure location	❑	❑	❑

_____

_____

_____

_____

CALCULATION

Total Possible Points: _____

Total Points Earned: _____ Multiplied by 100 = _____ Divided by Total Possible Points = _____ %

PASS **FAIL** **COMMENTS:**
❑ ❑

Student's signature _____ Date _____

Partner's signature _____ Date _____

Instructor's signature _____ Date _____

CHAPTER 42

Hematology

LEARNING OUTCOMES

COG Cognitive Domain*

1. Spell key terms
2. *Identify the following related to body systems:*
   a. *medical terms*
   b. *abbreviations*
3. *Identify CLIA-waived tests associated with common diseases*
4. List the parameters measured in the complete blood count and their normal ranges
5. State the conditions associated with selected abnormal complete blood count findings
6. *Identify normal and abnormal results as reported in:*
   a. *graphs*
   b. *tables*

PSY Psychomotor Domain*

1. Perform hemoglobin determination (Procedure 42-1)
   a. *Collect specimens and perform CLIA-waived hematology test*
   b. *Instruct and prepare a patient for a procedure or treatment*
   c. *Perform quality control measure*

   d. *Document patient care accurately in the medical record*
2. Perform microhematocrit determination (Procedure 42-2)
   a. *Collect specimens and perform CLIA-waived hematology test*
   b. *Instruct and prepare a patient for a procedure or treatment*
   c. *Perform quality control measures*
   d. *Document patient care accurately in the medical record*

AFF Affective Domain*

1. *Demonstrate critical thinking skills*
2. *Reassure patients*
3. *Demonstrate empathy for patients' concerns*
4. *Demonstrate active listening*
5. *Respect diversity*
6. *Recognize personal boundaries*
7. *Demonstrate tactfulness*
8. *Demonstrate self-awareness*
9. Protect the integrity of the medical record

MAERB Standards are Italicized.

ABHES Competencies

1. Practice quality control
2. Dispose of biohazardous materials
3. Collect, label, and process specimens: 1). Perform venipuncture 2). Perform capillary puncture
4. Perform selected CLIA-waived tests that assist with diagnosis and treatment: Hematology testing
5. Follow documentation guidelines
6. Adapt care to address the developmental stages of life
7. Display effective interpersonal skills with patients and healthcare team members
8. Demonstrate cultural awareness
9. Make adaptations for patients with special needs (psychological or physical limitations)
10. Make adaptations to care for patients across their lifespan

Name: _____   Date: _____   Grade: _____

COG MULTIPLE CHOICE

Circle the letter preceding the correct answer.

1. Leukocytosis is most likely caused by:
   a. chemical toxicity.
   b. inflammation.
   c. nutritional deficiencies.
   d. infection.
   e. anticoagulant therapy.

2. What indicates a vitamin B_{12} deficiency?
   a. The presence of bands
   b. Macrocytosis or a mean corpuscular volume (MCV) of higher than 100 fL
   c. High numbers of lymphocytes
   d. Erythrocytes that lack a nucleus
   e. Microcytosis or a mean cell volume (MCV) less than 80 fL

3. Which white blood cells produce antibodies?
   a. Neutrophils
   b. Eosinophils
   c. Monocytes
   d. Lymphocytes
   e. Basophils

4. Where in the body are red blood cells produced?
   a. Bone marrow
   b. Fatty tissue
   c. Liver
   d. Kidney
   e. Heart

5. A parasitic infection is indicated by increased numbers of which leukocytes?
   a. Neutrophils
   b. Lymphocytes
   c. Eosinophils
   d. Monocytes
   e. Basophils

6. Which condition could be caused by chemotherapy?
   a. Anemia
   b. Folate deficiency
   c. Leukocytosis
   d. Monocytosis
   e. Thrombocytopenia

7. One symptom of vitamin K deficiency is:
   a. left shift.
   b. macrocytosis.
   c. prolonged ESR.
   d. prolonged PT.
   e. thrombocytosis.

8. ESR tests should be read:
   a. after 1 minute.
   b. at 15 minutes.
   c. at 30 minutes.
   d. at 60 minutes.
   e. at any time; the exact time is not important.

9. Microcytosis indicates:
   a. iron deficiency.
   b. the presence of gamma globulins.
   c. liver disorders.
   d. B_{12} deficiency.
   e. sickle cell anemia.

10. Patients with iron deficiencies should be encouraged to eat:
    a. dairy.
    b. fish.
    c. fruit.
    d. tofu.
    e. liver.

11. Erythropoiesis is driven by chemical signals from:
    a. the brain.
    b. the kidneys.
    c. the liver.
    d. the marrow.
    e. the spleen.

12. What is the most direct measurement of the blood's ability to deliver oxygen available in the CBC?
    a. RBC count
    b. Hemoglobin (Hgb) determination
    c. Hematocrit (Hct) determination
    d. Mean cell volume (MCV)
    e. Mean corpuscular hemoglobin (MCH)

13. A patient has a platelet count of 75,000/mm³. What visible symptom might appear on the patient?
    a. Circular rash
    b. Edema
    c. Bruising
    d. Sloughing of skin
    e. Hair loss

14. Which is a normal platelet count?
    a. 4,300 to 10,800 /µL
    b. 150,000 to 400,000/µL
    c. 4.2 to 5.4 million/µL
    d. 4.6 to 6.2 million/µL
    e. 27 to 31 million/µL

15. Which is the normal RBC count for women?
    a. 4,300 to 10,800/mm³
    b. 200,000 to 400,000/mm³
    c. 3.9 to 5.2 million/mm³
    d. 4.4 to 5.8 million/mm³
    e. 27 to 31 million/mm³

⬤OG MATCHING

Match each key term with its definition.

Key Term

16. _____ band
17. _____ basophil
18. _____ complete blood count
19. _____ eosinophil
20. _____ erythrocytes
21. _____ erythrocyte indices
22. _____ erythrocyte sedimentation rate
23. _____ erythropoietin
24. _____ hematocrit
25. _____ hemoglobin
26. _____ leukocytes
27. _____ monocyte
28. _____ morphology
29. _____ neutrophil
30. _____ differential

Definition

a. red blood cells or RBCs
b. white blood cells or WBCs
c. the functioning unit of the red blood cell
d. influences RBC production when it is released from the kidneys
e. cell type that makes up only a small portion of the number of white blood cells but are important parts of the body's immune response
f. cells active at the end of allergic responses and of parasite elimination
g. third most abundant leukocyte that engulfs foreign material
h. cell that defends against foreign invaders by engulfing them
i. a younger, less-mature version of the neutrophils
j. contains WBC count and differential, RBC count, hemoglobin (Hgb) determination, hematocrit (Hct) determination, mean cell volume (MCV), mean corpuscular hemoglobin (MCH), mean corpuscular hemoglobin concentration (MCHC), and platelet count
k. WBCs are counted, tallied according to type, and reported as percentages
l. how cells appear under the microscope
m. percentage of RBCs in whole blood
n. measurements indicating the size of the RBC and how much hemoglobin the RBC holds
o. the rate in millimeters per hour at which RBCs settle out in a tube

⬤OG FILL IN THE BLANK

List the parameters measured in the complete blood count and their normal ranges

Test	Reference Interval
31.	
32.	
33.	
34.	
35.	
36.	
37.	
38.	

OOG MATCHING

Grade: _____

Match each condition with the correct abnormal finding.

Conditions	Abnormal Findings
39. _____ Increased bleeding	**a.** hemoglobin of 10 g/dL
40. _____ Infection	**b.** thrombocytopenia
41. _____ Anemia	**c.** hematocrit of 55%
42. _____ Low iron level	**d.** leukocytosis
43. _____ Dehydration	**e.** macrocytosis
44. _____ Liver disorders	**f.** red cell count of 3.9 million/mL
45. _____ Microcytic anemia	**g.** MCH of 22 picograms/red cell

OOG IDENTIFICATION

Grade: _____

Indicate whether following cell function is that of a red blood cell (RBC), a white blood cell (WBC), or a platelet (PLA).

46. _____ body's primary defense against bacteria found inside cells

47. _____ contribute to inflammatory reactions

48. _____ critical elements of clot formation

49. _____ defend against foreign invaders by engulfing them

50. _____ important parts of the body's immune response

51. _____ may indicate any of a variety of acute conditions that necessitate immediate attention

52. _____ plug can arrest bleeding

53. _____ process the antigens and through a series of cell transitions, produce the antibodies that can now fight that antigen in the body

54. _____ release carbon dioxide that was picked up from the tissues and then bind oxygen

55. _____ signal of a viral infection

OOG FILL IN THE BLANK

Grade: _____

56. Fill in the blanks in this description of the purpose of testing for the erythrocyte sedimentation rate.

The reference interval for men under 50 years of age is _____, and for women under 50 years, it is _____. Elevations in ESR values are _____ _____ for any disorder but indicate either _____ or any other condition that causes increased or altered _____ in the blood (e.g., rheumatoid arthritis). The more _____ the RBCs fall in the column, the greater the degree of inflammation. The ESR can be elevated with infection and _____.

OOG FILL IN THE BLANK

Grade: _____

List the leukocytes seen normally in the blood and their functions.

White Blood Cell Type	Function
57.	
58.	
59.	
60.	
61.	

OOG ANALYSIS

Grade: _____

62. Analyze a graph in the interpretation of healthcare results.

You have centrifuged your capillary collection tubes to calculate the patient's hematocrit.

a. Which tube is placed correctly on the measurement grid? (Place the letter identifying the correct tube in the space provided.) _____

b. How did you verify the correct placement of the tube on the grid?

_____

_____

_____

_____

c. Because this graph is difficult to interpret, estimate the approximate hematocrit for this patient. _____

COG IDENTIFICATION

Grade: _____

Indicate whether each laboratory result is normal (N) or abnormal (A).

63. _____ Platelet count = 110,000/μL

64. _____ Hemoglobin in a male = 16 g/dL

65. _____ Hematocrit in a male = 49%

66. _____ MCV = 75 fL

67. _____ MCH = 29 picograms

68. _____ MCHC = 35 g/dL

69. _____ RBC in a female = 3.71 million/mm^3

70. _____ ESR = 5 mm/hour

AFF CASE STUDIES FOR CRITICAL THINKING

Grade: _____

71. Men over age 35 and alcoholics frequently have difficulty absorbing vitamin B. What symptoms would you expect to see in an older male who drinks, and how could these be best addressed?

_____

_____

_____

_____

72. A trauma patient arrives in the hospital with extensive bleeding and internal injuries. The next day, you are asked to run lab tests on this patient's bloodwork. How do you expect her results to differ from those of a healthy patient?

_____

_____

_____

_____

73. Your patient presents with a persistent headache and nasal congestion. His WBC count is normal, but the eosinophil count is high. What is the probable cause of the patient's complaint?

_____

_____

_____

_____

74. You are performing an erythrocyte sedimentation rate. After 60 minutes, you look at the tube to report the test results. You cannot determine the separation between the cells and the plasma. The separation is not straight, and there are bubbles in the tube. What are the probable causes of your problem?

_____

_____

_____

_____

75. You are preparing to collect a fingerstick specimen from your patient for a PT and INR test. The puncture wound continues to bleed heavily after the specimen is completed. How do you stop the bleeding and reassure the patient?

_____

_____

_____

_____

76. Explain the rationale used when explaining a procedure to the patient within parameters set by the physician.

_____

_____

_____

_____

77. Your patient arrives for a fingerstick hematocrit test. She tells you she is worried because she continues to have anemia and treatment does not seem to be helping. How do you show awareness of the patient's feelings within the scope of practice of a medical assistant?

_____

_____

_____

_____

PSY PROCEDURE 42-1 Performing a Hemoglobin Determination

Name: _____ Date: _____ Time: _____ Grade: _____

EQUIPMENT/SUPPLIES: Hemoglobin meter, applicator sticks, whole blood, hand disinfectant, surface disinfectant, gloves, biohazard container, medical record

STANDARDS: Given the needed equipment and a place to work, the student will perform this skill with _____ % accuracy in a total of _____ minutes. *(Your instructor will tell you what the percentage and time limits will be before you begin practicing.)*

KEY: 4 = Satisfactory   0 = Unsatisfactory   NA = This step is not counted

PROCEDURE STEPS	SELF	PARTNER	INSTRUCTOR
1. Check the physician order and wash your hands. Put on personal protective equipment	❏	❏	❏
2. Assemble the necessary equipment and supplies. Check the expiration dates on supplies that require this and ensure the equipment is in good working order. Perform any calibration or quality control procedures as required per the manufacturer and office policy	❏	❏	❏
3. Take the equipment and supplies to the patient examination room or take the patient to the phlebotomy station, if available	❏	❏	❏
4. Greet and identify the patient and yourself, including your title. Explain the procedure and put on gloves	❏	❏	❏
5. Explain how you would respond to an elderly patient	❏	❏	❏
6. Obtain a blood specimen from the patient by capillary puncture	❏	❏	❏
7. Place well-mixed whole blood into the hemoglobinometer chamber or place the blood specimen on the reagent strip as described by the manufacturer	❏	❏	❏
8. Slide the chamber into the hemoglobinometer or process the specimen using the CLIA-waived machine as required by the manufacturer. Slide the chamber into the hemoglobin meter	❏	❏	❏
9. Record the hemoglobin level from the digital readout	❏	❏	❏
10. Dispose of the contaminated supplies into a biohazard waste receptacle according to office policy and procedure. Clean the work area with surface disinfectant. Remove gloves and wash your hands *Note:* This procedure may vary with the instrument	❏	❏	❏

(continues)

11. Log into the Electronic Medical Record (EMR) using your username and secure password OR obtain the paper medical record from a secure location and assure it is kept away from public access. Record the procedure, noting the date, time, site of the venipuncture, test results for CLIA-waived POC procedures or the name of the lab where the specimen was sent, and your name	❑	❑	❑
12. When finished, log out of the EMR and/or replace the paper medical record in an appropriate and secure location	❑	❑	❑

_____

_____

_____

_____

CALCULATION

Total Possible Points: _____

Total Points Earned: _____ Multiplied by 100 = _____ Divided by Total Possible Points = _____ %

PASS   FAIL   COMMENTS:
❑   ❑

Chart Documentation _____ Date _____

Student's signature _____ Date _____

Partner's signature _____ Date _____

Instructor's signature _____ Date _____

PSY PROCEDURE 42-2 **Performing a Microhematocrit Determination**

Name: _____ Date: _____ Time: _____ Grade: _____

EQUIPMENT/SUPPLIES: Microcollection tubes, sealing clay, microhematocrit centrifuge, microhematocrit reading device, hand disinfectant, surface disinfectant, gloves, biohazard container, sharps container, medical record

STANDARDS: Given the needed equipment and a place to work, the student will perform this skill with _____ % accuracy in a total of _____ minutes. *(Your instructor will tell you what the percentage and time limits will be before you begin practicing.)*

KEY: 4 = Satisfactory 0 = Unsatisfactory NA = This step is not counted

PROCEDURE STEPS	SELF	PARTNER	INSTRUCTOR
1. Check the physician order and wash your hands	❏	❏	❏
2. Assemble the equipment and supplies. Check the expiration dates on supplies that require this and ensure the equipment is in good working order. Perform any calibration or quality control procedures as required per the manufacturer and office policy	❏	❏	❏
3. Take the equipment and supplies to the patient examination room or take the patient to the phlebotomy station, if available	❏	❏	❏
4. Greet and identify the patient and yourself, including your title. Explain the procedure and put on gloves	❏	❏	❏
5. Explain how you would respond to a patient who does not speak English as their first language	❏	❏	❏
6. Obtain a blood specimen from the patient by capillary puncture. Draw blood into the capillary tube by holding the capillary micro-hematocrit tube horizontally and touching one end of the tube to the blood coming from the capillary puncture. Allow the tube to fill to ¾ or the indicated mark on the capillary tube	❏	❏	❏
7. With the microhematocrit tube in a horizontal position, place your forefinger over the opposite end of the tube, lift it up, and push the tube into the clay sealant with the blood side in the clay	❏	❏	❏
8. Draw a second specimen in the same manner using a second microhematocrit tube	❏	❏	❏
9. Place the tubes, clay-sealed end out, in the radial grooves of the microhematocrit centrifuge opposite each other. Put the lid on the grooved area and tighten by turning the knob clockwise. Close the centrifuge lid. Spin for 5 minutes or as directed by the centrifuge manufacturer	❏	❏	❏
10. Remove the tubes from the centrifuge and read the results; instructions are printed on the device. Results should be within 5% of each other. Take the average and report as a percentage	❏	❏	❏

(continues)

PSY PROCEDURE 42-2 | **Performing a Microhematocrit Determination** (continued)

11. Dispose of the contaminated supplies into a biohazard waste receptacle according to office policy and procedure. Clean the work area with surface disinfectant. Dispose of equipment and supplies appropriately. Remove gloves and wash your hands *Note:* Some microhematocrit centrifuges have the scale printed in the machine at the radial grooves	❑	❑	❑
12. Log into the Electronic Medical Record (EMR) using your username and secure password OR obtain the paper medical record from a secure location and assure it is kept away from public access. Record the procedure, noting the date, time, site of the venipuncture, test results for CLIA-waived POC procedures or the name of the lab where the specimen was sent, and your name	❑	❑	❑
13. When finished, log out of the EMR and/or replace the paper medical record in an appropriate and secure location	❑	❑	❑

_____

_____

_____

_____

CALCULATION

Total Possible Points: _____

Total Points Earned: _____ Multiplied by 100 = _____ Divided by Total Possible Points = _____ %

PASS   **FAIL**   **COMMENTS:**
  ❑   ❑

Chart Documentation _____ Date _____

Student's signature _____ Date _____

Partner's signature _____ Date _____

Instructor's signature _____ Date _____

CHAPTER 43

Clinical Chemistry

LEARNING OUTCOMES

COG Cognitive Domain*

1. Spell key terms
2. *Identify the following related to body systems:*
   a. *medical terms*
   b. *abbreviations*
3. List the common electrolytes and explain the relationship of electrolytes to acid–base balance
4. Describe the nonprotein nitrogenous compounds and name conditions with abnormal values
5. *Identify CLIA-waived tests associated with common diseases*
6. *Identify normal and abnormal results as reported in*
   a. *graphs*
   b. *tables*
7. List and describe the substances commonly tested in liver function assessment
8. Describe glucose use and regulation and the purpose of the various glucose tests
9. Describe the function of cholesterol and other lipids and their correlation to heart disease
10. *Identify quality assurance practices in health care*

PSY Psychomotor Domain*

1. Perform blood glucose testing (Procedure 43-1)
   a. *Collect specimens and perform CLIA-waived chemistry test*
   b. *Instruct and prepare a patient for a procedure or treatment*
   c. *Perform quality control measure*
   d. *Document patient care accurately in the medical record*
2. Perform blood cholesterol testing (Procedure 43-2)
   a. *Collect specimens and perform CLIA-waived chemistry test*
   b. *Instruct and prepare a patient for a procedure or treatment*
   c. *Perform quality control measures*
   d. *Document patient care accurately in the medical record*

AFF Affective Domain*

1. *Demonstrate critical thinking skills*
2. *Reassure patients*
3. *Demonstrate empathy for patients' concerns*
4. *Demonstrate active listening*
5. *Respect diversity*
6. *Recognize personal boundaries*
7. *Demonstrate tactfulness*
8. *Demonstrate self-awareness*
9. Protect the integrity of the medical record

MAERB Standards are Italicized.

ABHES Competencies

1. Practice quality control
2. Dispose of biohazardous materials
3. Collect, label, and process specimens: 1). Perform venipuncture 2). Perform capillary puncture
4. Perform selected CLIA-waived tests that assist with diagnosis and treatment: Chemistry testing
5. Follow documentation guidelines
6. Adapt care to address the developmental stages of life
7. Display effective interpersonal skills with patients and healthcare team members
8. Demonstrate cultural awareness
9. Make adaptations for patients with special needs (psychological or physical limitations)
10. Make adaptations to care for patients across their lifespan

Name: _____   Date: _____   Grade: _____

OOG AFF MULTIPLE CHOICE

Circle the letter preceding the correct answer.

1. Sodium is used to maintain:
   a. blood urea nitrogen.
   b. TSH stimulation.
   c. waste materials.
   d. fluid balance.
   e. blood oxygen.

2. An enzyme is a(n):
   a. cell that speeds up the production of proteins.
   b. protein that quickens chemical reactions.
   c. chemical reaction that ionizes electrolytes.
   d. ion that has an electrical charge.
   e. specialized cell that deals with blood levels.

3. Which of the following is formed in the liver?
   a. Urea
   b. TSH
   c. Creatinine
   d. Lipase
   e. Amylase

4. A patient's blood work shows her amylase level is high. What other substance would indicate pancreatitis?
   a. Hemoglobin
   b. Triglycerides
   c. Potassium
   d. Lipase
   e. Lipoproteins

5. The function of LDLs is to:
   a. transport enzymes to the heart and lungs.
   b. assist in the production of lipoproteins.
   c. store energy in adipose tissue.
   d. move cholesterol from the liver to the arteries.
   e. carry cholesterol from the cells to the liver.

6. Chloride, bicarbonate, and electrolytes are all a part of:
   a. maintaining thyroid function.
   b. bile formation.
   c. red blood cell maturation.
   d. glucose storage.
   e. acid-base balance.

7. Women are screened for gestational diabetes:
   a. before they conceive.
   b. during the first month of pregnancy.
   c. during the second trimester.
   d. during the third trimester.
   e. after the baby is born.

8. When blood sugar levels go below 45 mg/dL, a person may experience:
   a. trembling.
   b. vomiting.
   c. diarrhea.
   d. chills.
   e. a high temperature.

9. If you are testing for a substance only found in serum, what should you do with a blood specimen?
   a. Use reagent strips to check for serum presence.
   b. Create a slide and analyze it under a microscope.
   c. Put the clotted specimen in the centrifuge to separate.
   d. Allow the specimen a few days to sit and separate.
   e. Run tests without doing anything to the specimen.

10. What is the body's normal blood pH range?
    a. 7.35 to 7.45
    b. 6.9 to 7.35
    c. 7.0 to 7.5
    d. 6.0 to 6.5
    e. 7.45 to 8.25

11. Hemoglobin A1C is tested to measure the patient's:
    a. fasting glucose.
    b. level of anemia.
    c. glucose that is attached to hemoglobin molecules.
    d. hemoglobin attached to glucose molecules.
    e. glucose tolerance.

12. Why is fasting required to accurately measure lipid levels?
    a. To evaluate how the body handles fat intake
    b. To establish fasting glucose levels
    c. To measure how much water is in body fat
    d. To limit the action of digestion on increasing lipid levels
    e. To lower HDL levels

COG MATCHING

Grade: _____

Match each key term with the correct definition.

Key Terms
13. _____ acidosis
14. _____ alkalosis
15. _____ amylase
16. _____ azotemia
17. _____ bicarbonate
18. _____ buffer systems
19. _____ creatinine
20. _____ electrolyte
21. _____ enzyme
22. _____ ions
23. _____ lipase
24. _____ lipoproteins
25. _____ urea

Definitions
a. electrically charged atoms
b. any substance-containing ions
c. an electrolyte with a negative charge formed when carbon dioxide dissolves in the blood
d. keeps the pH changes balanced
e. blood pH is below 7.4 caused by too much acid or too little base
f. blood pH is above 7.4 caused by too much base or too little acid
g. waste product from the body's metabolism of protein
h. abnormally high levels of nitrogen-containing compounds
i. a protein produced by living cells that speeds up chemical reactions
j. helps in the digestion of fats
k. breaks down starch into sugar
l. substances composed of lipids and proteins
m. a waste product from making the energy muscles used to function

COG IDENTIFICATION

Grade: _____

Identify the electrolyte by the stated relationship to acid–base balance.

Relationship	Electrolyte
26. It causes the most problems when its level is not stable	
27. When the level is extremely low, it becomes difficult for the patient to breathe	
28. Can be made unstable if the patient is suffering diabetic ketoacidosis and metabolic acidosis	
29. Most important electrolyte used in acid–base balance	
30. Low levels are seen in patients experiencing a long-term severe illness	
31. Low levels result from inadequate absorption from the diet, GI losses, electrolyte shifts, and endocrine disorders	
32. A waste product of oxygen metabolism	

COG IDENTIFY

Grade: _____

The following table lists nonprotein nitrogenous compound descriptions and associated abnormal conditions. Identify the nonprotein nitrogenous compound that is described.

Compound	Description	Abnormal Condition
33.	Waste product from the body's metabolism of protein	Dehydration, renal disease, inadequate dialysis, azotemia
34.	Waste product from making the energy muscles use to function	Kidney damage, kidney disease
35.	Waste product from breaking down protein	Gout, kidney stones

COG FILL IN THE BLANK

Grade: _____

36. _____ is elevated in MI.

37. _____ Most of the CK is located in _____ muscle.

38. _____ CK has three parts: _____, _____, and _____.

39. The _____ _____ is present in both cardiac and skeletal muscle.

40. The _____ _____ is much more specific for cardiac muscle.

41. The CKMB fraction increases within _____ following MI.

42. Troponins will begin to rise following MI within _____.

43. _____ levels are the best indicator of MI.

44. Rise in myoglobin can help to determine the _____ of an infarction.

45. Because inflammation is part of MI, _____ _____ is tested to predict the diagnosis of MI.

COG SHORT ANSWER

Grade: _____

46. What is pancreatitis, and what two enzymes are elevated in this condition?

_____

_____

_____

_____

47. The pancreas makes two endocrine hormones that are important in diabetes. What are they and what do they do?

_____

_____

_____

_____

48. What are the two hormones that regulate the process of storing glucose as glycogen?

a. _____

b. _____

49. What glucose test is used for screening?

_____

_____

_____

_____

50. What glucose test is used to monitor insulin therapy?

_____

_____

_____

_____

51. How does hemoglobin A1C give the physician a picture of the patient's glucose levels over the past 3 months?

_____

_____

_____

_____

52. What are the four fats measured in a lipid panel?

_____

_____

_____

_____

AFF **CASE STUDIES FOR CRITICAL THINKING**

Grade: _____

53. Your patient is a 5-year-old girl. The physician has ordered a fingerstick glucose. The mother of the child accompanied her to the office and gave the child a piece of candy because she thought her sugar might be low. You collect the specimen and run the test. The glucose is 60 mg/dL. You realize that you forgot to help the child wash her hands before the test. How could the result be affected if traces of the candy were on the child's finger? What do you do? What will make it difficult to do the right thing? How do you manage the parent and the child?

_____

_____

_____

_____

54. Your patient, Sarah Ingle, had an electrolyte panel ordered by Dr. Willis. The results are back from the reference lab, and your job includes screening test results. What are the reference intervals (normal ranges) you expect to see for these tests: sodium, potassium, chloride, and CO_2? You find that the potassium level is 6.0 mmol/L. What action do you take, and how do you document your action?

_____

_____

_____

_____

55. Estimate Melissa Woermann had a glucose tolerance test, and her fasting glucose was 90 mg/dL. At 1 hour after drinking the glucose solution it was 170 mg/dL, at 2 hours 140 mg/dL, and at 3 hours 125 mg/dL. What are the criteria proposed by the National Diabetes Data Group and the World Health Organization and endorsed by the ADA for a diagnosis of diabetes? Does it appear that Ms. Woermann could be diagnosed with diabetes?

_____

_____

_____

_____

PSY PROCEDURE 43-1   **Perform Blood Glucose Testing**

Name: _____   Date: _____   Time: _____   Grade: _____

EQUIPMENT/SUPPLIES: Glucose meter, glucose reagent strips, control solutions, capillary puncture device, personal protective equipment, gauze, paper towel, adhesive bandage, lancet, alcohol pad, hand sanitizer, surface sanitizer, contaminated waste container

NOTE: These are generic instructions for using a glucose meter. Refer to the manufacturer's instructions shipped with the meter for instructions specific to the instrument in use

STANDARDS: Given the needed equipment and a place to work, the student will perform this skill with _____ % accuracy in a total of _____ minutes. *(Your instructor will tell you what the percentage and time limits will be before you begin practicing.)*

KEY: 4 = Satisfactory   0 = Unsatisfactory   NA = This step is not counted

PROCEDURE STEPS	SELF	PARTNER	INSTRUCTOR
1. Check the physician order and wash your hands	❏	❏	❏
2. Assemble the equipment and supplies	❏	❏	❏
3. Review the instrument manual for your glucose meter	❏	❏	❏
4. Turn on the instrument and verify that it is calibrated	❏	❏	❏
5. Perform the test on the quality control (QC) material. Record results. Determine whether QC is within control limits. If yes, proceed with patient testing. If no, take corrective action and recheck controls. Document corrective action. Proceed with patient testing when acceptable QC results are obtained	❏	❏	❏
6. Remove one reagent strip, lay it on the paper towel, and recap the container	❏	❏	❏
7. **AFF** Greet and identify the patient. Identify yourself, including your title. Explain the procedure. Ask for and answer any questions	❏	❏	❏
8. Have the patient wash hands in warm water. Put on gloves	❏	❏	❏
9. Cleanse the selected puncture site (finger) with alcohol	❏	❏	❏
10. Perform a capillary puncture and wipe away the first drop of blood	❏	❏	❏
11. Turn the patient's hand, palm down, and gently squeeze the finger to form a large drop of blood	❏	❏	❏
12. Bring the reagent strip up to the finger and touch the pad to the blood **a.** Do not touch the finger **b.** Completely cover the pad or fill the testing chamber with blood	❏	❏	❏
13. Insert the reagent strip into the analyzer **a.** Meanwhile, apply pressure to the puncture wound with gauze **b.** The meter will continue to incubate the strip and measure the reaction	❏	❏	❏

(continues)

PSY PROCEDURE 43-1	Perform Blood Glucose Testing (continued)		
14. The instrument reads the reaction strip and displays the result on the screen in mg/dL	❏	❏	❏
15. Apply a small adhesive bandage to the patient's fingertip	❏	❏	❏
16. Properly care for or dispose of equipment and supplies	❏	❏	❏
17. Clean the work area. Remove personal protective equipment and wash your hands	❏	❏	❏
18. Log into the Electronic Medical Record (EMR) using your username and secure password OR obtain the paper medical record from a secure location and assure it is kept away from public access. Record the procedure noting the date, time, test results for CLIA-waived POC procedure, and your name	❏	❏	❏
19. When finished, log out of the EMR and/or replace the paper medical record in an appropriate and secure location	❏	❏	❏

_____
_____
_____
_____

CALCULATION

Total Possible Points: _____

Total Points Earned: _____ Multiplied by 100 = _____ Divided by Total Possible Points = _____ %

PASS   FAIL   COMMENTS:
  ❏   ❏

Student's signature _____ Date _____

Partner's signature _____ Date _____

Instructor's signature _____ Date _____

PSY PROCEDURE 43-2 **Perform Blood Cholesterol Testing**

Name: _____ Date: _____ Time: _____ Grade: _____

EQUIPMENT/SUPPLIES: Cholesterol meter and supplies or test kit, control solutions, capillary puncture equipment or blood specimen as indicated by manufacturer, personal protective equipment, hand sanitizer, surface sanitizer, contaminated waste container

NOTE: These are generic instructions for using a cholesterol meter or test kit. Refer to the manufacturer's instructions shipped with the testing tool for instructions specific for the instrument in use.

STANDARDS: Given the needed equipment and a place to work, the student will perform this skill with _____ % accuracy in a total of _____ minutes. *(Your instructor will tell you what the percentage and time limits will be before you begin practicing.)*

KEY: 4 = Satisfactory 0 = Unsatisfactory NA = This step is not counted

PROCEDURE STEPS	SELF	PARTNER	INSTRUCTOR
1. Check the physician order and wash your hands	❏	❏	❏
2. Assemble the equipment and supplies	❏	❏	❏
3. Review the instrument manual for your cholesterol meter or kit. Put on gloves	❏	❏	❏
4. Perform the test on the quality control material. Record results. Determine whether QC is within control limits If yes, proceed with patient testing. If no, take corrective action and recheck controls. Document corrective action. Proceed with patient testing when acceptable QC results are obtained	❏	❏	❏
5. Follow manufacturer's instructions in using a patient specimen obtained by capillary puncture or from tube evacuation	❏	❏	❏
6. Follow manufacturer's instructions for applying the sample to the testing device and inserting the device into the analyzer. Record results	❏	❏	❏
7. Properly care for or dispose of equipment and supplies	❏	❏	❏
8. Clean the work area. Remove personal protective equipment and wash your hands	❏	❏	❏
9. AFF Log into the Electronic Medical Record (EMR) using your username and secure password OR obtain the paper medical record from a secure location and assure it is kept away from public access. Record the procedure, noting the date, time, test results for CLIA-waived POC procedure, and your name	❏	❏	❏
10. When finished, log out of the EMR and/or replace the paper medical record in an appropriate and secure location	❏	❏	❏

(continues)

PSY PROCEDURE 43-2 **Perform Blood Cholesterol Testing** (continued)

_____

_____

_____

_____

CALCULATION

Total Possible Points: _____

Total Points Earned: _____ Multiplied by 100 = _____ Divided by Total Possible Points = _____ %

PASS   FAIL   COMMENTS:
❏   ❏

Student's signature _____ Date _____

Partner's signature _____ Date _____

Instructor's signature _____ Date _____

© YASHARADA/Shutterstock

CHAPTER 44

Microbiology and Immunology

LEARNING OUTCOMES

COG Cognitive Domain*

1. Spell the key terms
2. *Identify the following related to body systems:*
   a. *medical terms*
   b. *abbreviations*
3. *Identify CLIA-waived tests associated with common diseases*
4. *Identify normal and abnormal results as reported in*
   a. *graphs*
   b. *tables*
5. List major types of infectious agents
6. *Identify quality assurance practices in healthcare*

PSY Psychomotor Domain*

1. Collect throat specimens (Procedure 44-1)
   a. *Collect specimens and perform CLIA-waived microbiology test*
   b. *Instruct and prepare a patient for a procedure or treatment*
   c. *Perform quality control measures*
   d. *Document patient care accurately in the medical record*
2. Collect nasopharyngeal specimens (Procedure 44-2)
   a. *Collect specimens and perform CLIA-waived microbiology and immunology test*
   b. *Instruct and prepare a patient for a procedure or treatment*
   c. *Perform quality control measures*
   d. *Document patient care accurately in the medical record*

3. Collect wound specimens (Procedure 44-3)
   a. *Collect specimens and perform CLIA-waived microbiology test*
   b. *Instruct and prepare a patient for a procedure or treatment*
   c. *Perform quality control measures*
   d. *Document patient care accurately in the medical record*
4. Collect stool specimen for ova and parasites (Procedure 44-4)
   a. *Collect specimens and perform CLIA-waived microbiology test*
   b. *Instruct and prepare a patient for a procedure or treatment*
   c. *Perform quality control measures*
   d. *Document patient care accurately in the medical record*
5. Inoculate a culture (Procedure 44-5)
   a. *Collect specimens and perform CLIA-waived microbiology test*
   b. *Instruct and prepare a patient for a procedure or treatment*
   c. *Perform quality control measures*
   d. *Document patient care accurately in the medical record*
6. Perform mononucleosis testing (Procedure 44-6)
   a. *Collect specimens and perform CLIA-waived microbiology test*
   b. *Instruct and prepare a patient for a procedure or treatment*
   c. *Perform quality control measures*
   d. *Document patient care accurately in the medical record*

7. Perform HCG pregnancy testing (Procedure 44-7)
   a. *Collect specimens and perform CLIA-waived microbiology test*
   b. *Instruct and prepare a patient for a procedure or treatment*
   c. *Perform quality control measures*
   d. *Document patient care accurately in the medical record*
8. Perform rapid group A strep testing (Procedure 44-8)
   a. *Collect specimens and perform CLIA-waived microbiology test*
   b. *Instruct and prepare a patient for a procedure or treatment*
   c. *Perform quality control measures*
   d. *Document patient care accurately in the medical record*

AFF Affective Domain*

1. *Demonstrate critical thinking skills*
2. *Reassure patients*
3. *Demonstrate empathy for patients' concerns*
4. *Demonstrate active listening*
5. *Respect diversity*
6. *Recognize personal boundaries*
7. *Demonstrate tactfulness*
8. *Demonstrate self-awareness*
9. Protect the integrity of the medical record.

* MAERB Standards are Italicized.

ABHES Competencies

1. Practice quality control
2. Dispose of biohazardous materials

3. Collect, label, and process specimens: 1). Perform venipuncture 2). Perform capillary puncture
4. Instruct patients in the collection of sputum or fecal specimens
5. Perform selected CLIA-waived tests that assist with diagnosis

and treatment: Microbiology and Immunology testing
6. Follow documentation guidelines
7. Adapt care to address the developmental stages of life
8. Display effective interpersonal skills with patients and healthcare team members

9. Demonstrate cultural awareness
10. Make adaptations for patients with special needs (psychological or physical limitations)
11. Make adaptations to care for patients across their lifespan

Name: _____   Date: _____   Grade: _____

⬤⬤G MULTIPLE CHOICE

Circle the letter preceding the correct answer.

1. A pregnancy test detects the presence of:
   a. RhoGAM.
   b. protein.
   c. genetic defects.
   d. HCG.
   e. immune-D serum.

2. Where will the medical assistant find instructions for the correct method for collecting and transporting microbiology specimens?
   a. The test requisition
   b. The patient's chart
   c. A textbook
   d. The laboratory's procedure manual
   e. The physician

3. The result of a laboratory test is only as good as:
   a. the physician.
   b. the medical assistant.
   c. the laboratory equipment.
   d. the specimen.
   e. the patient.

4. Sensitivity tests monitor the microorganism's sensitivity to:
   a. RhoGAM.
   b. antibiotics.
   c. light.
   d. color.
   e. other microorganisms.

5. Bacilli can be recognized by their:
   a. globular shape.
   b. long, spiral shape.
   c. rigid, spiral shape.
   d. comma-like shape.
   e. rod-like shape.

6. Why is it important to transport or process microbiology specimens as soon as possible?
   a. So the organism does not die
   b. To get the results to the physician as soon as possible
   c. To start the patient on antibiotics
   d. So normal flora bacteria do not overgrow the specimen
   e. So the infection will not be contagious

7. Antigens are:
   a. proteins the body creates as a defensive measure against foreign substances.
   b. foreign substances that cause the body to initiate a defense response.
   c. reagents used to detect the presence of antibodies in a culture dish.
   d. media used to create an environment suitable for organism growth.
   e. dyes used to stain cells that are prepared for microscope slides.

8. How long is a culture incubated to verify that there is no bacterial growth from the specimen?
   a. 8 hours
   b. 12 hours
   c. 24 hours
   d. 48 hours
   e. 72 hours

9. Which of these conditions is caused by a virus?
   a. Impetigo
   b. Tuberculosis
   c. Strep throat
   d. Ringworm
   e. Rabies

10. What organism results in Lyme disease?
    a. *Clostridium botulinum*
    b. *Clostridium tetani*
    c. *Chlamydia trachomatis*
    d. *Borrelia burgdorferi*
    e. Bacteroides species

OOG **MATCHING**

Grade: _____

Match each key term with the correct definition.

Key Terms

11. _____ aerobes
12. _____ agar
13. _____ anaerobes
14. _____ bacilli (singular, bacillus)
15. _____ broth
16. _____ cocci
17. _____ culture
18. _____ differential stain
19. _____ diplococci
20. _____ Gram negative
21. _____ Gram positive
22. _____ Gram stain
23. _____ immunity
24. _____ isolate
25. _____ media
26. _____ mordant
27. _____ mycology
28. _____ normal flora
29. _____ nosocomial infection
30. _____ resistant
31. _____ sensitive
32. _____ sensitivity testing
33. _____ smear
34. _____ specificity
35. _____ spirochetes

Definitions

a. bacteria that require oxygen to survive
b. bacteria that require a lack of oxygen to survive
c. an environment that provides the bacteria with a place to grow
d. liquid media in glass tubes or bottles
e. the most widely used solid media
f. stain used to identify differences in cells
g. bacteria that will lose the purple color in a Gram stain and stain red with safranin
h. bacteria that are spherical in shape
i. spherical cocci in pairs
j. bacteria that are rod shaped and are usually aerobic
k. bacteria that normally live on the body and do not cause disease
l. infections acquired in a medical setting
m. a mixture of substances that nourish pathogens to support the growth of microorganisms for identification
n. materials that have been dried on a glass slide
o. primary stain used in the microbiology lab
p. bacteria that keep the purple color even when exposed to the ethyl alcohol step of the Gram stain
q. Gram's iodine is one, used to fix the dye on the smear to make it more intense
r. long, spiral, flexible organisms
s. testing to determine if an antibiotic will be effective in stopping growth of an organism (also identifies antibiotics that will not stop the growth of an organism)
t. organisms that are inhibited by an antimicrobial agent
u. organisms that grow even in the presence of an antimicrobial agent
v. separate from any other microorganisms present
w. the study of fungi
x. the response to foreign bodies
y. an antibody combines with only one antigen

OOG **MATCHING**

Grade: _____

Match each category of organisms to its description.

Key Terms

36. _____ rickettsia
37. _____ chlamydia
38. _____ mycoplasma
39. _____ viruses
40. _____ eukaryotic microorganisms
41. _____ fungi
42. _____ protozoa and helminths
43. _____ nematodes
44. _____ arthropods
45. _____ prokaryotic cells

Definitions

a. cause blindness, pneumonia, and lymphogranuloma venereum
b. cause atypical pneumonia and genitourinary infections
c. cells with no nuclei including bacteria
d. lice, fleas, and ticks
e. not susceptible to antibiotics and are extremely difficult to treat
f. pathogens include the groups fungi, algae, protozoans, and parasites
g. small organisms like bacteria with the potential to produce disease in susceptible hosts
h. parasites
i. round worm parasites
j. organisms carried on arthropods

OOG **FILL IN THE BLANK**

46. If the specimen is not fully and correctly labeled, the laboratory may be required to _____ of the specimen.

47. Use the appropriate _____ media, if indicated.

48. Transport specimens at the _____ temperature.

49. Correct steps are important for keeping the pathogen _____ until it reaches the laboratory.

50. Handle all specimens as if _____. Follow standard precautions.

OOG AFF **IDENTIFICATION**

51. List six autoimmune diseases.

_____

_____

_____

_____

52. How is an antigen–antibody reaction identified?

_____

_____

_____

_____

53. Using immunoassay test kits, how is a positive antigen indicated?

_____

_____

_____

_____

54. How does the medical assistant assure the accuracy of testing with an immunoassay test kit?

_____

_____

_____

_____

55. How are normal and abnormal test results identified using immunoassay test kits?

_____

_____

_____

_____

COG **AFF** **CASE STUDIES FOR CRITICAL THINKING** _____ Grade: _____

56. Your patient is concerned that others may learn of the results of her laboratory test. How do you reassure her that this will not happen?

_____

_____

_____

_____

57. Your patient is a little girl being evaluated for sexual abuse by her father. How do you display sensitivity to the mother regarding her distress about collecting the specimens? How do you explain the rationale for performing the procedure? How do you demonstrate your awareness of the patient's concerns regarding perceptions related to the procedure being performed? How do you demonstrate empathy in communicating with the patient and her mother? How will you use active listening skills in this scenario? How will you demonstrate awareness of the territorial boundaries of the child and her mother? How will you demonstrate your sensitivity to the situation?

_____

_____

_____

_____

58. Your patient is a 7-year-old boy. The doctor has ordered a throat culture, and the boy is obviously apprehensive. How do you use body language and other nonverbal skills to reassure the boy and also collect a good specimen?

_____

_____

_____

_____

PSY PROCEDURE 44-1 Collect a Throat Specimen

Name: _____ Date: _____ Time: _____ Grade: _____

EQUIPMENT/SUPPLIES: Tongue blade, light source, sterile specimen container and swab, personal protective equipment, hand sanitizer, surface sanitizer and biohazard transport bag (if it is to be sent to the laboratory for analysis)

STANDARDS: Given the needed equipment and a place to work, the student will perform this skill with _____ % accuracy in a total of _____ minutes. *(Your instructor will tell you what the percentage and time limits will be before you begin practicing.)*

KEY: 4 = Satisfactory   0 = Unsatisfactory   NA = This step is not counted

PROCEDURE STEPS	SELF	PARTNER	INSTRUCTOR
1. Check the physician order. Wash your hands	❏	❏	❏
2. Assemble the equipment and supplies	❏	❏	❏
3. Apply gloves	❏	❏	❏
4. **AFF** Greet and identify the patient. Identify yourself, including your title. Explain the rationale for the performance of the collection to the patient	❏	❏	❏
5. **AFF** If the patient is hearing-impaired, you need to speak clearly and distinctly in front of the patient's face	❏	❏	❏
6. **AFF** Use active listening to observe patients' body language and detect a lack of understanding of instructions. Obtain assistance when you realize that you are not able to communicate with the patient	❏	❏	❏
7. **AFF** Allow time for the adult patient or caregiver (if the patient is a child) to ask questions	❏	❏	❏
8. **AFF** Display empathy for the patient and family	❏	❏	❏
9. Have the patient sit with a light source directed at the throat	❏	❏	❏
10. Carefully remove the sterile swab from the container. If performing both the rapid strep and culture or confirming negative results with a culture, swab with two swabs held together	❏	❏	❏
11. Have the patient say "Ah" as you press down on the midpoint of the tongue with the tongue depressor. If the tongue depressor is placed too far forward, it will not be effective; if it is placed too far back, the patient will gag unnecessarily	❏	❏	❏
12. Swab the mucous membranes, especially the tonsillar area, the crypts, and the posterior pharynx in a "figure 8" motion. Turn the swab to expose all of its surfaces to the membranes. Avoid touching teeth, sides of mouth, and uvula	❏	❏	❏
13. Maintain the tongue depressor position while withdrawing the swab from the patient's mouth	❏	❏	❏

(continues)

PSY PROCEDURE 44-1   **Collect a Throat Specimen** (continued)

14. Follow the instructions on the specimen container for transferring the swab or processing the specimen in the office using a commercial kit. Label the specimen with the patient's name, the date and time of collection, and the origin of the material	❏	❏	❏
15. Properly dispose of the equipment and supplies in a biohazard waste container. Remove PPE and wash your hands	❏	❏	❏
16. Route the specimen or store it appropriately until routing can be completed	❏	❏	❏
17. AFF Log into the Electronic Medical Record (EMR) using your username and secure password OR obtain the paper medical record from a secure location and assure it is kept away from public access. Record the procedure noting the date, time, specimen collected, and specimen processing procedure (i.e., sent to the lab, tested using CLIA-waived test, etc.). Include your name and title according to office policy and procedure	❏	❏	❏

_____

_____

_____

_____

CALCULATION

Total Possible Points: _____

Total Points Earned: _____ Multiplied by 100 = _____ Divided by Total Possible Points = _____ %

PASS   FAIL   COMMENTS:
❏   ❏

Student's signature _____ Date _____

Partner's signature _____ Date _____

Instructor's signature _____ Date _____

PSY PROCEDURE 44-2 Collect a Nasopharyngeal Specimen

Name: _____ **Date:** _____ **Time:** _____ **Grade:** _____

EQUIPMENT/SUPPLIES: Penlight, tongue blade, sterile flexible wire swab, transport media, personal protective equipment, hand sanitizer, surface sanitizer and biohazard transport bag (if it is to be sent to the laboratory for analysis)

STANDARDS: Given the needed equipment and a place to work, the student will perform this skill with _____ % accuracy in a total of _____ minutes. *(Your instructor will tell you what the percentage and time limits will be before you begin practicing.)*

KEY: 4 = Satisfactory 0 = Unsatisfactory NA = This step is not counted

PROCEDURE STEPS	SELF	PARTNER	INSTRUCTOR
1. Check the physician order. Wash your hands	❑	❑	❑
2. Assemble the equipment and supplies	❑	❑	❑
3. Put on gloves	❑	❑	❑
4. **AFF** Greet and identify the patient. Identify yourself, including your title. Explain the rationale of the performance of the collection to the patient	❑	❑	❑
5. **AFF** If your patient is developmentally challenged, have the individual who transported the patient to the office assist you with communicating with the patient. The developmentally challenged patient may struggle if you have to proceed with something they do not understand. Have another medical assistant available to help you if extra support is necessary to support the patient	❑	❑	❑
6. **AFF** Leave time for the adult patient or caregiver of a child to ask questions	❑	❑	❑
7. Position the patient with his head tilted back	❑	❑	❑
8. Using a penlight, inspect the nasopharyngeal area	❑	❑	❑
9. Gently pass the swab through the nostril and into the nasopharynx, keeping the swab near the septum and floor of the nose. Rotate the swab quickly and then remove it and place it in the transport media	❑	❑	❑
10. Label the specimen with the patient's name, the date and time of collection, and the origin of the specimen	❑	❑	❑
11. Properly dispose of the equipment and supplies in a biohazard waste container. Remove gloves and wash your hands	❑	❑	❑

(continues)

PSY PROCEDURE 44-2 **Collect a Nasopharyngeal Specimen** (continued)

12. Route the specimen or store it appropriately until routing can be completed	❏	❏	❏
13. **AFF** Log into the Electronic Medical Record (EMR) using your username and secure password OR obtain the paper medical record from a secure location and assure that it is kept away from public access. Record the procedure noting the date, time, specimen collected, and specimen processing procedure (i.e., sent to the lab, tested using CLIA-waived test, etc.). Include your name and title according to office policy and procedure	❏	❏	❏

_____

_____

_____

_____

_____

CALCULATION

Total Possible Points: _____

Total Points Earned: _____ Multiplied by 100 = _____ Divided by Total Possible Points = _____ %

PASS   FAIL   COMMENTS:
❏   ❏

Student's signature _____ Date _____

Partner's signature _____ Date _____

Instructor's signature _____ Date _____

PSY PROCEDURE 44-3 — Collect a Wound Specimen

Name: _____ Date: _____ Time: _____ Grade: _____

EQUIPMENT/SUPPLIES: Sterile swab, transport media, personal protective equipment, hand sanitizer, surface sanitizer, and biohazard transport bag (if it is to be sent to the laboratory for analysis)

STANDARDS: Given the needed equipment and a place to work, the student will perform this skill with _____ % accuracy in a total of _____ minutes. *(Your instructor will tell you what the percentage and time limits will be before you begin practicing.)*

KEY: 4 = Satisfactory 0 = Unsatisfactory NA = This step is not counted

PROCEDURE STEPS	SELF	PARTNER	INSTRUCTOR
1. Check the physician order. Wash your hands	❏	❏	❏
2. Assemble the equipment and supplies	❏	❏	❏
3. Put on gloves	❏	❏	❏
4. **AFF** Greet and identify the patient. Identify yourself, including your title. Explain the procedure	❏	❏	❏
5. **AFF** If your patient is struggling with dementia, be prepared to gently repeat yourself as necessary until you have collected your specimen. You may have to physically adjust your patient as necessary to collect the specimen. Be gentle but remember to speak to the patient as an adult	❏	❏	❏
6. If dressing is present, remove it and dispose of it in a biohazard container. Assess the wound by observing color, odor, and amount of exudate. Remove contaminated gloves and put on clean gloves	❏	❏	❏
7. Use the sterile swab to sample the exudate. Saturate swab with exudate, avoiding the skin edge around the wound	❏	❏	❏
8. Place swab back in container and crush the ampule of transport medium	❏	❏	❏
9. Label the specimen with the patient's name, the date and time of collection, and the origin of the specimen	❏	❏	❏
10. Route the specimen or store it appropriately until routing can be completed	❏	❏	❏
11. Clean the wound and apply a sterile dressing using sterile technique	❏	❏	❏

(continues)

PSY PROCEDURE 44-3 **Collect a Wound Specimen** (continued)

12. Properly dispose of the equipment and supplies in a biohazard waste container. Remove gloves and wash your hands	❏	❏	❏
13. **AFF** Log into the Electronic Medical Record (EMR) using your username and secure password OR obtain the paper medical record from a secure location and assure it is kept away from public access. Record the procedure noting the date, time, specimen collected, and specimen processing procedure (i.e., sent to lab, tested using CLIA-waived test, etc.). Include your name and title according to office policy and procedure	❏	❏	❏

_____

_____

_____

_____

CALCULATION

Total Possible Points: _____

Total Points Earned: _____ Multiplied by 100 = _____ Divided by Total Possible Points = _____ %

PASS **FAIL** **COMMENTS:**
❏ ❏

Student's signature _____ Date _____

Partner's signature _____ Date _____

Instructor's signature _____ Date _____

PSY PROCEDURE 44-4 **Collect a Stool Specimen for Ova and Parasites**

Name: _____ Date: _____ Time: _____ Grade: _____

EQUIPMENT/SUPPLIES: Specimen container dependent on test ordered (sterile container or Para-Pak collection system for C&S or ova and parasites, tongue blade or wooden spatula, personal protective equipment, hand sanitizer, surface sanitizer, and biohazard transport bag

STANDARDS: Given the needed equipment and a place to work, the student will perform this skill with _____ % accuracy in a total of _____ minutes. *(Your instructor will tell you what the percentage and time limits will be before you begin practicing.)*

KEY: 4 = Satisfactory 0 = Unsatisfactory NA = This step is not counted

PROCEDURE STEPS	SELF	PARTNER	INSTRUCTOR
1. Check the physician order. Wash your hands	❏	❏	❏
2. Assemble the equipment and supplies	❏	❏	❏
3. **AFF** Greet and identify the patient. Identify yourself, including your title. Explain the procedure	❏	❏	❏
4. **AFF** If you are in a significantly different generation than the patient, you will need to take extra precautions with communication. First, remember that collecting a stool specimen is embarrassing for most patients. Watch the patient's facial expressions to note if they are understanding your instructions. This is one of the times you may find that your patient does not understand professional terminology	❏	❏	❏
5. When obtaining a stool specimen for C&S or ova and parasites, the patient should collect an amount of the first and last portion of the stool after the bowel movement with the wooden spatula or tongue blade and place it in the specimen container without contaminating the outside of the container. Fill Para-Pak until fluid reaches "fill" line and recap the container	❏	❏	❏
6. Upon receipt of the specimen, you should put on gloves and place the specimen in the biohazard bag for transport to the reference laboratory. Fill out a laboratory requisition slip to accompany the specimen	❏	❏	❏
7. Label the specimen with the patient's name, the date and time of collection, and the origin of the specimen	❏	❏	❏
8. Transport the specimen to the laboratory or store the specimen as directed. Refer to the laboratory procedure manual since some samples require refrigeration, others are kept at room temperature, and some must be placed in an incubator at a laboratory as soon as possible after collecting	❏	❏	❏

(continues)

PSY PROCEDURE 44-4	Collect a Stool Specimen for Ova and Parasites (continued)		
9. Properly dispose of the equipment and supplies in a biohazard waste container. Remove gloves and wash your hands	❏	❏	❏
10. **AFF** Log into the Electronic Medical Record (EMR) using your username and secure password OR obtain the paper medical record from a secure location and assure it is kept away from public access. Record the procedure, noting the date, time, specimen collected, and specimen processing procedure (i.e., sent to lab, tested using CLIA-waived test, etc.). Include your name and title according to office policy and procedure	❏	❏	❏

_____

_____

_____

_____

CALCULATION

Total Possible Points: _____

Total Points Earned: _____ Multiplied by 100 = _____ Divided by Total Possible Points = _____ %

PASS   FAIL   COMMENTS:
❏   ❏

Student's signature _____ Date _____

Partner's signature _____ Date _____

Instructor's signature _____ Date _____

PSY PROCEDURE 44-5 | **Inoculating a Culture**

Name: _____ Date: _____ Time: _____ Grade: _____

EQUIPMENT/SUPPLIES: Specimen on a swab, permanent laboratory marker, Petri dish, gloves, hand sanitizer, surface sanitizer, biohazard waste container

STANDARDS: Given the needed equipment and a place to work, the student will perform this skill with _____ % accuracy in a total of _____ minutes. *(Your instructor will tell you what the percentage and time limits will be before you begin practicing.)*

KEY: 4 = Satisfactory 0 = Unsatisfactory NA = This step is not counted

PROCEDURE STEPS	SELF	PARTNER	INSTRUCTOR
1. Check the physician order. Wash your hands	❑	❑	❑
2. Assemble the equipment and supplies, checking expiration dates	❑	❑	❑
3. Put on gloves	❑	❑	❑
4. Label the medium side of the plate with the permanent marker. Include the patient's name, identification number, source of specimen, time collected, time inoculated, your initials, and date	❑	❑	❑
5. Remove the Petri dish from the cover (the Petri dish is always stored with the cover down), and place the cover on the work surface with the opening up. Do not open the cover unnecessarily	❑	❑	❑
6. Using a rolling and sliding motion, streak the specimen swab across one fourth of the plate, starting at the top and working to the center. Dispose of the swab in a biohazard container. The specimen will spread in gradually thinning colonies of bacteria	❑	❑	❑
7. Use a disposable sterile loop and turn the plate a quarter turn from its previous position. Pass the loop a few times in the original inoculum and then across the medium approximately a quarter of the surface of the dish. Do not enter the originally streaked area after the first few sweeps	❑	❑	❑
8. Turn the dish another quarter turn so that now it is 180 degrees to the original smear. Working in the previous manner, draw the loop at right angles through the most recently streaked area. Again, do not enter the originally streaked area after the first few sweeps	❑	❑	❑
9. Place the prepared culture with the lid on in an incubator per office policy and procedure. Properly dispose of the contaminated supplies in a biohazard waste container. Remove gloves and wash your hands	❑	❑	❑
10. **AFF** Log into the Electronic Medical Record (EMR) using your username and secure password OR obtain the paper medical record from a secure location and assure it is kept away from public access. Record the procedure noting the date, time, specimen collected, and specimen processing procedure (i.e., sent to lab, tested using CLIA-waived test, etc.). Include your name and title according to office policy and procedure	❑	❑	❑

(continues)

| PSY | PROCEDURE 44-5 | **Inoculating a Culture** (continued) |

_____

_____

_____

_____

CALCULATION

Total Possible Points: _____

Total Points Earned: _____ Multiplied by 100 = _____ Divided by Total Possible Points = _____ %

PASS   FAIL   COMMENTS:
❏   ❏

Student's signature _____ Date _____

Partner's signature _____ Date _____

Instructor's signature _____ Date _____

PSY PROCEDURE 44-6 **Mononucleosis Testing**

Name: _____ Date: _____ Time: _____ Grade: _____

EQUIPMENT/SUPPLIES: Patient's labeled specimen (whole blood, plasma, or serum, depending on the kit), CLIA-waived mononucleosis kit (slide or test strip) with instructions, stopwatch or timer, gloves, hand sanitizer, surface sanitizer, biohazard waste container

STANDARDS: Given the needed equipment and a place to work, the student will perform this skill with _____ % accuracy in a total of _____ minutes. *(Your instructor will tell you what the percentage and time limits will be before you begin practicing.)*

KEY: 4 = Satisfactory   0 = Unsatisfactory   NA = This step is not counted

PROCEDURE STEPS	SELF	PARTNER	INSTRUCTOR
1. Check the physician order. Wash your hands	❏	❏	❏
2. Assemble the equipment and ensure that the materials in the kit and the patient specimen are at room temperature	❏	❏	❏
3. Label the test pack or test strip (depending on type of kit) with the patient's name, positive control, and negative control. Use one test pack or strip per patient and control	❏	❏	❏
4. Put on gloves. Collect the blood specimen according to the test kit instructions	❏	❏	❏
5. Perform the test as directed. Also, perform the controls according to the kit instructions	❏	❏	❏
6. Set timer for the period indicated in the package insert	❏	❏	❏
7. Read reaction results at the end of the time period	❏	❏	❏
8. Verify the results of the controls before documenting the patient's results. Log the QC and patient information on any worksheet required per the office policy and procedure manual	❏	❏	❏
9. Properly dispose of the equipment and supplies in a biohazard waste container	❏	❏	❏
10. Remove your gloves and wash your hands	❏	❏	❏
11. **AFF** Log into the Electronic Medical Record (EMR) using your username and secure password OR obtain the paper medical record from a secure location and assure it is kept away from public access. Record the procedure noting the date, time, specimen collected, and specimen processing procedure (i.e., sent to lab, tested using CLIA-waived test, etc.). Include your name and title according to office policy and procedure	❏	❏	❏

(continues)

PSY PROCEDURE 44-6   **Mononucleosis Testing** (continued)

_____

_____

_____

_____

CALCULATION

Total Possible Points: _____

Total Points Earned: _____ Multiplied by 100 = _____ Divided by Total Possible Points = _____ %

PASS   FAIL   COMMENTS:
❑   ❑

Student's signature _____   Date _____

Partner's signature _____   Date _____

Instructor's signature _____   Date _____

PSY PROCEDURE 44-7	**Perform HCG Pregnancy Test**

Name: _____ Date: _____ Time: _____ Grade: _____

EQUIPMENT/SUPPLIES: Patient's labeled urine specimen, CLIA-waived HCG pregnancy kit, timer, gloves, hand sanitizer, surface sanitizer, biohazard waste container

STANDARDS: Given the needed equipment and a place to work, the student will perform this skill with _____ % accuracy in a total of _____ minutes. *(Your instructor will tell you what the percentage and time limits will be before you begin practicing.)*

KEY: 4 = Satisfactory   0 = Unsatisfactory   NA = This step is not counted

PROCEDURE STEPS	SELF	PARTNER	INSTRUCTOR
1. Check the physician order. Wash your hands	❑	❑	❑
2. Assemble the equipment and supplies	❑	❑	❑
3. Verify that the urine specimen is for the correct patient. Verify the HCG test kit is not expired	❑	❑	❑
4. Perform the test as indicated on the test kit package insert directions	❑	❑	❑
5. Sample the positive and negative controls as directed for the test kit	❑	❑	❑
6. Set the timer for running the test as indicated in the package insert	❑	❑	❑
7. Read reaction results at the end of the prescribed period of time	❑	❑	❑
8. Verify the results of the controls before documenting the patient's results. Log controls and patient information on the worksheet according to the office policy and procedure	❑	❑	❑
9. Properly dispose of the equipment and supplies in a biohazard waste container	❑	❑	❑
10. Remove gloves and wash your hands	❑	❑	❑
11. **AFF** Log into the Electronic Medical Record (EMR) using your username and secure password OR obtain the paper medical record from a secure location and assure it is kept away from public access. Record the procedure noting the date, time, specimen collected, and specimen processing procedure (i.e., sent to lab, tested using CLIA-waived test, etc.). Include your name and title according to office policy and procedure	❑	❑	❑

_____
_____
_____
_____

(continues)

PSY PROCEDURE 44-7 | **Perform HCG Pregnancy Test** (continued)

CALCULATION

Total Possible Points: _____

Total Points Earned: _____ Multiplied by 100 = _____ Divided by Total Possible Points = _____ %

PASS   FAIL   COMMENTS:
❑   ❑

Student's signature _____   Date _____

Partner's signature _____   Date _____

Instructor's signature _____   Date _____

PSY PROCEDURE 44-8 **Rapid Group A Strep Testing**

Name: _____ Date: _____ Time: _____ Grade: _____

EQUIPMENT/SUPPLIES: CLIA-waived Group A strep kit (controls may be included, depending on the kit), timer, gloves, hand sanitizer, surface sanitizer, biohazard waste container

STANDARDS: Given the needed equipment and a place to work, the student will perform this skill with _____ % accuracy in a total of _____ minutes. *(Your instructor will tell you what the percentage and time limits will be before you begin practicing.)*

KEY: 4 = Satisfactory   0 = Unsatisfactory   NA = This step is not counted

PROCEDURE STEPS	SELF	PARTNER	INSTRUCTOR
1. Check the physician order. Wash your hands	❏	❏	❏
2. Assemble the equipment including the test kit. Familiarize yourself with the instructions before obtaining the specimen and performing the procedure	❏	❏	❏
3. Apply gloves. Obtain the throat specimen from the patient after assuring you have the correct patient. Use the swabs that come with the testing kit	❏	❏	❏
4. Follow the directions for the kit. Add the appropriate reagents and drops to each of the extraction-appropriate test tubes	❏	❏	❏
5. Insert the patient swab into the labeled extraction tube	❏	❏	❏
6. Add the appropriate controls to each of the labeled extraction tubes	❏	❏	❏
7. Set the timer for the appropriate time to ensure accuracy	❏	❏	❏
8. Add the appropriate reagent and drops to each of the extraction tubes	❏	❏	❏
9. Use the swab to mix the reagents. Then press out any excess fluid on the swab against the inside of the tube	❏	❏	❏
10. Add the appropriate number of drops from the well-mixed extraction tube to the sample window of the strep A test unit. Do the same for each control	❏	❏	❏
11. Set the timer for the time indicated in the kit package insert	❏	❏	❏
12. Depending on the test kit used, a positive result may appear as a line in the result window within 5 minutes. The strep A test unit or strip has an internal control; if a line appears in the control window, the test is valid			
13. Read a negative result at exactly 5 minutes or as per the test kit instructions to avoid a false negative			
14. Verify results of the controls before recording or reporting test results. Log the controls and the patient's information on the worksheet according to office policy and procedure			

(continues)

15. Properly dispose of the equipment and supplies in a biohazard waste container	❏	❏	❏
16. Remove your gloves and wash your hands	❏	❏	❏
17. **AFF** Log into the Electronic Medical Record (EMR) using your username and secure password OR obtain the paper medical record from a secure location and assure it is kept away from public access. Record the procedure noting the date, time, specimen collected, and specimen processing procedure (i.e., sent to lab, tested using CLIA-waived test, etc.). Include your name and title according to office policy and procedure	❏	❏	❏

_____

_____

_____

_____

CALCULATION

Total Possible Points: _____

Total Points Earned: _____ Multiplied by 100 = _____ Divided by Total Possible Points = _____ %

PASS   **FAIL**   **COMMENTS:**
 ❏   ❏

Student's signature _____ Date _____

Partner's signature _____ Date _____

Instructor's signature _____ Date _____

CHAPTER 45

Urinalysis

LEARNING OUTCOMES

COG Cognitive Domain*

1. Spell key terms
2. Identify the following related to body systems:
   a. medical terms
   b. abbreviations
3. Identify CLIA-waived tests associated with common diseases
4. Identify normal and abnormal results as reported in
   a. graphs
   b. tables
5. Identify quality assurance practices in healthcare
6. Describe the methods of urine collection
7. List and explain the physical and chemical properties of urine
8. Describe the components that can be found in urine sediment and describe their relationships to chemical findings
9. Explain the procedures in urine drug testing, including chain of custody

PSY Psychomotor Domain*

1. Obtaining a clean-catch midstream urine specimen (Procedure 45-1)

a. Collect specimens and perform CLIA-waived urinalysis test
b. Instruct and prepare a patient for a procedure or treatment
c. Perform quality-control measure
d. Document patient care accurately in the medical record

2. Perform a physical and chemical urinalysis (Procedure 45-2)
   a. Collect specimens and perform CLIA-waived urinalysis test
   b. Instruct and prepare a patient for a procedure or treatment
   c. Perform quality control measures
   d. Document patient care accurately in the medical record

AFF Affective Domain*

1. Demonstrate critical thinking skills
2. Reassure patients
3. Demonstrate empathy for patients' concerns
4. Demonstrate active listening
5. Respect diversity
6. Recognize personal boundaries

7. Demonstrate tactfulness
8. Demonstrate self-awareness
9. Protect the integrity of the medical record

MAERB Standards are Italicized.

ABHES Competencies

1. Practice quality control
2. Dispose of biohazardous materials
3. Instruct patients in the collection of clean-catch urine specimens
4. Practice quality control
5. Perform selected CLIA-waived tests that assist with diagnosis and treatment
6. Follow documentation guidelines
7. Adapt care to address the developmental stages of life
8. Display effective interpersonal skills with patients and healthcare team members
9. Demonstrate cultural awareness
10. Make adaptations for patients with special needs (psychological or physical limitations)
11. Make adaptations to care for patients across their lifespan

Name: _____   Date: _____   Grade: _____

COG MULTIPLE CHOICE

Circle the letter preceding the correct answer.

1. What color will be observed on the reagent pad if nitrites are present in urine?
   a. Blue
   b. Pink
   c. Red
   d. Yellow
   e. Green

2. Why is a 24-hour collection a better indicator of some values than a random specimen?
   a. Some substances are excreted with diurnal variation
   b. Some bacteria do not develop fully for 24 hours
   c. A 24-hour collection gives the physician a more accurate idea of the patient's diet
   d. The higher the volume of urine tested, the more accurate the result
   e. Some substances are excreted only at night

3. The most common method of urine collection is:
   a. suprapubic aspiration.
   b. clean-catch midstream.
   c. random specimen.
   d. first morning void.
   e. postprandial specimen.

4. Which of these conditions may cause a patient's urine to smell sweet?
   a. Urinary tract infection
   b. Kidney infection
   c. Diabetes
   d. Dehydration
   e. Yeast infection

5. What is the specific gravity of a normal urine specimen?
   a. 0.900–1.000
   b. 1.001–1.035
   c. 1.100–1.135
   d. 1.500–1.635
   e. 2.000–2.001

6. What is the expected pH range for urine?
   a. 3.0–6.0
   b. 4.0–7.0
   c. 5.0–8.0
   d. 6.0–9.0
   e. 7.0–10.0

7. Increased numbers of epithelial cells in urine may indicate that:
   a. there is an irritation, such as inflammation, somewhere in the urinary system.
   b. the patient is overly hydrated.
   c. the patient is pregnant.
   d. the urine sample has sat for too long before examination.
   e. the testing was not performed correctly.

8. Which group of people is most at risk of developing galactosuria?
   a. Teenagers
   b. Newborns
   c. Pregnant women
   d. Older adult men
   e. Older adult women

9. A patient with uric acid crystals in their urine possibly has:
   a. osteoarthritis.
   b. a urinary tract infection.
   c. hepatitis.
   d. gout.
   e. gallbladder cancer.

10. Which of these should be included on a chain-of-custody document?
    a. The results of the urine test
    b. The reason for the chain of custody
    c. Instructions for providing a specimen
    d. The date the specimen was collected or transferred
    e. The volume of urine in the specimen

11. Which biological pigment gives urine its color?
    a. Melanin
    b. Hemoglobin
    c. Myoglobin
    d. Beta-carotene
    e. Urochrome

12. Why is a urine test preferable to a blood test for a routine drug test?
    a. It is less invasive and has national standards for testing
    b. It is less expensive
    c. There is less risk of contamination
    d. It requires less equipment
    e. A urine specimen will stay fresh longer than a blood sample

13. Strenuous physical exercise may cause:
    a. increased protein in urine.
    b. decreased amounts of epithelial cells.
    c. increased quantities of ketones.
    d. increased glucose in urine.
    e. decreased concentration of phosphates.

14. Cast formation occurs in the:
    a. liver.
    b. small intestine.
    c. bladder.
    d. pathways of the digestive tract.
    e. tubules of the nephron.

⬢ MATCHING

Match each key term with the correct definition.

Key Terms

15. _____ bacteriuria
16. _____ bilirubinuria
17. _____ chain-of-custody procedure
18. _____ conjugated bilirubin
19. _____ diurnal variation
20. _____ glycosuria
21. _____ hematuria
22. _____ ketoacidosis
23. _____ ketones
24. _____ microhematuria
25. _____ proteinuria
26. _____ pyuria
27. _____ sediment
28. _____ specific gravity
29. _____ supernatant
30. _____ turbidity

Definitions

a. variation during a 24-hour period
b. presence of glucose in the urine
c. group of chemicals produced during fat and protein metabolism
d. blood in urine
e. bilirubin in the urine
f. the written policy for maintaining an accurate written record to track the possession, handling, and location of samples and data from collection through reporting
g. too much ketone in the blood and urine
h. type of bilirubin that does dissolve in the bloodstream
i. presence of bacteria in urine
j. cloudiness
k. reflects the ability of the kidney to concentrate or dilute the urine
l. increased amounts of protein in the urine
m. white cells in urine
n. the amount of blood in the urine is so small that the color of the specimen is not affected
o. the button of cells and other particulate matter that collects in the bottom of the tube when centrifuging a urine specimen
p. urine above the sediment when the tube of urine is centrifuged

⬢ MATCHING

Match each type of specimen collection method with the correct description.

Collection Methods

31. _____ Random specimen
32. _____ First morning void
33. _____ Postprandial specimen
34. _____ Clean-catch urine specimen
35. _____ Suprapubic aspiration
36. _____ 24-hour collection

Descriptions

a. A specimen that is collected 2 hours after a patient consumes a meal
b. A specimen that is voided into a sterile container after the urinary meatus and surrounding skin have been cleansed
c. A specimen that is formed over a 6- to 8-hour period
d. A specimen voided into a clean, dry container
e. A specimen consisting of all urine voided over a 24-hour period
f. A specimen that is taken directly from the bladder using a needle

OOG AFF MATCHING

Grade: _____

Read the descriptions of five patients. From your knowledge of chemical and physical properties of urine, match each patient with Dr. Philbin's diagnosis.

Patients

37. _____ Mr. Himmel is a 45-year-old father who is suffering from a stomach upset. His urine sample has a high specific gravity and is a deep yellow color.

38. _____ Mrs. Lincoln is a 33-year-old receptionist. Her urine sample is alkaline and contains leukocytes and a small amount of blood.

39. _____ Mr. Ackton is a 60-year-old gardener. His urine sample is dark yellow and contains bilirubin.

40. _____ Mrs. Franklin is a 75-year-old widow. Her urine sample has a high specific gravity, contains a high level of glucose, and is very acidic.

41. _____ Mrs. Taylor is a 29-year-old surgeon who has little time to exercise. She has a large quantity of protein in her urine.

42. _____ Ms. Sheffield is a 20-year-old college student. She has a large quantity of ketones in her urine.

43. _____ Mrs. Kotizky is a 43-year-old homemaker. Her urine is cloudy with a positive nitrite reaction.

44. _____ Mr. Kubik is a 67-year-old retiree. He has been a heavy drinker for 30 years and has increased his intake of alcohol significantly since retirement. His urine has an elevated urobilinogen level.

Diagnoses
a. Urinary tract infection
b. Diabetes mellitus
c. Dieting until protein breakdown
d. Pregnancy
e. Cirrhosis
f. Dehydration
g. Hepatitis

OOG IDENTIFICATION

Grade: _____

List and explain the physical and chemical properties of urine.

Property	Explanation
45.	
46.	
47.	
48.	
49.	
50.	
51.	
52.	
53.	
54.	
55.	

COG MATCHING

Grade: _____

As a medical assistant, you'll probably be asked to assist in the urinalysis procedure. Study the list of tasks below and decide which duties are within the scope of practice for a medical assistant. Place a check mark in the "Yes" box for tasks you would complete yourself and in the "No" box for tasks that would be completed by another member of the team.

Task	Yes	No
56. Prepare urine sediment for microscopic examination		
57. Instruct the patient on how to provide urine sample		
58. Perform microscopic examination of urine sediment		
59. Ensure that urine is tested or refrigerated within the correct time period		
60. Use suprapubic aspiration to collect a urine sample		
61. Perform confirmatory tests on urine samples		
62. Label specimens for clear identification		
63. Assemble equipment needed for urinalysis procedures		

COG AFF SHORT ANSWER

Grade: _____

64. A patient provides a sample of urine for testing. You know that everyone in the medical office is extremely busy and that it will not get tested for at least 3 hours. What should you do with the sample?

_____

_____

_____

_____

65. A patient gives a urine sample at 11 AM, and the physician asks you to perform a urinalysis on the specimen. Before you can analyze the sample, there is an emergency situation in the office, and you become distracted. At 2 PM you remember that the specimen has still not been analyzed, and it is in a container that is not refrigerated. What should you do? Explain your answer.

_____

_____

_____

_____

66. A severely underweight 15-year-old girl comes into the physician's office to give a urine sample. The test reveals that there are ketones in the patient's urine. Explain why this may be the case.

_____

_____

_____

_____

67. A urine sample has tested positive for protein. What procedure would be used to confirm the reagent strip reaction? Explain how the procedure works.

_____

_____

_____

_____

68. You are instructing your female patient how to collect a clean-catch specimen. She says she has diarrhea and is concerned about contaminating the specimen. How do you instruct her to collect the specimen? How do you use this information to coach her about her ongoing general health?

_____

_____

_____

_____

COG IDENTIFICATION

Grade: _____

The chain-of-custody process is used to ensure that all urine specimens are identifiable and have not been tampered with. Read the scenarios in the table below and decide whether the correct chain-of-custody patient screening and procedure have taken place. Place a check mark in the appropriate box.

Scenario	Correct Procedure Used	Possibility of Contamination
69. A patient faxes you her identification in advance to save time at the reception desk		
70. A patient enters the bathroom to give a urine sample wearing jeans and a T-shirt		
71. A patient selects his own sealed collection container from the cupboard		
72. A patient empties her pockets and enters the bathroom to give a urine sample while carrying a bottle of water		
73. A patient enters the bathroom to give a urine sample wearing cargo pants, a sweater, and a baseball cap		
74. A patient washes and dries his hands before entering the bathroom to give a urine sample		
75. A patient has forgotten her ID, but an employer representative verifies that she is the correct person		

COG PSY AFF **CASE STUDIES FOR CRITICAL THINKING**   Grade:_____

76. One of your patients needs to provide a 24-hour urine collection. She has never done it before and is unsure about how to carry out the procedure. Write the patient a list of instructions, explaining what she should do in order to provide an accurate specimen. Why is it important that the patient thoroughly understands and complies with your instructions?

_____

_____

_____

_____

77. You instruct a patient on how to perform a clean-catch midstream urine specimen. When you test the sample, you discover that the urine is cloudy, with a pH level of 7.5, and contains traces of red blood cells, nitrites, and leukocytes. How would you document this information on the patient's chart?

_____

_____

_____

_____

78. A patient asks you what types of drugs can be detected in urine. Two weeks later, the same patient comes into the office to provide a urine specimen. He appears to be acting suspiciously and you think you see him pick up a bottle before entering the bathroom. What should you do next?

_____

_____

_____

_____

79. Your patient, Sharon, has never collected a clean-catch midstream urine specimen before. As you describe the procedure, her facial expressions begin to change, and she becomes aloof. What are the possible reasons for her response? How do you adjust your behavior to support the patient's understanding of the procedure? How do you demonstrate empathy to this patient?

_____

_____

_____

_____

80. The results have come back from the testing laboratory on a drug screen test you collected. The medical assistant working in the front office comes to you asking about this patient's test results. She says the woman babysits her children after school, and she wants to know if the patient is taking drugs. How do you respond?

_____

_____

_____

_____

PSY PROCEDURE 45-1	Obtaining a Clean-Catch Midstream Urine Specimen

Name: _____ **Date:** _____ **Time:** _____ **Grade:** _____

EQUIPMENT/SUPPLIES: Sterile urine container labeled with patient's name, cleansing towelettes (two for males, three for females), gloves if you are to assist patient, hand sanitizer

STANDARDS: Given the needed equipment and a place to work, the student will perform this skill with _____ % accuracy in a total of _____ minutes. *(Your instructor will tell you what the percentage and time limits will be before you begin.)*

KEY: 4 = Satisfactory 0 = Unsatisfactory NA = This step is not counted

PROCEDURE STEPS	SELF	PARTNER	INSTRUCTOR
1. Check the physician order. Wash your hands	❑	❑	❑
2. Assemble the equipment and supplies	❑	❑	❑
3. ☰ Identify the patient and explain the procedure. Identify, yourself, including your title. Explain the rationale for performance of a procedure to the patient	❑	❑	❑
4. ☰ If the patient is hearing impaired, you may need to face the person and speak clearly, not loudly. You should have an easy-to-read instruction guide for the patient to follow and have them point out where there are questions. If the patient can sign and you cannot, have someone proficient in sign language assist you in instructing the patient	❑	❑	❑
5. If the patient is to perform the procedure, provide the necessary supplies	❑	❑	❑
6. Have the patient perform the procedure properly with the following instructions: **A.** Male patients: 　**i.** If uncircumcised, expose the glans penis by retracting the foreskin, then clean the meatus with an antiseptic wipe. The glans should be cleaned in a circular motion away from the meatus. A new wipe should be used for each cleaning sweep 　**ii.** Keeping the foreskin retracted, initially void a few seconds into the toilet or urinal 　**iii.** Bring the sterile container into the urine stream and collect a sufficient amount (about 30 to 60 mL). Instruct the patient to avoid touching the inside of the container with the penis 　**iv.** Finish voiding into the toilet or urinal **B.** Female patients: 　**i.** Kneel or squat over the toilet bowl. Spread the labia minora widely to expose the meatus. Using an antiseptic wipe, cleanse on either side of the meatus, and then cleanse the meatus itself. Use a wipe only once in a sweep from the anterior to the posterior surfaces, and then discard it 　**ii.** Keeping the labia separated, initially void a few seconds into the toilet 　**iii.** Bring the sterile container into the urine stream and collect a sufficient amount (about 30 to 60 mL) 　**iv.** Finish voiding into the toilet	❑	❑	❑

PSY PROCEDURE 45-1	**Obtaining a Clean-Catch Midstream Urine Specimen** (continued)			
7. Cap the filled container and place it in a designated area		❏	❏	❏
8. Transport the specimen in a biohazard container for testing or test the urine specimen according to office policy and procedure		❏	❏	❏
9. Properly care for or dispose of equipment and supplies. Clean the work area. Remove gloves and wash your hands		❏	❏	❏
10. **AFF** Log into the Electronic Medical Record (EMR) using your username and secure password OR obtain the paper medical record from a secure location and assure it is kept away from public access. Record the procedure noting the date, time, specimen collected, and specimen processing procedure (i.e., sent to lab, tested using CLIA-waived test, etc.). Include your name and title according to office policy and procedure		❏	❏	❏

_____

_____

_____

_____

CALCULATION

Total Possible Points: _____

Total Points Earned: _____ Multiplied by 100 = _____ Divided by Total Possible Points = _____ %

PASS   FAIL   COMMENTS:
❏   ❏

Student's signature _____ Date _____

Partner's signature _____ Date _____

Instructor's signature _____ Date _____

PSY PROCEDURE 45-2 | **Perform a Physical and Chemical Urinalysis**

Name: _____ Date: _____ Time: _____ Grade: _____

EQUIPMENT/SUPPLIES: Gloves, patient's labeled urine specimen, chemical reagent strips (such as Multistix™ or Chemstrip™), hand disinfectant, biohazard waste container

STANDARDS: Given the needed equipment and a place to work, the student will perform this skill with _____ % accuracy in a total of _____ minutes. *(Your instructor will tell you what the percentage and time limits will be before you begin.)*

KEY: 4 = Satisfactory　　　0 = Unsatisfactory　　　NA = This step is not counted

PROCEDURE STEPS	SELF	PARTNER	INSTRUCTOR
1. Check the physician order. Wash your hands	❑	❑	❑
2. Assemble the equipment	❑	❑	❑
3. Put on gloves	❑	❑	❑
4. Verify the name on the specimen container and the physician order	❑	❑	❑
5. In bright light against a white background, examine the color of the specimen. The most common colors are straw (very pale yellow), yellow, dark yellow, and amber (brown–yellow).	❑	❑	❑
6. Determine clarity. Hold the specimen container in front of a printed surface. If you see the image or print clearly (not obscured), record as clear. If you see the image or print but they are not well delineated, record as hazy. If you cannot see the image or print at all, record as cloudy	❑	❑	❑
7. Remove the reagent strip from its container and replace the lid to prevent deterioration of the strips by humidity	❑	❑	❑
8. Immerse the reagent strip in the urine completely, immediately remove it, sliding the edge of the strip along the lip of the container to remove excess urine. Pooling of excess urine on the dipstick causes cross-contamination among the reactions, possibly obscuring accurate color detection	❑	❑	❑
9. Start your stopwatch or timer immediately	❑	❑	❑
10. Compare the reagent pads to the color chart, determining results at the intervals stated by the manufacturer. Example: Glucose is read at 30 seconds. To determine results, examine that pad 30 seconds after dipping and compare with color chart for glucose	❑	❑	❑
11. Read all reactions at the times indicated and record the results	❑	❑	❑
12. Discard the reagent strips in the biohazard receptacle. Discard urine	❑	❑	❑

(continues)

PSY PROCEDURE 45-2	**Perform a Physical and Chemical Urinalysis** (continued)		
13. Remove your gloves and wash your hands	❏	❏	❏
14. **ARF** Log into the Electronic Medical Record (EMR) using your username and secure password OR obtain the paper medical record from a secure location and assure it is kept away from public access. Record the procedure noting the date, time, specimen collected, and specimen processing procedure (i.e., sent to lab, tested using CLIA-waived test, etc.). Include your name and title according to office policy and procedure	❏	❏	❏

_____

_____

_____

_____

CALCULATION

Total Possible Points: _____

Total Points Earned: _____ Multiplied by 100 = _____ Divided by Total Possible Points = _____ %

PASS   FAIL   COMMENTS:
  ❏   ❏

Student's signature _____   Date _____

Partner's signature _____   Date _____

Instructor's signature _____   Date _____

Career Strategies

Competing in the Job Market

CHAPTER 46

Making the Transition: Student to Employee

LEARNING OUTCOMES

COG Cognitive Domain

1. Spell and define the key terms
2. Explain the purpose of experiential learning
3. List your professional responsibilities during practicum
4. List personal and professional attributes necessary to ensure a successful practicum
5. Determine your best career direction based on your skills and strengths
6. Identify the steps necessary to apply for the right position and be able to accomplish those steps
7. List guidelines for an effective interview that will lead to employment
8. Explain the process for recertification of medical assisting credentials
9. Describe the importance of membership in a professional organization
10. *Identify professional behaviors of a medical assistant*
11. *Identify legal and illegal applicant interview questions*

PSY Psychomotor Domain

1. Write a résumé to properly communicate skills and strengths (Procedure 46-1)
2. *Using technology, compose clear and correct correspondence (Procedure 46-1)*

AFF Affective Domain

1. Apply local, state, and federal healthcare legislation
2. *Demonstrate self-awareness of professional behaviors as a medical assistant*

*MAERB Standards are italicized.

ABHES Competencies

1. Comply with federal, state, and local health laws and regulations
2. Describe the current employment outlook for the medical assistant
3. Demonstrate professional behaviors
4. Perform the essential requirements for employment, such as résumé writing, effective interviewing, dressing professionally, time management, and following up appropriately

Name: _____   Date: _____   Grade: _____

COG **MULTIPLE CHOICE**

1. Most practicums range from:
   a. 160 to 240 hours a semester.
   b. 80 to 160 hours a semester.
   c. 200 to 240 hours a semester.
   d. 240 to 300 hours a semester.
   e. 260 to 300 hours a semester.

2. Practicum site supervisors are typically:
   a. physicians.
   b. nurses.
   c. graduate medical assistants.
   d. academic instructors.
   e. other students.

3. When responding to an online advertisement, you should:
   a. mail your résumé and a portfolio.
   b. send your résumé by email.
   c. phone right away to inquire about the job.
   d. follow the instructions in the advertisement.
   e. call to schedule an interview.

4. A CMA wishing to recertify must either retake the examination or complete:
   a. 60 hours of continuing education credits.
   b. 50 hours of continuing education credits.
   c. 100 hours of continuing education credits.
   d. 30 hours of continuing education credits.
   e. 75 hours of continuing education credits.

5. Two standard ways of listing experience on a résumé are:
   a. functional and chronologic.
   b. functional and alphabetical.
   c. alphabetical and chronologic.
   d. chronologic and referential.
   e. referential and alphabetical.

6. During your practicum, it is a good practice to arrive:
   a. a few minutes early.
   b. half an hour early.
   c. right on time.
   d. with enough time to beat traffic.
   e. as early as you can.

7. What is the appropriate length of a résumé?
   a. One page
   b. Two pages
   c. Three pages
   d. As long as it needs to be
   e. Check with the potential employer first

8. In addition to providing proof of general immunizations, what other vaccinations may be required before you begin your practicum?
   a. Vaccination for strep throat
   b. Vaccination for cancer
   c. Vaccination for hepatitis B
   d. Vaccination for hepatitis C
   e. Vaccination for HIV

9. During your practicum, you are expected to perform as:
   a. the student you are; your site supervisor will teach you the same skills as in the classroom.
   b. an experienced professional; your site supervisor will expect you to perform every task perfectly.
   c. an entry-level employee; your site supervisor will expect you to perform at the level of a new employee in the field.
   d. a patient; you have to see what it feels like to be on the receiving end of treatment.
   e. independently as possible; your site supervisor will not have time to answer many questions.

10. Checking for telephone messages and arranging the day's appointments should be done:
   a. during your lunch break.
   b. at the close of the business day.
   c. after the office has opened.
   d. before the scheduled opening.
   e. between patients.

11. Fingernails should be kept short and clean to avoid:
   a. making your supervisor upset.
   b. accidentally scratching or harming a patient.
   c. transferring pathogens or ripping gloves.
   d. getting nail polish chips in lab samples.
   e. infecting sterile materials or surfaces.

12. Which document provides proof that tasks are performed and learning is taking place?
   a. Timesheet
   b. Journal
   c. Survey
   d. Evaluation
   e. Personal interview

13. Which document is used to improve performance and services offered to students?
   a. Timesheet
   b. Journal
   c. Survey
   d. Evaluation
   e. Personal interview

14. Membership in your professional medical assistant organization proves:
  a. that you are an allied health student.
  b. your level of professionalism and seriousness of purpose.
  c. that you will become a medical professional in 2 years.
  d. your willingness to network with other professionals.
  e. your interest in the medical field.

15. Which question should you avoid asking during an interview?
  a. Is there access to a 401(k) plan?
  b. Is tuition reimbursement available?
  c. How many weeks of vacation are available in the first year?
  d. Are uniforms or lab coats worn?
  e. What are the responsibilities of this position?

16. If you decide to leave your job, it is a good idea to:
  a. tell your employer the day before you plan to leave.
  b. make sure your new job will pay more.
  c. get contact information for all of the new friends you made.
  d. finish all duties and tie up any loose ends.
  e. criticize employees during an exit interview.

17. If you are having a problem performing your assigned job duties, it is best to:
  a. volunteer for extra hours.
  b. inform your site supervisor and instructor.
  c. ask for less-challenging work.
  d. ask for a different externship site.
  e. switch your course of studies.

18. When anticipating calls from prospective employers, avoid:
  a. leaving silly or cute messages on your answering machine.
  b. telling family members or roommates that you are expecting important telephone calls.
  c. keeping a pen near the telephone at all times.
  d. checking messages on a regular basis.
  e. calling them every day after submitting your résumé.

19. If bilingual applicants are encouraged to apply for a position you want, you should:
  a. learn simple greetings and act as if you can speak several languages.
  b. learn simple greetings and admit that you know a few words but are not fluent.
  c. do nothing; being bilingual is not important.
  d. avoid applying since you do not fluently speak another language.
  e. learn how to answer possible interview questions in two different languages.

20. Being a lifelong learner is a must for all medical professionals because:
  a. medical professionals have to recertify every 5 years.
  b. medical professionals are widely respected.
  c. changes in procedures, medical technologies, and legal issues occur frequently.
  d. changes in medical technologies are decreasing the need for medical professionals.
  e. medical professionals are required to change legal statutes once a year.

⬡⬡⬡ MATCHING

Grade: _____

Match the following key terms to their definitions:

Key Terms
21. _____ practicum
22. _____ networking
23. _____ portfolio
24. _____ site supervisor
25. _____ résumé

Definitions
  a. someone who oversees another; one who gives direction, as in a technical matter
  b. an educational course that allows the student to obtain hands-on experience
  c. a system of personal and professional relationships through which to share information
  d. a document summarizing an individual's work experience or professional qualifications
  e. a portable case containing documents

COG SHORT ANSWER

Grade: _____

26. What is the purpose of a practicum?

_____

_____

_____

_____

27. List three responsibilities you will have during a practicum.

a. _____

b. _____

c. _____

28. How will the site supervisor assist you in your practicum?

_____

_____

_____

_____

29. List five traditional sources of information for job openings.

a. _____

b. _____

c. _____

d. _____

e. _____

AFF PSY REFLECTION

Grade: _____

30. Write a list of your strengths and weaknesses as discussed in the chapter. Critically evaluate what you are able to contribute to the job and address your weaknesses. How can you work with these weaknesses to make them strengths? Now evaluate what kind of medical assisting job would work best with what you are already good at and how you would like to continue to grow in your professional development. Identify for yourself what type of job would be ideal for you.

_____

_____

_____

_____

31. Practice interviewing with a fellow student. Make sure that you take turns asking questions so that you can both get to experience being on each side of the interview.

COG IDENTIFICATION

Grade: _____

32. Below are items that could be included on a résumé. Circle all that are appropriate.

   a. Contact information

   b. Race

   c. Relevant volunteer work

   d. Birth date

   e. Experience

   f. Picture of yourself

   g. List of professional goals

   h. Education

   i. Credit history

   j. References

   k. Date of high school graduation

Action Words

| generates | ensures | implements and maintains | interviews | records | articulates |
| draws and collects | prepares | selects | measures | assists | composes |

Choose a more accurate action word from the box to replace the words in bold.

33. **Helps** in examination and treatment of patients under the direction of a physician

_____

34. **Talks to** patients, **takes** vital signs (i.e., pulse rate, temperature, blood pressure, weight, and height), and **writes** information on patients' charts _____

35. **Gets** blood samples from patients and prepares specimens for laboratory analysis

_____

36. **Sets up** treatment rooms for examination of patients _____

37. Read each of the following tips for completing a job application. Circle all appropriate best practices for completing an application.

   a. Read through the application completely before beginning.

   b. Follow the instructions exactly.

   c. In the line for wage or salary desired, write highest pay possible.

   d. Answer every question. If the question does not apply to you, draw a line or write "N/A" so that the interviewer will know that you did not overlook the question.

   e. Use your best cursive writing.

   f. Highlight important information in red ink.

   g. Ask for two applications. Use the first one for practice.

38. From the list of questions below, circle all that would be appropriate for a job applicant to ask a prospective employer.

a. What are the responsibilities of the position offered?

b. What is the benefit package? Is there access to a 401(k) plan or other retirement plan? Health insurance? Life insurance?

c. Is it acceptable to take 3 weeks off during the holiday season?

d. How does the facility feel about continuing education? Is time off offered to employees to upgrade their skills? Does the facility subsidize the expense?

e. Do I have to work with physicians who have bad attitudes?

f. How many potlucks and happy hours does this office usually have?

g. Is there a job performance or evaluation process?

COG EXPLANATION

Grade: _____

39. Explain what it means to be a lifelong learner.

_____

_____

_____

_____

40. How can you prepare for the process of recertification?

_____

_____

_____

_____

41. List two professional organizations you could join while you are a student.

a. _____

b. _____

AFF WHAT WOULD YOU DO?

Grade: _____

42. The office manager at your practicum site does not allow CMAs to give injections. At an office meeting, the employees ask her why not. Her reply is, "it is illegal." The employees tell her that it is not illegal for medical assistants to give injections in your state. She is surprised to hear this and asks the group to prove it to her. Because you are a student and have skills in researching topics, they ask you to find the legislation and bring it to the office manager. Choose all appropriate actions from the list below.

   a. Go to the state website and search "general assembly."

   b. Search for the information on the AAMA website by entering key words, "CMA scope of practice."

   c. Search for the information in general statutes by entering key words, "health care legislation in [name of your state]."

   d. Search for the information by entering key words, "unlicensed health personnel" under *general assembly* in your state.

   e. Search for the information by entering key words, "practice of medicine."

43. While working as a practicum at a family care provider, you encounter an older adult patient who is uncomfortable with the fact that you as a student are participating in her care. What would you say to help her feel more comfortable?

   _____
   _____
   _____
   _____

44. There are multiple gaps in your work history, and your interviewer asks you to explain why. One of the gaps is from relocation, and other gaps are from taking time off to evaluate what you wanted to be doing. How would you explain this to your interviewer?

   _____
   _____
   _____
   _____

45. During an interview, you are asked to explain why your grades were low last semester. How would you answer this question honestly while still speaking about yourself fairly and objectively?

   _____
   _____
   _____

COG **TRUE OR FALSE?**

Grade: _____

Determine whether the following statements are true or false. If false, explain why.

46. When you see dangerous practices, it is usually best to confront the employee first.

_____

_____

47. Problems encountered at a practicum site are best handled by site employees who have experience working with the office manager.

_____

_____

48. It is a good idea to include hobbies and personal interests on your résumé.

_____

_____

49. It is a good idea to write a long and detailed cover letter.

_____

_____

AFF **CASE STUDIES FOR CRITICAL THINKING**

Grade: _____

It is the first day of your medical assisting practicum.

50. Your practicum site supervisor has said that you cannot receive permission to draw blood and perform other phlebotomy procedures. However, you know this is an area that you are required to complete. Circle all of the appropriate actions from the list below.

   a. Tell your practicum coordinator from your college at her next site visit.

   b. Tell the site supervisor that you must perform these tasks and leave.

   c. Call your practicum coordinator immediately.

   d. Call a classmate and ask her what to do.

51. Your school will likely request that you fill out an evaluation form to determine if your practicum site was effective for training. This helps the school decide if it is a good site for future practicums. Review the list of questions below and circle all you should consider when filling out your site evaluation form on your practicum.

   a. Was the overall experience positive or negative?

   b. Was my site supervisor fun to be around?

   c. Did the office have a good cafeteria or break room?

   d. Were opportunities for learning abundant and freely offered or hard to obtain?

e. Was my site supervisor flexible about taking personal time during the day for phone calls and breaks?

f. Were staff personnel open and caring or unwelcoming?

g. Was the site supervisor available and easily approachable or preoccupied and distant?

52. Choose all appropriate ways to dress for your practicum from the list below.

a. Burgundy and navy scrubs along with a set of bangle bracelets, your favorite gemstone rings, and a pair of comfortable white clogs

b. The required scrubs with a pair of clean white sneakers. Dreadlocks placed in a neat ponytail above the shoulders

c. The required uniform and a pair of dark walking shoes. Hair with the tips of a spiked Mohawk dyed burgundy to match

d. The required uniform with white sneakers and college name tag

e. Street clothes with lab coat and required name tag

f. Long sleeves to cover the tattoo on your arm

PORTFOLIO

Grade: _____

Design and compile a portfolio to present at your upcoming job interviews. Refer to Chapter 46 for a list of possible contents of the portfolio. Remember, the purpose of a portfolio is to impress an interviewer. You have worked hard to earn your medical assisting certificate, diploma, or degree. This is your opportunity to show off your professional skills, abilities, and accomplishments.

PSY PROCEDURE 46-1 | Writing a Résumé

Name: _____ **Date:** _____ **Time:** _____ **Grade:** _____

EQUIPMENT/SUPPLIES: Word processor, paper, personal information

STANDARDS: Given the needed equipment and a place to work, the student will perform this skill with _____ % accuracy in a total of _____ minutes. *(Your instructor will tell you what the percentage and time limits will be before you begin practicing)*

KEY: 4 = Satisfactory 0 = Unsatisfactory NA = This step is not counted

PROCEDURE STEPS	SELF	PARTNER	INSTRUCTOR
1. At the top of the page, center your name, address, and phone numbers	❏	❏	❏
2. List your education, starting with the most current and working back. List graduation dates and areas of study. It is not necessary to go all the way back to elementary school	❏	❏	❏
3. Using the chronological format, list your prior related work experience with dates, responsibilities, company, and supervisor's name	❏	❏	❏
4. List any volunteer work with dates and places	❏	❏	❏
5. List skills you possess, including those acquired in your program and on your practicum	❏	❏	❏
6. List any certifications or awards received	❏	❏	❏
7. List any information relevant to a certain position (e.g., competence in spreadsheet applications for a job in a patient billing department)	❏	❏	❏
8. After obtaining permission and/or notifying the people, prepare a list of references with their addresses and phone contact information	❏	❏	❏
9. Carefully proofread the résumé for accuracy and typographical errors	❏	❏	❏
10. Have someone else proofread the résumé for errors other than content	❏	❏	❏
11. Print the résumé on high-quality paper	❏	❏	❏
12. **AFF** You had only one job before finishing your medical assisting program. Should you try to "pad" your résumé by listing some anyway? Why or why not?	❏	❏	❏

_____

_____

_____

_____

PSY PROCEDURE 46-1 **Writing a Résumé** (continued)

CALCULATION

Total Possible Points: _____

Total Points Earned: _____ Multiplied by 100 = _____ Divided by Total Possible Points = _____ %

PASS   FAIL   COMMENTS:
❏   ❏

Student's signature _____   Date _____

Partner's signature _____   Date _____

Instructor's signature _____   Date _____

CHAPTER 47

Comprehensive Final Examination

CAPSTONE ACTIVITIES: APPLYING WHAT YOU HAVE LEARNED

Working in a medical office means dealing with situations as they arise in a professional, nonjudgmental manner. Your education and training has provided you with the information and tools to give you administrative competence as well as the clinical skills necessary to function in the medical office, but you must also use professional judgment and critical thinking when making decisions and interacting with patients, families, and staff. This chapter will provide opportunities for you to practice using professional judgment and critical thinking skills as would a practicing medical assistant in the physician's office. Each section, containing documentation and active learning exercises, provides real-life scenarios followed by questions for you to think about and respond to according to directions from your instructor. Be sure to read carefully and, as usual, have fun!

COG PSY **DOCUMENTATION**
_____ Grade: _____

CHAPTER 1

Christopher Guest is waiting to see the physician, who has been called to the emergency room. You explain the situation to the patient, and he asks if you can perform his physical instead. You explain your scope of practice. Write a chart note to record the conversation.

_____

_____

_____

_____

CHAPTER 2

Your physician asks you to write a letter to Jean Mosley, a patient who has continued to be noncompliant. She wants to formally terminate the patient's care and refer her elsewhere. Write a note in the patient's chart documenting your actions.

_____

_____

_____

_____

CHAPTER 3

You are checking in a new patient who is obviously in acute pain. He is crying and pacing the floor. You take him to a private area to carry out the patient interview and help him complete his medical questionnaire. Write a note in the patient's chart documenting the fact that you assisted the patient with the questionnaire.

_____

_____

_____

_____

CHAPTER 4

Julia is an 8-year-old patient who has been diagnosed with juvenile diabetes. You supply the patient and her mother with educational materials about Julia's condition and how to manage her blood sugar. Write a chart note to document the conversation and actions.

_____

_____

_____

_____

CHAPTER 5

Megan O'Conner is a patient who was discharged from the hospital a few hours ago. She calls the office to report that she is now feeling woozy and nauseous. She thinks it might be a side effect of the pain medication she was given. Per your office protocol, she is advised to stop taking the medication, and you will have the doctor prescribe a different medication. Ms. O'Conner is obviously very upset. She is crying and says she just wants to go back to the hospital. You reassure her. Write a note about the conversation to be included in the chart.

_____

_____

_____

_____

CHAPTER 6

Mr. Sheffield did not show up for his appointment. You call him, and he says he forgot. You reschedule his appointment for the next day at 10:00 AM. Write a note to document this in the chart.

_____

_____

_____

_____

CHAPTER 7

The physician asks you to write a note to a patient, Nancy Chesnutt, informing her of her normal lab results. Construct the note that would be included as a copy in the patient's chart.

_____

_____

_____

_____

CHAPTER 8

A patient requests release of his records to another physician. What documentation is necessary for this release? Write a note to document the release in the patient's chart.

_____

_____

_____

_____

CHAPTER 9

You receive an email from Mr. Hagler saying that his medication is working out well and is not causing any side effects. He will be in for this appointment next Tuesday. How do you document this information in Mr. Hagler's medical record?

_____

_____

_____

_____

CHAPTER 10

During a routine visit, Carlos Delgado, a 55-year-old male, slips in the exam room and strikes his right forearm on the exam table causing a small laceration. The physician examines the patient's arm and determines it is nothing significant, but he cleans and applies a sterile dressing to it. The patient is also given a tetanus booster and instructions to change the dressing and clean the wound again this evening and was told to contact the office if he has any further problems with it. Use the space below to record the incident in the chart.

_____

_____

_____

_____

CHAPTER 11

Theo Smith, a 7-year-old male patient, needs to have his tonsils removed. The surgery was ordered by Dr. Kyle Dunn. His father, Ted Smith, has a PPO insurance plan that has denied preauthorization for a tonsillectomy due to _lack of medical necessity_. The patient has had recurrent throat infections during the last 12 months (a total of eight) with six testing positive for a streptococcus infection. He has tonsil hypertrophy and obstructive sleep apnea. Write a letter to the insurance company appealing the preauthorization denial.

_____

_____

_____

_____

CHAPTER 12

An 18-year-old woman is seen for a college physical. While being examined, she tells the physician's assistant that her boyfriend is abusive on occasion. The visit becomes predominantly counseling for the next 20 minutes of her 30-minute visit. How would you document this in the chart so that the visit can be coded accurately?

_____

_____

_____

_____

CHAPTER 13

Laila Hildreath is a 4-year-old girl who needs to have tubes in her ears after failing conservative treatment for recurrent ear infections. Her father is a member of an HMO that requires preauthorization for surgery. You call the HMO and receive authorization for the inpatient procedure. You are given the following preauthorization number: 67034598 AB. Record your actions for the patient's financial record.

_____

_____

_____

_____

CHAPTER 14

Tonya Sushkin's insurance company paid $25.00 for an office visit on the 20th of last month. Your physician is a participating provider for this company. Your initial charge was $75.00 for the date of service on the 2nd of last month. Post the payment and adjustment on a blank patient account ledger. Ms. Sushkin's previous balance is $75.00.

_____

_____

_____

_____

CHAPTER 15

Ms. Bailey has a large balance, and she is in today to see the doctor. You have a conversation with her about her unpaid bill. She promises to send $50.00 on the fifth of each month beginning next month. Write a note to record this agreement for her financial record.

_____

_____

_____

_____

CHAPTER 16

A 40-year-old woman comes to talk to the physician because she would like to start a new exercise routine and change her diet to lose 15 pounds. She is currently 25 pounds overweight, so this is a great idea and a good move toward healthy living. The physician asks you to discuss exercise and diet changes with the patient. Write a narrative patient note describing your interaction with the patient to include in her chart.

_____

_____

_____

_____

CHAPTER 17

Although you always take care to protect yourself from exposure to biohazardous materials, you spill a tube of a patient's blood while performing hematology testing. You have a fresh cut on your hand that came into contact with the blood. Following your office's exposure control plan, you clean up and then document the incident. What information will you make sure to include in your report?

_____

_____

_____

_____

CHAPTER 18

You are interviewing a young patient during an assessment when you notice that he has three small burn marks on his arm. The burns are round and less than a centimeter in diameter. When you ask the patient about the burns, he suddenly turns solemn and avoids answering the question. You suspect that the patient has been abused. How should you document this interaction on the patient's chart?

_____

_____

_____

_____

CHAPTER 19

How should you record an axillary temperature, and why is it important to record it differently from other temperatures?

_____

_____

_____

_____

CHAPTER 20

A 45-year-old patient comes into the office for a routine physical examination. He has high blood pressure and is considerably overweight. The patient asks you for advice on healthy eating, and you provide him with several pamphlets and advise him to cut down on fatty foods. How would you document this interaction in the patient's chart?

_____

_____

_____

_____

CHAPTER 21

The autoclave in your office has not been working properly. It takes twice as long for the steam in the autoclave to reach an adequate temperature for sterilization. You realize that this may affect daily procedures within the office and could lead to bigger problems with the autoclave. You decide to have the autoclave serviced by a professional. What documentation will be needed in connection with this service request?

_____

_____

_____

_____

CHAPTER 22

A patient is recovering from a Caesarian section and returns to the office to have her staples removed. The physician asks you to remove the staples and apply adhesive skin closures over the incision site. The patient asks you when the strips should be removed, and you tell her that they should fall off on their own within 10 days. How would you document this interaction in the patient's chart?

_____

_____

_____

_____

CHAPTER 23

The physician has prescribed a patient 250 mg of amoxicillin for an ear infection.
The patient should take this medication three times a day by mouth for 9 days.
Write a note to document this in the patient's chart.

_____

_____

_____

_____

CHAPTER 24

The physician has asked you to prepare an administration of gr iii Haldol IM for a patient. The dispenser is labeled in milligrams. How do you convert this dosage to the metric system, and how many milligrams of Haldol should you dispense? Write the preparation as a chart note.

_____

_____

_____

_____

CHAPTER 25

You have just taken a chest x-ray to rule out pneumonia. Write a narrative note detailing this procedure to be included in the patient's chart.

_____

_____

_____

_____

CHAPTER 26

A patient received penicillin for a sexually transmitted infection, and this was the last event documented in the patient's chart. Fifteen minutes later, the patient began wheezing and gasping and within 5 minutes was clearly suffering anaphylactic shock. A first injection of epinephrine administered SC at that time was ineffective, and the patient was in respiratory arrest when EMS arrived. Mask-to-mouth respirations were given with supplemental oxygen at 15 L per minute for 2 minutes before EMS assumed care of the patient. How would you document this interaction in the patient's chart?

_____

_____

_____

_____

CHAPTER 27

Your patient is a 9-year-old girl who suffers from severe eczema. The physician has recommended that she wear bandages at night to protect against scratching. You demonstrate to the patient's mother how to apply the bandages. The patient's mother asks how often she should apply ointment to her daughter's skin, and you repeat the physician's instructions to use it twice a day. How would you document this interaction in the patient's chart?

_____

_____

_____

_____

CHAPTER 28

Your patient is an older adult man. The physician has determined that the patient requires an ambulatory assist device. You first attempt to teach the patient to use a cane. The patient is unsteady while using the cane, so you instead teach the patient to use a walker. The patient successfully learns how to use the walker and demonstrates stability and control. You explain to the patient how to use the aid safely, including how to maintain the aid and what changes the patient should make at home to operate the aid safely. The patient verbalizes that he is comfortable using the walker and that he understands his maintenance responsibilities. How would you document this interaction on the patient's chart?

_____

_____

_____

_____

CHAPTER 29

A patient has come in for ceruminosis treatment. Document the steps that were taken to complete this procedure as well as any complications that might have arisen during the procedure. Be sure to include any instructions that were given to the patient after the procedure.

_____

_____

_____

_____

CHAPTER 30

Write a patient care note for a patient recovering from bacterial pneumonia. Explain what her symptoms are as well as what remedies the physician recommends/prescribes. Also, indicate how these remedies are intended to combat specific elements of the disease. You do not need to explain the details of how a remedy works, only what it is intended to do (i.e., a glucocorticoid is prescribed to reduce inflammation).

_____

_____

_____

_____

CHAPTER 31

When interviewing a patient prior to a physical examination of the cardiovascular system, what should you ask the patient and document in his chart?

_____

_____

_____

_____

CHAPTER 32

A patient is being scheduled for a colonoscopy. You explain the preparation to him. Document your actions for inclusion in the patient's chart.

_____

_____

_____

_____

CHAPTER 33

A father brings in his 8-year-old daughter because she fell and hit her head while rollerblading. She was not wearing a helmet and seems to have lost consciousness for just a few seconds. The father is concerned about a possible traumatic brain injury. After a physical examination, the physician finds that the child has suffered a mild concussion. She is sent home, and you give her father instructions regarding her treatment. Write a narrative note documenting this visit for inclusion in the patient's chart.

_____

_____

_____

_____

CHAPTER 34

You have just spoken with a 20-year-old patient about cystitis and have given her tips on how to avoid cystitis in the future. Record what you would write in the woman's chart, and make a note of any handout materials you might give the patient.

_____

_____

_____

_____

CHAPTER 35

Ms. Molly Espinoza is a 43-year-old female patient. Dr. Cord ordered a routine screening mammogram for this patient. You confirm with her that she is not pregnant and explain the procedure. Then you prepare the patient, and two radiographs are taken of each breast, with repositioning the patient between each image. All four radiographs are developed and are readable and accurate. Record the incident in the chart.

_____

_____

_____

_____

CHAPTER 36

John Suiker is an athletic 38-year-old man scheduled for a routine visit. He arrives disoriented and appears to be drunk and unsteady on his feet. He presents with pale, moist skin; rapid, bounding pulse; and shallow breathing. You notify the physician, Dr. Burns, of the patient's condition, and she orders an immediate blood glucose test. The patient's blood glucose is 48 mg/dL. The patient is still conscious, so you provide him with fruit juice, which he accepts. Recovery is immediate. Record the incident in the chart.

_____

_____

_____

_____

CHAPTER 37

Rose Ryan is a 24-month-old girl visiting your office for a well-child visit. The physician directs you to obtain her length, weight, and head and chest circumference. You find the child measures 92 cm tall and weighs 15 kg. Her head circumference is 50 cm, and her chest circumference is 52 cm. Document these procedures. Use the space below to record the procedure in the chart. How would you document the above scenario on the child's chart? Be sure to document the interaction, as well as the education that was provided during her visit, and any scheduled follow-up appointments. How would you record the procedure in the chart?

_____

_____

_____

_____

CHAPTER 38

A 78-year-old patient visits the physician's office to ask about treatment for arthritis in his knees. While you are talking to the patient, you notice that his hearing has decreased considerably since the last time he was in the physician's office. How would you document this information in the patient's chart?

_____

_____

_____

_____

CHAPTER 39

How would you document the collection of a blood specimen and prepare it to be sent out for testing?

_____

_____

_____

_____

CHAPTER 40

You have just completed maintenance on the glucose meter. Document this maintenance as you would in the laboratory instrument maintenance log.

_____

_____

_____

_____

CHAPTER 41

Nicole Patton is a 35-year-old female inpatient receiving both a Lovenox injection and oral Coumadin. You are directed to obtain blood specimens by evacuated tube for platelet count, prothrombin time, and partial thromboplastin time tests. Document your collection as you would in the patient's chart. Include the type(s) of specimens you collected.

CHAPTER 42

You perform an ESR test on an older adult male patient with rheumatoid arthritis. You measure a rate of 16 mL/hour. How would you document the results of this test in the patient's chart?

CHAPTER 43

You instruct a patient on how to perform a clean-catch midstream urine specimen. When you test the sample, you discover that the urine is cloudy, with a pH level of 7.5, and contains traces of red blood cells, nitrites, and leukocytes. Your office does not use laboratory report forms. How would you document this information in the patient's chart?

CHAPTER 44

The physician has ordered an influenza test for your patient. The influenza test requires a nasopharyngeal specimen. You collect the specimen. Document the collection as you would in a patient's chart.

CHAPTER 45

Dr. Ashanti asks you to perform a blood cholesterol test on a patient. The results are 282 mg/dL. Write a note to document this test and its results in the patient's chart as you would if your office does not use laboratory report forms.

_____

_____

_____

_____

CHAPTER 46

You just completed an interview with the office manager of a large family practice. Write a thank you note to the interviewer.

_____

_____

_____

_____

PSY ACTIVE LEARNING

CHAPTER 1

Talk with a grandparent or another older adult and ask them to tell you about a medical discovery that they remember well. Create a "before and after" chart, explaining what life was like before the discovery and the changes and benefits that came about after the discovery.

CHAPTER 2

Go to the Health and Human Services website, http://www.hhs.gov/ocr/privacy. What is the mission statement of the Office for Civil Rights regarding the HIPAA Privacy Rule?

CHAPTER 3

Do a web search for "anger management techniques." Are there suggestions that could help you communicate with an angry patient? Record your findings. Cite websites used.

CHAPTER 4

Go to the Council on Aging's website, http://www.ncoa.org. Describe the plan included in the _Falls Free Coalition_ outlined in the Safety of Seniors Act of 2008.

CHAPTER 5

Go the Americans with Disabilities website, https://ada.gov. Go to the Primer for Small Businesses. Who is covered by the ADA?

CHAPTER 6

Memorize the days of the week in Spanish. Recite them for your classmates.

CHAPTER 7

When writing, it is important to know your audience. The way you write for a physician is different from the way you write for a patient. In the case of a physician, you can assume they understand medical terminology, but this is not so for a patient. Do some Internet research to better understand the possible digestive side effects of a common medication like simvastatin (Zocor) or esomeprazole (Nexium). Then, write two letters discussing the side effects, one to a physician and one to a patient. Think about what you must do differently when writing to a patient.

CHAPTER 8

If you were opening a new medical facility, consider whether you would want staff members using abbreviations in patient records. Next, create a list of acceptable abbreviations that may be used in your new facility. Then create a "Do Not Use" list for abbreviations that may be confusing and should not be included in records. Visit the website for the Joint Commission (http://www.jointcommission .org) and include all of those abbreviations in addition to five other abbreviations of your own choice.

CHAPTER 9

Go to WebMD (http://www.webmd.com). Scroll down to the Symptom Checker. Think back to your last illness or pick an illness and answer the questions about the symptoms. What do you have?

CHAPTER 10

Prepare a list of emergency contacts in the area, including the contact information of local hospitals, poison control centers, and emergency medical services.

CHAPTER 11

Call two collection agencies in your local area. Compare services and fees. Record your findings.

CHAPTER 12

Research the banking services offered by your local bank. Gather brochures outlining the services. Share with classmates to compare services.

CHAPTER 13

When did ICD-10 CM codes go into effect and when do new codes become effective? Search http://www.aapc.com/ICD-10 for the answer.

CHAPTER 14

Find the ICD-10-CM codes for the following diseases:

a. Acute gastric ulcer with hemorrhage and perforation without obstruction _____

b. Meningococcal pericarditis _____

c. Impetigo _____

d. Benign essential hypertension _____

CHAPTER 15

Research the subject of Current Procedural Coding. Write a paragraph describing the origin of the CPT codes. What was the original purpose of CPT coding?

CHAPTER 16

The Centers for Disease Control and Prevention (CDC) offers a body mass calculator on its website. Visit http://www.cdc.gov and search for the BMI calculator. Determine whether your BMI is within normal limits for your gender, age, and height. Describe at least three things you can do to either maintain your current weight or lose/gain weight if necessary.

CHAPTER 17

You have been asked to select the best hand soap for use throughout the urgent care center where you work. Do Internet research to identify different types of antibacterial agents that are commonly used in hand soaps. Cite any evidence you can find as to the effectiveness of the agents. Determine which soap you believe is best. Write a letter to the office manager that gives your recommendation, clearly explaining why you chose that soap.

CHAPTER 18

Conduct a patient interview with a family member or friend. Use a sample patient history form such as the one found in this chapter from your textbook. Be sure to perform the interview in person so that you can observe the physical and mental status of your patient. When you are finished, ask your patient for feedback, such as demeanor and professionalism or comfort level of the patient. Use their comments to set one goal for yourself regarding your skills conducting patient interviews.

CHAPTER 19

With a partner, practice taking body temperature measurements with all of the types of thermometers to which you have access. For those you cannot access, mime the process so that you at least have the steps down the first time you are faced with the real thermometer. For all methods, go through all of the steps from picking up the thermometer to returning it to the disinfectant or returning the unit to the charging base.

CHAPTER 20

Even though the physician is the person who is responsible for using most of the instruments discussed in this chapter, you should still be familiar with how all of the instruments are used. Working with a partner, access at least three of the following instruments: tongue depressor, percussion hammer, tuning fork, nasal speculum, otoscope, and stethoscope. If you do not have access to these instruments, ask your teacher if they can assist you. Once you have the instruments, identify the main use of those instruments during a physical exam.

CHAPTER 21

Using the library and the Internet, research the instruments and equipment commonly used by the following medical specialties: endocrinology, rheumatology, palliative care, and radiology. Add to the list found in Chapter 21 of your text with the information you find. Include images of some of the instruments and equipment.

CHAPTER 22

One of the most common minor surgeries performed in your office is the excision of skin lesions and moles, often related to the possibility of skin cancer. Skin cancer is prevalent today, and you feel that it is important to educate young people on the importance of taking proper precautions to protect skin from harmful sunrays. You have been asked to prepare a one-page patient education handout highlighting the dangers of skin cancer and prevention techniques designed especially for young adults.

- Do Internet research to identify the leading causes of skin cancer and the dangers associated with harmful sun exposure. Gather any statistics that are available from reputable websites.
- Outline steps that can be taken to protect the skin when outside.
- Highlight issues that are especially important to teens (e.g., summer jobs as lifeguards and outdoor sports practice during the day).
- Create a one-page handout to be given to teens in the office explaining how to protect their skin from the sun.

CHAPTER 23

You have just begun working in a medical office and are getting yourself acquainted with the types of medications that the physician frequently prescribes. You know that many medications interact with food; however, you don't know a lot about specific food–drug interactions. Choose 10 common drugs from different therapeutic classifications in Table 23-1 and then research any possible food interactions. Make a chart for patients showing how common drugs and foods interact with one another.

CHAPTER 24

Accidental needlesticks are one of the most frightening occupational hazards you will encounter as a medical assistant. The greatest fear is centered on human immunodeficiency virus (HIV) and hepatitis B (HBV). Research the incubation, signs and symptoms, treatment, and prognosis associated with these two diseases. Prepare a one-page handout on each.

CHAPTER 25

Research the current recommendations by the American Cancer Society for mammography. At what age does the ACS recommend that women get their first mammogram? What other important information do women need to know about breast cancer?

CHAPTER 26

Some medical professionals live on the front line of emergency medical care. Locate an EMT-Basic (EMT-B) textbook at a library, bookstore, or other source. Make a list of some basic emergency care that is expected of the EMT-B that may also be expected of the practicing medical assistant. Are there any skills that are similar? Different?

CHAPTER 27

Use the Internet to research the major causes of fungal infections and find out how they can be prevented. Produce a poster to display in the office, educating patients about the main types of fungal infection, how they are spread, and how patients can protect their families from outbreaks.

CHAPTER 28

School children, especially girls, are commonly screened for scoliosis. Research the methods used for this screening using the Internet or the library. Then prepare a patient education pamphlet for school children who are about to undergo the screening. Explain the procedure in a way that will calm any anxieties. Include information about scoliosis as well as preventative measures the children can take and warning signs they should look for in the years following their school screening.

CHAPTER 29

The composer Beethoven was afflicted with hearing loss that left him completely deaf. Many music lovers today suffer from hearing loss as well, and they rely on the available technology to help them enjoy the subtle tones that are written into compositions. Research the new programs and software that are being installed in hearing aids that are specifically aimed at listening to music. List differences between listening to music and listening to speech, and make a note of tips for listening to music that physicians can give to patients with hearing aids.

CHAPTER 30

Most people are aware of the dangers of smoking. However, it is still important to educate children about the long-term dangers of smoking. Create a pamphlet outlining the dangers of smoking to be presented to a group of middle school children.

CHAPTER 31

Pretend you are a patient who is keeping a Holter monitor diary. Create a diary based on experiences a patient is likely to have. What kinds of activities do you participate in during the day? How are these activities influencing your symptoms?

CHAPTER 32

One of the deadliest types of cancer is pancreatic cancer, which kills most patients within a year of diagnosis. Research the latest information about the suspected causes of pancreatic cancer on the Internet. Try to find out which treatments are proving the most effective and whether there have been any recent developments.

- Use the information you find to create an informational poster about pancreatic cancer, educating high-risk patients on how they can lower their chances of developing pancreatic cancer.
- Write a one-page leaflet for physicians, informing them of the latest treatments for pancreatic cancer.

CHAPTER 33

Safe use of car seats can reduce brain and spinal cord injuries in infants and young children. Research the guidelines for car seat use. Then research car seat ratings and find five car seats that receive high safety ratings in each category. Create a handout for parents of young children to promote car seat safety awareness.

CHAPTER 34

Prostate cancer is most common in men over age 50 years and, like many other cancers, it is best treated in the early stages. Testicular cancer is another form of cancer, but it occurs most often in younger men, ages 15 to 34 years. Go online and research more information about these diseases. Design a presentation to be educational for both your classmates and patients. Be sure to include information about the causes, the symptoms, the ways to diagnose them, and the treatments available.

CHAPTER 35

With so many prenatal tests, procedures, and appointments at the physician's office, a pregnant patient can feel overwhelmed. Create a packet that can be distributed to a patient during the first prenatal visit. Include the schedule of prenatal visits and the procedures that will be done at each of these visits. Also include important information for the patient to consult throughout the duration of the pregnancy. Especially include a list of signs and symptoms that may indicate a problematic condition.

CHAPTER 36

Make a list of common foods for a diabetes sufferer to avoid. Then create a poster to display in the office, highlighting your findings. Be sure to stress the importance of proper nutrition.

CHAPTER 37

The physician has asked that you make a poster for the waiting room that shows important hygienic tips for children, such as washing hands, covering the mouth and nose while sneezing, etc. Come up with a list of five hygienic tips that could be illustrated and design the poster. Use visuals so that children who are too young to read can understand the concepts being displayed.

CHAPTER 38

Research the latest information about Alzheimer's disease on the Internet. Produce an informative poster to display in a physician's waiting room, educating people about the early warning signs of Alzheimer's disease. Include information about the stages of Alzheimer's disease and what friends and families can expect if a loved one develops it.

CHAPTER 39

Patient confidentiality is always an important part of your job, but so is safety. Research your state's rules and regulations with regard to the rights of a patient and the rights of the public. For instance, is someone with HIV/AIDS required by law to report their condition to their employer? What about other illnesses? After you have run a test and found a patient who tested positive for a specific disease, what are the obligations of your office in dealing with this?

CHAPTER 40

You perform an HCG pregnancy test for your patient. She has a weak positive result, which fails the QC, so you must administer the test again. The second time, the test shows a positive result, and the QC is acceptable. Document the QC results as you would in the office QC log.

CHAPTER 41

Familiarize yourself with phlebotomy equipment and draw a diagram of your blood-drawing station; detail on your diagram where supplies are kept. Think, in terms of safety, about where your blood station should be positioned in the office. Think about how the organization of your station will assist you in phlebotomy procedures and minimize the likelihood of accidents.

CHAPTER 42

White blood cells are the body's defense against foreign substances and objects that enter the bloodstream. However, there are cancers, diseases, and other ailments that attack white blood cells and their production. Research one of these diseases. How many people are reported to have this disease? Is there current treatment or therapy? What are some of the cures that are being developed to stop these diseases and to rebuild the immune system? After you have gathered the information, prepare a report on this disease to present to the class.

CHAPTER 43

Identify common features that patients can take note of in their own urine (e.g., dark color = possible dehydration). Make a brochure to raise patients' awareness of how their physical health can be reflected in the color and clarity of their urine.

CHAPTER 44

Many soaps and cleaning products today are antibacterial, meaning that they work to kill bacteria. People use these antibacterial products to wash and sanitize their hands as well as their homes, especially the kitchen and bathroom. Some studies have shown that the rise in popularity of antibacterial products may be creating strains of bacteria that are resistant to antibiotics. Perform research on this topic and present it to the class.

CHAPTER 45

A new patient says there is a history of heart attacks in his family, and he wants to know what he can do to prevent it. He is middle aged and slightly overweight; however, he has a healthy diet and exercises regularly. Search the Internet and list websites that could contain credible information for the patient. Compile a brochure for the prevention of heart disease.

CHAPTER 46

Do an Internet search of medical assisting job opportunities in your area. Now broaden your search to check jobs in any large metropolitan area. What are the differences and similarities in your local opportunities and those in the other city?

Index